MEDICAL RADIOLOGY

Diagnostic Imaging

Editors:
A. L. Baert, Leuven
M. Knauth, Göttingen

J. Stoker · S. A. Taylor · J. O. L. DeLancey (Eds.)

Imaging Pelvic Floor Disorders

2nd Revised Edition

With Contributions by

P. Abrams · C. I. Bartram · A. E. Bharucha · A. C. de Bruijne-Dobben · J. O. L. DeLancey
H. P. Dietz · A. V. Emmanuel · J. G. Fletcher · D. S. Hale · S. Halligan · F. Housami
M. Oelke · J.-P. Roovers · S. Shawki · H. Siddiki · J. Stoker · S. A. Taylor · W. H. Umek
D. B. Vodušek · C. Wallner · S. D. Wexner

Foreword by

A. L. Baert

With 212 Figures in 276 Separate Illustrations, 68 in Color and 23 Tables

Springer

Jaap Stoker, MD, PhD
Professor of Radiology
Department of Radiology
Academic Medical Center
University of Amsterdam
Meibergdreef 9
1105 AZ Amsterdam
The Netherlands

Stuart A. Taylor, MD, MRCP, FRCR
Senior Lecturer in Radiology
Department of Specialist X-Ray
University College Hospital
2F Podium, 235 Euston Road
London NW1 2BU
UK

John O. L. DeLancey, MD
Norman F. Miller Professor of Gynecology
Director, Pelvic Floor Research Group
Director, Fellowship in Female Pelvic Medicine and
Reconstructive Surgery
L4000 Women's Hospital
University of Michigan
1500 E. Medical Center Drive
Ann Arbor, Mi 48109-0276
USA

Medical Radiology · Diagnostic Imaging and Radiation Oncology
Series Editors:
A. L. Baert · L. W. Brady · H.-P. Heilmann · M. Knauth · M. Molls · C. Nieder

Continuation of Handbuch der medizinischen Radiologie
Encyclopedia of Medical Radiology

ISBN 978-3-540-71966-3 e-ISBN 978-3-540-71968-7

DOI 10.1007 / 978-3-540-71968-7

Medical Radiology · Diagnostic Imaging and Radiation Oncology ISSN 0942-5373

Library of Congress Control Number: 2007942181

Cover Design and Layout: PublishingServices Teichmann, 69256 Mauer, Germany

Printed on acid-free paper

9 8 7 6 5 4 3 2 1

springer.com

Foreword

Pelvic floor disorders represent an increasingly important clinical problem due to the aging of the population.

Recent technical progress in cross-sectional imaging with ultrasound as well as with MRI now enables us to obtain totally new insights into the anatomy and pathophysiology of the complex pelvic floor structures.

This second edition has been fully updated to represent the current state of the art and provide an excellent and comprehensive overview of the techniques to be applied in a focused study of the pelvic floor. It also offers expert guidance in modern management of the various clinical conditions related to the dysfunction of specific components of the pelvic floor.

J. Stoker and S. A. Taylor have joined J. O. L. DeLancey as editors for this second edition. They are internationally recognized leaders in the field and I am very much indebted to them for their judicious choice of topics and collaborating authors, as well as for the expedient and rapid preparation of this superb volume.

I am convinced that this second edition will again be met with great interest by radiologists and all other clinicians involved in the care of patients with pelvic disorders.

Leuven

Albert L. Baert

Preface

Disorders of the pelvic floor are very common, particularly affecting the female population. Although not life-threatening, the impact of these disorders on the quality of life of those affected cannot be understated, and indeed may be devastating. Imaging plays an important role in the management of these disorders, its utility further increased with the new and valuable insights provided by current techniques.

The aim of this book is to provide those practitioners with an interest in the imaging, diagnosis and treatment of pelvic floor dysfunction with a thorough update of this rapidly evolving field. As in the first edition, this volume is written by a combination of radiologists and clinicians (urogynaecologists, surgeons, urologists), reflecting the importance of a multidisciplinary approach when considering pelvic floor disorders in both clinical practice and research.

Based on the success of the first edition, edited by our friend and colleague Clive Bartram, the overall structure of this new edition remained largely unchanged. Introductory chapters on anatomy and (patho)physiology are followed by chapters on state-of-the-art imaging techniques and their application in pelvic floor dysfunction. The closing chapters describe modern clinical management of pelvic floor disorders with specific emphasis on the integration of diagnostic and treatment algorithms. All existing chapters have been rewritten or updated to reflect the rapid developments in this field, and chapters on several new topics have been added, including perineal ultrasound and MRI of the levator muscles.

We thank the contributing authors for their valuable contribution to this book. We are very fortunate to have so many distinguished experts in the field contributing to this volume. Professor Baert has our thanks for his invitation to contribute a second edition of Imaging Pelvic Floor Disorders to the renowned Medical Radiology series. We also thank Ursula Davis and her colleagues at Springer for the very effective production process and polite, timely communication.

Amsterdam — Jaap Stoker
London — Stuart A. Taylor
Ann Arbor — John O. L. DeLancey

Contents

The Anatomy of the Pelvic Floor and Sphincters

1

Jaap Stoker and Christian Wallner

CONTENTS

1.1 Introduction

The pelvic floor supports the visceral organs, is crucial in maintaining continence, facilitates micturition and evacuation and in women forms part of the birth canal. This multifunctional unit is a complex of muscles, fasciae and ligaments that have numerous interconnections and connections to bony structures, organs and the fibroelastic network within fat-containing spaces. A detailed appreciation of the pelvic floor is essential to understand normal and abnormal function. The embryology of the pelvic floor is included to help explain certain anatomical features.

J. Stoker, MD, PhD
Professor of Radiology, Department of Radiology, Academic Medical Center, University of Amsterdam, Meibergdreef 9, 1105 AZ Amsterdam, The Netherlands
C. Wallner, MSc
Department of Anatomy and Embryology, Academic Medical Center, University of Amsterdam, Meibergdreef 69–71, 1105 BK Amsterdam, The Netherlands

The anatomy of the pelvic floor is described in an integrated manner, with special attention to the connections between structures that are crucial for a proper function of the pelvic floor. Apart from line drawings, T2-weighted magnetic resonance imaging (MRI) is used to illustrate normal anatomical structures.

The structure of the pelvic floor and its attachments to pelvic bones are an evolutionary adaptation to our upright position, which requires greater support for the abdominal and pelvic organs overlying the large pelvic canal opening. The initial evolutionary step was the development of a pelvic girdle, as found in amphibians, which were the first vertebrates adapted to living on land. The second was adaptation of the pelvic floor muscles. Pelvic organ support in early primates was controlled by contraction of the caudal muscles pulling the root of the tail forward against the perineum. With the gradual introduction of upright posture and loss of the tail, this mechanism became inadequate, and further adaptive changes occurred with the caudal muscles becoming more anterior, extra ligamentous support (coccygeus and sacrospinous ligament), and the origin of the iliococcygeus muscle moving inferiorly to arise from the arcus tendineus levator ani with some associated changes in the bony pelvis (Lansman and Robertson 1992). Partial loss of contact of the pubococcygeus with the coccyx led to the development of the pubovisceralis (puborectalis).

1.2 Embryology

The embryology of the pelvic floor and related structures remains unclear, and new concepts are continually being introduced, e.g. the fusion of the urogenital septum and cloacal membrane (Nievelstein et al. 1998). This brief overview may be supplemented by more detailed texts (Arey 1966; Hamilton and Mossman 1972; Moore and Persaud 1998).

1.2.1 Cloaca and Partition of the Cloaca

The earliest stage in the development of the pelvic floor, comprising the urogenital, anorectum and perineal regions, is the invagination of the yolk sac 4 weeks after fertilization to form the foregut, midgut and hindgut. A diverticulum, the allantois, develops from the hindgut. The part of the hindgut connected to the allantois is called the cloaca (Figs. 1.1, 1.2). The cloaca is joined laterally by the nephric (later mesonephric) ducts. At the angle of the allantois and hindgut there is a coronal rim of endoderm and mesenchyme proliferation – the urogenital septum (or cloacal septum), which develops from the sixth week (Fig. 1.1). The septum grows in the direction of the cloacal membrane while fork-like extensions produce lateral cloacal infolding. At the margins of the cloacal membrane, mesenchyme migrates from the primitive streak to form lateral (genito- or labioscrotal) folds and a midline genital tubercle (precursor of the phallus) (Hamilton and Mossman 1972). By the seventh week, the urogenital septum divides the endodermal lined cloaca in a larger anterior urogenital sinus (including the vesicourethral canal) continuous with the allantois, and a smaller posterior anorectal canal (Bannister et al. 1995). The nodal centre of division of the cloacal plate is the future perineal body. A recent experimental study demonstrated that the cloacal sphincter muscles develop from migrating cells from the embryonic hind limb muscle mass (Valasek et al. 2005).

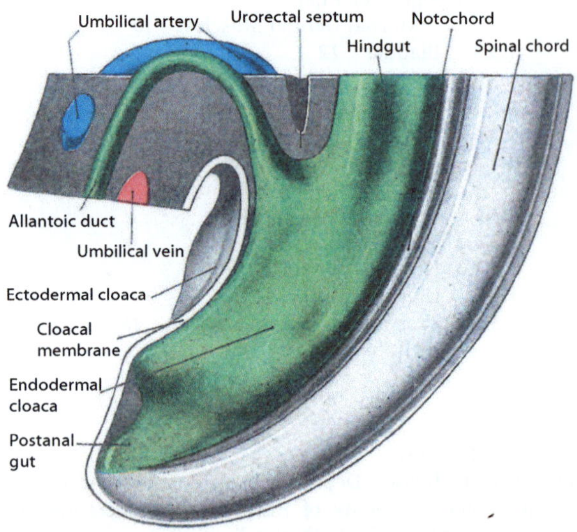

Fig. 1.1. The tail end of a human embryo, about 4 weeks old. Reprinted from Bannister et al. (1995, p. 206), by permission of Churchill Livingstone

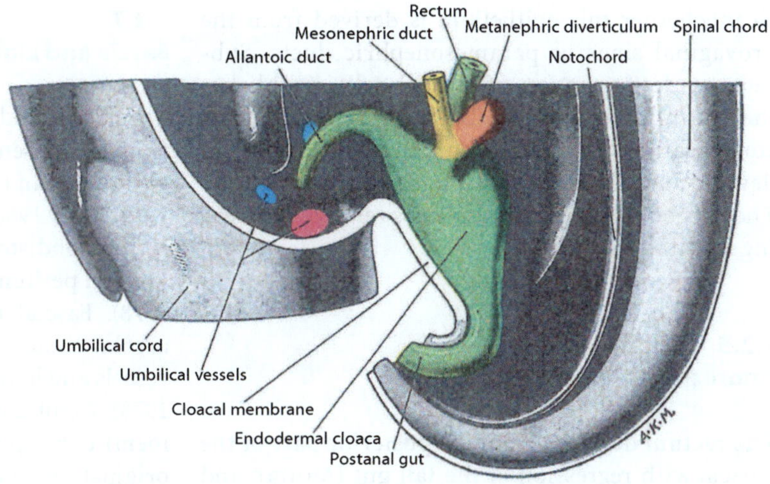

Fig. 1.2. The caudal end of a human embryo, about 5 weeks old. Reprinted from Bannister et al. (1995, p. 207), by permission of Churchill Livingstone

1.2.2 Bladder

The cylindrical vesicourethral canal is a part of the primitive urogenital sinus superior to the opening of the mesonephric ducts. The canal has a dilated upper portion and a relatively narrow lower part, representing the primitive bladder and urethra. The upper part of the bladder is continuous with the allantois, which regresses early on into the urachus, a fibrous cord attached to the apex of the bladder and the umbilicus. The mucosa of the bladder primarily develops from the endodermal lining of the vesicourethral canal, the bladder musculature from the surrounding splanchnic mesenchyme, and the ureteric orifices from dorsal outgrowths of the mesonephric ducts. During the developmental process the mesonephric ducts are absorbed into the bladder wall and contribute to the trigone (Bannister et al. 1995).

1.2.3 Urethra

In women the urethra is derived mostly from its primitive counterpart, whereas in men this develops into the superior part of the prostatic urethra extending from the internal urethral orifice to the entrance of the common ejaculatory ducts. In men the mesonephric ducts also contribute to the proximal urethra. The connective tissue and smooth muscle develop from the adjacent splanchnic mesenchyme. Striated muscle fibres form around the smooth muscle, initially anterior, and later encircling the smooth muscle. The epithelium of the remainder of the prostatic and the membranous urethra in males is derived from the endoderm of the urogenital sinus. Fusion of the urogenital swellings with primary luminization gives rise to the penile urethra, whereas the glandular part of the urethra is formed through secondary luminization of the epithelial cord that is formed during fusion of the arms of the genital tubercle, i.e. the glans. In both fusion processes, apoptosis plays a key role (van der Werff et al. 2000). The consequence of fusion of the urogenital swellings is that their mesodermal cores unite on the ventral aspect of the penile urethra, where they differentiate into the integumental structures.

1.2.4 Vagina

The paramesonephric ducts play a major role in the development of the uterus and vagina. The uterus is formed from the cranial part of the paramesonephric ducts, while the caudal vertical parts of the paramesonephric ducts fuse to form the uterovaginal primordium (Bannister et al. 1995). From this primordium part of the uterus and the vagina develop. The primordium extends to the urogenital sinus and at the dorsal wall of the urogenital sinus an epithelium proliferation develops (sinovaginal bulb), the site of the future hymen. Progressive proliferation superiorly from the sinovaginal bulb results in a solid plate in the uterovaginal primordium, which develops into a solid cylindrical structure. It is not clear whether this epithelium is derived from the urovaginal sinus or paramesonephric ducts. Subsequent desquamation of central cells establishes the central vaginal lumen. The tubular mesodermal condensation of the uterovaginal primordium will develop into the fibromuscular wall of the vagina. The urogenital sinus demonstrates relative shortening forming the vestibule.

1.2.5 Anorectum

The rectum develops from the posterior part of the cloaca, with regression of the tail gut (Moore and Persaud 1998). The upper two-thirds of the anal canal is endodermal from the hindgut; the lower one-third is epithelial from the proctoderm. The proctoderm is formed by mesenchymal elevations around the anal membrane, which originate from the primitive streak and migrate between the ectoderm and endoderm. The dentate line represents the junction of these epithelial and endodermal tissues and is the site of the anal membrane. Inferior to the dentate line is the anocutaneous line where there is a transition from columnar to stratified keratinized epithelium. At the outer verge, the anal epithelium is continuous with the skin around the anus. The arterial, venous, lymphatic and nerve supply of the superior two-thirds of the anus is of hindgut origin, compared to the inferior one-third, which is of proctodermal origin.

1.2.6 Pelvic Floor Muscles

The pelvic floor comprises several muscle groups of different embryological origin, some developing from the cloacal sphincter and others from the sacral myotomes (Hamilton and Mossman 1972). The urogenital septum divides the cloacal sphincter into anterior and posterior parts. The external anal sphincter develops from the posterior part, and the superficial transverse perineal muscle, bulbospongiosus and ischiocavernosus from the anterior part (Moore and Persaud 1998; Hamilton and Mossman 1972), thus explaining their common innervation by the pudendal nerve. The levator ani muscle and coccygeus muscle develop from the first to the third sacral segments (myotomes) (Hamilton and Mossman 1972).

1.2.7 Fascia and Ligaments

The fascia and ligaments of the pelvic floor arise from the mesenchyme between and surrounding the various organ rudiments (Hamilton and Mossman 1972; Arey 1966). The mesenchyme may develop into either nondistensible or distensible fascia (e.g. the visceral peritoneal fascia of the pelvic viscera) (Last 1978). Fascial tissues arise from condensations of areolar tissue surrounding the branches of the iliac vessels and hypogastric plexuses to the viscera (Last 1978). Genital ligaments (e.g. in females broad ligament) develop from loose areolar tissue precursors originating from the mesenchymal urogenital ridge (Arey 1966). The vagina and uterus develop from paired paramesonephric ducts. These ducts, with their mesenterium attached to the lateral wall, migrate and fuse medially, carrying the vessels that supply the ovary, uterus and vagina. Tissue around these vessels condenses into the cardinal and sacrouterine ligaments that attach the cervix and upper vagina to the lateral pelvic walls. Fusion of the embryological cul-de-sac creates the single layered Denonvilliers' fascia in men (van Ophoven and Roth 1997).

1.2.8 Perineum

As the cloacal membrane disappears, a sagittal orientated external fissure between the labioscrotal folds develops, except where the urogenital septum is fused. This fold, covered by encroaching ectoderm and marked by a median raphe, is the primary perineum (Arey 1966). Later in development of male embryos, the perineal raphe becomes continuous with the scrotal raphe, the line of fusion of the labioscrotal swellings. The perineal body, the tendineus centre of the perineum, is formed at the junction of the urogenital septum and the cloacal membrane.

1.2.9 Newborn

The pelvic anatomy is almost complete at birth, although some changes occur from birth to adulthood. These relate to organ maturation as well as responses to other effects, such as respiration and an increased intraabdominal pressure. Notable are the pelvis changing from its funnel shape in newborns, and the straight sacrum becoming curved (Lansman and Robertson 1992), and nerve endings at the dentate line as part of the continence mechanism developing after birth (Li et al. 1992).

1.3 Anatomy

The pelvic floor is attached both directly and indirectly to the pelvis. Its layers, from superior to inferior, are the endopelvic fascia, the muscular pelvic diaphragm, the perineal membrane (urogenital diaphragm), and a superficial layer comprising the superficial transverse perineal, bulbospongiosus (bulbocavernous) muscle and ischiocavernous muscles. The pelvic floor is traversed by the urethra and anal sphincters, and in women the vagina. As the majority of patients with pelvic floor disorders are women, emphasis will be on the female anatomy.

Most of the MRI figures in this chapter were obtained at a field strength of 1.5 T with phased array coils, and a few with an endoluminal coil (used either endovaginally or endoanally), as indicated in the legend. All are T2-weighted images (turbo spin-echo sequences), where the bony pelvis exhibits a relatively hyperintense marrow with hypointense cortex. Fascia, tendons and striated muscles have a relatively hypointense signal intensity. Smooth muscles (e.g. internal anal sphincter) are relatively hyperintense. Fat and most vessels are relatively hyperintense.

1.3.1 Pelvic Wall

The bony pelvic wall is the site of attachment of pelvic floor structures. Pelvic floor structures attach directly to bone at the pubic bones, ischial spines, sacrum and coccyx, and indirectly by fascia. The muscles attached directly to the bony pelvic wall are the primary components of the pelvic diaphragm: the anterior part of the levator ani (the anterior part of the pubococcygeus muscle, including the pubovisceralis) and the coccygeus muscle. The periosteum of the posterior surface of the pubic bone at the lower border of the pubic symphysis is the site of origin of the pubococcygeus and pubovisceralis muscles (Figs. 1.3, 1.4). The tip of the ischial spine is the origin of the coccygeus muscle (Figs. 1.3, 1.4), which inserts into the lateral aspect of the coccyx and the lowest part of the sacrum. The sacrospinous ligament is a triangular-shaped ligament at the posterior margin of the coccygeus muscle, separating the sciatic notch in the greater sciatic foramen, containing the piriformis muscle and pudendal nerve, and, together with the sacrotuberous ligament, the lesser sciatic foramen, which transmits amongst others the internal obturator tendon muscle and the pudendal nerve (Fig. 1.3).

The internal obturator muscle forms the major constituent of the pelvic sidewall (Fig. 1.5). It originates from the obturator membrane (covering the obturator foramen), the margins of the obturator foramen and the pelvic surfaces of the ilium and ischium (Tobias and Arnold 1981). The obturator tendon inserts into the greater trochanter of the femur. A tendineus ridge of the obturator fascia, the arcus tendineus levator ani, forms the pelvic sidewall attachment for the levator ani (Figs. 1.6, 1.7, 1.8). The piriformis is a flat triangular-shaped muscle arising from the second to fourth sacral segments inserting into the greater trochanter of the femur. It lies directly above the pelvic floor and is the largest structure in the greater sciatic foramen

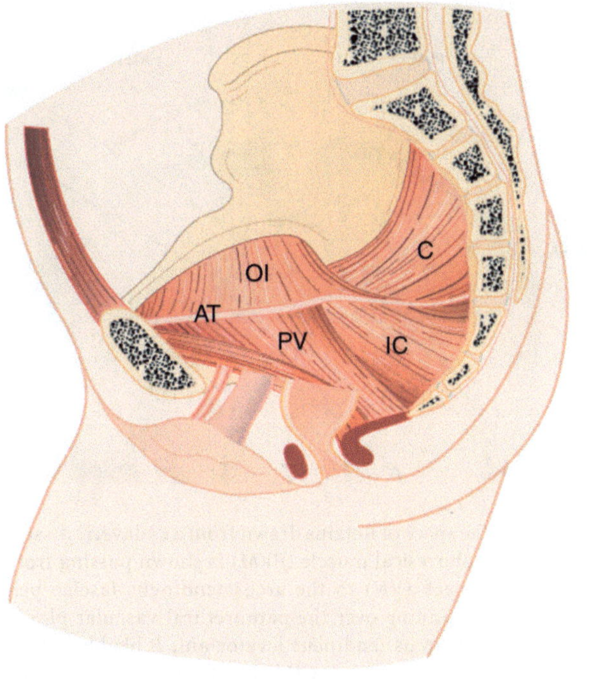

Fig. 1.3. Diagram of the levator ani showing the pubovisceralis (*PV*), iliococcygeus (*IC*), coccygeus (*C*), and the arcus tendineus (*AT*) arising from the obturator internus (*OI*) fascia

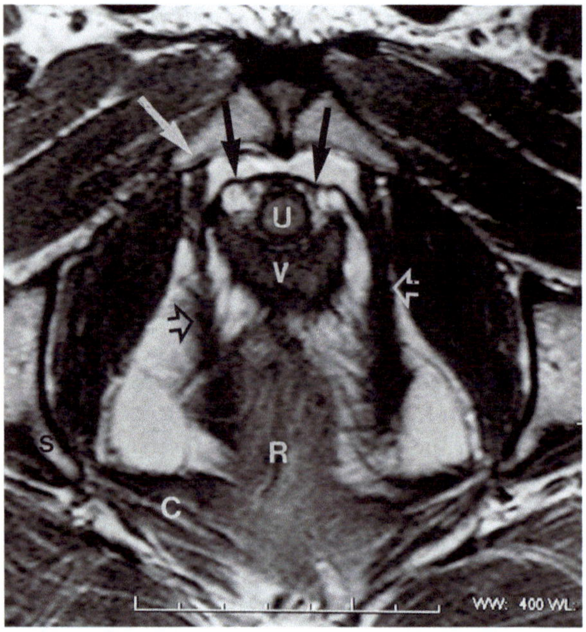

Fig. 1.4. Axial oblique T2-weighted turbo spin-echo. Note the attachment of the pubovesicalis (*black arrows*) to the levator ani (*open arrows*) (*U*=urethra, *V*=vagina, *R*=rectum, *S*=ischial spine, *C*=coccygeus). Note the attachment of pubococcygeus to pubic bone (*white arrow*)

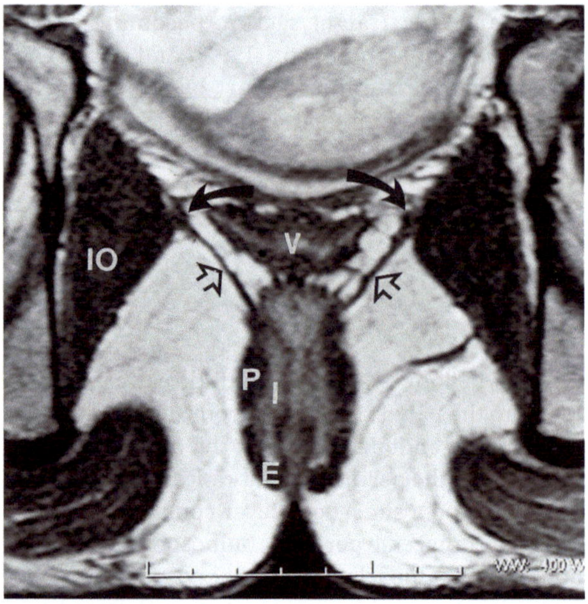

Fig. 1.5. Coronal oblique T2-weighted turbo spin-echo parallel to the axis of the anal canal in a woman (*I*=internal anal sphincter, *E*=external anal sphincter, *P*=puborectalis, *V*=vagina). The iliococcygeus (*open arrows*) inserts into the arcus tendineus levator ani (ATLA, *curved arrows*) formed from fascia over the internal obturator muscle (*IO*)

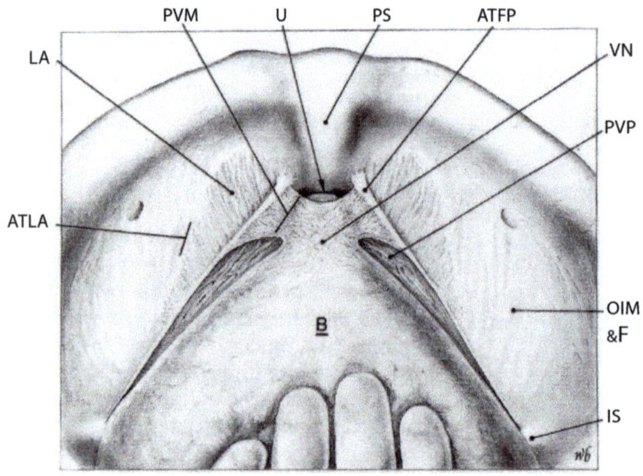

Fig. 1.6. The space of Retzius drawn from a cadaveric dissection. The pubovesical muscle (*PVM*) is shown passing from the vesical neck (*VN*) to the arcus tendineus fasciae pelvis (*ATFP*), running over the paraurethral vascular plexus (*PVP*) (*ATLA* arcus tendineus levator ani, *B* bladder, *IS* ischial spine, *LA* levator ani, *OIM&F* obturator internus muscle and fascia, *PS* pubic symphysis, *U* urethra). Reprinted from Cardozo (1997, p. 36), by permission of the publisher Churchill Livingstone

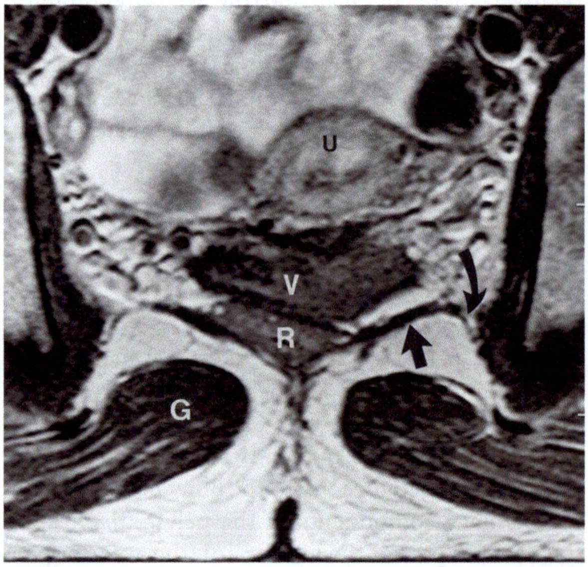

Fig. 1.7. Coronal oblique T2-weighted turbo spin-echo posterior to the anal canal of a woman. The iliococcygeus part of the levator ani muscle (*black arrow*) has its origin at the arcus tendineus levator ani. The lateral part of the iliococcygeus is relatively thin and membranous (*curved arrow*) (*R*=rectum, *V*=vagina, *U*=uterus, *G*=gluteus maximus)

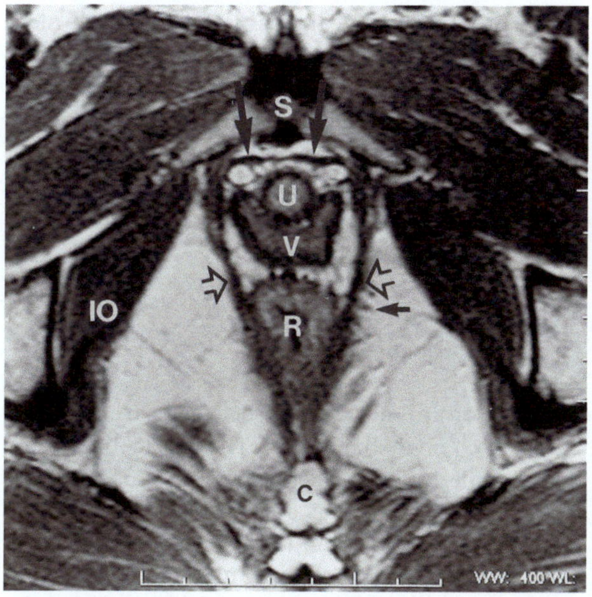

Fig. 1.8. Axial oblique T2-weighted turbo spin-echo in a woman (*black arrows* pubovesical muscle, *U*=urethra, *V*=vagina, *R*=rectum, *S*=pubic symphysis, *IO*=internal obturator muscle, *C*=coccyx, *open arrows* transition between the pubococcygeus (anterior) and iliococcygeus (posterior), at the borders of the urogenital hiatus). Note fibres of the iliococcygeus extending towards the pelvic sidewall (*small solid arrow*)

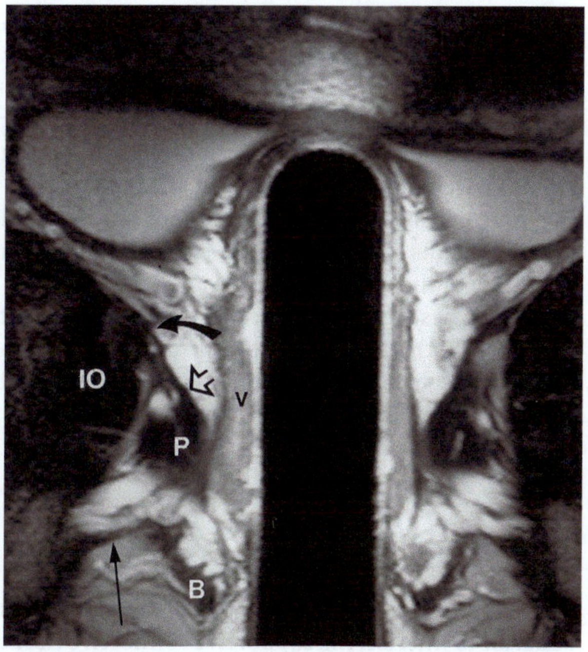

Fig. 1.9. Endovaginal coronal oblique T2-weighted turbo spin-echo parallel to the vaginal axis (*V*=vaginal wall, *B*=bulbospongiose muscle, *long arrow* perineal membrane, *P*=pubovisceralis). The levator ani (iliococcygeus) (open arrow) has its origin from the arcus tendineus levator ani (*curved arrow*) formed from the fascia of the internal obturator muscle (*IO*). Note the attachment of the lateral vaginal wall to the pubovisceralis. Reprinted with permission from Tan et al. (1998)

(Fig. 1.3). The sacral plexus is formed on the pelvic surface of the piriformis fascia. The fascia of the pelvic wall is a strong membrane covering the surface of the internal obturator and piriform muscles with firm attachments to the periosteum (Last 1978).

1.3.1.1
Tendineus Arcs

The arcus tendineus levator ani and the arcus tendineus fascia pelvis are oblique sagittal-orientated linear dense, pure connective tissue structures at the pelvic sidewall. These structures have well-organized fibrous collagen and are histologically akin to the tendons and ligaments of the peripheral musculoskeletal system. The arcus tendineus levator ani is a condensation of the obturator fascia, extending to the pubic ramus anteriorly and to the ischial spine posteriorly. Most of the levator ani muscle arises from it (Figs. 1.5, 1.6, 1.9).

The posterior half of the arcus tendineus fascia pelvis joins with the arcus tendineus levator ani, whereas the anterior half has a more inferior and

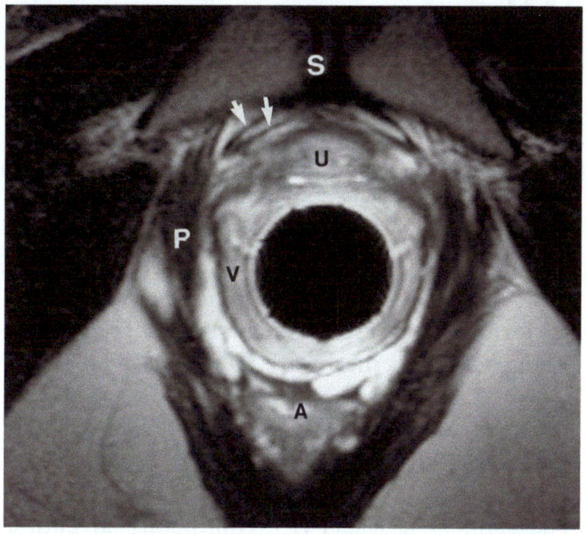

Fig. 1.10. Endovaginal axial oblique T2-weighted turbo spin-echo in a woman (*S*=pubic symphysis, *small arrows* arcus tendineus fascia pelvis, *U*=urethra, *V*=vaginal wall, *A*=anus, *P*=puborectalis). Reprinted with permission from Tan et al. (1998)

medial course than the arcus tendineus levator ani (Fig. 1.6) attaching to the pubis close to the pubic symphysis (DeLancey and Starr 1990) (Fig. 1.10).

These tendineus arcs are reinforced by a four stellate-shaped tendineus structure originating from the ischial spine (Mauroy et al. 2000), including the tendineus arcs, sacrospinous and ischial arch ligaments. The latter is the transition between the fascia of the piriform muscle and the pelvic diaphragm. These tendineus arcs form the attachment for several structures: the levator ani muscle, endopelvic fascia (anterior vaginal wall), pubovesical muscle, and other supportive structures.

1.3.2 Pelvic Floor

The pelvic floor comprises four principal layers: from superior to inferior, the supportive connective tissue of the endopelvic fascia and related structures, the pelvic diaphragm [levator ani (iliococcygeus, pubococcygeus) and coccygeus muscles], the perineal membrane (urogenital diaphragm) and the superficial layer (superficial transverse perineal muscle, bulbospongiosus and ischiocavernous muscles). The pelvic floor gives active support by the muscular contraction and passive elastic support by fascia and ligaments.

1.3.2.1 Supportive Connective Tissue (Endopelvic Fascia)

The connective tissue of the pelvis and pelvic floor is a complex system important for the passive support of visceral organs and pelvic floor. The connective tissue comprises collagen, fibroblasts, elastin, smooth muscle cells and neurovascular and fibrovascular bundles (Norton 1993; Strohbehn 1998). The connective tissue is present in several anatomical forms (e.g. fascia, ligaments) and levels, constituting a complex meshwork (De Caro et al. 1998).

1.3.2.1.1 Endopelvic Fascia

The endopelvic fascia is a continuous adventitial layer covering the pelvic diaphragm and viscera. This expansile membrane is covered by parietal peritoneum. The structure of the endopelvic fascia varies considerably in different areas of the pelvis. For example, primarily perivascular connective tissue is present at the cardinal ligaments with more fibrous tissue and fewer blood vessels at the rectal pillars. The endopelvic fascia envelops the pelvic organs, including the parametrium and paracolpium, giving support to the uterus and upper vagina. Ligamentous condensations within this fascia are primarily aggregations of connective tissue surrounding neurovascular bundles.

1.3.2.2 Pelvic Diaphragm

The levator ani muscle and coccygeus are the muscles of the pelvic diaphragm. The pelvic diaphragm acts as a shelf supporting the pelvic organs (Fig. 1.8). It has been described as a basin based on observations at dissection when the muscles are flaccid or surgery without normal tone. However, the constant muscle tone of the levator ani and coccygeus muscles by type I striated muscle fibres combined with fascial stability results in a dome-shaped form of the pelvic floor in the coronal plane, and also closes the urogenital hiatus. This active muscular support prevents the ligaments becoming over-stretched and damaged by constant tension (DeLancey 1994a).

1.3.2.2.1 Coccygeus Muscle

The coccygeus arises from the tip of the ischial spine, along the posterior margin of the internal obturator muscle (Figs. 1.3, 1.4). This shelf-like musculotendinous structure forms the posterior part of the pelvic diaphragm. The fibres fan out and insert into the lateral side of the coccyx and the lowest part of the sacrum. The sacrospinous ligament is at the posterior edge of the coccygeus muscle and is fused with this muscle. The proportions of the muscular and ligamentous parts may vary. The coccygeus is not part of the levator ani, having a different function and origin, being the homologue of a tail muscle (m. agitator caudae). The coccygeus muscle is innervated by the third and fourth sacral spinal nerves on its superior surface.

1.3.2.2.2 Levator Ani Muscle

The iliococcygeus, pubococcygeus and puboviscerralis form the levator ani muscle and may be differentiated by their lines of origin and direction (Fig. 1.8). The iliococcygeus muscle and pubococcygeus muscle arise from the ischial spine, the tendineus arc of the levator ani muscle and the pubic bone.

The iliococcygeus arises from the posterior half of the tendineus arc (Fig. 1.7) inserting into the last two segments of the coccyx and the midline anococcygeal raphe. An accessory slip may extend to the sacrum (iliosacralis). The anococcygeal raphe extends from the coccyx to the anorectal junction and represents the interdigitation of iliococcygeal fibres from both sides (LAST 1978). The iliococcygeus forms a sheet like layer and is often largely aponeurotic.

The pubococcygeus arises from the anterior half of the tendineus arc and the periosteum of the posterior surface of the pubic bone at the lower border of the pubic symphysis, its fibres directed posteriorly inserting into the anococcygeal raphe and coccyx.

The pubovisceralis forms a sling around the urogenital hiatus. The puborectalis is the main part of this "U"-shaped sling and goes around the anorectum where it is attached posteriorly to the anococcygeal ligament. Other slings have been identified: the puboanalis is a medially placed slip from this that runs into the anal sphincter providing striated muscle slips to the longitudinal muscle layer. The puboprostaticus in men (or puboperineus) and pubovaginal muscle in women. The former forms a sling around the prostate to the perineal body and the latter passes along the vagina to the perineal body with attachments to the lateral vaginal walls (SAMPSELLE and DELANCEY 1998; DELANCEY and RICHARDSON 1992) (Figs. 1.9, 1.11). Both interdigitate widely. Contraction of the pubovisceralis lifts and compresses the urogenital hiatus.

During vaginal delivery the levator ani muscle is under great mechanical stress. A computer model study of levator ani stretch during vaginal delivery estimated that the different portions of the levator ani muscle stretch up to 326% (LIEN et al. 2004). Recent imaging studies have demonstrated that levator ani muscle injury can occur during vaginal delivery (TUNN et al. 1999, HOYTE et al. 2001, DIETZ and LANZARONE 2005, KEARNEY et al. 2006). Defects often occur near the origin of the muscle at the pubic bone. In the case of de novo stress urinary incontinence, use of forceps, anal sphincter laceration, and episiotomy increased the odds ratio for levator muscle injury by 14.7-, 8.1- and 3.1-fold, respectively (KEARNEY et al. 2006).

The levator ani muscle is innervated from its superior side by the levator ani nerve. This nerve originates from sacral segments S3 and/or S4 (WALLNER

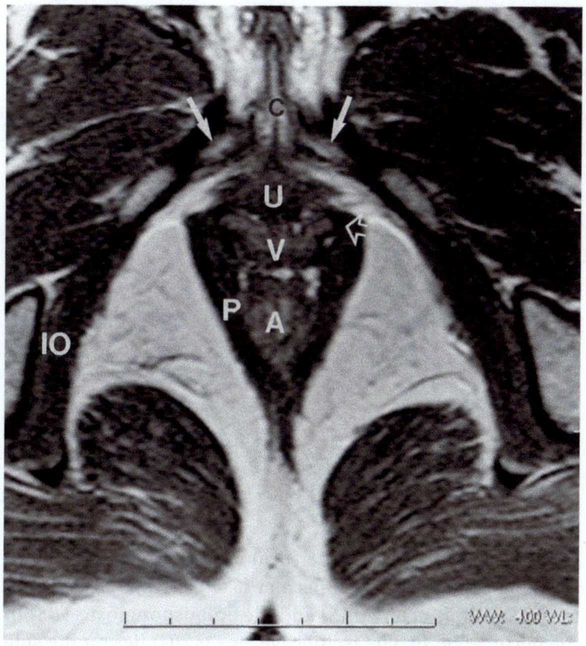

Fig. 1.11. Axial oblique T2-weighted turbo spin-echo in a woman (*U*=external urethral meatus, *V*=vagina, A=anus, *P*=pubovisceralis, white arrows ischiocavernous muscle, *IO*=internal obturator muscle, *C*=clitoris). Note the attachment of the vagina lateral walls to the pubovisceralis (*open arrow*)

et al. 2006a, WALLNER et al. 2006b). The pudendal nerve has a minor contribution. It only innervates the the levator ani muscle (from its inferior surface) in approximately 50% of the investigated cases (WALLNER et al. in print).

1.3.2.3
Perineal Membrane (Urogenital Diaphragm)

The perineal membrane, also named the urogenital diaphragm, is a fibromuscular layer directly below the pelvic diaphragm. The diaphragm is triangular in shape and spans the anterior pelvic outlet, and is attached to the pubic bones (Fig. 1.12). The urogenital diaphragm is crossed by the urethra and vagina. In men it is a continuous sheet, whereas in women it is attached medially to lateral vaginal walls.

Classically it is described as a trilaminar structure with the deep transverse perineal muscles sandwiched between the superior and inferior fascia. However, the superior fascia is now discounted, and even the existence of the deep transverse perinei has been questioned in cadaveric and MRI studies (OELRICH 1983; DORSCHNER et al. 1999). It is likely that these are really muscle fibres from the compres-

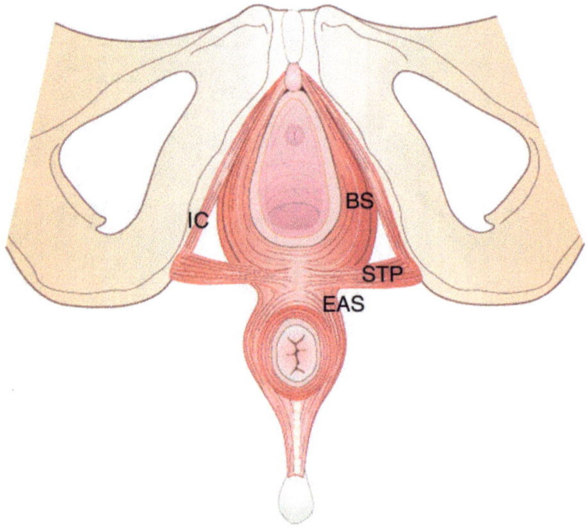

Fig. 1.12. Diagram of the perineal muscles in a female with the superficial transverse perinei (*STP*) fusing with the external anal sphincter (*EAS*) and the bulbospongiosus (*BS*) in the perineal body. The ischiocavernosus (*IC*) lies on the side wall of the perineal membrane

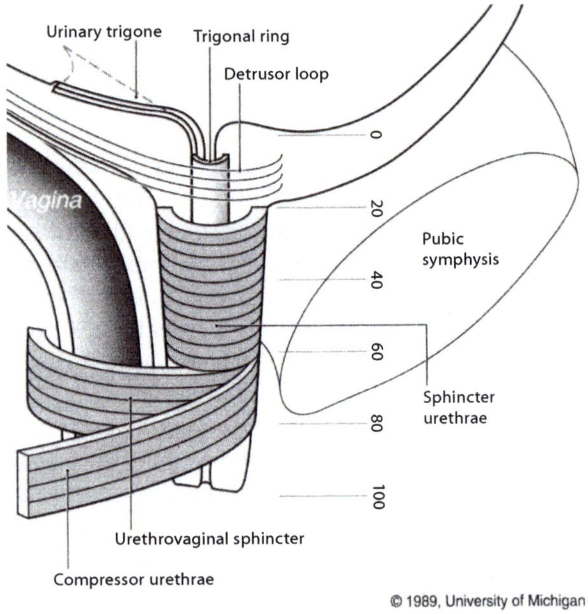

Fig. 1.13. The internal and external urethral sphincteric mechanisms and their locations. The sphincter urethrae, urethrovaginal sphincter and compressor urethrae are all parts of the striated urogenital sphincter muscle. Reprinted from CARDOZO (1997, p. 34), by permission of the publisher Churchill Livingstone

sor urethrae and urethrovaginalis part of the external urethral sphincter muscle (Figs. 1.13, 1.14) (see Sect. 1.3.4.3 Urethral Support), which lie above the perineal membrane, or transverse fibres inserting into the vagina (OELRICH 1983) that can be identified at this level on MRI (TAN et al. 1998) (Fig. 1.9).

1.3.2.4 Superficial Layer (External Genital Muscles)

At the most superficial of the four layers of the pelvic floor lie the external genital muscles, derived from the cloacal sphincter, comprising the superficial transverse perinei, the bulbospongiosus and the ischiocavernosus (Fig. 1.12). The former is supportive; the other two play a role in sexual function.

In females, the bulbospongiosus courses from the clitoris along the vestibulum to the perineal body (Figs. 1.4–1.12, 1.15–1.17). The ischiocavernosus originates from the clitoris, covers the crus of the clitoris that has a posterolateral course and terminates at the ischiopubic ramus (Figs. 1.15, 1.18). Both muscles compress the venous return of the clitoris (and crus of the clitoris), leading to erection of the clitoris. In males both muscles have a similar erectile function. The male bulbospongiosus (bul-

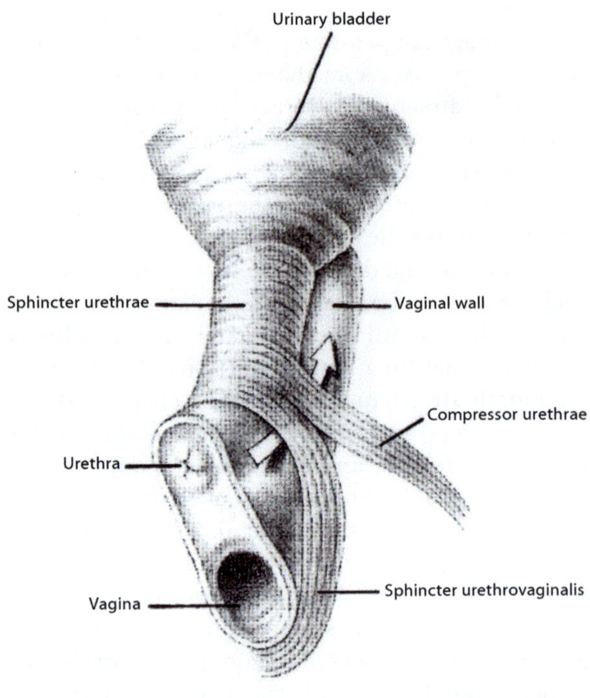

Fig. 1.14. Urethrovaginal sphincter, compressor urethrae and urethral sphincter (sphincter urethrae). Reprinted from BANNISTER et al. (1995, p. 834), by permission of Churchill Livingstone

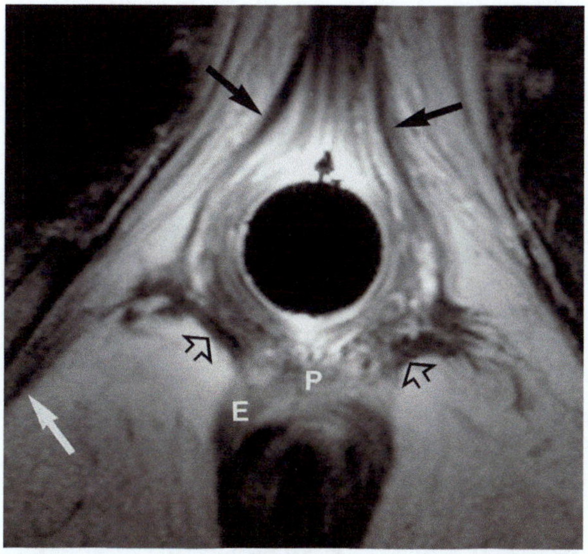

Fig. 1.15. Endovaginal axial oblique T2-weighted turbo spin-echo (*black arrows* bulbospongiosus, *open arrows* transverse perinei, *P*=perineal body, *E*=external anal sphincter, *white arrow* insertion of the ischiocavernous). Reprinted with permission from Tan et al. (1998)

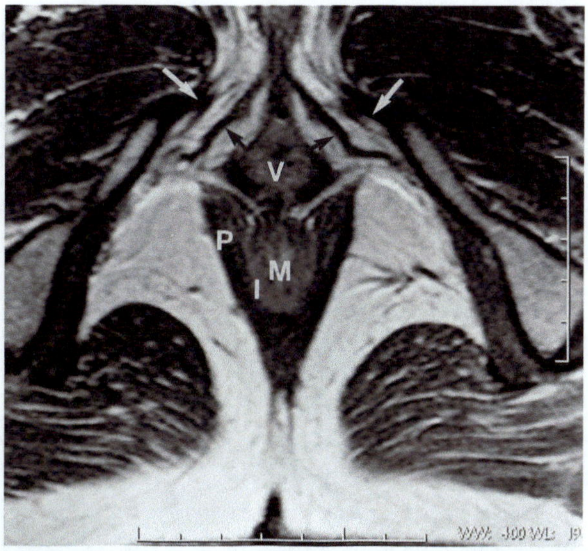

Fig. 1.17. Axial oblique T2-weighted turbo spin-echo in a woman (*I*=internal anal sphincter, *M*=mucosa/submucosa, *P*=pubovisceralis, *V*=vagina, *black arrows* bulbospongiosus, *white arrows* ischiocavernous)

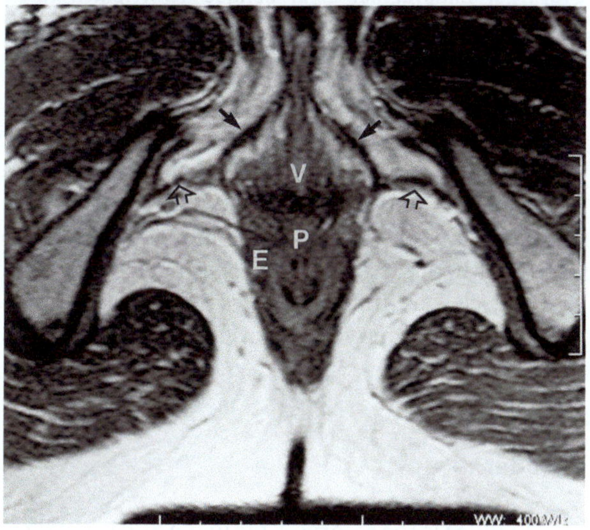

Fig. 1.16. Axial oblique T2-weighted turbo spin-echo in a woman (*E*=external anal sphincter, *P*=perineal body, *V*=vagina, *black arrows* bulbospongiosus, *open arrows* transverse perinei)

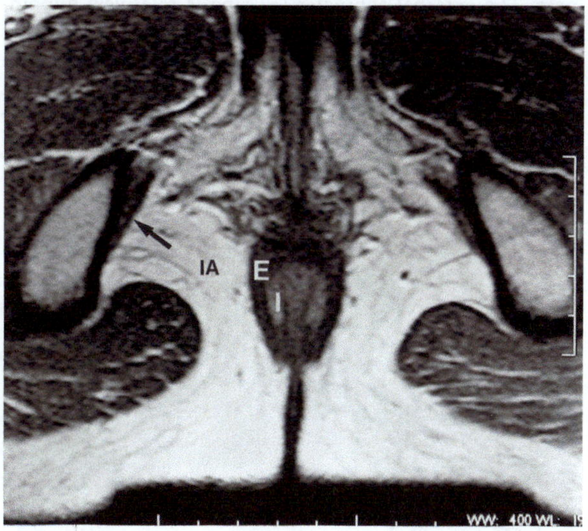

Fig. 1.18. Axial oblique T2-weighted turbo spin-echo in a woman (*E*=external anal sphincter, *I*=internal anal sphincter, *IA*=ischioanal space, *arrow* ischiocavernosus insertion)

bocavernous) covers the bulb of the penis and is attached to the perineal body. The male ischiocavernosus covers the crus of the penis and, as in the female, terminates at the ischiopubic ramus. The bulbospongiosus and ischiocavernosus muscles are innervated by the perineal branch of the pudendal nerve (Schraffordt et al. 2004).

1.3.2.4.1 Transverse Perineal Muscles

The superficial transverse perinei span the posterior edge of the urogenital diaphragm (Figs. 1.12, 1.15, 1.16, 1.19, 1.20), inserting into the perineal body and external sphincter. In men this is into the cen-

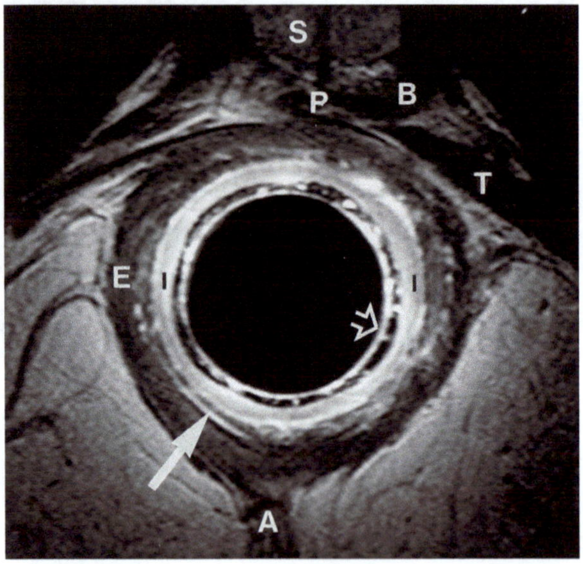

Fig. 1.19. Endoanal axial oblique T2-weighted turbo spin-echo orthogonal to the axis of the anal canal in a male volunteer (inferior to Fig. 1.30). The mucosa/submucosa is relatively hyperintense (*open arrow*) with hypointense muscularis submucosae ani. The internal anal sphincter (*I*) is relatively hyperintense and forms a ring of uniform thickness. The external sphincter (*E*) ring is relatively hypointense. In between the internal and external anal sphincter is the fat-containing hyperintense intersphincteric space with the relatively hypointense longitudinal layer (*white arrow*). The external sphincter (*E*), transverse perinei (*T*) and the bulbospongiosus (*B*) attach to the perineal body (*P*). Spongiose body of the penis (*S*). The external anal sphincter has a posterior attachment to the anococcygeal ligament (*A*)

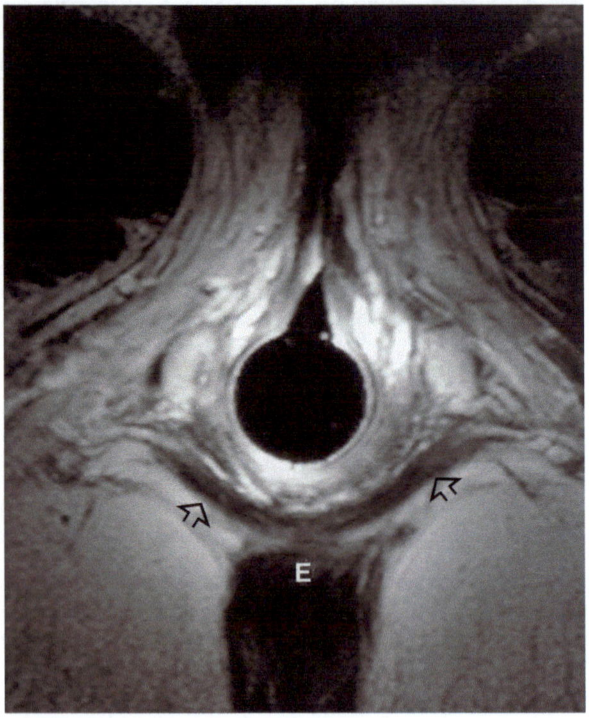

Fig. 1.20. Endovaginal axial oblique T2-weighted turbo spin-echo through the vaginal introitus. The transverse perinei (*open arrows*) course posterior to the vagina and anterior to the external anal sphincter (*E*)

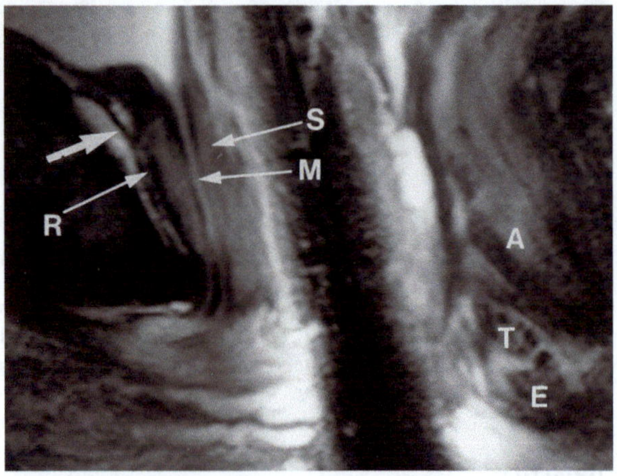

Fig. 1.21. Endovaginal sagittal oblique T2-weighted turbo spin-echo (*white arrow* pubovesicalis, *R* outer striated urethral muscle (rhabdosphincter), *S*=inner smooth urethral sphincter, *M*=urethral mucosa/submucosa, *A*=anus). The transverse perinei (*T*) and external anal sphincter (*E*) are part of the midline perineal body. Reprinted with permission from Tan et al. (1998)

tral point of the perineum, with a plane of cleavage between this and the external sphincter. There is no such plane in women as the fibres decussate directly with the external anal sphincter (Fig. 1.21). The muscles are innervated by the perineal branch of the pudendal nerve (Schraffordt et al. 2004).

1.3.3 Bladder

The bladder is the reservoir for urine and crucial for proper lower urinary tract function. It lies posterior to the pubic bones and is separated from the pubic bones by the retropubic space (space of Retzius), containing areolar tissue, veins and supportive ligaments. The wall has three layers: an inner mucous membrane, a smooth muscle layer–the detrusor–and an outer adventitial layer in part covered by peritoneum. The lax, distensible mucosal membrane of the bladder comprises transitional epithelium supported by a layer of loose fibroelastic connective tissue, the lamina propria. No real muscularis mucosae is present. At the trigone of the bladder the mucosa is adherent to the underlying muscle layer. Laterally at the trigone the ureteric orifices are present, with the ureteric folds. The internal urethral orifice is at the apex of the trigone, posteriorly bordered by the uvula in men (elevation caused by the median prostate lobe). During distension the trigone remains relatively fixed as the dome of the bladder rises into the abdomen.

1.3.3.1 Detrusor

The detrusor is the muscular wall of the bladder. The smooth muscle bundles are arranged in whorls and spirals, with the fibres of more circular orientation in the middle layer, and more longitudinal in the inner and outer layers. Functionally the detrusor acts as a single unit. Some of the outer longitudinal fibres of the detrusor are continuous with the pubovesical muscles (ligaments), the capsule of the prostate in men and the anterior vaginal wall in women (Bannister et al. 1995). Some bundles, the rectovesicalis, are continuous with the rectum. At the trigone two muscular layers can be identified. The deep layer is the continuation of the detrusor muscle, while the superficial layer is composed of small-diameter bundles of smooth muscle fibres, continuous with the muscle of the intramural ureters as well as with the smooth muscle of the proximal urethra in both sexes. More recent work has shown that the superficial layer constitutes two muscular structures, a musculus interuretericus and a sphincter trigonalis or sphincter vesicae (Bannister et al. 1995; Dorschner et al. 1999). The latter surrounds the urethral orifice, is reported not to extend into the urethra, and a dual role in men is hypothesized: preventing urinary incontinence and retrograde ejaculation.

1.3.3.2 Adventitia

The adventitia of the bladder is loose, except behind the trigone. At this site the bladder is anchored to the cervix uteri and anterior fornix in women. In men this part of the fascia is the upper limit of the rectovesical fascia (fascia of Denonvilliers). At the base of the bladder, condensations of areolar tissue envelop the inferior vesical artery, lymphatics, nerve supply and the vesical veins, forming the lateral ligaments or pillars of the bladder. The upper surface of the bladder is covered by peritoneum, while the rest of the bladder is surrounded by areolar tissue.

1.3.3.3 Bladder Support

The bladder is supported by several ligaments and by connections to surrounding structures. Anteriorly, the fibromuscular pubovesical muscle (ligament) is a smooth muscle extension of the detrusor muscle of the bladder to the arcus tendineus fascia pelvis and the inferior aspect of the pubic bone (DeLancey and Starr 1990). Based on a cadaver study, others have considered this structure as a ligament, anterior part of the hiatal membrane of the levator hiatus (Shafik 1999). This muscle is closely related to the pubourethral ligaments in females and puboprostatic ligaments in males. The pubovesical muscle (ligament) has been identified at MRI and may assist in opening the bladder neck during voiding (Strohbehn et al. 1996). Apart from the pubovesical muscle, other condensations of connective tissue around neurovascular structures can be found. The bladder neck position is influenced by connections between the pubovisceral (puborectal) muscle, vagina and proximal urethra. At the apex of the bladder is the median umbilical ligament, a remnant of the urachus. Posteroinferior support to the trigone in women is given by the lateral ligaments of the bladder, and attachments to the cervix uteri and to the anterior vaginal fornix. In men posteroinferior support is from the lateral ligaments and attachment to the base of the prostate. The base of the bladder rests on the pubocervical fascia, part of the endopelvic fascia, suspended between the arcus tendineus fasciae.

1.3.3.4 Neurovascular Supply

The innervation of the bladder (detrusor) is complex, involving parasympathetic and sympathetic nerve components (Chai and Steers 1997). Sympathetic fibres from the hypogastric nerves (lumbar splanchnic or presacral nerves) reach the bladder via the pelvic plexuses. The parasympathetic nerve supply is via the pelvic splanchnic nerves (nervi erigentes, S2 to S4) via the pelvic plexuses and innervates the detrusor. For the efferent sympathetic innervation there are differences in receptors. At the bladder neck and urethra a-adrenergic sympathetic innervation is predominant, leading to contraction. At the bladder dome there is predominant b-adrenergic sympathetic innervation leading to relaxation. Sympathetic stimulation from the spinal cord (T10–L2) via the hypogastric plexus with parasympathetic inhibition causes relaxation of the bladder dome and neck, with urethral contraction. In micturition the opposite mechanism, i.e. bladder contraction, relaxation of bladder neck and urethra, is established by parasympathetic activity and sympathetic inhibition. The ultimate control of the lower urinary function is in the central nervous system (CNS), including regions in the sacral spinal cord (S2–S4; Onuf), pons and cerebral cortex.

1.3.4 Urethra and Urethral Support

The control of micturition depends on a complex interaction between sphincteric components of the urethra, supportive structures, and CNS coordination.

1.3.4.1 Female Urethra

The female urethra has a length of approximately 4 cm. The wall of the female urethra comprises an inner mucous membrane and an outer muscular coat. The latter consists of an inner smooth muscle coat (lissosphincter) and an outer striated muscle sphincter (rhabdosphincter) (Figs. 1.21, 1.22). This outer striated muscle is anatomically separated from the adjacent striated muscle of the pelvic diaphragm. On T2-weighted MRI the urethra is seen embedded in the adventitial coat of the anterior vaginal wall, which is attached to the arcus tendineus fascia by the endopelvic fascia. In women the urethra is attached anteriorly to the pubic bone by the pubovesical ligaments, which are bordered laterally by the pubovaginal muscle (Last 1978).

Urethral closure pressure depends on the resting tone of the smooth and striated urethral muscles, and on a process of coaptation of the vascular plexus to form a complete mucosal seal.

1.3.4.1.1 Urethral Mucosa

The mucosal membrane of the urethra comprises epithelium and underlying lamina propria. The lumen of the urethra at rest is crescentic and slit-like in shape in the transverse plane, with a posterior midline ridge (urethral crest, crista urethralis). The proximal epithelium of the female urethra is tran-

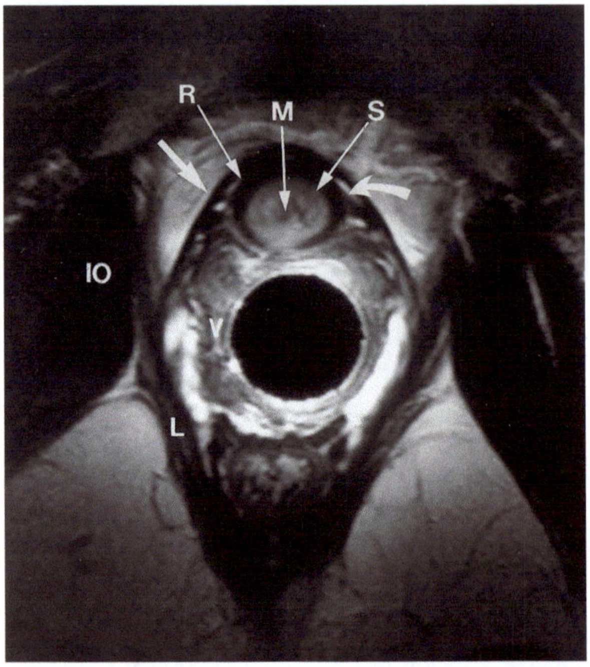

Fig. 1.22. Endovaginal axial oblique T2-weighted turbo spin-echo through the superior part of the urethra (*white arrow* pubovisceralis, *curved arrow* urethral supports, *R* = outer striated urethral muscle (rhabdosphincter), *S* = inner smooth urethral muscle, *M* = mucosa/submucosa, *V* = vagina, *L* = levator ani muscle, *IO* = internal obturator muscle). Reprinted with permission from Tan et al. (1998)

sitional epithelium, changing to non-keratinizing stratified epithelium for the major portion of the urethra. At the external meatus the epithelium becomes keratinized and is continuous with the vestibular skin. The lamina propria is a supportive layer of loose tissue underlying the epithelium and consists of collagen fibrils and longitudinally and circularly orientated elastic fibres and numerous veins. The rich vascular supply of the lamina propria has a function in urethral closure by coaptation of the mucosal surfaces (mucosal seal), a mechanism influenced by oestrogen levels. Pudendal nerve branches are found in the lamina propria. Afferent pathways transmit the sensation of temperature and urine passage via the pudendal nerve.

1.3.4.1.2 Smooth Muscle Urethral Coat

The smooth muscle urethral coat is in the form of a cylinder and present along the length of the female urethra. The fibres have a predominantly oblique or longitudinal orientation, although at the outer border circularly orientated fibres are present that intermingle with the inner fibres of the external urethral sphincter. The circular orientation of these fibres and the outer striated muscle suggest a role in constricting the lumen at contraction. Strata of connective tissue have been described dividing the smooth muscles of the proximal two-thirds of the female urethra into three layers and thin fibres of the pelvic plexus course to this part of the urethra (Colleselli et al. 1998). These layers comprise a thin inner longitudinal layer, thinning out to the external meatus, a thicker transverse layer and an outer longitudinal layer. The smooth muscles have primarily a parasympathetic autonomic nerve supply originating from the pelvic plexus. The innervation and fibre orientation make a role for this muscle coat during micturition more likely than in preserving continence.

1.3.4.1.3
External Urethral Sphincter

The external urethral sphincter has circularly disposed slow-twitch fibres forming a sleeve that is thickest at the middle of the urethra (rhabdosphincter). At this level the external urethral sphincter is a continuous ring, although it is relatively thin and largely devoid of muscle fibres posteriorly (Colleselli et al. 1998) (Fig. 1.22). This is the level of maximal closure pressure. At the superior and inferior part of the urethra the external urethral sphincter is deficient posteriorly. The external sphincter slow-twitch fibres exert a constant tone upon the urethral lumen and play a role in active urethral closure at rest. During raised abdominal pressure additional closure force is provided by fast-twitch fibres. There is a close relationship with the smooth muscle urethral coat The striated sphincter muscle is closely related to the perineal membrane (urogenital diaphragm) and is separate from the adjacent striated muscle of the levator ani muscle (Yucel and Baskin 2004). At the distal end the rhabdosphincter consists of two additional elements: the compressor urethrae and urethrovaginal sphincter. The anatomy of the external urethral sphincter muscle was described in detail by Oelrich 1983 (see Sect. 1.3.4.3 Urethral Support). With advancing age, a progressive and age-dependent decrease of the density of striated muscle cells can be observed in the external sphincter (Strasser et al. 1999). Controversy exists about whether the external urethral sphincter has both a somatic and autonomic innervation. The somatic innervation of the external sphincter is through the pudendal nerve (second to fourth sacral nerve) (Yucel et al. 2004). Whether the autonomic nerve fibres from the pelvic plexus, which innervate the smooth muscle of the inner smooth muscle coat, also contribute to the external sphincter innervation remains questionable.

1.3.4.2
Male Urethra

The male urethra extends from the internal orifice (meatus) to the external urethral orifice (meatus) beyond the navicular fossa. The length is approximately 18–20 cm. In general the male urethra is considered in four parts: preprostatic, prostatic, membranous and spongiose. In this chapter on anatomy of the pelvic floor emphasis is on the former three as part of the lower urinary tract.

1.3.4.2.1
Lining of the Male Urethra

The preprostatic and proximal prostatic urethra is lined by urothelium that is continuous with the bladder lining as well as with the ducts entering this part of the urethra (e.g. ducts of the prostate). Below the ejaculatory ducts the epithelium changes into (pseudo)stratified columnar epithelium lining the membranous urethra and part of the penile urethra. The distal part of the urethra is lined with stratified squamous epithelium.

1.3.4.2.2
Preprostatic Urethra

The preprostatic urethra is approximately 1–1.5 cm in length. Superficial smooth muscle fibres surrounding the bladder neck are continuous around the preprostatic urethra and the prostatic capsule. The smooth muscle fibres surrounding the preprostatic urethra form bundles including connective tissue with elastic fibres. These bundles have been identified as an internal sphincter at the bladder neck, the musculus sphincter trigonalis, or musculus sphincter vesicae (Bannister et al. 1995; Gilpin and Gosling 1983). The rich sympathetic adrenergic supply of this smooth muscle sphincter has been suggested as indicative of a function in preventing retrograde ejaculation.

1.3.4.2.3
Prostatic Urethra

The prostatic urethra is embedded within the prostate, emerging just anterior to the apex of the prostate. In the posterior midline the urethral crest is present, with the verumontanum. At this level the ejaculatory ducts and prostatic ducts enter. The lower part of the prostatic urethra has a layer of smooth muscle fibres and is enveloped by striated muscle fibres continuous with the external urethral sphincter of the membranous part of the urethra.

1.3.4.2.4
Membranous Urethra and Spongiose Urethra

The membranous urethra extends from the prostatic urethra to the bulb of the penis and is approximately 2 cm long. The urethra transverses the perineal membrane with a close relationship with the membrane, especially laterally and posteriorly. Under the lining of membranous urethra is fibroelastic tissue that is bordered by smooth muscle. This smooth muscle is continuous with the smooth muscle of the prostatic urethra. Outside this smooth muscle layer is a prominent circular layer of slow-twitch striated muscle fibres, the external urethral sphincter. The fibres of the external urethral sphincter are capable of prolonged contraction, resulting in muscle tone and urethral closure, important for continence. A study using dissection of cadavers and MRI in volunteers has indicated the presence of an outer striated muscle and inner smooth muscle part of the rhabdosphincter, introducing the terms musculus sphincter urethrae transversostriatus and musculus sphincter urethrae glaber (Dorschner et al. 1999). The innervation of the external urethral sphincter is from S2 to S4. The spongiose urethra commences below the perineal membrane and is within the spongiose body.

1.3.4.3
Urethral Support

Urethral support is complex and not fully elucidated, although importantly more insight has been gained in recent decades. In females the urethra is supported by numerous structures, including the endopelvic fascia, the anterior vagina and arcus tendineus fascia pelvis. The endopelvic fascia (also named pubocervical fascia at this location) is attached at both lateral sides to the arcus tendineus fascia pelvis (primarily attached to the levator ani muscle as well to the pubic bone) (Fig. 1.10) and superiorly continuous with the sacrouterine and cardinal ligaments. This layer of anterior vaginal wall and pubocervical fascia suspended between the tendineus arcs at both sides forms a "hammock" underlying and supporting the urethra (DeLancey 1994b) (Figs. 1.6, 1.23). Contraction of the levator ani muscles elevates the arcus tendineus fascia pelvis and thereby the vaginal wall. This leads to compression of the urethra by the hammock of supportive tissue. Close to the midline a pair of fibromuscular ligaments – pubourethral ligaments – anchor the urethra and vagina (Fig. 1.24), which can also be visualized using MRI (El-Sayed et al. 2007). These pubourethral ligaments contain smooth muscle fibres, an inferior extension of the detrusor muscle. The ligaments give support to the bladder neck and urethra (Papa Petros 1998), and this may be enhanced by contraction of the smooth muscle fibres in the ligaments.

Anterior to the urethra a sling-like structure can be identified (Figs. 1.4, 1.8, 1.21–1.23, 1.25). This structure courses just anterior to the urethra and has lateral attachments to the levator ani muscle (Tan et al. 1998; Tunn et al. 2001). This structure has been identified as the inferior extension of the pubovesical muscle, originating from the vesical neck (Tunn et al. 2001) and has also been named the periurethral ligament (Tan et al. 1998). The aspect of the structure resembles the configuration of the compressor urethrae (see below), but the pubovesical muscle has a higher position, namely at the superior urethra. At high resolution endovaginal MRI, urethral support structures (paraurethral ligaments) originating from the urethra and vaginal surface of the urethra seem to attach to this sling-like structure (Fig. 1.22). This structure seems to have an intimate relationship with the inferior urethral supportive structures (Figs. 1.21, 1.25).

The urethra is in females at the level of the pelvic diaphragm bordered by the most medial part of the pubococcygeus muscle (i.e. pubovaginal muscle), which inserts posteroinferiorly into the perineal body. The pubococcygeus (pubovaginal) muscle is not directly attached to the urethra, but with contraction the proximity and orientation results in a closing force on the urethral lumen. In males, the medial part of the pubococcygeus muscle (puboperineales) has a close relationship, but no direct attachments to the urethra. Contraction of this muscle has an occlusive effect on the urethra to a certain extent and is considered important in the quick stop of micturition (Myers et al. 2000).

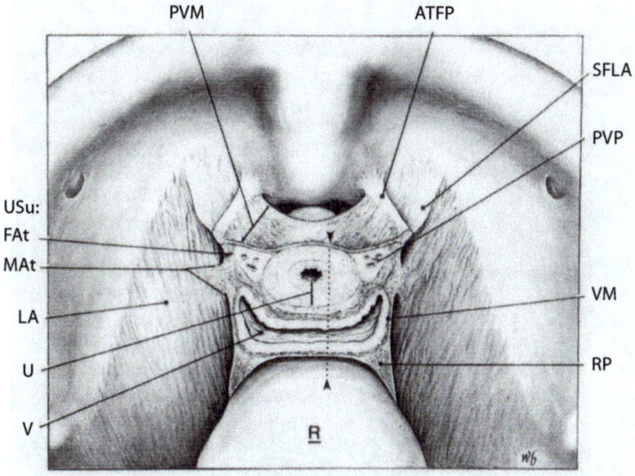

Fig. 1.23. Cross-section of the urethra (*U*), vagina (*V*), arcus tendineus fasciae pelvis (*ATFP*) and superior fascia of the levator ani muscle (*SFLA*) just below the vesical neck (drawn from cadaveric dissection). The pubovesicalis (*PVM*) lies anterior to the urethra, and anterior and superior to the paraurethral vascular plexus (*PVP*). The urethral supports (*USu*) attach the vagina and vaginal surface of the urethra to the levator ani (*LA*) muscles (*MAt* muscular attachment) and to the superior fascia of the levator ani muscle (*FAt*=fascial attachment) (*R*=rectum, *RP*=rectal pillar, VM=vaginal wall muscularis). Reprinted from Cardozo (1997, p. 36), by permission of the publisher Churchill Livingstone

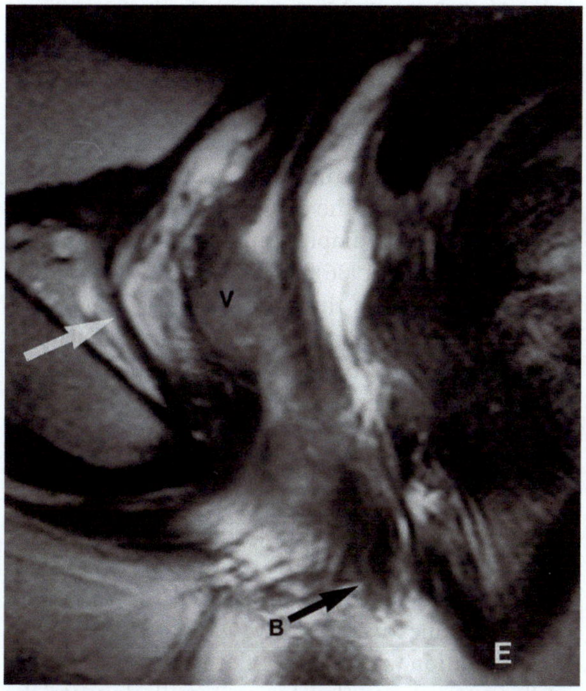

Fig. 1.25. Endovaginal parasagittal oblique T2-weighted turbo spin-echo parallel to the vaginal axis (*white arrow* pubovesicalis, *V*=vagina). The bulbospongiosus (*B*) and external anal sphincter (*E*) course to the midline perineal body. Reprinted with permission from Tan et al. (1998)

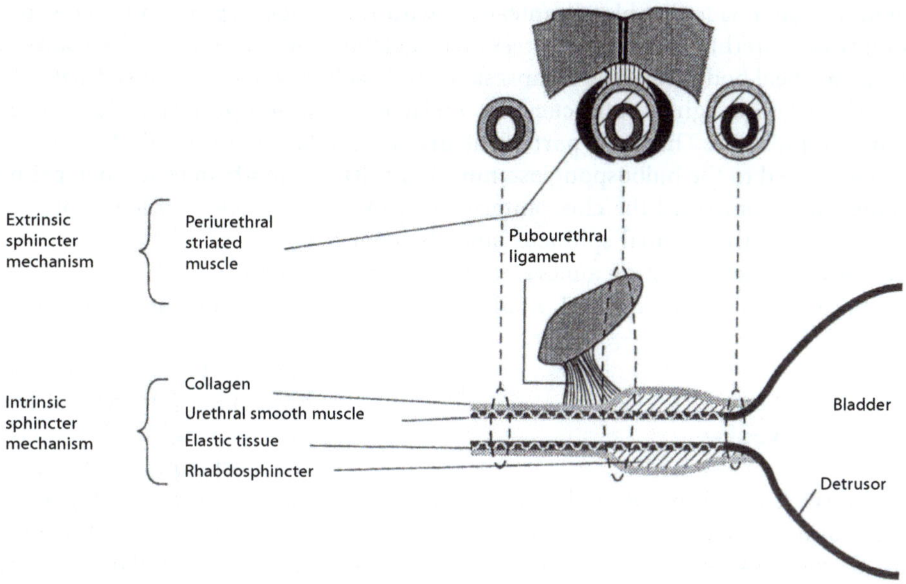

Fig. 1.24. Schematic representation of the urethra sphincter. Reprinted from Cardozo (1997, p. 35), by permission of the publisher Churchill Livingstone

At the inferior half of the urethra, the striated muscle of the external urethral sphincter exists of two additional elements: the compressor urethrae and urethrovaginal sphincter (Oelrich 1983) (Fig. 1.14). These muscles were previously described as part of the deep transverse perineal muscle. The slow-twitch fibres of the compressor urethrae insert into the urogenital diaphragm near the ischiopubic rami (DeLancey 1986), forming a broad arching muscular sheet with the contralateral counterpart. The most anterior part is in the midline ventral to the urethra. It has been described as being below the sphincter urethrae and has been reported to be approximately 6 mm wide (Oelrich 1983). The superior edge lies within the urogenital hiatus of the pelvic diaphragm and is continuous with the lower fibres of the anterior rhabdosphincter. The compressor urethrae compresses the urethra. As it is orientated at an angle of 130° to the urethra, it can pull the external meatus inferiorly (Oelrich 1983). This, in combination with bladder elevation by other pelvic floor structures (levator ani), will elongate the urethra. Visualization of the compressor urethrae at MRI is not fully elucidated. A sling-like structure can be identified, although this has a relatively superior position and also has been identified as the pubovesical muscle (Tunn et al. 2001) (Figs. 1.4, 1.8, 1.22). Other striated muscle fibres encircle the vagina, forming the urethrovaginal sphincter (Fig. 114). The urethrovaginal sphincter can be identified as a low signal intensity fibrous structure at MRI (Tan et al. 1998) (Fig. 1.26). This structure is a thin flat muscle up to 5 mm wide that blends anteriorly with the compressor urethrae. Posterior fibres may extend to the perineal body. Both the compressor urethrae and the urethrovaginal sphincter are variable in form and presence. The distal part of the urethra is closely related to the bulbospongiose muscles. MRI studies have confirmed the close anterior relationship of the urethrovaginal sphincter and the compressor urethrae presenting a more or less anterior sheet (Tan et al. 1998) (Figs. 1.21, 1.25).

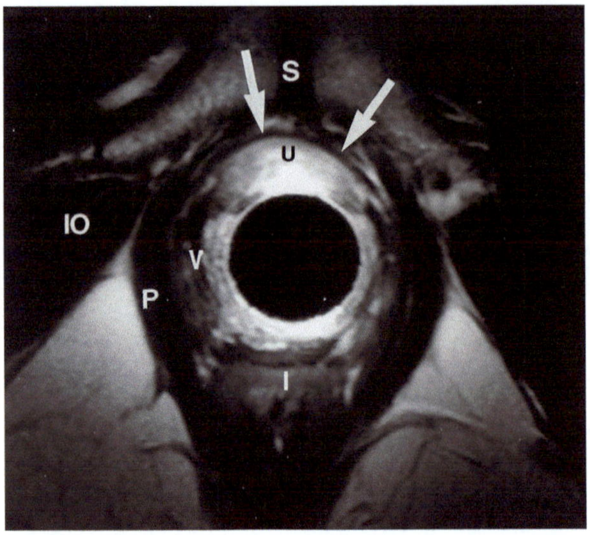

Fig. 1.26. Endovaginal axial oblique T2-weighted turbo spin-echo (*S*=pubic symphysis, *white arrows* urethrovaginal sphincter, *U*=external urethral meatus, *V*=vaginal wall, *P*=pubovisceralis, *I*=internal anal sphincter, *IO*=internal obturator). Reprinted with permission from Tan et al. (1998)

1.3.5 Uterus and Vagina

The uterus is a midline visceral organ, pear-shaped and mainly horizontal in orientation. The upper two-thirds constitute the body and the lower one-third the uterine cervix. In general, the cervix is tilted forward from the coronal plane (anteversion), while the body is slightly flexed on the cervix (anteflexion). The uterus is above the pelvic diaphragm.

The vagina transverses the pelvic floor in a sagittal oblique plane, parallel to the pelvic inlet. The vagina is a fibromuscular sheath extending from the uterine cervix to the vestibule. The unstretched length is approximately 7.5 cm anteriorly and 8.5 cm posteriorly. The vagina is lined by stratified squamous epithelium. The mucous coat is corrugated by transverse elevations, the vaginal rugae. The walls are collapsed with the lumen flattened in the anteroposterior plane (H-shape) in the lower third, while the vestibular entrance is a sagittal cleft. The smooth muscle coat primarily has a longitudinal and oblique orientation.

1.3.5.1 Uterus and Vaginal Support

Support to the uterus and vagina artificially can be divided into several levels. The endopelvic fascia covering the parametrium (broad ligament) is the most superior, first layer of pelvic support. The parametrium enveloped by endopelvic fascia gives lateral support. At the anterior side of the parametrium the round ligament gives accessory support in maintaining anteversion of the uterus. The endopelvic fascia covering the parametrium is continuous with the endopelvic fascia supporting the paracolpium and has been indicated as level I vaginal support (DeLancey 1993) (Figs. 1.6, 1.23).

The second level of support is at the uterine cervix and primarily concerns the uterosacral and cardinal ligaments. The uterosacral ligaments are attached to the posterolateral aspect of the cervix, form the lateral margins of the pouch of Douglas and insert fan-like at the presacral fascia at the level of the second to fourth sacral foramen. The cardinal ligament arises from the area of the greater sciatic foramen and courses to the uterine cervix. Both the cardinal and sacrouterine ligaments surround the cervix forming a pericervical ring and have attachments to the bladder base. The ligaments also envelop the superior part of the vagina. Both ligaments have a vertical orientation, suspending the cervix and upper vagina, and act as a single unit (DeLancey 1994a). The cardinal ligaments comprise perivascular connective tissue and the sacrouterine ligaments are predominantly smooth muscle and connective tissue (DeLancey and Richardson 1992).

One level inferiorly, support is given by several structures. The cardinal and sacrouterine ligaments have downward extensions forming the pubocervical fascia and rectovaginal fascia, both with attachment to the pelvic side wall (DeLancey 1988; DeLancey 1994a). These fasciae (all part of the endopelvic fascia) act as a single unit, just as the sacrouterine and cardinal ligaments. The fasciae give lateral support and have been indicated as level II support (DeLancey 1993). The anteromedial part of the vagina is suspended by the pubocervical fascia. This fascia is embedded with smooth muscles fibres and is attached to the arcus tendineus fascia pelvis. The attachment of the anterior vaginal wall to the tendineus arcs at both sides forms a supportive "hammock" of vaginal tissue and endopelvic fascia underneath the urethra (Fig. 1.23). The rectovaginal fascia of the rectovaginal septum supports the posterior part of the vagina. This septum is a sheet of fibromuscular tissue with an abundant venous supply. The rectovaginal fascia is suspended by attachments to the cardinal and sacrouterine ligaments and is laterally attached to the superior fascia of the pelvic diaphragm (DeLancey and Richardson 1992). The rectovaginal fascia has attachments to the perineal body. The vagina also has lateral support from the medial part of the levator ani (level III support), just caudal to the arcus tendineus fasciae pelvis (Figs. 1.9, 1.11), and from the perineal membrane (DeLancey and Starr 1990; DeLancey 1993, 1994a). This support has been described as attachment and has also been identified as a separate part of the levator ani: the pubovaginal muscle. The perineal body and its attachments give inferior support.

1.3.6 Perineum and Ischioanal Fossa

The perineum is the region below the pelvic diaphragm extending to the perineal skin. The region is bordered from anterior to posterior by the pubic arch, the inferior pubic ramus, ischial tuberosity, ischial ramus, sacrotuberous ligament and the coccyx. Often the term perineum is used in a more restrictive manner, indicating the region of the perineal body and overlying skin.

1.3.6.1 Perineal Body

The perineal body (also named the central perineal tendon) is a pyramidal fibromuscular node located at the midline between the urogenital region and the anal sphincter. At this centre numerous striated muscles and fascia converge and interlace: the longitudinal muscle of the anorectum, the pubovaginal (puboprostaticus) part of the pubococcygeus muscle, the perineal membrane, the superficial transverse perineal muscle, the bulbospongiosus and the external anal sphincter (Figs. 1.15, 1.16, 1.19, 1.21). In men, this structure is more like a central point and may be named the central perineal tendon. In women the insertion is larger, and the imbrication of the muscle fibres is more pronounced; therefore, it is often described as the perineal body. The involvement of numerous muscles with their attachments to several parts of the pelvic ring (for example, the anal sphincter is connected to the coccyx by the anococcygeal ligament) gives the perineal body an important function in the complex interaction of the pelvic floor muscles.

1.3.6.2 Ischioanal Fossae

The fat-containing space lying below the levator ani between the pelvic side wall and the anus (Figs. 1.18, 1.27) is properly termed the ischioanal fossa. The ischioanal fossa is a wedge-shaped region, extending from the perineal skin to the under-surface of the pelvic diaphragm. The base of the fossa is at

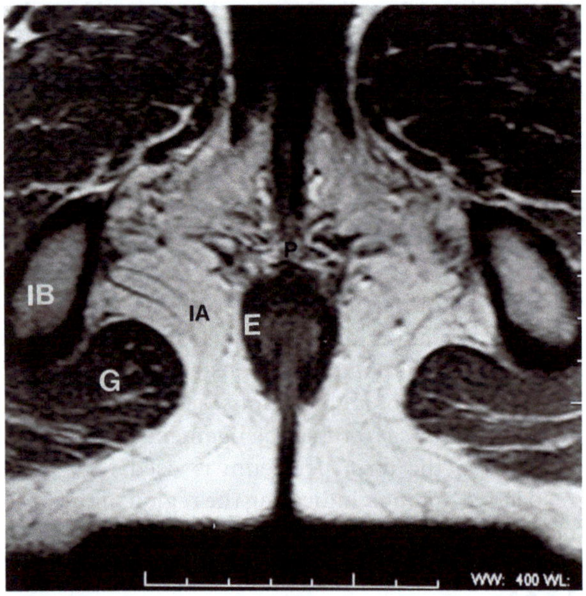

Fig. 1.27. Axial oblique T2-weighted turbo spin-echo through the lower edge of the anal sphincter in a woman (*E*=external anal sphincter, *P*=perineum, *IA*=ischioanal space, *IB*=ischial bone, *G*=gluteal musculature)

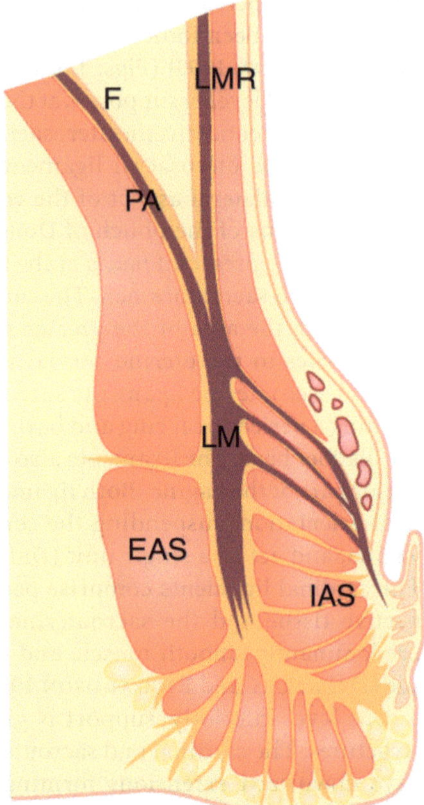

Fig. 1.28. Diagram of the anal sphincter in coronal section showing the contributions of the longitudinal muscle of the rectum (*LMR*), fascia (*F*) and puboanalis (*PA*) to form the longitudinal muscle (*LM*) running between the external anal sphincter (*EAS*) and the internal anal sphincter (*IAS*)

the perineum and the apex is superior. The lateral margin is the internal obturator fascia and posteriorly the fossa is bordered by the gluteus fascia. The anterior margin is the perineal membrane, with a recess at each side extending anteriorly. The ischioanal fossa is lined by the deep perineal fascia. This fascia is attached to the ischiopubic rami, the posterior margin of the perineal membrane and the perineal body. The pudendal canal with the pudendal nerve and vessels lies at the lateral wall of the ischioanal fossa

1.3.6.3 Perianal Connective Tissue

The superficial perineal fascia envelops a pad of fat tissue filling a large part of the ischioanal space. A network of fibroelastic connective tissue fibres traverses the perianal fat. This arises from the connective tissue within the longitudinal layer (conjoined longitudinal coat) (Haas and Fox 1977) (Fig. 1.28) and permeates through the sphincters, interlacing with each other as well as with the perimysium and endomysium to the pelvic side wall to connect with the caudal levator fascia and to the perianal skin, thus anchoring the anus within the pelvic cavity.

1.3.7 Rectum

The rectum commences where the taeniae coli fuse to form a continuous longitudinal muscular coat. The intraperitoneal rectum is related anteriorly in women to the upper vagina and uterus, and in men to the seminal vesicles with the pouch of Douglas in between. Anterior to the extraperitoneal rectum are the posterior vaginal wall and rectovaginal septum in women and the prostate and seminal vesicles in men. The ampullary portion of the rectum rests on the pelvic diaphragm. At this level the tube turns backward and downward at about a 90° angle at the anorectal junction. The inferior rectum has no mesentery, but is enveloped in fat (mesorectum) and is bordered by the mesorectal fascia. The length of the rectum is approximately 12 cm. The rectum has three lateral curves, the rectal valves of Houston, often two on the left and one on the right.

1.3.7.1
Rectal Wall

The epithelium of the upper rectum is continuous with the colon. The lining comprises columnar cells, goblet (mucous) cells and microfold cells overlying lymphoid follicles. Within the mucosa are distension-sensitive nerve endings, while in the muscular wall nerve endings are more sensitive to the intensity of distension (Hobday et al. 2001). The lining is supported by the lamina propria, composed of connective tissue. Below this layer are the muscularis mucosae (with longitudinal and circular layers) and submucosa.

The muscularis propria of the rectum comprises an outer longitudinal layer and an inner circular layer. This layer is uniform except for some thickening of the longitudinal layer anteriorly and posteriorly (anterior and posterior bands). The inner circular layer thickens at the anorectal junction, forming the internal sphincter. The longitudinal layer continues as the longitudinal layer of the anal sphincter. Some anterior fibres of the longitudinal layer run into the perineal body as the musculus rectourethralis (Bannister et al. 1995).

1.3.7.2
Rectal Support

The rectum is supported by several condensations of the rectal fascia (ligaments) and by the pelvic floor. The rectum is surrounded by fat and the mesorectal fascia. It is fixed to the sacrum posteriorly by the presacral fascia (fascia of Waldeyer). Lateral condensations of the endopelvic fascia, as also present at the bladder and vagina, give lateral support: the lateral rectal ligaments (or pillars). The lateral ligaments course from the posterolateral pelvic wall at the level of the third sacral vertebra to the rectum. The ligaments have a divergent spiral course, being posterior at the rectosigmoid junction and anterolateral at the lower third of the rectum (Muntean 1999). Within these ligaments run nerves and the middle rectal vessels. The lateral ligaments divide the loose connective tissue-containing pelvirectal space in an anterior and posterior region. In men, the posterior layer of the rectovesical fascia is continuous with the prostatic fascia and the peritoneum of the rectovesical pouch (prostatoperitoneal membrane, Denonvilliers' fascia) giving some anterior support (Muntean 1999). In women the rectovaginal fascia gives anterior support.

1.3.7.3
Neurovascular Supply of the Rectum

The arterial supply of the rectal mucosal membrane is by the superior rectal branch of the inferior mesenteric artery (hindgut artery), with arterial supply also to the superior anal sphincter. The muscularis propria also receives branches of the middle rectal artery, coursing through the lateral rectal ligament. Small branches of the median sacral artery are also part of the arterial supply of the posterior rectum and anorectal junction (Last 1978; Bannister et al. 1995). Venous return follows the arterial supply, although there is an extensive anastomosis between the venous tributaries. Lymphatic drainage follows the arterial sources of supply. The superior rectal vessels are enveloped in a sheet, the fascia of Waldeyer. There are above the level of the pelvic floor at both sides of the rectum condensations of areolar tissue, the lateral ligament (pillar). These condensations include the middle rectal artery and branches of the pelvic plexuses.

The nerve supply of the rectum is by the autonomic system. Sympathetic supply is by branches of the superior hypogastric plexus and by fibres accompanying the inferior mesenteric and superior rectal arteries from the coeliac plexus. Parasympathetic (motor) supply is from S2–S4 to the inferior hypogastric plexuses by the pelvic splanchnic nerves (nervi erigentes). These fibres give sensory supply (crude sensation and pain) and have a role in discriminating between flatus and faeces.

1.3.8
Anal Sphincter

The anal sphincter envelops the anal canal and is tilted anteriorly in the sagittal plane with the cranial part forward. The canal is 4–6 cm (average 5 cm) in length (Rociu et al. 2000; Beets-Tan et al. 2001).

The anal sphincter is composed of several cylindrical layers (Fig. 1.19). The innermost layer is the subepithelium that seals off the anal canal (anal cushions) (Gibbons et al. 1986). The next layer is the cylindrical smooth muscle of the internal sphincter, often separated from the longitudinal layer by a thin fat-containing layer that represents the surgical intersphincteric space. The outermost layer is the striated muscle of the external sphincter. The cranial part of the external sphincter has a close anatomical relationship with the puborectalis (Fig. 1.29). The sphincter is surrounded by the ischioanal fossae. The anococcygeal ligament lies posteriorly in the midline and attaches the external sphincter to the coccyx (Figs. 1.19, 1.30). The anococcygeal raphe is situated superior to this ligament.

1.3.8.1 Lining of the Anal Canal

The lining of the anal canal varies according to embryological origin. There is variation in the relative contribution between the various linings in individuals and a transitional zone is present (Fenger 1988).

The upper part of the anus is lined by mucosa that is colonic in type. The uppermost part still has muscularis mucosae so that there is a true submucosa present, but there is no muscularis in most of the canal, so that "subepithelium" is used. The mucosa is arranged into six to ten vertical folds, called the anal columns, which are separated by grooves (Woodburne 1983). A small crescentic mucous fold, the anal valves, join the caudal ends of each column. The submucosal anal glands open just above the valves. The valves are situated at the dentate line, which may represent the junction of the endoderm and ectoderm (anal membrane), although this is disputed.

The anal cushions are three specialized vascular engorgements of the submucosa that act as seals for the anal canal. The lining directly below the anal columns is smooth hairless skin of the about 1-cm-wide transitional zone, the dentate line. The dentate line separates the neurovascular supply of the upper and lower part of the anus; above is auto-

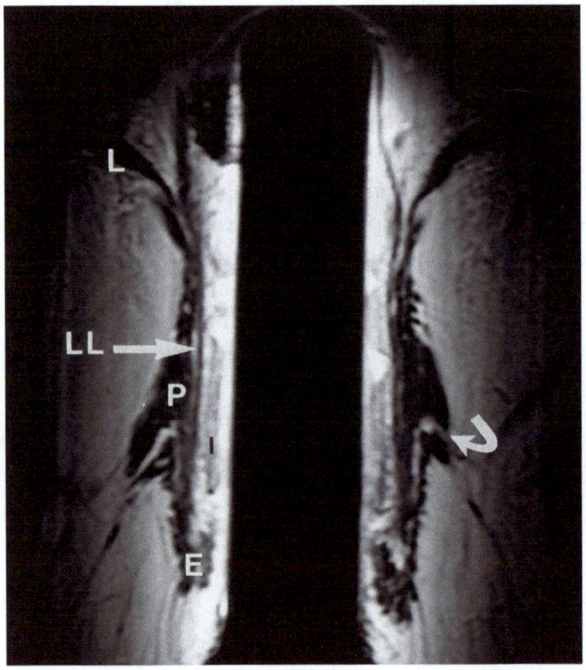

Fig. 1.29. Endoanal coronal oblique T2-weighted turbo spin-echo at the midanal canal in a 45-year-old man (posterior to Fig. 1.33) [I=internal sphincter with some internal haemorrhoids at the upper half of the sphincter, LL=longitudinal layer in the intersphincteric space, E=external sphincter, P=pubovisceralis (puborectalis), L=levator ani (iliococcygeus) muscle]. Note the close relationship of the deep part of the external sphincter and the puborectalis (*curved arrow*)

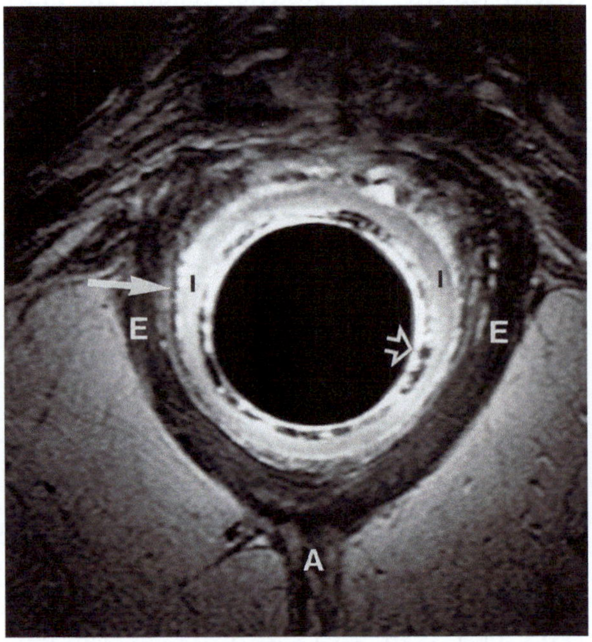

Fig. 1.30. Endoanal axial oblique T2-weighted turbo spin-echo in a male volunteer (superior to Fig. 1.19) (*open arrow* mucosa/submucosa with hypointense submucosal muscularis ani, I=internal anal sphincter, *white arrow* intersphincteric space with the relatively hypointense longitudinal muscle, E=external sphincter, A=anococcygeal ligament). The external anal sphincter shortest longitudinal dimension is anterior, and at this level, the ring is incomplete anteriorly (see also Fig. 1.33)

nomic, below is somatic. There is a portosystemic venous connection at this level. The lining is non-keratinized cuboidal epithelium, and this region is richly supplied with sensory nerve endings (both free and organized nerve endings), important in the continence mechanism (Fenger 1988). The lowest part of the anal canal is lined by keratinized stratified squamous epithelium with underlying subcutis with sweet and sebaceous glands similar to and continuous with the perianal dermis.

The muscularis submucosae ani is derived from the longitudinal muscle and forms a thin band of smooth muscle in the subepithelial layer. Fibres are orientated downwards towards the dentate line and are not seen in the lower canal.

1.3.8.2 Internal Anal Sphincter

The internal sphincter is the continuation of the circular layer of the muscularis propria of the rectum. This layer increases in thickness below the anorectal junction to form the circular internal sphincter. The internal sphincter is approximately 2.8 mm thick on endoluminal imaging (Rociu et al. 2000) (Figs. 1.19, 1.29, 1.30). The inferior border of the internal sphincter is approximately 1 cm above the inferior edge of the sphincter complex (i.e. inferior edge of the external sphincter). On MRI with a T2-weighted sequence the internal sphincter appears as a relatively hypertense circular structure with a homogeneous, uniform architecture (Fig. 1.19).

1.3.8.3 Intersphincteric Space

The intersphincteric space, is the plane of surgical dissection between the sphincters. This is presumed to be the thin sheet of fat containing loose areolar tissue seen as a bright line on T2-weighted MRI (Figs. 1.19, 1.29). It lays either between the internal sphincter and the longitudinal layer or between this layer and the external sphincter, or both. The width of this space varies considerably.

1.3.8.4 Longitudinal Layer

In the last decade several studies have increased our understanding of the complex anatomy of the longitudinal layer (Lunniss and Phillips 1992). The longitudinal layer (conjoint longitudinal layer or longitudinal muscle) is the continuation of the smooth muscle longitudinal layer of the rectum, with striated muscles from the levator ani, particularly the puboanalis (Lunniss and Phillips 1992), and a large fibroelastic element derived from the endopelvic fascia.

The layer is 2.5 mm thick (Rociu et al. 2000). Cranially it is predominantly muscular and fibroelastic caudally. The fibroelastic tissue forms a network throughout the sphincter and passes through the subcutaneous external sphincter as bundles or fibres to insert into the perianal skin. Some fibres running into the lower canal have been considered to form the corrugator cutis ani, though this is disputed, as is even the existence of any such muscle (Lunniss and Phillips 1992; Bannister et al. 1995). On T2-weighted MRI the longitudinal muscle layer is seen as a relatively hypointense layer within the hyperintense intersphincteric space (Figs. 1.19, 1.29, 1.30), with its termination into multiple bundles in the lower sphincter visible on MRI.

1.3.8.5 External Anal Sphincter

The external sphincter envelops the intersphincteric space and represents the inferior outer aspect of the anal sphincter. The external sphincter is approximately 2.7 cm high, while it is shorter anteriorly in women, approximately 1.5 cm (Rociu et al. 2000). The lateral part of the external sphincter is approximately 2.7 cm high. The external sphincter has a thickness of 4 mm on endoluminal imaging. The external sphincter extends approximately 1 cm beyond the internal sphincter (Figs. 1.29, 1.31–1.33). The muscle is a striated muscle under voluntary control and comprises predominantly slow-twitch muscle fibres, capable of prolonged contraction. There is with increasing age a shift towards more type II (rapid) fibres (Lierse et al. 1993). The action of the external sphincter is voluntary closure and reflex closure of the anal canal and it contributes to the sphincter tonus to some extent.

The concept of the anatomy of the external sphincter with respect to the pubovisceral (puborectal/puboanal) muscle has changed over time (Milligan and Morgan 1934; Goligher 1967; Oh and Kark 1972). Some consider the external sphincter to constitute the complete or largest part of the outer cylinder of the anal sphincter. The pubovisceral (puborectal/puboanal) muscle is described as being present at the level of the anorectal junction

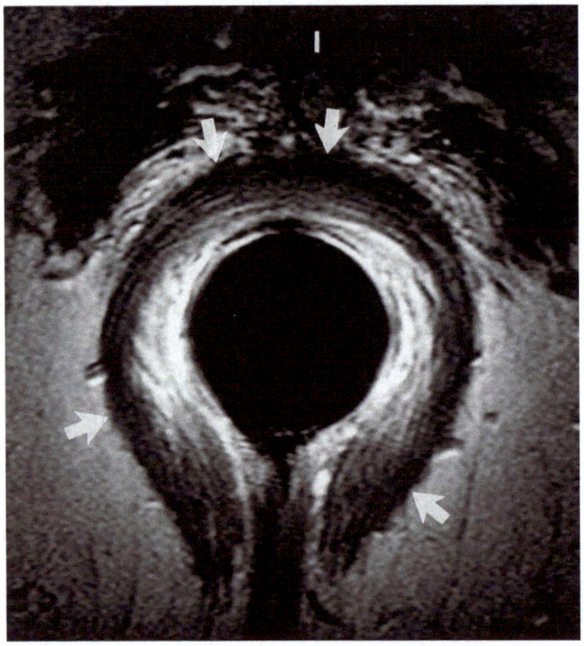

Fig. 1.31. Endoanal axial oblique T2-weighted turbo spin-echo in a woman through the lower aspect of the external sphincter (*arrows*) with a complete anterior ring (*I*=vaginal introitus)

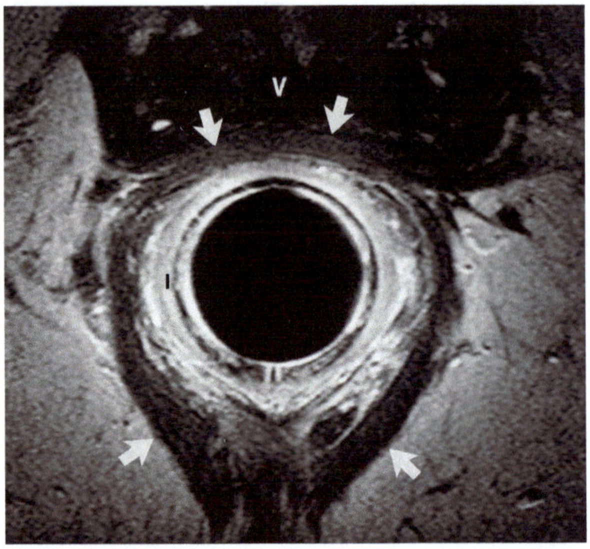

Fig. 1.32. Endoanal axial oblique T2-weighted turbo spin-echo through the lower edge of the internal sphincter (*I*) in a woman at a higher level than Figure 1.31 (*arrows* external sphincter, *V*=vagina)

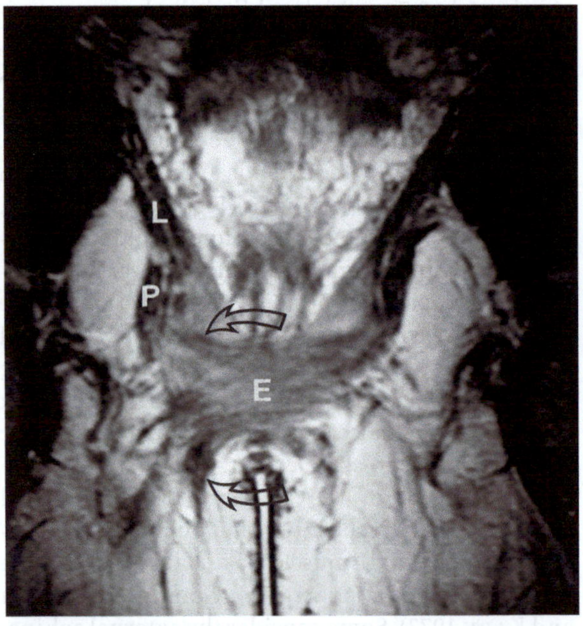

Fig. 1.33. Endoanal coronal oblique T2-weighted turbo spin-echo anterior to Figure 1.29, through the anterior part of the external anal sphincter. Note that the external sphincter (*curved arrows*) is shorter anteriorly than laterally (*P*=pubovisceralis, *L*=levator ani)

or most superior part of the anal sphincter. These concepts are based on findings at dissection and at surgery. Imaging studies, especially endoluminal MRI, have supported the concept that the pubovisceral (puborectal) muscle comprises approximately the upper outer half of the anal sphincter (Hussain et al. 1995; Rociu et al. 2000) (Figs. 1.29, 1.34). The pubovisceral muscle forms a sling around the upper half. Because of the sling form, no striated muscle is present anteriorly at this level. The pubovisceral (puboanal) muscle can be separated from the external sphincter muscle on imaging (MRI, endosonography) and cadaver studies (Hussain et al. 1995; Rociu et al. 2000; Fucini et al. 1999) (Fig. 1.29).

In the literature the external sphincter is often described as subdivided in the coronal plane: the subcutaneous, superficial and deep part. However, this concept is not supported by all studies and also single-layer and bilayer concepts have been described as well as a triple-loop concept (Bannister et al. 1995; Goligher 1967; Oh and Kark 1972; Shafik 1975; Garavoglia et al. 1993; Bogduk 1996). MRI studies have identified different aspects of the external sphincter at certain levels, which to some extent supports a multilayer anatomy (Rociu et al. 2000). Clefts between parts of the external sphincter can be identified at MRI in some individuals, although

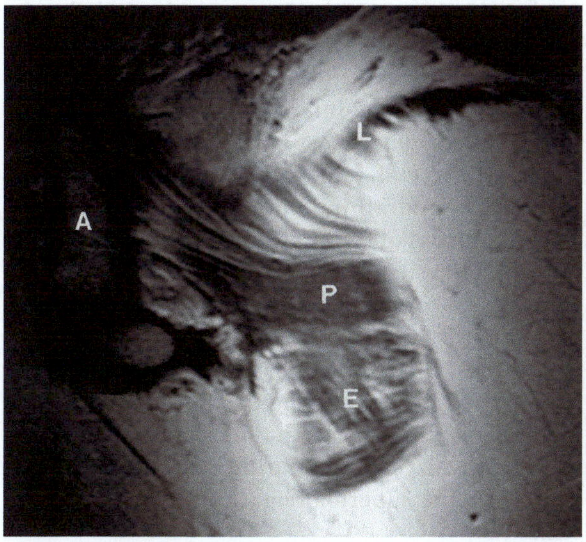

Fig. 1.34. Endoanal parasagittal oblique T2-weighted turbo spin-echo in a male volunteer. Note the difference in orientation of the external sphincter (*E*) and pubovisceralis (*P*) (*A*=anterior, *L*=levator ani)

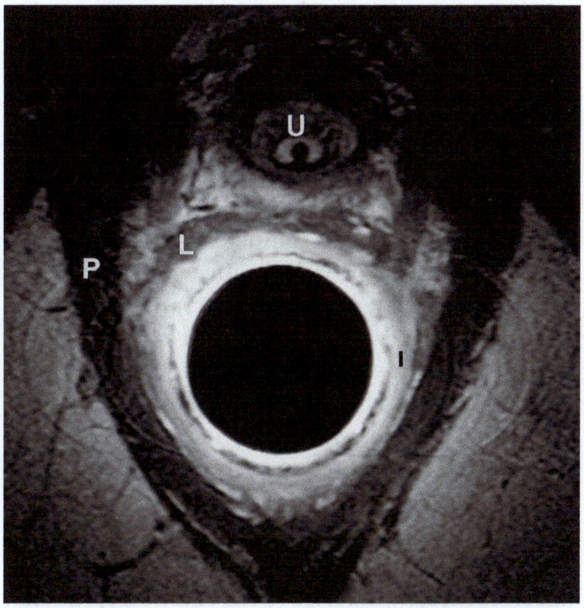

Fig. 1.35. Endoanal axial oblique T2-weighted turbo spin-echo in a male volunteer (superior to Fig. 1.30) (*P*=pubovisceralis, *L*=longitudinal layer, *I*=internal sphincter, *U*=urethra)

often only several bundles (also more than three) can be identified without clear clefts. The external sphincter has posterior fibres continuous with the anococcygeal ligament. Some of the anterior fibres decussate into the superficial transverse perineal muscle and perineal body. The deep part of the external sphincter is intimately related to the puborectal muscle (Fig. 1.29).

1.3.8.6 Pubovisceral (Puborectal) Muscle

The pubovisceral part of the levator ani comprises the puborectalis and pubococcygeus. The pubovisceral (puborectal) muscle is approximately 2.8 cm high and 5.6 mm thick when measured on endoanal MRI (Rociu et al. 2000) (Fig. 1.29). The sling-like puborectalis has a somewhat tilted transverse orientation with the open ends attached to the pubic bone (see Sect. 1.3.2.2 Pelvic Diaphragm) (Fig. 1.35). The puborectalis displays some resting tone, but contracts rapidly in response to any sudden increase in intraabdominal pressure to prevent incontinence. The urogenital hiatus with urethra, vagina and anus and supportive structures is bordered and supported by the puborectalis (see Sect. 1.3.2.2 Pelvic Diaphragm).

1.3.8.7 Anal Sphincter Support

The anal sphincter has numerous attachments. For anterior support the perineal body and its attachments are important, as well as other supportive structures in the anovaginal septum in females and the Denonvilliers' fascia in males. Lateral support is given by the levator ani muscle (pubovisceral muscle) and superficial transverse perineal muscle. Posterior support is given by the attachment of the anococcygeal ligament to the coccyx and superiorly by the continuity with the rectum. The fibroelastic network surrounding and involving the anal sphincter gives more general support.

1.3.8.8 Anal Sphincter Anatomy Variance and Ageing

Normal variants of anal sphincter anatomy have been identified, such as differing relationships between the superficial transverse perineal muscle and the external sphincter (Haas and Fox 1977). The inferior edge of the external sphincter may have a closed circular configuration or may be open anteriorly and posteriorly. After trauma (e.g. obstetric), the anal sphincter anatomy may be disturbed without clinical symptoms. These findings may possibly be related to late-onset incontinence.

Sex-related differences include a significantly shorter external sphincter in women than in men, especially anteriorly. The central perineal tendon in men is a central muscular insertion point; in women, it represents an area where muscle fibres imbricate. The external sphincter has a more horizontal orientation in women. In women, the longitudinal muscle terminates just cranial to the external sphincter, whereas in men it extends to the caudal part of the external sphincter. The superficial transverse perineal muscle is close to the external sphincter, and their relationship in the craniocaudal direction is different between the sexes. In women, the superficial transverse perineal muscle is directly superior to the external sphincter, often with some overlap (Fig. 1.21). In men, the superficial perineal muscle is directly anterior to the external sphincter. The central perineal tendon is an insertion common to all the striated muscles, which anchors the anal sphincter to the surrounding structures (superficial transverse perineal muscle, bulbospongiosus muscle, urogenital diaphragm). In men, this structure is more like a central point, whereas in women this insertion is larger, and the imbrication of the muscle fibres is more pronounced; therefore, it is often described as the perineal body.

Age-related variations included a significant decrease in the thickness of the longitudinal muscle and an increase in the thickness of the internal sphincter in both sexes (Rociu et al. 2000). A decrease in the thickness of the external sphincter in men with age has been demonstrated. In females this is also most likely in normal ageing; however when coinciding with external sphincter defects this may lead to incontinence. No significant age-related differences in the lengths of the anal canal, external sphincter and puborectalis are found.

1.3.8.9 Neurovascular Supply of the Anal Sphincter

The arterial, venous, lymphatic and nerve supply of the superior two-thirds of the anus (hindgut origin) is different from the inferior one-third (proctoderm origin) (Moore and Persaud 1998). The arterial supply of the superior two-thirds is mainly by the inferior rectal artery, a branch of the inferior mesenteric artery (hindgut artery). Small branches of the median sacral artery also are part of the arterial supply of the posterior anorectal junction (Bannister et al. 1995; Last 1978). Venous drainage is by the superior rectal vein, draining to the inferior mesenteric artery. For the inferior one-third of the anus, arterial supply is by inferior rectal branches of the internal pudendal artery and venous drainage by the inferior rectal vein, a tributary of the internal pudendal vein draining into the internal iliac vein. The submucosa of the anal canal is a junction of the portal and systemic venous systems. Longitudinal veins, cross-connecting at the anal valves, are connected to the veins of the transitional zone (dentate or pectineal line) and cutis and to radicles crossing the anal sphincters forming the inferior and middle rectal veins draining to the internal iliac vein and inferior caval vein. Ascending mucosal veins will drain into the superior rectal vein and portal system.

The lymphatics of the (cloacal) anus primarily follow the supplying and draining vessels, especially the superior rectal vessels to the inferior mesenteric nodes. Lymphatic drainage of the lowest (proctoderm) part of the anal sphincter is to the superficial inguinal nodes.

The autonomic nerve supply of the internal sphincter is by sympathetic fibres along the superior rectal artery via the inferior pelvic plexus and parasympathetic (inhibitory) fibres through the inferior pelvic plexus and splanchnic nerves (S2–S4). For the function of the internal sphincter, the enteric plexus and associated autonomic and visceral sensory nerves are involved. Afferent impulses (distension) pass through the parasympathetic nerves and pain impulses through sympathetic and parasympathetic nerves (Bannister et al. 1995). The external sphincter has nerve supply by the inferior rectal branch of the pudendal nerve (S2, S3) and the perineal branch of the fourth sacral nerve (S4). The puborectalis has a dual somatic innervation by the levator ani nerve from its superior surface (S3/S4) and by the pudendal nerve (inferior rectal nerve branch and/or perineal nerve branch). For both external sphincter and puborectalis, regulation is partly reflex (e.g. sudden increase in abdominal pressure) and partly voluntary through the visceral and somatic afferent and somatic efferent nerves. Important for proper function of the anal sphincter is the rich supply of sensory endings at the dentate line and proprioceptive fibres. Motor control and sensory input are processed at several levels of the central nervous system. Nerve supply to the superior two-thirds of the anal lining is by the autonomic nervous system, for the lower part by the inferior rectal nerve.

1.3.9
Nerve Supply of the Pelvic Floor

In this section the main nerve supply of the pelvic floor is described. The specific nerve supply for parts of the pelvic floor has been described in the sections describing these structures. The nerve supply to the pelvic floor and related organs is by branches of the sacral plexus – the pudendal nerve (coursing inferior to the pelvic floor), the levator ani nerve (coursing superior to the pelvic floor) and the parasympathetic pelvic splanchnic nerves (nervi erigentes) – and the sympathetic supply by the hypogastric nerve. Higher regulating levels of the central nervous system (e.g. pontine micturition centre, cerebral cortex) are crucial for proper function of the pelvic floor.

1.3.9.1
Somatic Nerve Supply

The pudendal nerve supplies the majority of the somatic innervation of the pelvic floor region. The pudendal nerve courses through the greater sciatic foramen, travelling dorsal to the ischial spine to the pudendal canal at the lateral side of the ischiorectal fossa (Colleselli et al. 1998). At the level of the pelvic floor the pelvic floor divides into the inferior rectal nerve, the perineal nerve and the dorsal nerve of the clitoris/penis. These branches give motoric supply to the the pelvic floor muscles and sphincters and additionally have a sensory contribution. The levator ani muscle is mainly innervated by the levator ani nerve on its superior surface (S3/S4). The pudendal nerve only has a contribution in approximately 50% of cases (Wallner et al. 2006a, Wallner et al. 2006b, Wallner et al. submitted).

1.3.9.2
Autonomic Nerve Supply

The pelvic parasympathetic supply (pelvic splanchnic nerves or nervi erigentes) arises from S2–S4. The sympathetic nerves arising from T10–T12 course through the sympathetic chain and preaortic plexus (superior hypogastric plexus) to the hypogastric nerve which subsequently approaches the pelvic plexus. Together, these parasympathetic and sympathetic nerves form the autonomic nerve plexus in the small pelvis (pelvic plexus or inferior hypogastric plexus).

The pelvic plexus is a coarse, flat meshwork, enlarged in places by ganglia and is situated laterally to the pelvic organs. It stretches from an area anterolateral to the rectum, passes the cervix and the vaginal fornix laterally and extends to the lateral vaginal wall and the base of the bladder. The course of the nerve plexus through the small pelvis follows the connective tissue plane which supports the uterine cervix, vagina and bladder (Maas et al. 1999).

The pelvic plexus is the pathway for sympathetic and parasympathetic nerves supplying the rectum, uterus, vagina, vestibular bulbs, clitoris, bladder and the urethra. The superior hypogastric plexus and hypogastric nerves are mainly sympathetic, and the pelvic splanchnic nerves are mainly parasympathetic. In urinary function, parasympathetic injury produces a hypocontractile or acontractile bladder with decreased sensation. Sympathetic denervation can result in a bladder with decreased compliance and a high storage pressure. In addition, sympathetic nerve injury may cause bladder neck incompetence and incontinence. Disruption of the autonomic nerves to the rectum would result in colorectal motility disorders (Maas et al. 1999). Moreover, the autonomic nerves are essential to a normal sexual function. Disruption of the sympathetic nerve supply to the pelvic plexus could lead to disturbed ejaculation in men and impaired vaginal lubrication in women. Damage to the parasympathetic nerve supply could lead to erectile dysfunction in men and to impairment of the vasocongestion response in women (Maas 2003).

References

Arey LB (1966) Developmental anatomy, 7th edn. Saunders, Philadelphia

Bannister LH, Berry MM, Collins P, Dyson M, Dussek JE, Ferguson MWJ (1995) Gray's anatomy, 38th edn. Churchill Livingstone, New York

Beets-Tan RGH, Morren GL, Beets G et al (2001) Measurement of anal sphincter muscles: endoanal US, endoanal MR imaging, or phased array MR imaging? A study with healthy volunteers. Radiology 220:81–89

Bogduk N (1996) Issues in anatomy: the external anal sphincter revisited. Aust N Z J Surg 66:626–629

Cardozo L (ed) (1997) Urogynecology. Churchill Livingstone, Edinburgh

Chai TC, Steers WD (1997) Neurophysiology of micturition and continence in women. Int Urogynecol J Pelvic Floor Dysfunct 8:85–97

Colleselli K, Stenszl A, Eder R, Strasser H, Poisel S, Bartsch G (1998) The female urethral sphincter: a morphological and topographical study. J Urol 160:49–54

De Caro R, Aragona F, Herms A, Guidolin D, Brizzi E, Pagano F (1998) Morphometric analysis of the fibroadipose tissue of the female pelvis. J Urol 160:707–713
DeLancey JOL (1986) Correlative study of paraurethral anatomy. Obstet Gynecol 68:91–97
DeLancey JOL (1988) Structural aspects of the extrinsic continence mechanism. Obstet Gynecol 72:296–301
DeLancey JOL (1993) Anatomy and biomechanics of genital prolapse. Clin Obstet Gynecol 36:897–909
DeLancey JOL (1994a) Functional anatomy of the female pelvis. In: Kursh ED, McGuire EJ (eds) Female urology, 1st edn. Lippincott, Philadelphia
DeLancey JOL (1994b) Structural support of the urethra as it relates to stress urinary incontinence: the hammock hypothesis. Am J Obstet Gynecol 170:1713–1723
DeLancey JOL, Richardson AC (1992) Anatomy of genital support. In: Benson JT (ed) Female pelvic floor disorders: investigation and management, 1st edn. Norton Medical Books, New York
DeLancey JOL, Starr RA (1990) Histology of the connection between the vagina and levator ani muscles. Implications for urinary tract function. J Reprod Med 35:765–771
Dietz HP, Lanzarone V (2005). Levator trauma after vaginal delivery. Obstet Gynecol 106: 707–712
Dorschner W, Biesold M, Schmidt F, Stolzenburg JU (1999) The dispute about the external sphincter and the urogenital diaphragm. J Urol 162:1942–1945
El-Sayed RF, Morsy MM, El-Mashed SM, Abdel-Azim MS (2007) Anatomy of the urethral supporting ligaments defined by dissection, histology, and MRI of female cadavers and MRI of healthy nulliparous women. Am J Roentgenol 189:1145–1157
Fenger C (1988) Histology of the anal canal. Am J Surg Pathol 12:41–55
Fucini C, Elbetti C, Messerini L (1999) Anatomic plane of separation between external anal sphincter and puborectalis muscle. Clinical implications. Dis Colon Rectum 42:374–379
Garavoglia M, Borghi F, Levi AC (1993) Arrangement of the anal striated musculature. Dis Colon Rectum 36:10–15
Gibbons CP, Trowbridge EA, Bannister JJ, Read NW (1986) Anal cushions. Lancet 8486:886–887
Gilpin SA, Gosling JA (1983) Smooth muscle in the wall of the developing human urinary bladder and urethra. J Anat 137:503–512
Goligher J (1967) Surgery of the anus, rectum and colon, 2nd edn. Baillière Tindall, London
Haas PA, Fox TA (1977) The importance of the perianal connective tissue in the surgical anatomy and function of the anus. Dis Colon Rectum 20:303–313
Hamilton WJ, Mossman HW (1972) Hamilton, Boyd and Mossman's human embryology, 4th edn. Williams and Wilkins, Baltimore
Hobday DI, Aziz Q, Thacker N, Hollander I, Jackson A, Thompson DG (2001) A study of the cortical processing of ano-rectal sensation using functional MRI. Brain 124:361–368
Hoyte L, Schierlitz L, Zou K, Flesh G, Fielding JR (2001). Two- and 3-dimensional MRI comparison of levator ani structure, volume, and integrity in women with stress incontinence and prolapse. Am J Obstet Gynecol 185:13–19
Hussain SM, Stoker J, Laméris JS (1995) Anal sphincter complex: endoanal MR imaging of normal anatomy. Radiology 197:671–677
Kearney R, Miller JM, Ashton-Miller JA, DeLancey JO (2006). Obstetric factors associated with levator ani muscle injury after vaginal birth. Obstet Gynecol 107:144–149
Lansman HH, Robertson EG (1992) Evolution of the pelvic floor. In: Benson JT (ed) Female pelvic floor disorders: investigation and management, 1st edn. Norton Medical Books, New York
Last RJ (1978) Anatomy. Regional and applied, 6th edn. Churchill Livingstone, Edinburgh
Li L, Li Z, Huo HS, Wang HZ, Wang LY (1992) Sensory nerve endings in the puborectalis and anal region of the fetus and newborn. Dis Colon Rectum 35:552–559
Lien K, Morgan D, Delancey J, Ashton-Miller J (2004) Pudendal nerve stretch during vaginal birth. A 3D computer simulation. Am J Obstet Gynecol 192:1669–1676
Lierse W, Holschneider AM, Steinfeld J (1993) The relative proportions of type I and type II muscle fibres in the external sphincter ani muscle at different ages and stages of development – observations on the development of continence. Eur J Pediatr Surg 3:28–32
Lunniss PJ, Phillips RKS (1992) Anatomy and function of the anal longitudinal muscle. Br J Surg 79:882–884
Maas CP, DeRuiter MC, Kenter GG, Trimbos JB (1999) The inferior hypogastric plexus in gynecologic surgery. J Gynecol Tech 5: 55–62
Maas CP (2003) Nerve sparing radical pelvic surgery. PhD Thesis, Leiden University, The Netherlands
Mauroy B, Goullet E, Stefaniak X, Bonnal JL, Amara N (2000) Tendinous arch of the pelvic fascia application to the technique of paravaginal colposuspension. Surg Radiol Anat 22:73–79
Milligan ETC, Morgan CN (1934) Surgical anatomy of the anal canal. Lancet 2:1150–1156
Moore K, Persaud TVN (1998) The developing human: clinically oriented embryology, 6th ed. Saunders, Philadelphia
Muntean V (1999) The surgical anatomy of the fasciae and the fascial spaces related to the rectum. Surg Radiol Anat 21:319–324
Myers RP, Cahill DR, Kay PA et al (2000) Puboperineales: muscular boundaries of the male urogenital hiatus in 3D from magnetic resonance imaging. J Urol 164:1412–1415
Nievelstein RAJ, van der Werff JFA, Verbeek FJ et al (1998) Normal and abnormal development of the anorectum in human embryos. Teratology 57:70–78
Norton PA (1993) Pelvic floor disorders: the role of fascia and ligaments. Clin Obstet Gynecol 36:926–938
Oelrich TM (1983) The striated urogenital muscle in the female. Anat Rec 205:223–232
Oh C, Kark AE (1972) Anatomy of the external anal sphincter. Br J Surg 1972:717–723
Papa Petros PE (1998) The pubourethral ligaments. An anatomical and histological study in the live patient. Int Urogynecol 9:154–157
Rociu E, Stoker J, Eijkemans MJC, Laméris JS (2000) Normal anal sphincter anatomy and age- and sex-related variations at high spatial resolution endoanal MR imaging. Radiology 217:395–401
Sampselle CM, DeLancey JO (1998) Anatomy of female continence. J Wound Ostomy Continence Nurs 25:63–74
Schraffordt SE, Tjandra JJ, Eizenberg N, Dwyer PL (2004) Anatomy of the pudendal nerve and its terminal branches: a cadaver study. ANZ J Surg 74:23–26

Shafik A (1976) A new concept of the anatomy of the anal sphincter mechanism and the physiology of defecation. III. The longitudinal muscle: anatomy and role in anal sphincter mechanism. Invest Urol 13:271–277

Shafik A (1999) Levator ani muscle: new physioanatomical aspects and role in the micturition mechanism. World J Urol 17:266–273

Strasser H, Tiefenthaler M, Steinlechner M, Bartsch G, Konwalinka G (1999) Urinary incontinence in the elderly and age-dependent apoptosis of rhabdosphincter cells. Lancet 354:918–919

Strohbehn K, Ellis J, Strohbehn JA, DeLancey JOL (1996) Magnetic resonance imaging of the levator ani with anatomic correlation. Obstet Gynecol 87:277–285

Strohbehn K (1998) Normal pelvic floor anatomy. Obstet Gynecol Clin North Am 25:683–705

Tan IL, Stoker J, Zwamborn AW, Entius KAC, Calame JJ, Laméris JS (1998) Female pelvic floor. Endovaginal MR imaging of normal anatomy. Radiology 206:777–783

Tobias PV, Arnold M (1981) Man's anatomy, 3rd ed. Witwatersrand University Press, Johannesburg

Tunn R, DeLancey JO, Howard D, Thorp JM, Ashton-Miller JA, Quint LE (1999) MR Imaging of levator ani muscle recovery following vaginal delivery. Int Urogynecol J 10:300–307

Tunn R, DeLancey JOL, Quint EE (2001) Visibility of pelvic organ support system structures in magnetic resonance images without an endovaginal coil. Am J Obstet Gynecol 184:1156–1163

Valasek P, Evans DJ, Maina F, Grim M, Patel K (2005) A dual fate of the hindlimb muscle mass: cloacal/perineal musculature develops from leg muscle cells. Development 132:447–458

Van der Werff JFA, Nievelstein RAJ, Brands E et al (2000) Normal development of the male anterior urethra. Teratology 61:172–183

Van Ophoven A, Roth S (1997) The anatomy and embryological origins of the fascia of Denonvilliers: a medico-historical debate. J Urol 157:3–9

Wallner C, Maas CP, Dabhoiwala NF, Lamers WH, DeRuiter MC (2006a) Innervation of the pelvic floor muscles: a reappraisal for the levator ani nerve. Obstet Gynecol 108:529–534

Wallner C, Maas CP, Dabhoiwala NF, Lamers WH, DeRuiter MC (2006b) Evidence for the innervation of the puborectalis muscle by the levator ani nerve. Neurogastroenterol Motil 18:1121–1122

Wallner C, van Wissen J, Maas CP, Dabhoiwala NF, DeRuiter MC, Lamers WH (in print) The contribution of the levator ani nerve and the pudendal nerve to the innervation of the levator ani muscles; a study in human fetuses. Eur Urol. doi:10.1016/j.eururo.2007.11.015 (in print)

Woodburne RT (1983) Essentials of human anatomy, 7th ed. Oxford University Press, New York

Yucel S, Baskin LS (2004). An anatomical description of the male and female urethral sphincter complex. J Urol 171:1890–1897

Yucel S, De Souza A Jr, Baskin LS (2004) Neuroanatomy of the human female lower urogenital tract. J Urol 172:191–195

Functional Anatomy of the Pelvic Floor

2

John O. L. DeLancey

CONTENTS

2.1 Introduction

Pelvic organ prolapse and urinary incontinence are debilitating problems that prevent one in nine women from enjoying a full and active life (Olsen et al. 1997). They arise due to injuries and deterioration of the muscles, nerves and connective tissue that support and control normal pelvic organ function.

Although it is clear that incontinence and prolapse increase with age (Olsen et al. 1997), there is no hour during a woman's life when these structures are more vulnerable than during the time a woman delivers a child. Vaginal birth confers a 4- to 11-fold increase in risk of developing pelvic organ prolapse (Mant et al. 1997).

This chapter addresses the functional anatomy of the pelvic floor in women. The anal sphincter and intestinal tract are discussed in Section 4 of this book. This chapter focuses specifically on how the pelvic organs are held in their normal positions and how pelvic visceral function affects urinary continence and prolapse of the vagina and uterus. The basic anatomy of the female pelvic floor is covered in Chapter 1, but short reviews of pertinent material are provided here to assist in orientation before describing the functional aspects of those anatomical structures.

2.2 Support of the Pelvic Organs

The pelvic organs, when removed from the body, exist only as a limp and formless mass. Their shape and position in living women is determined by their attachments to the pubic bones through the muscles and connective tissue of the pelvis. The actions of their sphincters and muscles require connection to the peripheral and central nervous systems. The structures of the pelvic organ supports are important to understanding pelvic floor dysfunction. In this chapter the term pelvic floor is used broadly to include all the structures supporting the abdominal and pelvic cavity rather than the restricted use of this term to refer to the levator ani group of muscles.

J. O. L. DeLancey, MD
Norman F. Miller Professor of Gynecology, L4000 Women's Hospital, University of Michigan, 1500 E. Medical Center Drive, Ann Arbor, MI 48109-0276, USA

The pelvic floor consists of several components lying between the pelvic peritoneum and the vulvar skin. These are (from above downward) the peritoneum, pelvic viscera and endopelvic fascia, levator ani muscles, perineal membrane and external genital muscles. The eventual support for all of these structures comes from their connection to the bony pelvis and its attached muscles. The viscera are often thought of as being supported by the pelvic floor, but are actually a part of it. The viscera play an important role in forming the pelvic floor through their connections to the pelvis by such structures such as the cardinal and uterosacral ligaments.

The phenomenon of prolapse can be understood by analogy (Fig. 2.1). Bonney (1934) pointed out that the vagina is in the same relationship to the abdominal cavity as the in-turned finger of a surgical glove is to the rest of the glove. If the pressure in the glove is increased, it forces the finger to protrude downwards in the same way that increases in abdominal pressure force the vagina to prolapse. Figure 22 demonstrates this phenomenon and the strategies the body uses to prevent prolapse. Figure 2.2a and Figure 2.2b provide a schematic illustration of this phenomenon of prolapse. In Figure 22c, the lower end of the vagina is held closed by the pelvic floor muscles preventing prolapse by constriction. Figure 2.2d shows suspension of the vagina to the pelvic walls. Figure 2.2e demonstrates that spatial relationships are important. This is a flap valve closure where the suspending fibers hold the vagina in a position against the supporting walls of the pelvis so that increases in pressure force the vagina against

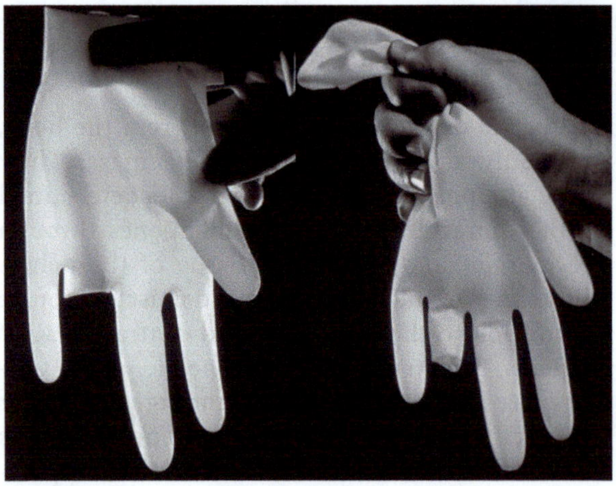

Fig. 2.1. Bonney's analogy of the eversion of an inturned surgical glove finger by increasing pressure in the glove simulating prolapse of the vagina (DeLancey 2002, with permission)

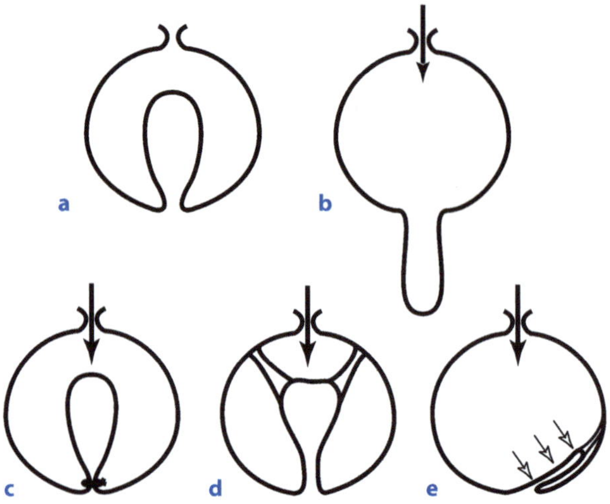

Fig. 2.2a–e. Diagrammatic display of vaginal support strategies. **a** Invaginated area in a surrounding compartment; **b** what happens when the pressure (*arrow*) is increased; **c** muscle action where closing the bottom of the vagina prevents its descent; **d** ligament suspension; **e** flap valve closure where a tethering suspension holds the vagina in such a position where it is pressed against the wall and pinned in place (DeLancey 2002, with permission)

the wall, thereby pinning it in place. Vaginal support is a combination of constriction, suspension and structural geometry.

Because the supportive tissues attach the pelvic organs to the pelvic walls, the female pelvis can naturally be divided into anterior and posterior compartments (Fig. 2.3). The levator ani muscles form the bottom of the pelvis. The organs are attached to the levator ani muscles when they pass through the urogenital hiatus and are supported by these connections.

2.2.1 Endopelvic Fascia

On each side of the pelvis the endopelvic fascia attaches the cervix and vagina to the pelvic wall (Fig. 2.4). This fascia forms a continuous sheet-like mesentery – extending from the uterine artery at its cephalic margin to the point at which the vagina fuses with the levator ani muscles below. The part that attaches to the uterus is called the parametrium and that which attaches to the vagina, the paracolpium (DeLancey 1992).

The vagina is attached laterally to the pelvic walls forming a single divider in the middle of the pelvis that determines the nature of prolapse. Cystoceles

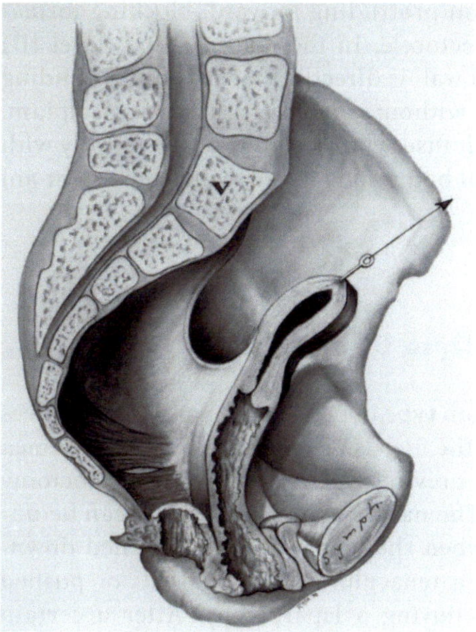

Fig. 2.3. Compartments of the pelvis. The vagina, connected laterally to the pelvic walls, divides the pelvis into an anterior and posterior compartment (DeLancey 1998, with permission; based on Sears 1933)

and rectoceles occur from the front or the back. There are no "lateroceles". The division of clinical problems into cystoceles, rectoceles and apical prolapse reflects the nature of these lateral connections. Therefore, there are three types of movement that occur in patients with pelvic organ prolapse: (1) the cervix or vaginal apex can move downward between the anterior and posterior supports; (2) the anterior vaginal wall can protrude through the introitus; and (3) the posterior wall can protrude through the introitus. These different types of support loss arise because of the location of the genital tract's connection to the pelvic sidewall. The location of connective tissue damage determines whether a woman has a cystocele, rectocele, or vaginal vault prolapse, and understanding the different characters of this support helps understand the different types of prolapse that can occur.

2.2.2 Uterovaginal Support

The attachments of the cervix and uterus to the pelvic walls are comprised of the cardinal and uterosacral ligaments (Campbell 1950; Range and Woodburne 1964), tissues that can be referred to together as the parametrium (Fig. 2.4). This tissue continues downward over the upper vagina to attach it to the pelvic walls and is called the paracolpium here (DeLancey 1992). These tissues provide support for the vaginal apex following hysterectomy (Fig. 2.5). This paracolpium has two portions. The upper portion (level I) consists of a relatively long sheet of tissue that suspends the vagina by attaching it to the pelvic wall whether or not the cervix

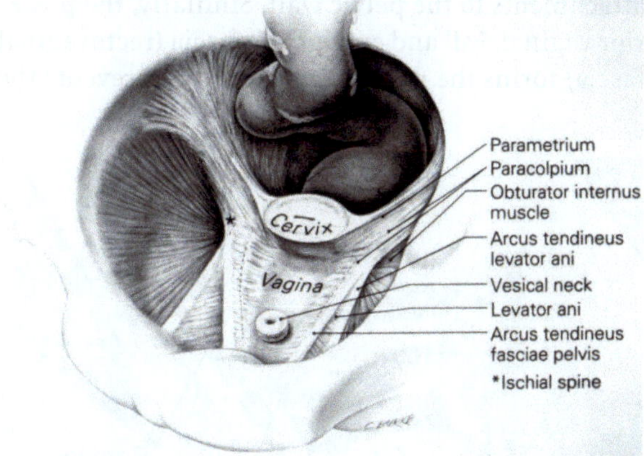

Fig. 2.4. Attachments of the cervix and vagina to the pelvic walls demonstrating different regions of support with the uterus in situ. Note that the uterine corpus and the bladder have been removed (DeLancey 2002, with permission)

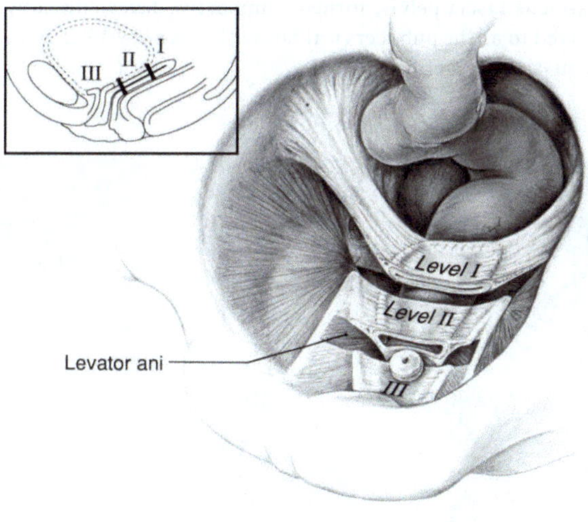

Fig. 2.5. Levels of vaginal support after hysterectomy. *Level I* (suspension) and *level II* (attachment). In *level I* the paracolpium suspends the vagina from the lateral pelvic walls. Fibers of *level I* extend both vertically and also posteriorly towards the sacrum. In *level II* the vagina is attached to the arcus tendineus fasciae pelvis and the superior fascia of levator ani (DeLancey 1992, with permission)

is present. In the mid-portion of the vagina, the paracolpium attaches the vagina laterally and more directly to the pelvic walls (level II). This attachment stretches the vagina transversely between the bladder and rectum and has functional significance. The structural layer that supports the bladder ("pubocervical fascia") is composed of the anterior vaginal wall and its attachment through the endopelvic fascia to the pelvic wall (Fig. 2.6). It is not a separate layer from the vagina as sometimes inferred, but is a combination of the anterior vaginal wall and its attachments to the pelvic wall. Similarly, the posterior vaginal wall and endopelvic fascia (rectovaginal fascia) forms the restraining layer that prevents the rectum from protruding forward, blocking formation of a rectocele. In the distal vagina (level III) the vaginal wall is directly attached to surrounding structures without any intervening paracolpium. Anteriorly it fuses with the urethra, posteriorly with the perineal body, and laterally with the levator ani muscles.

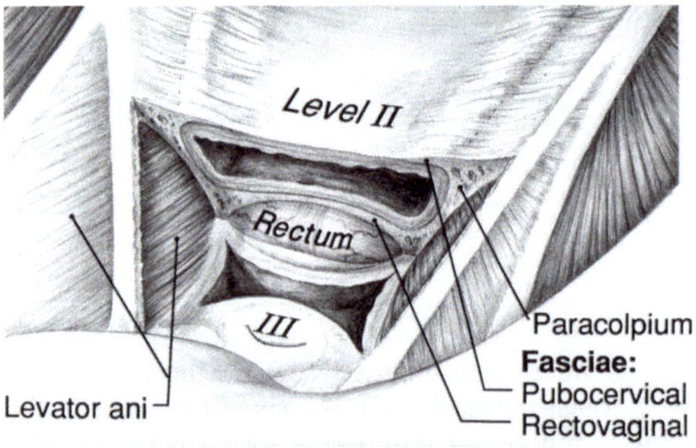

Fig. 2.6. Close-up of the lower margin of *level II* after a wedge of vagina has been removed (*inset*). Note how the anterior vaginal wall, through its connections to the arcus tendineus fascia pelvis, forms a supportive layer clinically referred to as the pubocervical fascia (DeLancey 1992, with permission)

2.2.3 Apical Prolapse; Uterus or Vaginal Apex

One common type of pelvic organ prolapse involves descent of the uterus or the vaginal apex in women that have previously undergone a hysterectomy (Fig. 2.7). The nature of uterine support can be understood when the uterine cervix is pulled downward with a tenaculum during a D&C or pushed downward during a laparoscopy. After a certain amount of descent within the elastic range of the fascia, the parametria become tight and arrest further cervical descent. Similarly, downward descent of the vaginal apex after hysterectomy is resisted by the paracolpia. The fact that these ligaments do not limit the downward movement of the uterus in normal healthy women is attested to by the observation that the cervix may be drawn down to the level of the hymen with little difficulty (Bartscht and DeLancey 1988). The same can be said of the vaginal apex after hysterectomy.

Damage to the upper suspensory fibers of the paracolpium causes uterine or vaginal vault prolapse (Fig. 2.8) and damage to the level II and III supports

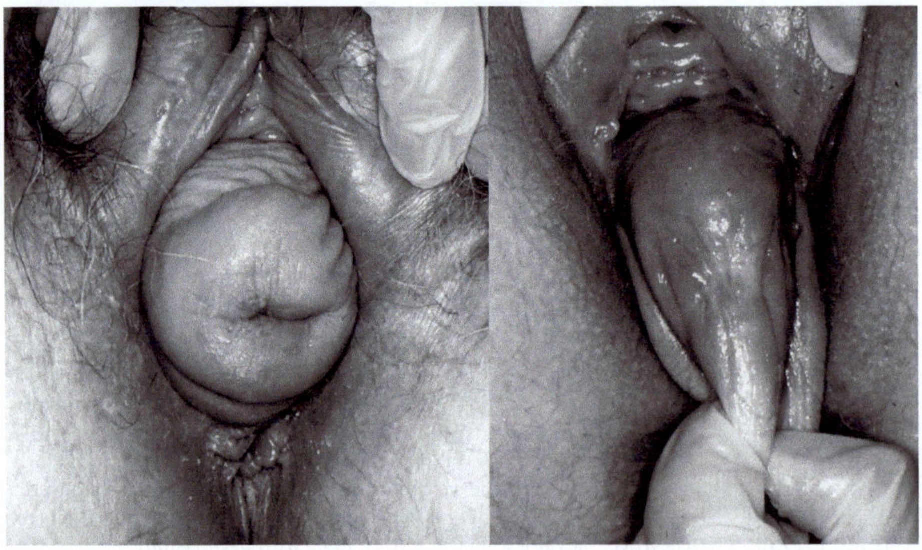

Fig. 2.7. Uterine prolapse (*left*) showing the cervix protruding from the vaginal opening and vaginal prolapse (*right*) where the puckered scar from where the cervix used to be and upper vagina are prolapsed (DeLancey 2002, with permission)

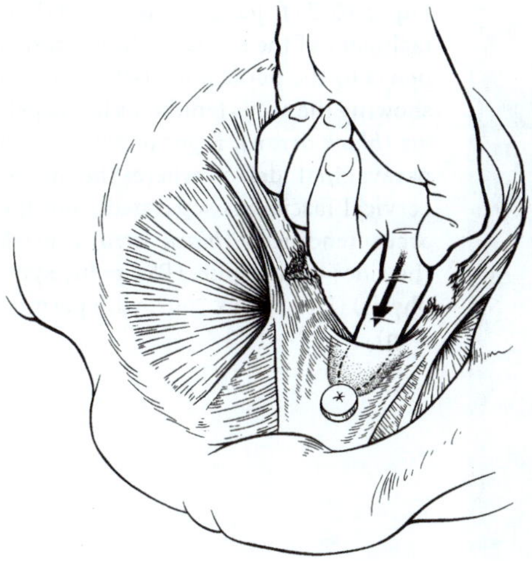

Fig. 2.8. Damage to the suspensory ligaments that can lead to eversion of the vaginal apex when subjected to downward force (DeLancey 2002, with permission)

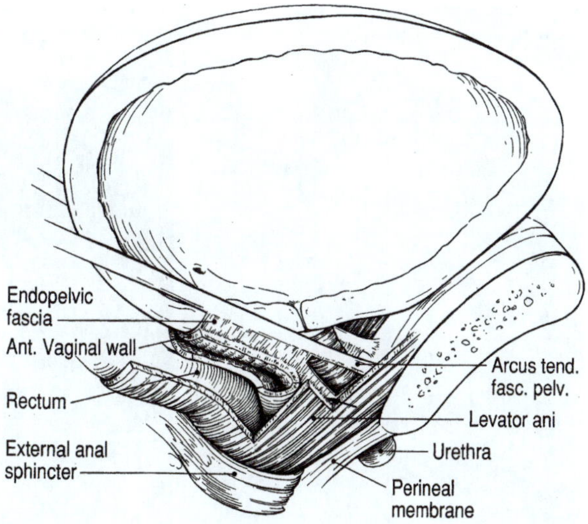

Fig. 2.9. Lateral view of the pelvic floor structures related to urethral support seen from the side in the standing position, cut just lateral to the midline. Note that windows have been cut in the levator ani muscles, vagina, and endopelvic fascia so that the urethra and anterior vaginal walls can be seen (DeLancey 2002, with permission; redrawn after DeLancey 1994)

of the vagina, resulting in cystocele and rectocele. These defects occur in varying combinations and this variation is responsible for the diversity of clinical problems encountered within the overall spectrum of pelvic organ prolapse.

2.2.4 Anterior Wall Support and Urethra

The position and mobility of the anterior vaginal wall, bladder and urethra are important to urinary continence and cystocele (Ala-Ketola 1973). Fluoroscopic examination has shown that the upper urethra and vesical neck are normally mobile structures while the distal urethra remains fixed in position (Muellner 1951; Westby et al. 1982). Both the pelvic floor muscles and the pelvic fasciae therefore, determine the support and fixation of the urethra, and the activity of the muscles has significant impact on urethral support (Miller et. al. 2001).

The anterior vaginal wall and urethra are intimately connected. Failure of this supportive system results in downward descent of the anterior vaginal wall. Their support depends not on attachments of the urethra itself to adjacent structures, but upon the connection of the vagina and periurethral tissues to the muscles and fascia of the pelvic wall (Fig. 2.9). On either side of the pelvis, the arcus tendineus fasciae pelvis is found as a band of connective tissue attached at one end to the lower sixth of the pubic bone, 1 cm from the midline, and at the other end to the ischial spine. The anterior portion of this band lies on the inner surface of the levator ani muscle that arises some 3 cm above the arcus tendineus fasciae pelvis.

The layer of tissue that provides urethral support has two lateral attachments; a fascial attachment and a muscular attachment (Fig. 2.9) (DeLancey 1994). The fascial attachment of the urethral supports connects the periurethral tissues and anterior vaginal wall to the arcus tendineus fasciae pelvis and has been called the paravaginal fascial attachments by Richardson et al. (1981). They observed that it is a lateral detachment of the connections of the pubocervical fascia from the pelvic wall that is associated with stress incontinence and cystourethrocele (Fig. 2.10). The muscular attachment connects these same periurethral tissues to the medial border of the levator ani muscle. These attachments allow the levator ani muscle's normal resting tone to maintain the position of the vesical neck, supported by the fascial attachments. When the muscle relaxes at the onset of micturition, it allows the vesical neck to rotate downward to the limit of the elasticity of the fascial attachments, and then contraction at the end of micturition allows it to resume its normal position.

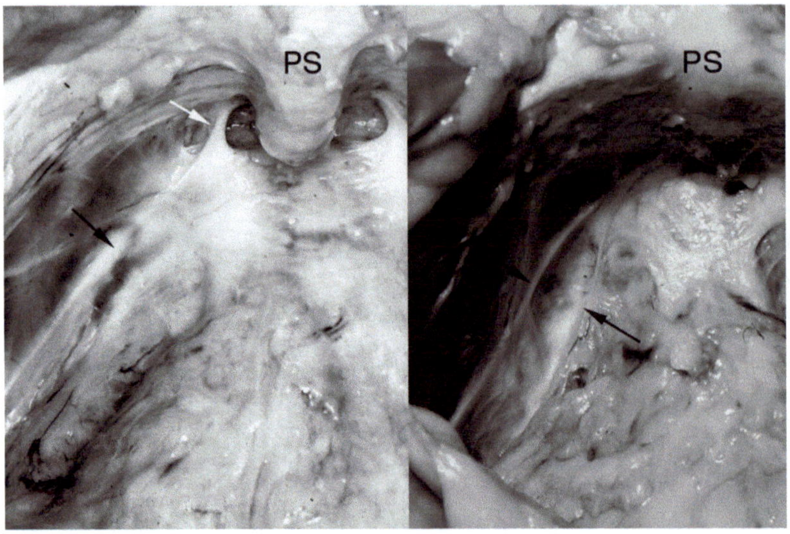

Fig. 2.10. *Left panel* shows normal attachment of the arcus tendineus fascia pelvis to the pubic bone (*white arrow*) showing the arcus tendineus fascia pelvis (*black arrow*). *Right panel* shows a paravaginal defect where the pubocervical fascia has separated from the arcus tendineus (*black arrows* mark the sides of the split) (*PS*=pubic symphysis) (DeLancey 2002, with permission)

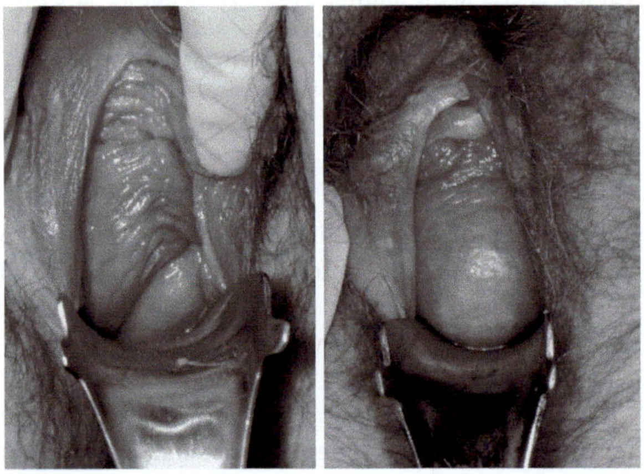

Fig. 2.11. *Left* Displacement cystocele where the intact anterior vaginal wall has prolapsed downward due to paravaginal defect. Note that the right side of the patient's vagina and cervix has descended more than the left because of a larger defect on this side. *Right* Distension cystocele where the anterior vaginal wall fascia has failed and the bladder is distending the mucosa (DeLancey 2002, with permission)

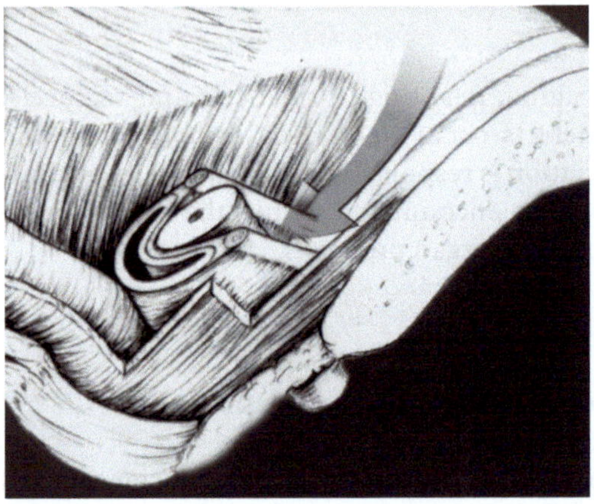

Fig. 2.12. Lateral view of pelvic floor with the urethra, vagina and fascial tissues transected at the level of the vesical neck drawn indicating compression of the urethra by downward force (*arrow*) against the supportive tissues indicating the influence of abdominal pressure on the urethra (DeLancey 1994, with permission)

Loss of anterior vaginal support results in what gynecologists call a cystocele or anterior wall prolapse (Fig. 2.11). This can occur either because of lateral detachment of the anterior vaginal wall at the pelvic side wall, referred to as a displacement cystocele, or as a central failure of the wall ("pubocervical fascia") itself that results in a distension cystocele.

The urethral support mechanism influences stress incontinence, not by determining how high or how low the urethra is, but by how it is supported. In examining anatomic specimens, simulated increases in abdominal pressure reveal that the urethra lies in a position where it can be compressed against the supporting hammock by rises in abdominal pressure (Fig. 212) (DeLancey 1994). In this hypothesis, it is the stiffness of this supporting layer under the urethra rather than the height of the urethra that would influence stress continence. In an individual with a firm supportive layer the urethra would be compressed between abdominal pressure and pelvic fascia in much the same way that you can stop the flow of water through a garden hose by stepping on it and compressing it against an underlying sidewalk. If, however, the layer under the urethra becomes unstable and does not provide a firm backstop for abdominal pressure to compress the urethra against, the opposing force that causes closure is lost and the occlusive action diminished. This latter situation is similar to trying to stop the flow of water through a garden hose by stepping on it while it lays on soft soil.

2.2.5 Posterior Support

The posterior vaginal wall is supported by connections between the vagina, the bony pelvis and the levator ani muscles (DeLancey 1999). The lower one-third of the vagina is fused with the perineal body (Fig. 2.13). This structure is the attachment between the perineal membranes on either side. This connection prevents downward descent of the rectum in this region. If the fibers that connect one side with the other rupture, then the bowel can protrude downward. (Fig. 2.14)

The mid-posterior vaginal wall is connected to the inside of the levator ani muscles by sheets of endopelvic fascia (Fig. 2.15). These connections prevent the ventral movement of the vagina during increases in abdominal pressure. These paired sheets are sometimes called the rectal pillars. In the upper one-third of the vagina, the vaginal wall is connected laterally by the paracolpium and in this region there is a single attachment for the vagina and there is not a separate system for the anterior and posterior vaginal walls. This is essentially the same support provided by level I.

When abdominal pressure forces the posterior vaginal wall downward towards the introitus, these attachments between the posterior vaginal wall and the levator muscles prevent this downward movement. The uppermost area of the posterior wall is suspended and descent of this area is most closely associated with the clinical problem of enterocele and vaginal vault prolapse. The lateral connections in the mid-vagina hold this portion of the vaginal

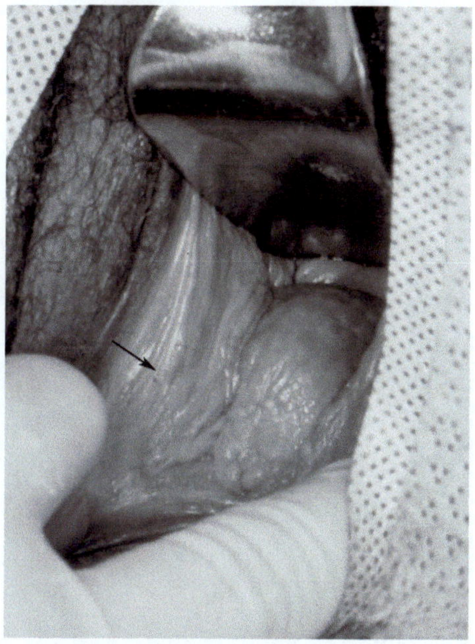

Fig. 2.14. Rectocele due to separation of the perineal body. Note the end of the hymenal ring that lies laterally on the side of the vagina, no longer united with its companion on the other side (DeLancey, with permission)

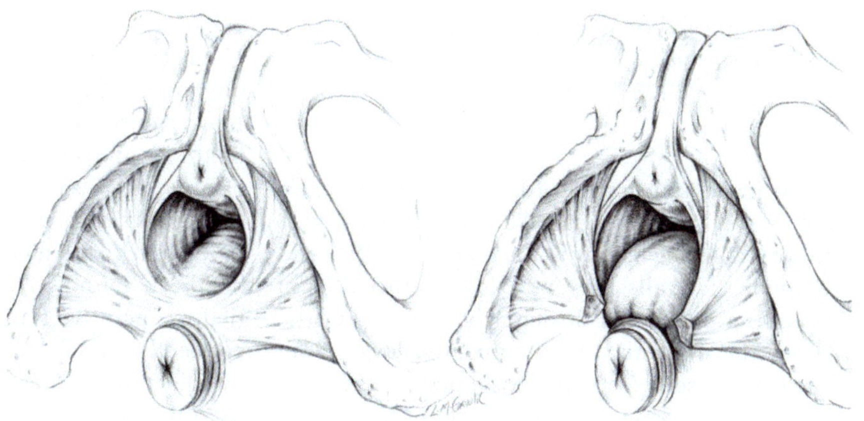

Fig. 2.13. The perineal membrane spans the arch between the ischiopubic rami with each side attached to the other through their connection in the perineal body. Note that separation of the fibers in this area leaves the rectum unsupported and results in a low rectocele (DeLancey 1999, with permission)

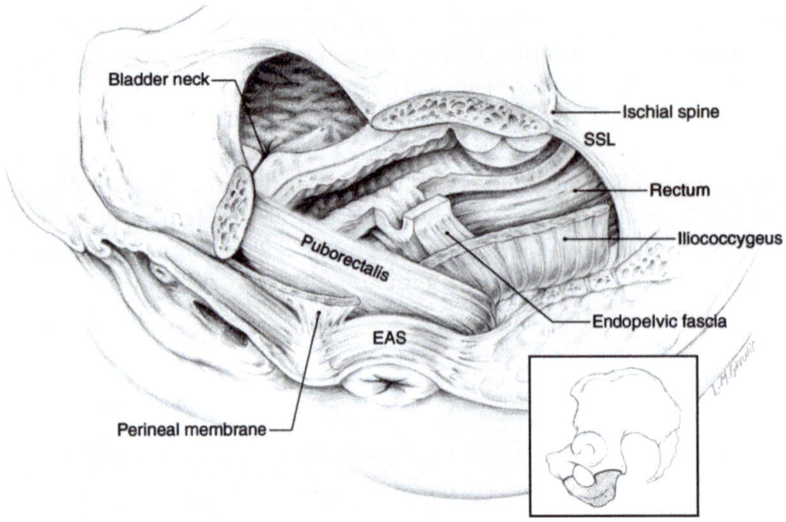

Fig. 2.15. Lateral view of the pelvis showing the relationships of the puborectalis, iliococcygeus and pelvic floor structures after removal of the ischium below the spine and sacrospinous ligament (*SSL*) (*EAS*=external anal sphincter). The bladder and vagina have been cut in the midline yet the rectum left intact. Note how the endopelvic fascial "pillars" hold the vaginal wall dorsally preventing its downward protrusion (DeLancey 1999, with permission)

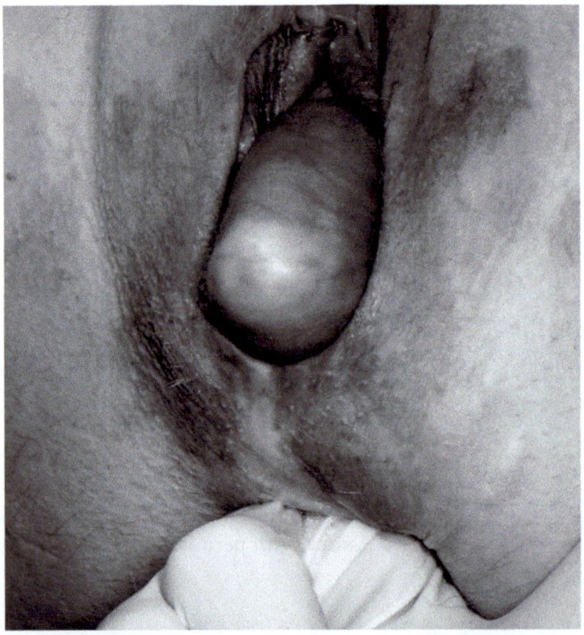

Fig. 2.16. Mid-vaginal rectocele that protrudes through the introitus despite a normally supported perineal body (DeLancey, with permission)

wall in place and prevent a mid-vaginal rectocele from occurring (Fig. 216). The multiple connections of the perineal body to the levator muscles and the pelvic sidewalls prevent a low rectocele from descending downward through the opening of the vagina (the urogenital hiatus and the levator ani muscles). These defects in the support at the level of the perineal body most frequently occur during vaginal delivery and are the most common type of posterior vaginal wall support problem.

The attachment of the levator ani muscles into the perineal body is important and damage to this part of the levator ani muscle during birth is one of the unrepairable aspects of pelvic floor dysfunction. Recent magnetic resonance imaging has vividly depicted these defects and will add greatly to our understanding of pelvic organ prolapse etiology. It is the author's personal belief that this muscular damage is one of the important factors that results in recurrence. An individual with muscles that do not function properly has a problem that is not surgically correctable. A more complete understanding of the biomechanics of this region will be needed for us to fully appreciate the importance of this injury.

2.2.6 Levator Ani Muscles

The levator ani muscles play a critical role in supporting the pelvic organs (Halban and Tandler 1907, summarized in Porges and Porges 1960; Berglas and Rubin 1953). Not only has evidence of this been seen in magnetic resonance scans (Kirschner-Hermanns et al. 1993; Tunn et al. 1998) but histological evidence of muscle damage has been found as well (Koelbl et al. 1989) and tied to operative failure (Hanzal et al. 1993). Any connective tissue within the body may be stretched by subjecting it to a constant force. Skin expanders used in plastic surgery stretch the dense and resistant dermis to extraordinary degrees and flexibility exercises practiced by dancers and athletes elongate leg ligaments with as little as 10 min of stretching a day. Both of these observations underscore the malleable nature of connective tissue when subjected to force over time. If the ligaments and fasciae within the pelvis were subjected to the continuous stress imposed on the pelvic floor by the great force of abdominal pressure, they would stretch. This stretching does not occur because the constant tonic activity of the pelvic floor muscles (Parks et al. 1962) closes the pelvic floor and carries the weight of the abdominal and pelvic organs, preventing constant strain on the ligaments.

Below the fascial layer is the levator ani group of muscles (Lawson 1974). (Fig. 2.17). They have a connective tissue covering on both superior and inferior surfaces called the superior and inferior fasciae of the levator ani. When these muscles and their fasciae are considered together, the combined structure is called the pelvic diaphragm.

The opening within the levator ani muscle through which the urethra and vagina pass (and through which prolapse occurs), is called the urogenital hiatus of the levator ani. The rectum also passes through this opening, but because the levator ani muscles attach directly to the anus it is not included in the name of the hiatus. The hiatus, therefore, is bounded ventrally (anteriorly) by the pubic bones, laterally by the levator ani muscles and dorsally (posteriorly) by the perineal body and external anal sphincter. The normal baseline activity of the levator ani muscle keeps the urogenital hiatus closed (Taverner 1959). It squeezes the vagina, urethra and rectum closed by compressing them against the pubic bone and lifts the floor and organs in a cephalic direction.

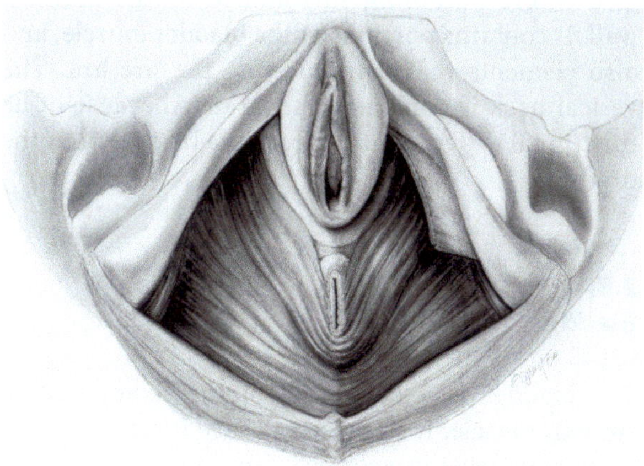

Fig. 2.17. Levator ani muscles seen from below. The cut edge of the perineal membrane ("urogenital diaphragm") can be seen on the left of the specimen (DeLancey, with permission)

There are two basic regions of the levator ani muscle. One, the iliococcygeal portion, forms a relatively flat, horizontal shelf that spans the pelvic opening from one pelvic sidewall to the other. The second portion of the pubovisceral muscle is a sling of muscle that arises from the pubic bone on either side forming a sling around and behind the pelvic organs and also attaches to the walls of the pelvic organs. This includes what is generally referred to as the pubococcygeus and the puborectalis portions. This medial portion has constant activity and is responsible for holding the pelvic floor closed by constricting the urogenital hiatus in the levator ani muscles.

The constant activity of the levator ani muscle is similar to other postural muscles. This continuous contraction is similar to the continuous activity of the external anal sphincter muscle and closes the lumen of the vagina in a way similar to the way in which the anal sphincter closes the anus. This constant action eliminates any opening within the pelvic floor through which prolapse could occur and forms a relatively horizontal shelf on which the pelvic organs are supported (Nichols et al. 1970).

2.2.7 Pelvic Floor Muscles and Endopelvic Fascia Interactions

The interaction between the pelvic floor muscles and the supportive ligaments is critical to pelvic organ support. As long as the levator ani muscles function properly the pelvic floor is closed and the ligaments and fasciae are under no tension. The fasciae simply act to stabilize the organs in their position above the levator ani muscles. When the pelvic floor muscles relax or are damaged, the pelvic floor opens and the vagina lies between the high abdominal pressure and low atmospheric pressure. In this situation it must be held in place by the ligaments. Although the ligaments can sustain these loads for short periods of time, if the pelvic floor muscles do not close the pelvic floor then the connective tissue must carry this load for long periods of time and will eventually fail to hold the vagina in place.

This support of the uterus has been likened to a ship in its berth floating on the water attached by ropes on either side to a dock (Paramore 1918). The ship is analogous to the uterus, the ropes to the ligaments, and the water to the supportive layer formed by the pelvic floor muscles. The ropes function to hold the ship (uterus) in the center of its berth as it rests on the water (pelvic floor muscles). If, however, the water level were to fall far enough that the ropes would be required to hold the ship without the supporting water, the ropes would all break. The analogous situation in the pelvic floor involves the pelvic floor muscles supporting the uterus and vagina that are stabilized in position by the ligaments and fasciae. Once the pelvic floor musculature becomes damaged and no longer holds the organs in place, the connective tissue fails.

2.2.8 Perineal Membrane and External Genital Muscles

In the anterior pelvis, below the levator ani muscles, is a dense triangularly shaped membrane called the perineal membrane (urogenital diaphragm). It lies at the level of the hymenal ring, and attaches the urethra, vagina, and perineal body to the ischiopubic rami (Fig. 2.18). Associated with the upper surface of the perineal membrane are the compressor urethrae and urethrovaginal sphincter muscles.

The term perineal membrane replaces the old term urogenital diaphragm, reflecting more accurate recent anatomical information (Oelrich 1983). Previous concepts of the urogenital diaphragm show two fascial layers, with a transversely oriented muscle in between (the deep transverse perineal muscle). Observations based on serial histology and gross dissection, however, reveal a single connective tissue membrane, with muscle lying immediately above. The correct anatomy explains the observation that pressures during a cough are greatest in the distal urethra (Hilton and Stanton 1983; Constantinou 1985) where the compressor urethra and urethrovaginal sphincter can compress the lumen closed in anticipation of a cough (DeLancey 1986, 1988).

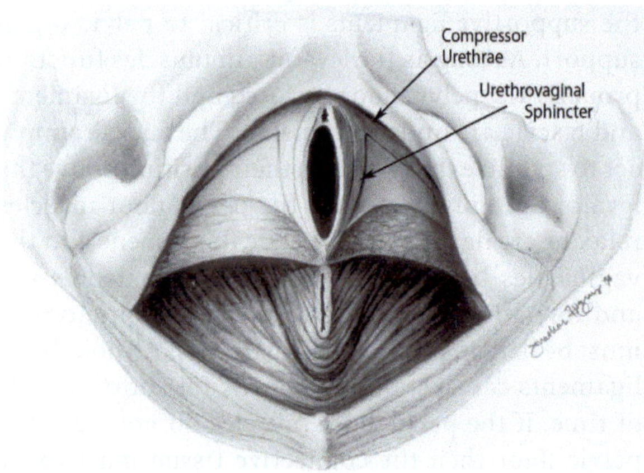

Fig. 2.18. Position of the perineal membrane and its associated components of the striated urogenital sphincter, the compressor urethra and the urethrovaginal sphincter (DeLancey, with permission)

2.3 Functional Anatomy of the Lower Urinary Tract

The inseparable link between structure and function found in living organisms is one of the common themes found in biology. The anatomy and clinical behavior of the lower urinary tract exemplify this immutable link. The following descriptions are intended to offer a brief overview of some clinically relevant aspects of lower urinary tract structure that help us understand the normal and abnormal behavior of this system. The lower urinary tract can he divided into the bladder and urethra (Figs. 2.19, 2.20). At the junction of these two continuous, yet discrete structures, lies the vesical neck. This hybrid structure represents that part of the lower urinary tract where the urethral lumen traverses the bladder wall before becoming surrounded by the urethral wall. It contains portions of the bladder muscle, and also elements that continue into the urethra. The vesical neck is considered separately because of its functional differentiation from the bladder, and the urethra.

2.3.1 Bladder

The bladder is a bag-like structure composed of smooth muscle. It relaxes to receive incoming urine so that increasing volumes can be stored with no appreciable increase in intravesical pressure. At a certain point, determined by multiple physiological and psychological factors, cerebral inhibition of the detrusor muscles' relaxation is released and a reflex

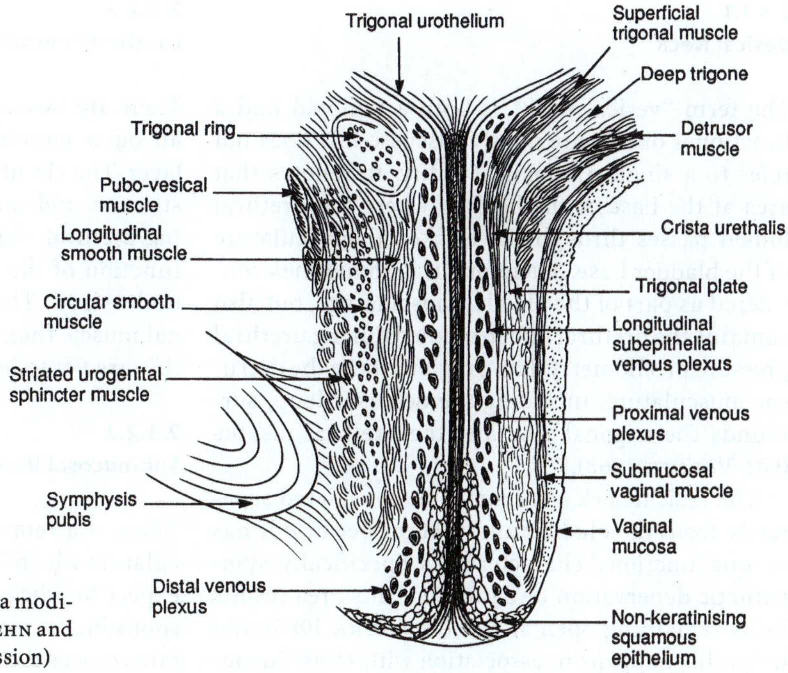

Fig. 2.19. Cross-section of the mid-urethra modified from Huisman (1983). From Strohbehn and DeLancey (1997) (Saunders, with permission)

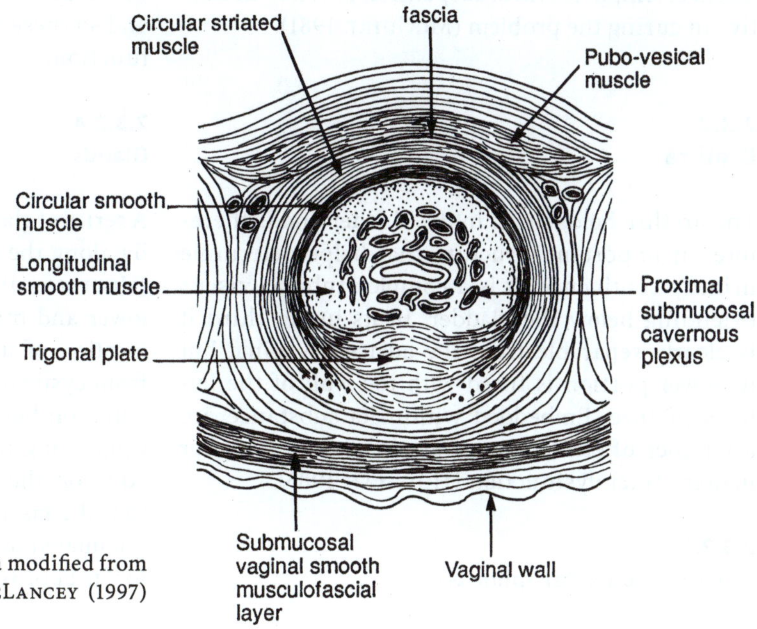

Fig. 2.20. Sagittal section of the mid-urethra modified from Huisman (1983). From Strohbehn and DeLancey (1997) (Saunders, with permission)

voiding contraction initiated. The complex interactions between environmental, societal, personal, and physiological factors that determines this storage and periodic release are the subject of active clinical investigation in the field of urinary incontinence as it relates to the clinical problem of detrusor instability. From a structural standpoint, however, this has not been a particularly active area of investigation other than some studies noting the relationship between bladder wall thickness and voiding dysfunction. Bladder diverticula which can extend between fascicles of the interlacing detrusor muscles do have clinical importance and are easily documented either radiographically or cystoscopically.

2.3.1.1 Vesical Neck

The term "vesical neck" is both a regional and a functional one as previously discussed. It does not refer to a single anatomical entity. It denotes that area at the base of the bladder where the urethral lumen passes through the thickened musculature of the bladder base. Therefore, it is sometimes considered as part of the bladder musculature, but also contains the urethral lumen studied during urethral pressure profilometry. It is a region where the detrusor musculature, including the detrusor loop, surrounds the trigonal ring and the urethral meatus (Gil Vernet 1968).

The vesical neck has come to be considered separately from the bladder and urethra because it has unique functional characteristics. Specifically, sympathetic denervation or damage of this area results in its remaining open at rest (McGuire 1986) and when this happens in association with stress incontinence, simple urethral suspension is often ineffective in curing the problem (McGuire 1981).

2.3.2 Urethra

The urethra holds urine in the bladder and is therefore an important structure that helps determine urinary continence. It is a complex tubular viscus extending below the bladder. In its upper third it is clearly separable from the adjacent vagina, but its lower portion is fused with the wall of the latter structure. Embedded within its substance are a number of elements that are important to lower urinary tract dysfunction (Huisman 1983).

2.3.2.1 Striated Urogenital Sphincter

The striated urogenital sphincter muscle encircles the urethra in its mid portion. Distally under the arch of the pubic bone, these fibers diverge to insert into the walls of the vagina and the perineal membrane (compressor urethrae and urethrovaginal sphincter) (Fig. 2.18). This muscle is responsible for increasing intraurethral pressure during times of need and also contributes about a third of the resting tone of the urethra. Its composition primarily of slow-twitch fatigue-resistant muscle fibers belies its constant activity.

2.3.2.2 Urethral Smooth Muscle

There are two layers of the urethral smooth muscle, an outer circular layer and an inner longitudinal layer. The circular fibers contribute to urethral constriction and smooth muscle blockade reduces resting urethral closure pressure by about a third. The function of the longitudinal muscle is not entirely understood. There is considerably more longitudinal muscle than circular muscle and the reasons for this are yet to be determined.

2.3.2.3 Submucosal Vasculature

There is a remarkably prominent submucosal vasculature which is far more extensive than one would expect for such a small organ. This is probably responsible in part for the hermetic seal that maintains mucosal closure. Occlusion of arterial flow into this area decreases resting urethral closure pressure and so these vessels are felt to participate in closure function.

2.3.2.4 Glands

A series of glands are found in the submucosa primarily along the dorsal (vaginal) surface of the urethra (Huffman 1948). They are most concentrated in the lower and middle thirds, and vary in number. The location of urethral diverticula, which are derived from cystic dilation of these glands, follows this distribution being most common distally, and usually originating along the dorsal surface of the urethra. In addition, their origin within the submucosa indicates that the fascia of the urethra must be stretched and attenuated over their surface, and indicates the need for its approximation after diverticular excision.

References

Ala-Ketola L (1973) Roentgen diagnosis of female stress urinary incontinence. Roentgenological and clinical study. Acta Obstet Gynecol Scand Suppl 23:1–59

Bartscht KD, DeLancey JOL (1988) A technique to study cervical descent. Obstet Gynecol 72:940–943

Berglas B, Rubin IC (1953) Study of the supportive structures of the uterus by levator myography. Surg Gynecol Obstet 97:677–692

Bonney V (1934) The principles that should underlie all operations for prolapse. J Obstet Gynaecol Br Emp 41:669–683

Campbell RM (1950) The anatomy and histology of the sacro-uterine ligaments. Am J Obstet Gynecol 59:1–12

Constantinou CE (1985) Resting and stress urethral pressures as a clinical guide to the mechanism of continence in the female patient. Urol Clin North Am 12:247–258

DeLancey JOL (1986) Correlative study of paraurethral anatomy. Obstet Gynecol 68:91–97

DeLancey JOL (1988) Structural aspects of the extrinsic continence mechanism. Obstet Gynecol 72:296–301

DeLancey JOL (1992) Anatomic aspects of vaginal eversion after hysterectomy. Am J Obstet Gynecol 166:1717–1728

DeLancey JOL (1994) Structural support of the urethra as it relates to stress urinary incontinence: the hammock hypothesis. Am J Obstet Gynecol 170:1713–1720

DeLancey JOL (1999) Structural anatomy of the posterior compartment as it relates to rectocele. Am J Obstet Gynecol 180:815–823

Gil Vernet S (1968) Morphology and function of the vesico-prostato-urethral musculature. Edizioni Canova, Treviso

Halban J, Tandler J (1907) Anatomie und Aetiologie der Genitalprolapse beim Weibe. Braumuller, Vienna

Hanzal F, Berger F, Koelbl H (1993) Levator ani muscle morphology and recurrent genuine stress incontinence. Obstet Gynecol 81:426–429

Hilton P, Stanton SL (1983) Urethral pressure measurement by microtransducer: the results in symptom-free women and in those with genuine stress incontinence. Br J Obstet Gynaecol 90:919–933

Huffman J (1948) Detailed anatomy of the paraurethral ducts in the adult human female. Am J Obstet Gynecol 55:86–101

Huisman AB (1983) Aspects on the anatomy of the female urethra with special relation to urinary continence. Contrib Gynecol Obstet 10:1–31

Kirschner-Hermanns R, Wein B, Niehaus S, Schaefer W, Jakse G (1993) The contribution of magnetic resonance imaging of the pelvic floor to the understanding of urinary incontinence. Br J Urol 72:715–718

Koebl H, Strassegger H, Riss PA, Gruber H (1989) Morphologic and functional aspects of pelvic floor muscles in patients with pelvic relaxation and genuine stress incontinence. Obstet Gynecol 74:789–795

Lawson JO (1974) Pelvic anatomy. I. Pelvic floor muscles. Ann R Coll Surg Engl 54:244–252

Mant J, Painter R, Vessey M (1997) Epidemiology of genital prolapse: observations from the Oxford Family Planning Association study. Br J Obstet Gynaecol 104:579–585

McGuire EJ (1981) Urodynamic findings in patients after failure of stress incontinence operations. Prog Clin Biol Res 78:351–360

McGuire EJ (1986) The innervation and function of the lower urinary tract. J Neurosurg 65:278–285

Miller JM, Perucchini D, Carchidi LT, DeLancey JOL, Ashton-Miller J (2001) A pelvic floor muscle contraction during a cough decreases vesical neck mobility. Obstet Gynecol 97:255–260

Muellner SR (1951) Physiology of micturition. J Urol 65:805–810

Nichols DH, Milley PS, Randall CI (1970) Significance of restoration of normal vaginal depth and axis. Obstet Gynecol 36:251–256

Oelrich TM (1983) The striated urogenital sphincter muscle in the female. Anat Rec 205:223–232

Olsen AL, Smith VJ, Bergstrom JO, Coiling JC, Clark AL (1997) Epidemiology of surgically managed pelvic organ prolapse and urinary incontinence. Obstet Gynecol 89:501–506

Paramore RH (1918) The uterus as a floating organ. In: The statics of the female pelvic viscera. Lewis, London, pp 12–15

Parks AG, Porter NH, Melzak J (1962) Experimental study of the reflex mechanism controlling muscles of the pelvic floor. Dis Colon Rectum 5:407–414

Porges RF, Porges JC (1960) After office hours: the anatomy and etiology of genital prolapse in women (translated by J Halban and J Tandler). Obstet Gynecol 15:790–796

Range RL, Woodburne RT (1964) The gross and microscopic anatomy of the transverse cervical ligaments. Am J Obstet Gynecol 90:460–467

Richardson AC, Edmonds PB, Williams NL (1981) Treatment of stress urinary incontinence due to paravaginal fascial defect. Obstet Gynecol 57:357–362

Sears PS (1933) The fascia surrounding the vagina, its origin and arrangement. Am J Obstet Gynecol 25:484–492

Strohbehn K, DeLancey JOL (1997) The anatomy of stress incontinence. Oper Tech Gynecol Surg 2:5–16

Taverner D (1959) An electromyographic study of the normal function of the external anal sphincter and pelvic diaphragm. Dis Colon Rectum 2:153–160

Tunn R, Paris S, Fischer W, Hamm B, Kuchinke J (1998) Static magnetic resonance imaging of the pelvic floor muscle morphology in women with stress urinary incontinence and pelvic prolapse. Neurourol Urodyn 17:579–589

Westby M, Astumussen M, Ulmsten U (1982) Location of maximum intraurethral pressure related to urogenital diaphragm in the female subject as studied by simultaneous urethrocystometry and voiding urethrocystography. Am J Obstet Gynecol 144:408–412

Pelvic Floor Muscles-Innervation, Denervation and Ageing

3

David B. Vodušek

CONTENTS

3.1 Introduction

Striated muscle, including pelvic floor muscle (PFM) activity, is totally controlled by the nervous system. Although PFM are striated muscles and share many similarities with other striated muscles, they nevertheless differ in their control mechanisms from both limb and axial muscles, as they do not directly participate in interaction with the mechanical tasks in the external world, but rather participate in "visceral" activity.

D. B. Vodušek, PhD
Professor of Neurology, Medical Faculty, University of Ljubljana *and*
Medical Director, Division of Neurology, University Medical Centre, 1525 Ljubljana, Slovenia

PFM are involved in "sacral functions": functions of lower the urinary tract (LUT), the anorectum, and the sexual organs. Thus, as neural control of pelvic organs is affected by a unique co-ordination of somatic and autonomic motor nervous systems, this duality is reflected in the specific neural control of PFM.

Sensorimotor innervation and the neural control of PFM, as well as their involvement in sacral functions, are presented in this chapter. Changes in PFM with ageing and due to lesions of innervation and neural control are discussed and are related to sacral dysfunction. As both PFM and striated sphincter muscles are involved in visceral activity and are controlled by the lower sacral segments, both will be discussed; differences will be pointed out.

3.2 Innervation and Neural Control

The terms "innervation" and "neural control" are proposed to be two different and useful concepts in discussing the neurobiology of body organs and understanding the clinical issues related to their neuroanatomy and neurophysiology. "Innervation" means straightforward anatomical data. These are particularly relevant to surgical dissection. Anatomical data are of course the basis for discerning connectivity in the central nervous system and in the peripheral neuromuscular system. "Neural control" implies the physiological activity of the underlying anatomical connections. Thus, functional neural control is not same as integrity of anatomy. To study neural control, methods providing neuroanatomical data are not sufficient. Using the term "neural control" furthermore implies that a single "anatomical entity" is never functioning on its own, but always in concert with "significant others". Thus, for instance, it is utterly impossible to have voluntary or reflex activation of one single muscle – there is always co-activation of a "primary mover" and its helpers – to fine tune the action, to co-ordinate it with the rest of body activity, to adjust posture, etc.

3.2.1 Somatic Motor System

Muscle – like every tissue – consists of cells (muscle fibres). But the functional unit within striated muscle is not a single muscle cell, but a motor unit. A motor unit consists of one alpha (or "lower") motor neuron (from the motor nuclei in spinal cord) and all the muscle fibres this motor neuron innervates. The motor unit is thus the basic functional unit of the somatic motor system.

It is important to stress that PFMs (or the "levator ani") are not one muscle, not in the sense of anatomical morphology or in the sense of only one single function for the whole muscle bulk. Indeed, there are several components to the levator ani. The specific components are considered in the chapter on anatomy. Due to their different insertions, the "mechanical consequences" of contraction of these individual muscles differ. They do, however, act as a group, and there seems little possibility that physiologically the activation of isolated parts of PFM would be possible. In normal nulliparae, concomitant bilateral activation of pubococcygeus (pubovisceral) muscle is the rule (Deindl et al. 1993). The possibility of unilateral activation (or of activation of only one part of PFM) in some highly self-trained individuals performing circus feats with PFM and anal sphincters has not really been investigated.

Spinal motor neurons for an individual muscle in the anterior horn of the spinal cord are, as a rule, grouped together. The individual parts of PFM seem to be no exception. For the levator ani group of muscles, the motor nuclei are in segments S3–S5, ventromedially in the anterior horn of the spinal cord grey matter; there is some overlap between them (Barber et al. 2002). The PFM nuclei have been less researched than the dorsolatelly located group of motor neurons innervating the striated external urethral and anal sphincters called the Onuf's nucleus (Mannen et al. 1982), situated in humans in the S2–S3 and occasionally S1 segment (Schroder 1985). In squirrel monkeys, the levator ani muscle spinal cord nucleus is also quite separate from the striated sphincter (Onuf) nucleus. Interestingly, some contacts (dendritic processes?) from the levator ani nucleus seem to reach Onuf's nucleus. This was argued to be one of the possible substrates for close interaction of both muscles in visceral functions (Pierce et al. 2005). It has been demonstrated in animal spinal cords that the dendritic processes from PFM motor neurons have a U shape and reach the bladder nucleus on one hand, and other somatic muscles in same segments on the other, thus forming a substrate for coordination of somatic and visceral function (Pierce et al. 2005).

Sphincter motor neurons are uniform and smaller than other alpha motor neurons. They have high concentrations of aminoacid-, neuropeptide-, norephinephrin-, serotonin- and dopamin-containing terminals, which represent the substrate for the distinctive neuropharmacologic responses of these neurons, which differ from those of limb muscles, the pelvic floor muscles and the bladder. The axons from these sacral alpha motor neurons leave the spinal cord as ventral radices and combine with dorsal radices to constitute spinal nerves. After passing through to the intravertebral foramen, the spinal nerve divides into a dorsal ramus and a ventral ramus (Bannister 1995). The particular ventral rami from sacral segments form the "sacral plexus". The pudendal nerve is usually described as originating from S2–4 roots, but may have some contribution from the S1 root, and possibly little or no contribution from the S4 root (Marani et al. 1993). It has been well documented that the main innervation for the PFM is through direct branches from the sacral plexus (S3 and/or S4), or the levator ani nerve, rather than by branches of the pudendal nerve "from below" (Wallner et al. 2006) (Fig. 3.1). The levator ani nerve approaches PFM from their visceral side; interestingly, near the ischial spine it lies so close to the pudendal nerve (lying below the levator ani) that the distance measures only 6 mm (and the distance between the levator ani nerve and the site of entry of the needle for the pudendal blockade only 5 mm; Wallner et al. 2006). It can be argued that this closeness of both nerves was the reason for some of the claims of pudendal nerve innervating PFM (relying on indirect evidence); the closeness of both nerves means furthermore they are vulnerable to same trauma.

The pudendal nerve anatomically continues through the greater sciatic foramen and enters in a lateral direction through the lesser sciatic foramen into the ischiorectal fossa on the medial surface of

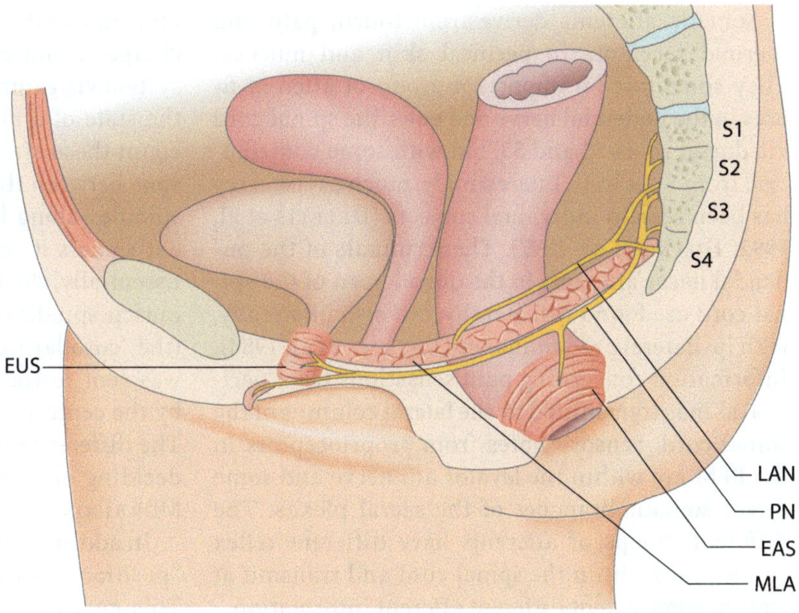

Fig. 3.1. The pudendal nerve (*PN*) is derived from dorsal and ventral rami of roots [(*S1*), *S2*, *S3*, (*S4*)]. The same rami (particularly *S3* and *S4*) contribute to the levator ani nerve (*LAN*) for the musculus levator ani (*MLA*). This muscle is thus as a rule innervated by direct branches from the sacral plexus "from above". The pudendal nerve "exits" the pelvis through the greater sciatic foramen and "enters" in a lateral direction into the ischiorectal fossa. Its muscular branches innervate the external anal sphincter (*EAS*) and the external urethral sphincter (*EUS*). Its sensory branch(es) innervate the perineal skin; its final sensory branch is the nervus dorsalis clitoridis (penis)

the internal obturator muscle (Alcock's canal). In the posterior part of the Alcock's canal, the pudendal nerve gives off the inferior rectal nerve, then it branches into the perineal nerve and the dorsal nerve of the penis/clitoris. The pudendal nerve supplies the striated anal and urethral sphincters.

The issue of (a)symmetry in striated sphincter innervation recently demonstrated by electrophysiological testing has been suggested to be a risk factor for incontinence when associated with childbirth-related sphincter injury (Wietek et al. 2007).

Most direct descending (efferent) connections to PFM and Onuf's nuclei are from the brainstem (raphe, ambiguous nuclei) and from the paraventricular hypothalamus. PET studies revealed activation of the (right) ventral pontine tegmentum (in the brainstem) during holding of urine in human subjects (Blok et al. 1997). This finding is consistent with the location of the "L region" in cats, proposed to control PFM nuclei.

PFM nuclei furthermore receive descending corticospinal input from the cerebral cortex. PET studies have revealed activation of the superomedial precentral gyrus during voluntary PFM contractions and of the right anterior cingulate gyrus during sustained pelvic floor muscle straining (Blok et al. 1997). PFM and striated perineal muscle contraction can be obtained by electrical or magnetic transcranial stimulation of the motor cortex in man (Vodušek 1996; Brostom 2003).

3.2.2 Sensory Control

Because PFM function is intimately connected to pelvic organ function, it is proposed that all sensory information from the pelvic region is relevant for PFM neural control. The sensory innervation of the pelvic region follows general principles. Primary sensory neurons – conveying information from the different type of receptors – are bipolar. Their cell bodies are in spinal ganglia. They send a long process to the periphery and a central process into the spinal cord where it terminates segmentally or – after branching for reflex connections – ascends in some cases as far as the brainstem (Bannister 1995). The afferent pathways from the anogenital region and pelvic region are divided into somatic and visceral components.

The visceral afferents accompany both parasympathetic and sympathetic efferents and also course through the pudendal nerves. The spinal pathways that transmit sensory information from the visceral afferent terminations in the spinal cord to more rostral structures can be found in the dorsal, lateral and ventral spinal cord columns. Information from perineal skin involves sexual sensation. In human spinal cord the pathway transmitting this information is situated superficially just ventral to the equator of the cord (within the spinothalamic tract) (Torrens and Morrison 1987).

Somatic afferents derive from touch, pain and thermal receptors in perineal skin and mucosa. They constitute an important group of afferent fibres in the pudendal nerve and enter the spinal cord via dorsal roots S2 and S3, but with some contribution from S1 as well. Interestingly, much asymmetry has been seen in individual subjects (Deletis et al. 1992; Huang et al. 1997). The terminals of the pudendal nerve afferents in the dorsal horn of the spinal cord are found ipsilaterally, but also bilaterally, with ipsilateral predominance (Ueyama et al. 1984). Information concerning pain sensations from perineal skin is transmitted by the lateral columns of the spinal cord. Sensory fibres from proprioceptors in the PFM are within the levator ani nerve and some direct somatic branches of the sacral plexus. The different groups of afferents have different reflex connections within the spinal cord and transmit at least to some extent different afferent information.

3.2.3 Sensory-Motor Integration in PFM Control

Proprioceptive afferent nerves arise particularly from muscle spindles; these are present in PFM, but most probably not in striated sphincters. Golgi tendon organs are only present in muscles with tendons. The proprioceptive afferents form synaptic contacts in the spinal cord and have collaterals ("primary afferent collaterals") that run ipsilaterally in the dorsal spinal columns to synapse in the gracilis (dorsal column) nuclei in the brainstem. This pathway transmits information about innocuous sensations from the pelvic floor muscles, such as proprioception from PFM adjacent to the rectum that probably contributes to sensation of rectal fullness.

Proprioceptors regulate the "basic motor control" of a particular muscle, but also provide the sensation of proprioception ("muscle awareness"). Proprioception is otherwise particularly important for sensing limb position (stationary proprioception) and limb movement (kinaesthetic proprioception). It relies on special mechanoreceptors in muscle tendons and joint capsules. In muscles there are specialised stretch receptors – muscle spindles, and in tendons there are Golgi tendon organs that sense the contractile force. Proprioceptive information is crucial for striated muscle motor control both in the "learning" phase of a certain movement and for later execution of learned motor behaviours. Proprioceptive information is influenced not only by the current state of the muscle, but also by the efferent discharge the muscle spindles receive from the nervous system via gamma efferents. In order to know about the state of a muscle, the brain must take into account these efferent discharges and make comparisons between the signals it sends out to the muscle spindles along the gamma efferents and the afferent signals it receives from the primary afferents. Essentially, the brain compares the signal from the muscle spindles with the copy of its motor command (the 'corollary discharge' or 'efferents copy') that was sent to the muscle spindle intrafusal muscles by the central nervous system via gamma efferents. The differences between the two signals are used in deciding on the state of the muscle (Torrens and Morrison 1987).

In addition, stretch-sensitive receptors signalling "position" information are also in the perineal skin. This cutaneous proprioception is particularly important for control of movements of muscles without bony attachment (lips, anal sphincter).

The functional status of a certain movement is represented in the brain by the afferent input just described. Muscle awareness reflects the amount of sensory information from various inputs (of which usually we are not "conscious"). Typically, feedback awareness on limb muscle function (acting at joints) is derived not only from muscle spindles and tendon receptors, but also from the skin sensation, from visual input, etc. The concept of the "awareness" thus in fact overlaps with the ability to voluntarily change the state of a muscle, as we have to have the appropriate brain "conceptualisation" of the particular movement before we execute it. This "concept" of a particular movement evolves through repeatedly (and appropriately) executed movements, probably resulting in facilitation of particular cortical motor areas (Gunnarsson et al. 1999).

In contrast to limb muscles, the pelvic floor muscles (and sphincters) lack several of the typical sensory input mechanisms we have described, and hence the brain is not "well informed" on their status. Additionally, there may be a gender difference, inasmuch as pelvic floor muscle awareness in females seems to be in general less as compared to males. (The author concludes this on the basis of long personal experience with PFM EMG in both genders; there seems to be no formal study on PFM activation patterns in man apart from ejaculation). Healthy males have no difficulties in voluntarily contracting the pelvic floor, but up to 30% of healthy women cannot do it readily on command. (cf. Fig. 3.2). The

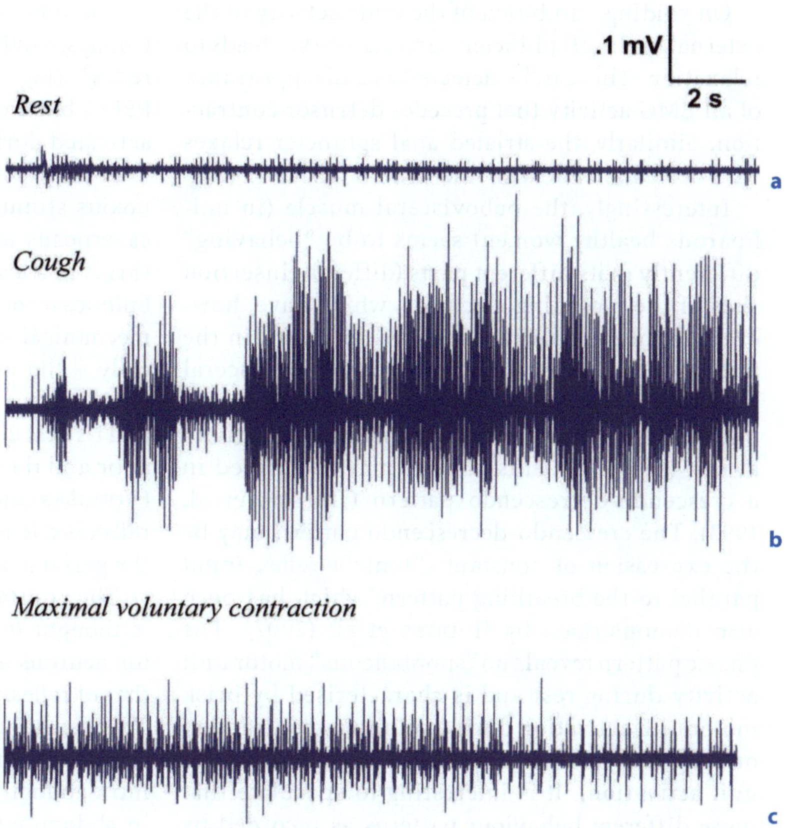

Fig. 3.2a–c. Kinesiological EMG (with a concentric needle electrode) recordings from levator ani muscle (in a 43-year-old continent neurologically healthy female): **a** ongoing activity of motor unit potentials during complete relaxation ("tonic" activity); **b** recruitment of motor units on reflex manoeuvre (activation during cough); **c** recruitment of motor units on command to contract (voluntary activation). Note that the voluntary activation cannot recruit the same number of motor units as coughing!

need for "squeezing out" the urethra at the end of voiding and the close relationship of penile erection and ejaculation to PFM contractions may be the origin of this gender difference.

3.2.4 Neural Control Manifesting as PFM Activity Patterns

Neural control mechanisms can be conceptualized to "produce" particular "muscle behaviour patterns", which can be observed by different recording techniques, particularly EMG. The activity patterns of PFM (within the overall behaviour of the individual) thus "serve" their function(s); these are probably not only the co-operation of PFM in sacral functions (see below), but also postural (Pool-Goudzwaart et al. 2004).

Most EMG studies have been performed for the striated sphincter muscles, which are also routinely examined during urodynamic testing. At rest, the striated sphincter muscles demonstrate continuous motor unit activity that persists even when subjects fall asleep during the examination (Chantraine 1973). This spontaneous activity of muscle may be called tonic and depends on prolonged activation of certain motor units (Vodušek 1982, 1994). As a rule tonic motor unit activity increases with bladder filling, and indeed any reflex or voluntary activation is mirrored first in an increase of the firing frequency of the "tonic" motor units. With any activity (e.g. coughing), and only for a limited length of time, new motor units are recruited. These may be called "phasic" motor units. As a rule, they have potentials of higher amplitudes, and their discharge rates are higher and irregular. A small percentage of motor units with an "intermediate" activation pattern can also be encountered (Vodušek 1982, 1994). It has to be stressed that the above typing of motor units is electrophysiological, and no direct correlation to histochemical typing of muscles has so far been achieved.

Tonic motor unit activity is as a rule not seen in the resting bulbocavernosus muscle (Vodušek 1982). However, spontaneous motor unit activity is encountered in most (but not all) detection sites for the levator ani muscle (Vodušek 1982; Deindl et al. 1993). In the pubococcygeus (pubovisceral) muscle of the normal female, there is some increase of activity during bladder filling.

On voiding, inhibition of the tonic activity of the external urethral sphincter – and also PFM – leads to relaxation. This can be detected as a disappearance of all EMG activity that precedes detrusor contraction. Similarly, the striated anal sphincter relaxes with defecation and also micturition (Read 1990).

Interestingly, the pubovisceral muscle (in nulliparous healthy women) seems to be "behaving" differently in its different parts (different insertion sites of the recording electrode, which have, however, not been visually monitored to ascertain the finer anatomical location within the pubovisceral muscle). In most insertion sites, the pubovisceral muscle demonstrates ongoing motor unit activity at rest (Fig. 3.2a). This activity may be formed in a crescendo-decrescendo pattern (Deindl et al. 1993). The crescendo-decrescendo pattern may be the expression of constant ("tonic") reflex input parallel to the breathing pattern, which has been also demonstrated by Hodges et al. (2007). The phasic pattern reveals no "spontaneous" motor unit activity during rest and is characterised by brisk motor unit activation during voluntary contraction or coughing (probably related to fast-twitch motor unit activation). It is interesting to speculate that these different behaviour patterns as recorded by EMG in different parts of the pubovisceral muscle relate to areas of relative prevalence of either slow- or fast-twitch motor units. It is known that there is histomorphological diversity of the levator ani, which consists of type-I (slow-twitch) and type-II (fast-twitch) muscle fibres, but in different proportions in different parts of the muscle (Critchley et al. 1980). It is interesting to speculate that within the apparent necessity of overall activation of PFM (due to the simple innervation by one nerve on each side), the neural control of PFM allows for the different anatomical divisions of the muscle to have differently fine-tuned "functions" on account of different thresholds of activation for different motor nuclei of the different muscle parts.

The human urethral and anal striated sphincters seem to have no muscle spindles; their reflex reactivity is thus intrinsically different from the levator ani muscle complex, in which muscle spindles and Golgi tendon organs have been demonstrated (Borghi et al. 1991). Thus, PFMs have the intrinsic proprioceptive "servo-mechanism" for adjusting muscle length and tension, while the sphincter muscles depend on afferents from skin and mucosa. Both muscle groups are integrated in reflex activity that incorporates pelvic organ function.

The reflex activity of PFM is clinically and electrophysiologically evaluated by eliciting the "cough reflex" (Fig. 32c); this is not exactly a "reflex of PFM", but a co-activation of several muscle groups activated during coughing as a co-ordinated group. PFM are to some extent activated by mechanical and noxius stimuli that are known to elicit the bulbocavernosus and anal reflex, respectively, although this is to a lesser degree than perineal muscles. The bulbocavernosus reflex is evoked on non-painful mechanical stimulation of the glans (or – electrically – the dorsal penile/clitoral nerve) (Vodušek 2002a). It is a complex electromyographic response, and its first component is thought to be an oligosynaptic and the latter component a polysynaptic reflex (Vodušek and Janko 1990). The (polysynaptic) anal reflex is elicited by painful (pinprick) stimulation in the perianal region.

The constant tonic activity of sphincter muscles is thought to be the result of "low-threshold" motor neurons and the constant (afferent) "inputs" either of reflex segmental or of suprasegmental origin. This constant activity is supported (or affected?) by cutaneous stimuli, by pelvic organ distension and by intra-abdominal pressure changes. Sudden increases in abdominal pressure as a rule lead to brisk PFM (reflex) activity, which has been called the "guarding reflex". It is organised at the spinal level, but the latter seems to be less important in various physiological manoeuvres as usually implied. It needs to be considered that "sudden increases in intra-abdominal pressure", if caused by an intrinsically driven manoeuvre (i.e. coughing, movement), include feed forward activation of PFM as part of the complex muscle activation pattern integrated by neural control networks and not simple "reflex responses" to some stimulus (Fig. 3.2c, normal recruitment of additional motor units during coughing). PFM and striated sphincter co-activation in advance arm movement has been described (Hodges et al. 2007), and the role of PFM in postural adjustments stressed. Their activation (also during quiet breathing) was more related to other muscle activity (for instance, abdominal muscles) than to increases of abdominal pressure. The observed PFM activation in the normal subject (as for instance during coughing) is thus a co-activation or possibly a compound of "feed-forward" and "reflex" activation of several muscle groups.

Another common stimulus leading an increase in PFM activity is pain. The typical phasic reflex response to a nociceptive stimulus is the anal reflex. It is commonly assumed that prolonged pain in pelvic organs is accompanied by an increase in the "reflex" PFM activity, which would indeed be manifested as "an increased tonic motor unit activity". This has so far not been formally studied. Whether such chronic PFM overactivity might itself generate a chronic pain state and even other dysfunctions may be a tempting hypothesis, but has not yet been explicitly demonstrated.

To correspond with their functional (effector) role as pelvic organ "supporters" (e.g. during coughing, sneezing), "sphincters" for the lower urinary tract (LUT) and anorectum, and as an effector in the sexual arousal response, orgasm and ejaculation, PFMs are also involved in very complex involuntary ("reflex") activity that co-ordinates behaviour of pelvic organs (smooth muscle) and several different groups of striated muscles. This activity is to be understood as originating from so-called "pattern generators" within the central nervous system, particularly the brainstem. These pattern generators ("reflex centres") are genetically inbuilt. Indeed, PFMs seem to be controlled by several integrated - and coordinated - neural networks.

Skilled movement of distal limb muscles requires individual motor units to be activated in a highly controlled manner by the primary motor cortex. By contrast, activation of axial muscles (necessary to maintain posture, etc.) - while also under voluntary control - depends particularly on vestibular nuclei and reticular formation to create predetermined "motor patterns". Similarities of PFM to axial muscles can be proposed as regards their neural control. This control can be best conceptualized as being part of the "emotional" motor system (Holstege 1998). Without doubt it is possible to voluntarily activate (Fig. 3.2b) or inhibit the firing of PFM and striated sphincter motor units (Sundin and Petersen 1975; Vodušek 1994) (although it is also true that a high percentage of normal women - without an "upper neuron lesion" - have difficulties in doing this).

3.3 Neural Control of Sacral Functions

PFM neural control mechanisms particularly serve the co-ordination of striated muscles with sacral functions (LUT; anorectal, and sexual). PFM and sphincters need to be controlled "within" a particular function (for instance, with bladder activity); single functions need to be neurally co-ordinated with each other (for instance, voiding and defecation; voiding and erection).

Activation of pelvic-floor and sphincter lower motor neurons is thus coordinated differently from other groups of motor neurons. In contrast to the reciprocal innervation that is common in limb muscles, the neurons innervating each side of the PFM have to work in harmony and synchronously. Indeed, sphincters may be morphologically considered to constitute "one" muscle - which is innervated by two nerves (left and right)! By concomitant activity PFMs act as the "closure unit" of the excretory tracts, the "support unit" for pelvic viscera and an "effector unit" in the sexual response. In general, muscles involved in the above functions from both sides of the body act as "one muscle": this has been demonstrated for pubococcygei muscles, but has not really been documented for the whole group of PFM and sphincters (Deindl et al. 1993). However, as each muscle in the pelvis has its own unilateral peripheral innervation, dissociated activation patterns are possible and have been reported between the two pubococcygei (Deindl et al. 1994) and between the levator ani and the urethral sphincter (Kenton and Brubaker 2002).

The differences in the evolutionary origin of the sphincter muscles and levator ani furthermore imply that unilateral activation may be less of an impossibility for the pelvic-floor muscles than for sphincters. It is clear, however, that the coordination between individual PFM can definitively suffer due to deranged neural control.

The sacral function neural control system is proposed to be a part of the "emotional motor system". This is a system derived from brain or brainstem structures belonging to the limbic system. It consists of the medial and a lateral component (Holstege 1998). The first represents diffuse pathways originating in the caudal brainstem and terminating on (almost all) spinal grey matter, using serotonin as its neurotransmitter. This system is proposed to "set the threshold" for overall changes in muscle activity, such as, for instance, in muscle tone under different physiological conditions (sleeping, etc.).

The lateral component of the emotional motor system consists of discreet areas in the hemispheres and the brainstem responsible for specific motor activities, such as micturition and mating. The pathways belonging to the lateral system use spinal premotor interneurons to influence motor neurons in somatic and autonomic spinal nuclei, thus allowing for confluent interactions of various inputs to modify the motor neuron activity.

3.3.1 Lower Urinary Tract Function and PFM

At rest urinary continence is assured by a competent sphincteric mechanism (including striated and smooth muscle sphincter, with PFM support) and an adequate bladder storage function. The kinesiological sphincter and PFM EMG recordings in normal individuals show continuous activity of motor units at rest (as defined by continuous firing of motor unit potentials), which increases with increasing bladder fullness. Reflexes mediating excitatory outflow to the sphincters are organised at the spinal level (the guarding reflex). The L region in the brainstem has also been called the "storage centre" (Blok et al. 1997). This area was active in PET studies of those volunteers who could not void, but contracted their PFM. The L region is thought to exert a continuous exciting effect on the Onuf's nucleus and thereby on the striated urinary sphincter during the storage phase; in humans it is probably part of a complex set of "nerve impulse pattern generators" for different coordinated motor activities, such as breathing, coughing, straining, etc.

During physical stress (e.g. coughing, sneezing), the baseline activity of the urethral and anal sphincter may not be sufficient to assure continence when the pressures arising in the abdominal cavity and hence within the bladder and lower rectum exceed these "resting" levels. Activation of the pelvic floor muscles is mandatory and may be perceived as occurring in two steps by two different activation processes:

Coughing and sneezing are thought to be generated by individual pattern generators within the brainstem, and thus activation of PFM is a preset co-activation – and not primarily a "reflex" reaction that occurs in response to increased abdominal pressure. Pelvic floor muscle activation has to be seen as a part of different pre-programmed movements. This can be thought of as a component of the anticipatory postural activity and respiratory activity (Hodges et al. 2007). In addition, there might be an additional reflex PFM response (due to distension of muscle spindles within pelvic floor muscles caused by a response to the increase in abdominal pressure). The PFM can, of course, also be voluntarily activated anticipating an increase in abdominal pressure. Such timed voluntary activity may be taught and learned as treatment for urinary incontinence (the "Knack procedure") (Miller et al. 1998).

Voluntary micturition is a behaviour pattern that starts with relaxation of the striated urethral sphincter and PFM. Areas rostral to the brainstem (the hypothalamus and other parts of the brain including the frontal cortex) are responsible for the timing of micturition. The pontine micturition centre co-ordinates the activity of motor neurons of the urinary bladder and the urethral sphincter (both nuclei located in the sacral spinal cord), receiving afferent input via the peri-aqueductal grey. The central control of lower urinary tract function is organised as an on-off switching circuit (or a set of circuits, rather) that maintains a reciprocal relationship between the urinary bladder and urethral outlet.

Without the pontine micturition centre and its spinal connections, co-ordinated bladder/sphincter activity is not possible. Thus, patients with such lesions demonstrate bladder sphincter disco-ordination (dyssynergia). Patients with lesions above the pons do not show detrusor-sphincter dyssynergia. They suffer from urge incontinence (due to bladder overactivity), demonstrate non-inhibited sphincter relaxation and have an inability to delay voiding to an appropriate place and time.

Voluntary PFM contraction during voiding can lead to a stop of micturition, probably because of collateral connections to detrusor control nuclei. Descending inhibitory pathways for the detrusor have been demonstrated (de Groat et al. 2001). Bladder contractions are also inhibited by reflexes, activated by afferent input from PFM, perineal skin and the anorectum (Sato et al. 2000).

3.3.2 Anorectal Function and PFM

Faeces stored in the colon are transported past the rectosigmoid into the normally empty rectum, which can store up to 300 ml of contents. Rectal distension causes regular contractions of the rectal wall, which is affected by the intrinsic nervous (myenteric) plexus, and prompts the desire to defecate (Bartolo et al. 2002). Stool entering the rectum is detected by stretch receptors in the rectal wall and PFM; their discharge leads to the sensation of a need to evacuate the rectum. It starts as an intermittent sensation that becomes more and more constant. Contraction of PFM may interrupt the process, probably by concomitant inhibitory influences to the defecatory neural "pattern generator", but also by "mechanical" insistence on sphincter contraction and the propelling of faeces back to the sigmoid colon (Bartolo et al. 2002).

PFMs are intimately involved in anorectal function. Apart from the "sensory" role of PFM and the external anal sphincter function, the puborectalis muscle is thought to maintain the "anorectal" angle associated with continence. Defecation requires increased rectal pressure co-ordinated with relaxation of the anal sphincters and PFM. Pelvic floor relaxation allows opening of the anorectal angle and perineal descent. However, observations by EMG and defecography suggest that the puborectalis may not always relax during defecation in healthy subjects (Fucini et al. 2001).

3.3.3 Sexual Behaviour and PFM

Complex postural changes are known for mating behaviour in animals, but have not been systematically studied in humans. PFM are definitely involved in the sexual response. In males the repetitive activation during ejaculation is responsible for the expulsion of semen from the urethra, particularly by the bulbocavernosus muscles (Petersen et al. 1955), and orgasm is accompanied by rhythmic contractions of the PFM/perineal muscles in both sexes.

During other parts of the human sexual response cycle, it is assumed that, apart from general changes in muscle tone set by the emotional motor system, it is the sacral reflex circuitry that governs much of the PFM activity during the sexual response cycle. The bulbocavernosus reflex behaviour would allow for reflex activation of PFM during genital stimulation (Vodušek 2002a). Tonic stimulation of the reflex is postulated to hinder venous outflow from the penis/clitoris, thus helping erection. PFM reflex contraction should conceivably contribute to the achievement of the "orgasmic platform" (contraction of the levator ani).

3.4 Ageing and PFM Changes

Pelvic floor disorders become more prevalent with increasing age. Normal ageing in humans is associated with a progressive decrease in skeletal muscle mass and strength. By the age of 70 years, the cross-sectional area of the range of muscles is reduced up to 30% and muscle strength up to 40%. In addition, ageing muscles are more susceptible to exercise-induced muscle damage (Close et al. 2005). This decline in strength is accompanied by a decrease in overall striated muscle mass, which falls by 25–30% by the seventh decade (Grimby and Saltin 1983). The changes due to ageing are not due to hypomobility; the atrophy of immobilisation can be reversed by training even in nonagenarians (Fiatarone et al. 1990).

It is generally accepted that the age-associated changes are a result of lower levels of anabolic hormones, oxidative damage, neuromuscular alterations and the general decrease in muscle protein turnover, but the details are far from elucidated. Loss of spinal cord motor neurons with age (with the resulting denervation of motor units) has been demonstrated and suggested as the main mechanism for losing muscle power and bulk. Denervation of single motor units leads to reinnervation (an adjacent motor neuron – usually a slow-twitch motor neuron – reinnervates at least some of the denervated muscle fibres); the result is "fibre-type grouping" as seen under the microscope. Skeletal muscle regenerative capacity has been shown to decline with age. This decline may be associated with a diminishing number of muscle progenitor ("satellite") cells and/or with their declining quality, but the issue is still open.

Age influences the proportion of muscle fibre types (which are characterized by their specific myosine heavy chain isoforms). A study on the vastus lateralis muscle demonstrated that between the ages of 20 and 80 there is about a 50% reduction in the total fibre number, the loss being faster after the age of 60. A selective loss of fast-twitch (type-II) fibres as compared to slow-twitch (type-I) fibres has been found (Lexell et al. 1986). Although there are indications that not all muscles have the same fate, the major quantitative changes in ageing muscles are loss of fibres, decrease in size, and fibre-type grouping (Brunner et al. 2007).

As stated, the main mechanism responsible for the loss of muscle fibres is loss of whole motor units, the responsible mechanism thus being neurogenic (Faulkner et al. 2007). The relative contribution of intrinsic ("myogenic") muscle changes as the underlying mechanism of functional decline in ageing muscle seems to be unclear, but "myopathic" histomorphological changes in muscles of normal individuals have been reported as rare. With different methods, the "neuropathic" changes in muscles of normal subjects have been demonstrated and attributed to ageing; particularly often used were electrophysiological tests (Campbell et al. 1973; Trontelj et al. 1979), but muscle fibre-type grouping (a typical "neurogenic" marker) was also histomorphologically demonstrated to increase with age (Tomlinson and Irving 1977). Thus, ageing was suggested to involve a continuous denervation/reinnervation process most likely caused by a loss of function of alpha motor neurons in the spinal cord (Lexell et al. 1986).

Age-related functional decline has also been demonstrated for PF and striated sphincter muscles. The nulliparous female urethral sphincter mechanism is significantly affected by age. Increasing age was associated with decreasing maximal urethral closure pressure; a 15-cmH_2O decrease in pressure per decade was found for a cohort of nulliparous women aged 21–70 years (Rodriguez Trowbridge et al. 2007). Similarly, most studies focussing on anal sphincter have documented age-related decline, for instance reduction of anal resting and squeeze pressures in asymptomatic women between 20 and 75+ years (Fox et al. 2006). Maximum resting pressure and maximum squeeze pressure of the anal sphincters were also significantly reduced with increasing age in a cohort of healthy women aged 20 to 83 years. Their results suggested gradual changes throughout adult life (Ryhammer et al. 1997). The calculated mean EMG values of three rapid contractions of the levator ani (as measured with the vaginal surface EMG probe) declined significantly with age in a cohort of women between 22 and 59 years (Aukee et al. 2003). Others (Rodriguez Trowbridge et al. 2007), however, could not demonstrate a change of levator ani function with increasing age (as measured by resting vaginal closure force or maximal voluntary contraction). This paradoxical lack of change of levator function with age was explained by a possible inability of women to maximally volitionally recruit the largest levator ani motor neurons at any age.

Apart from a decline in function of PF and striated sphincter muscles, structural changes were also found. External anal sphincter thinning with age has been demonstrated by high-spatial-resolution endoanal MR imaging (both in women and men; statistical significance was only reached for men); the thickness of the longitudinal muscle region significantly decreased with age for both genders (Rociu et al. 2000). The underlying decrease in urethral sphincter function was found to be the decrease of the relative volume of striated muscle (without change in the smooth muscle component) of the urethra (Carlile et al. 1988) and in the decrease in the number and density of urethral striated muscles with increasing age (Perucchini et al. 2002a,b). In the latter study, however, the effects of age and parity could not be well differentiated.

The cause of diminishing muscle bulk and failing function for PFM is generally accepted as being neurogenic. In a key study by Smith et al. (1989), single-fibre EMG changes in the pubococcygeus muscle were reported as not only due to parity, but also due to ageing. The results were interpreted as reflecting denervation and reinnervation. Rectal sensation also seems to be reduced with age (Fox et al. 2006). Unfortunately, few histopathological data focus specifically on ageing PFM. Histological studies were mostly concerned with consequences of parity, and if ageing was addressed, the methods focussed on general structural and functional changes (mentioned above). The one recent histological study reported age-related abnormalities in the levator ani as "myogenic", and – what is more – reported absence of neurogenic changes (Jundt et al. 2005)! The progressive histological changes in muscle were attributed to mechanical stress. In a previous study by the same group, the circumference of levator ani type-I fibres was reported as significantly larger in nulliparous women under 40 years of age compared to nulliparae older than 40 years (Dimpfl et al. 1998). A study in squirrel monkeys also revealed myogenic changes increased with age; neurogenic changes were only found in some multiparous monkeys (Pierce et al. 2007).

In an interesting study on a small number of subjects, Lierse et al. (1993) have demonstrated histological data on the developmental changes in the striated anal sphincter. In foetuses of up to 40 weeks' gestational age, there was first a predominance of type-II muscle fibres; this predominance subsequently diminished. Few-months-old infants showed a further increase in the proportion of type-I muscle fibres, which finally began to predominate (in two 5- and 8-year-old children and in adults up to 76 years of age). In older subjects (78–81 years old), the proportion of type-I fibres was again diminishing. The authors discussed this peculiarity of changing proportions of fibre types as an adaptation of PFM to the gradual change in posture of the infant towards sitting and standing.

More data on developmental histomorphological changes in PF and striated sphincter muscles, and more studies on ageing subjects, particularly women who have not had vaginal deliveries, are needed. This is particularly necessary as at present there seems to be a discrepancy of data related to PFM muscles (myopathic changes being mainly discussed as the consequence of ageing) and the rest of striated musculature (denervation being commonly accepted as the main consequence of ageing).

Although indeed many contributing factors are relevant for the ageing decline of skeletal muscles, at present, only exercise is proposed as a valuable preventive measure. Muscle training results in significant functional benefit also in the aged muscle, but the mechanisms of this protection are not fully understood (Close et al. 2005).

3.5 Vaginal Delivery and Neuromuscular Injury

Muscle activity is so dependent on neural control that denervated muscle (disconnected from its "lower motor neuron") not only stops contracting, but eventually atrophies and turns into fibrotic tissue. Partial lesions result in weakness. However, due to additional sensory lesions, the functional consequences seen in individuals may be more complex. Severe and clinically obvious PFM denervation can result from trauma or disease, but is relatively uncommon (if compared to the more "trauma exposed" limb muscles). Thus, clinically obvious PFM denervation results from sacral plexus/nerve lesions, which are – in this degree – an uncommon complication of vaginal delivery (Ismael et al. 2000). Interestingly, it seems that obvious – at least obvious to imaging methods – mechanical lesions to PFM are a more common sequel of vaginal delivery (Dietz and Lanzarone 2005).

Disconnection of the normally innervated muscle from "upper motor neuron" control disrupts integration of the particular muscle into "suprasegmentally" controlled activity patterns, which are paramount for the appropriate "function" of the muscle. This can result in weakness, change in muscle tone and particularly in disrupted co-ordination of the particular muscle within complex body actions/functions. The "central" motor control of PFM is not infrequently affected in neurological disease or trauma involving the spinal cord, brainstem and brain, but it cannot be a sequel of vaginal delivery. Any disco-ordination of PFM neural control after vaginal delivery would have to be explained by deranged afferent input (sensory denervation) or a change in the "peripheral conditions" of muscle (possibly mechanical injury).

The concept that relatively minor (partial) denervation of sphincter and PF muscles occurring at the time of vaginal delivery is central to discussions of the pathogenesis of several idiopathic sacral dysfunctions (particularly stress urinary and faecal incontinence and prolapse). Indeed, many studies using a variety of techniques have demonstrated both neurogenic and structural damage to PFM and sphincter muscles after vaginal delivery (cf. Vodušek 2002b). Muscle weakness has also been shown (Verelst and Leivseth 2004). In an animal model, the degree and duration of pressure and stretching during vaginal delivery can exceed thresholds for nerve and muscle damage (Lin et al. 1998). Older clinical neurophysiological studies (Allen et al. 1990) were confirmed by modern computer-assisted quantified EMG analysis; some abnormalities can be found also in the anal sphincter (Podnar et al. 2000) and PFM (Weidner et al. 2000). (It is a common experience that EMG changes after vaginal delivery are more pronounced in the urethral sphincter.) The concept of partial denervation due to the trauma of vaginal childbirth was supported by demonstration of neurogenic histomorphological changes (muscle -type grouping) in pelvic muscles (Kölbl et al. 1989; Gilpin et al. 1989; Dixon et al. 1994). However, others have not been able to find neurogenic histomorphological changes in PFM (Heit et al. 1996; Dimpfl et al. 1998). Nevertheless, there is a wide consensus on the aetiological significance of denervation injury induced by vaginal delivery inducing impairment of sphincter mechanisms and pelvic organ support, but considering also other possible (co-)factors (Bump and Cundiff 2000; Chaliha and Stanton 2000). Particularly interesting is the fact that mechanical lesions to PFM are common sequelae of vaginal delivery (DeLancey et al. 2003; Dietz and Lanzarone 2005). One of the important pathogenic mechanisms for this injury seems to be muscle stretch (Lien et al. 2004). It is interesting to note that tissue stretch was also invoked as the probable mechanism for nerve damage in combination with nerve compression. The relationship between the mechanical muscle injury and muscle denervation might be manifold. The stretch injury per se might induce a lesion both for muscle fibres and for intramuscular nerve endings; the mechanical and denervation injury may coexist and mutually exacerbate the ensuing functional disturbance;

the mechanical injury – although not accompanied by a significant denervation – might induce secondary dysfunction of neural control of the lesioned muscle, which has lost the normal mechanical properties and does not provide the adequate proprioceptive feedback to the central nervous system, not to mention the possibility that the pubovisceral muscle is mechanically injured, while the urethral sphincter (for instance) is denervated, leaving the woman with no spare continence mechanism. Indeed, the histomorphological study of Jundt et al. (2005) points to myopathic (and not neuropathic!) changes in the pubococcygeus muscles, increasing with age and parity, probably reflecting mechanical stress to the muscle itself. Studies paying attention to the different possible pathogenic factors in the same subject, keeping in mind that several muscle groups need to be studied concomitantly, have yet to be performed.

The neurogenic damage caused by vaginal delivery is acknowledged to be, to a large extent, repaired by regenerative processes, but may then recur in the long run (Snooks et al. 1990). Repetitive straining at stool due to constipation has been the main implicated pathogenic mechanism for such chronic progression of the neuromuscular lesion. Indeed, prolongation of PNTML has been demonstrated after 1 min of hard straining (Engel and Kamm 1994). Cumulative damage to the pudendal nerve may occur in severe chronic constipation, although our study in patients with mild chronic constipation failed to reveal anal sphincter abnormalities, as compared to non-constipated controls (Podnar and Vodušek 2000).

Physiologically, the relative importance of "simple" muscle weakness after (partial) denervation on one hand and the derangement of neural control (presenting as absence of appropriate, timely and co-ordinated muscle activation) on the other hand is unknown. Several aspects of "normal" pelvic floor muscle behaviour" in nulliparous continent women have already been described by kinesiological EMG (Deindl et al. 1993) and both by kinesiological EMG and ultrasound (Peschers et al. 2001). The latter study has shown that normal pelvic floor muscles stabilise the vesical neck and do not fatigue easily. Changes in muscular behaviour may originate from minor and repairable neuromuscular pelvic floor injury. With respect to muscle activation patterns, parous women with stress urinary incontinence are subjective to a number of possible changes, such as significant reduction of duration of motor unit recruitment, unilateral recruitment of reflex response in the pubococcygeal muscle and paradoxical inhibition of continuous firing of motor units in pelvic floor muscle activation on coughing (Deindl et al. 1994). The reasons for such persisting abnormalities are not clear and are difficult to explain by muscle denervation (which has been amply studied) alone. Although not proven in studies, it is reasonable to assume that motor denervation is accompanied also by sensory denervation of PFM. Structural lesions of PFM may contribute to disturbances of muscle activation patterns through failure of adequate proprioception feedback to muscle contraction.

3.6 Conclusion

PFMs are a deep-lying muscle group controlled by several integrated neural networks, akin to axial muscles, and under neural control of the emotional motor system. On the one hand, primarily the neural control allows for their co-ordinated activity in sacral functions and supports their as yet not fully clarified postural role. On the other hand, their voluntary control is possibly even more flimsy than for primarily postural muscles. The neural control of PFM "supporting function" may also be less robust due to the fact that upright stance is relatively recent philogenetically. Furthermore, there are fewer and less diversified sensory data contributing to the subject's awareness of her PFM, thus making it more difficult for her to compensate "automatically" partial loss of function.

Vaginal delivery – as the hopefully normal activity for the majority of females also in the human species – may lead to structural (myogenic, and neurogenic) changes in PF and striated sphincter muscles, but also to a secondary disruption of their activation patterns.

PF and sphincter muscles undergo age-related morphological changes that are reflected in a gradual loss of their function. It is at this point not clear to what extent these are different from changes in other striated muscles. Taken together, the non-robust/substandard neural control, the muscle changes due to wear, possible childbirth trauma and ageing may result in some loss of function, also reflected in the context of lower urinary tract, anorectal and possibly even sexual dysfunction. Muscle training is, at present, the only commonly accepted preventive measure to counteract the changes due to ageing.

Insofar as neural control is the primum movens of PFM, and is to some extent modifiable, focussing on improving dysfunctional neural control should be an advantageous target for conservative treatment of any sacral (pelvic organ) disorder that could be connected to PFM dysfunction.

References

Allen R, Hosker G, Smith A et al (1990) Pelvic floor damage and childbirth: a neurophysiological study. Brit J Obstet Gynaecol 97:770–779

Aukee P, Penttinen J, Airaksinen O (2003) The effect of aging on the electromyographic activity of pelvic floor muscles. A comparative study among stress incontinent patients and asymptomatic women. Maturitas 44:253–257

Bannister LH (ed) (1995) Gray's anatomy. The anatomical basis of medicine and surgery. 38th edn. Churchill Livingstone, New York, London

Barber MD, Bremer RE, Thor KB et al (2002) Innervation of the female levator ani muscles. Am J Obstet Gynecol 187:64–71

Bartolo DCC, Macdonald ADH (2002) Fecal continence and defecation. In: Pemberton JH, Swash M, Henry MM (eds) The pelvic floor. Its function and disorders. WB Saunders, London, pp 77–83

Blok BFM, Sturms LM, Holstege G (1997) A PET study on cortical and subcortical control of pelvic floor musculature in women. J Comp Neurol 389:535–544

Borghi F, Di Molfetta L, Garavoglia M et al (1991) Questions about the uncertain presence of muscle spindles in the human external anal sphincter. Panminerva Med 33:170–172

Brostrom S (2003) Motor evoked potentials from the pelvic floor. Neurourol Urodyn 22:620–637

Brunner F, Schmid A, Sheikhzadeh A et al (2007) Effects of aging on type II muscle fibers: A systematic review of the literature. J Aging Phys Activity 15:336–348

Bump RC, Cundiff GW (2000) Pelvic organ prolapse. In: Stanton SL, Monga AK (eds) Clinical urogynaecology, 2nd edn. Churchill Livingstone, London, pp 357-372

Campbell MJ, McComas AJ, Petito F (1973) Physiological changes in ageing muscles. J Neurol Neurosurg Psychiatr 36:174–182

Carlile A, Davies I, Rigby A et al (1988) Age changes in the human female urethra: a morphometric study. J Urol 139:532–535

Chaliha C, Stanton SL (2000) Urethral sphincter incompetence. In: Stanton SL, Monga AK (eds) Clinical urogynaecology, 2nd edn. Churchill Livingstone, London, pp 201–217

Chantraine A (1973) Examination of the anal and urethral sphincters. In: Desmedt JE (ed) New developments in electromyography and clinical neurophysiology, vol 2. Karger, Basel, pp 421–432

Close GL, Kayani A, Vasilaki A et al (2005) Skeletal muscle damage with exercise and aging. Sport Med 35:413–427

Critchley HOD, Dixon JS, Gosling JA (1980) Comparative study of the periurethral and perineal parts of the human levator ani muscle. Urol Int 35:226–232

de Groat WC, Fraser MO, Yoshiyama M et al (2001) Neural control of the urethra. Scand J Urol Nephrol Suppl 35–43, discussion:106–125

Deindl FM, Vodušek DB, Hesse U et al (1993) Activity patterns of pubococcygeal muscles in nulliparous continent women. Br J Urol 72:46–51

Deindl FM, Vodušek DB, Hesse U et al (1994) Pelvic floor activity patterns: comparison of nulliparous continent and parous urinary stress incontinent women. A kinesiological EMG study. Br J Urol 73:413–417

DeLancey JO, Kearney R, Chou Q et al (2003) The appearance of levator ani muscle abnormalities in magnetic resonance images after vaginal delivery. Obstetr Gynecol 101:46–53

Deletis V, Vodušek DB, Abbott R et al (1992) Intraoperative monitoring of dorsal sacral roots: minimizing the risk of iatrogrenic micturition disorders. Neurosurgery 30:72–75

Dietz HP, Lanzarone V (2005) Levator trauma after vaginal delivery. Obstet Gynecol 106:707–712

Dimpfl Th, Jaeger Ch, Mueller-Felber W et al (1998) Myogenic changes of the levator ani muscle in premenopausal women: the impact of vaginal delivery and age. Neurourol Urodynam 17:197–205

Dixon JS, Gosling JA (1994) Histomorphology of the pelvic floor muscle. In: Schüssler B, Laycock J, Norton P, Stanton SL (eds) Pelvic floor re-education: Principles and practice. Springer, Berlin, Heidelberg, New York, pp 28–33

Engel AF, Kamm MA (1994) The acute effect of straining on pelvic floor neurological function. Int J Colorect Dis 9:8–12

Faulkner JA, Larkin LM, Claflin DR et al (2007) Age-related changes in the structure and function of skeletal muscles. Clin Exp Pharmacol Physiol 34:1091–1096

Fiatarone MA, Marks EC, Ryan ND et al (1990) High-intensity strength training in nonagenarians. JAMA 263:3029–3034

Fox JC, Fletcher JG, Zinsmeister AR et al (2006) Effect of aging on anorectal and pelvic floor functions in females. Dis Colon Rectum 49:1726–1735

Fucini C, Ronchi O, Elbetti C (2001) Electromyography of the pelvic floor musculature in the assessment of obstructed defecation symptoms. Dis Colon Rectum 44:1168–1175

Gilpin SA, Gosling JA, Smith AR et al (1989) The pathogenesis of genitourinary prolapse and stress incontinence of urine. A histological and histochemical study. Br J Obstet Gynaecol 96:15–23

Grimby G, Saltin B (1983) The ageing muscle. Clin Phys 3:209–218

Gunnarsson M, Ahlmann S, Lindström S et al (1999) Cortical magnetic stimulation in patients with genuine stress incontinence: Correlation with results of pelvic floor exercises. Neurourol Urodynam 18:437–445

Heit M, Benson JT, Russell B et al (1996) Levator ani muscle in women with genitourinary prolapse: Indirect assessment by muscle histopathology. Neurourol Urodynam 15:17–29

Hodges PW, Spasford R, Pengel LHM (2007) Postural and respiratory functions of the pelvic floor muscles. Neurourol Urodyn 26:362–371
Holstege G (1998) The emotional motor system in relation to the supraspinal control of micturition and mating behavior. Behav Brain Res 92:103–109
Huang JC, Deletis V, Vodušek DB et al (1997) Preservation of pudendal afferents in sacral rhizotomies. Neurosurgery 41:411–415
Ismael SS, Amarenco G, Bayle B et al (2000) Postpartum lumbosacral plexopathy limited to autonomic and perineal manifestations:clinical and electrophysiological study of 19 patients. J Neurol Neurosurg Psychiatry 68:771–773
Jundt K, Kiening M, Fischer P et al (2005) Is the histomorphological concept of the female pelvic floor and its changes due to age and vaginal delivery correct? Uroneurol Urodyn 24:44–50
Kenton K, Brubaker L (2002) Relationship between levator ani contraction and motor unit activation in the urethral sphincter. Am J Obstet Gynecol 187:403–440
Kölbl H, Strasseger H, Riss P, Gruber H (1989) Morphologic and functional aspects of pelvic floor muscle in patients with pelvic relaxation and genuine stress incontinence. Obstet Gynecol 74:789–795
Lexell J, Downham D, Sjöström M (1986) Distribution of different types in human skeletal muscles. Type arrangement in m. vastus lateralis from three groups of healthy men between 15 and 83 years. J Neurol Sci 72:211–222
Lien KC, Mooney B, DeLancey JO et al (2004) Levator ani muscle stretch induced by simulated vaginal birth. Obstet Gynecol 103:31–40
Lierse W, Holschneider AM, Steinfeld J (1993) The relative proportions of type I and type II muscle fibers in the external sphincter ani muscle at different ages and stages of development–observations on the development of continence. Eur J Ped Surg 3:28–32
Lin AS, Carrier S, Morgan DM et al (1998) Effect of simulated birth trauma on the urinary continence mechanism in the rat. Urology 52:143–151
Mannen T, Iwata M, Toyokura Y et al (1982) The Onuf's nucleus and the external anal sphincter muscles in amyotrophic lateral sclerosis and Shy-Drager syndrome. Acta Neuropathol (Berlin) 58:255–260
Marani E, Pijl ME, Kraan MC et al (1993) Interconnections of the upper ventral rami of the human sacral plexus: a reappraisal for dorsal rhizotomy in neurostimulation operations. Neurourol Urodyn 12:585–598
Miller JM, Ashton-Miller JA, DeLancey JO (1998) A pelvic muscle precontraction can reduce cough-related urine loss in selected women with mild SUI. J Am Geriatr Soc 46:870–874
Perucchini D, DeLancey JOL, Ashton-Miller JA et al (2002a) Age effects on urethral striated muscle. Am J Obstet Gynecol 186:356–360
Perucchini D, DeLancey JOL, Ashton-Miller JA et al (2002b) Age effects on urethral striated muscle. I. Changes in number and diameter of striated muscle fibers in the ventral urethra. Am J Obstet Gynecol 186:351–355
Peschers UM, Fanger G, Schaer GN et al (2001) Bladder neck mobility in continent nulliparous women. Brit J Obstet Gynaecol 108:320–324
Petersen I, Franksson C, Danielson CO (1955) Electromyographic study of the muscles of the pelvic floor and urethra in normal females. Acta Obstet Gynecol Scand 34:273–285
Pierce LM, Baumann S, Rankin MR et al (2007) Levator ani muscle and connective tissue associated with pelvic organ prolapse, parity, and aging in the squirrel monkey: a histologic study. Am J Obstet Gynecol 197:60.e1–9
Pierce LM, Reyes M, Thor KB et al (2005) Immunohistochemical evidence for the interaction between levator ani and pudendal neurons in the coordination of pelvic floor and visceral activity in the squirrel monkey. Am J Obstet Gynecol 192:1506–1515
Podnar S, Vodušek DB (2000) Standardization of anal sphincter electromyography: effect of chronic constipation. Muscle Nerve 23:1748–1751
Podnar S, Lukanovi A, Vodušek DB (2000) Anal sphincter electromyography after vaginal delivery: Neuropathic insufficiency or normal wear and tear? Neurourol Urodynam 19:249–257
Pool-Goudzwaard A, van Dijke GH, van Gurp M et al (2004) Contribution of pelvic floor muscles to stiffnes of the pelvic ring. Clin Biomech (Bristol, Avon) 19:564–571
Read NW (1990) Functional assessment of the anorectum in faecal incontinence. Neurobiology of incontinence (Ciba Foundation Symposium 151). John Wiley, Chichester, New York, Brisbane, Toronto, Singapore, pp 119–138
Rociu E, Stoker J, Eijkemans MJC et al (2000) Normal anal sphincter anatomy and age- and sex-related variations at high-spatial-resolution endoanal MR imaging. Radiology 217:395–401
Rodriguez Trowbridge E, Wei JT, Fenner DE et al (2007) Effects of aging on lower urinary tract and pelvic floor function in nulliparous women. Obstet Gynecol 109:715–720
Ryhammer AM, Laurberg S, Sørensen FH (1997) Effects of age on anal function in normal women. Int J Colorect Dis 12:225–229
Sato A, Sato Y, Schmidt RF (2000) Reflex bladder activity induced by electrical stimulation of hind limb somatic afferents in the cat. J Auton Nerv Syst 1:229–241
Schroder HD (1985) Anatomical and pathoanatomical studies on the spinal efferent systems innervating pelvic structures. 1. Organization of spinal nuclei in animals. 2. The nucleus X-pelvic motor system in man. J Auton Nerv Syst 14:23–48
Smith AR, Hosker GL, Warrell DW (1989) The role of partial denervation of the pelvic floor in the aetiology of genitourinary prolapse and stress incontinence of urine. Brit J Obstet Gynaecol 96:24–28
Snooks SJ, Swash M, Mathers SE et al (1990) Effect of vaginal delivery in the pelvic floor: a 5-year follow-up. Br J Surg 77:1358–1360
Sundin T, Petersen I (1975) Cystometry and simultaneous electomyography from the striated uretheral and anal sphincters and from levator ani. Invest Urol 13:40–46
Tomlinson BE, Irving D (1977) The numbers of limb motor neurons in the human lumbosacral cord throughout life. J Neurol Sci 34:213–219
Torrens M, Morrison JFB (eds) (1987) The physiology of the lower urinary tract. Springer, London
Trontelj JV, Vodušek DB, Zidar J (1979) Neurogenic changes in short toe extensor in healthy young subjects. Zdrav Vestn 48:691–693
Ueyama T, Mizuno N, Nomura S et al (1984) Central distribution of afferent and efferent components of the pudendal nerve in cat. J Comp Neurol 222:38–46

Verelst M, Leivseth G (2004) Are fatigue and disturbances in pre-programmed activity of pelvic floor muscles associated with female stress urinary incontinence? Neurourol Urodyn 23:143–147
Vodušek DB (1982) Neurophysiological study of sacral reflexes in man (in Slovene). Institute of Clinical Neurophysiology. University E Kardelj in Ljubljana, pp 1–55
Vodušek DB (1994) Electrophysiology. In: Schuessler B, Laycock J, Norton P, Stanton S (eds) Pelvic floor re-education, principles and practice. Springer, London, pp 83–97
Vodušek DB (1996) Evoked potential testing. Urol Clin North Am 23:427–446
Vodušek DB (2002a) Sacral reflexes. In: Pemberton JH, Swash M, Henry MM (eds) Pelvic floor. Its functions and disorders. Saunders, London, pp 237–247
Vodušek DB (2002b) The role of electrophysiology in the evaluation of incontinence and prolapse. Curr Opin Obstet Gynecol 14:509–514
Vodušek DB, Janko M (1990) The bulbocavernosus reflex. A single motor neuron study. Brain 113 (Pt 3):813–820
Wallner C, Maas CP, Dabhoiwala NF et al (2006) Innervation of the pelvic floor muscles. A reappraisal for the levator ani nerve. Obstet Gynecol 108:529–534
Weidner AC, Barber MD, Visco AG et al (2000) Pelvic muscle electromyography of levator ani and external anal sphincter in nulliparous women and women with pelvic floor dysfunction. Am J Obstet Gynecol 183:1390–1401
Wietek BM, Hinninghofen H, Jehle EC et al (2007) Asymmetric sphincter innervation is associated with fecal incontinence after anal sphincter trauma during childbirth. Neurourol Urodynam 26:134–139

Imaging Techniques

4

4.1 Evacuation Proctography and Dynamic Cystoproctography

Stuart A. Taylor and Steve Halligan

CONTENTS

4.1.1 Evacuation Proctography

4.1.1.1 Introduction

Evacuation proctography is a simple radiological technique that images rectal voiding of a barium paste enema. Evacuating proctography serves two main purposes: It images rectal configuration throughout all phases of rectal evacuation and also provides an assessment of whether voiding is normal or difficult (which usually means prolonged). Thus, evacuation proctography provides both morphological and functional information.

Radiological studies of rectal evacuation have been performed for over 50 years (Wallden 1952), but it was the description in 1984 of a relatively simple technique along with parameters for interpretation that was the impetus for more general acceptance (Mahieu et al. 1984). Evacuation proctography is now widely disseminated, even though it remains predominantly confined to specialist centres. Although requested most by coloproctological surgeons, proctography is also useful to both urogynaecologists and gastroenterologists. Difficult rectal evacuation is by far the most common clinical indication for referral. The examination is frequently termed "defecography", and other terms are also occasionally used: videoproctography, cinedefecography, and dynamic rectal examination. Whatever the terminology, it should be remembered that the findings are based on voluntary rectal evacuation of a paste and not physiologic defecation of stool. The latter is accompanied by colonic contraction and complex coordination of anorectal reflexes, many of which are absent during proctographic examination. Because of this, the authors believe that terminology that implies physiologic defecation is best avoided.

4.1.1.2 Technique

There are possibly as many different techniques adopted as there are practitioners (Finlay 1988). Opinions differ as to the type of contrast used, its consistency, the volume instilled, imaging modality, manoeuvres taken, and the images acquired.

S. A. Taylor, MD, FRCR, MRCP
S. Halligan, MD, FRCR, MRCP
Department of Specialist Radiology, University College Hospital, 235 Euston Road, London, NW1 2BU, UK

Furthermore, the basic technique may be modified so that other pelvic organs are imaged at the same sitting, the ultimate expression of which is dynamic cystoproctography (see Sect. 4.1.2). The purpose of this section is to describe the basic proctographic technique, which the author feels should be as rapid and simple as possible.

Assessment of evacuation rate and completeness is an essential part of the examination, and very possibly the most important part (Halligan et al. 1995a). Because of this, the author prefers the rectum to be emptied before proctography, simply achieved in most subjects by inserting two glycerine suppositories and asking the patient to visit the lavatory after having retained these for approximately 20 min. Alternatively, an enema may be administered. The same volume of contrast (the authors use 120 cc) can then be used in all patients so that meaningful comparison of the rate and completeness of rectal evacuation can be made with established values derived from normal subjects (Kamm et al. 1989). Furthermore, a consistent standardised technique means that follow-up studies are comparable when clinically necessary, and comparisons between patients are possible for research. Alternatively, some investigators omit rectal emptying and instil contrast until an urge to evacuate is elicited. It has been suggested that this approach is more physiological, but, for the reasons described above, the entire examination is unphysiological irrespective of the technique used. Furthermore, an initially empty rectum is more acceptable to staff for obvious reasons; stool is not voided. It is also possible that stool may inhibit some findings, such as intussusception.

It is generally accepted that contrast consistency should be approximately the same as faeces. Mahieu et al. (1984) used barium suspension mixed with potato starch. Others have used methylcellulose, and preparations specifically designed for the purpose are now commercially available. However, there is good evidence that the consistency of the contrast used is largely irrelevant (Ickenberry et al. 1996), which is in accord with physiological studies of constipated patients that suggest evacuation is disordered regardless of the consistency of rectal content. Interestingly, large stools are actually easier to pass than small ones (Bannister et al. 1987).

The paste is administered with the patient in the left-lateral position on the fluoroscopy table. A simple approach is to fill two plastic bladder syringes (which have a wide-tipped nozzle) with 60 cc of contrast each and then to syringe the contrast directly into the rectum after lubricating the syringe tip. If the paste is very viscous, then a caulking gun can be used instead of a simple hand injection. The syringe is withdrawn towards the end of injection in order to mark the anal canal and verge.

The patient then steps off the table, which is then it is brought upright, and a commode placed on the footrest. Commercial commodes are available, although it is a simple task to build one. The commode should be comfortable, and the seat should be relatively radiolucent. Perspex or wood is commonly used. The commode also needs to be able to support a disposable plastic bag to collect voided material and must also incorporate some filtration underneath the seat to balance radiographic exposure and prevent screen flare, 4 mm of copper plate, for example (Fig. 4.1.1). Others have used water-filled rubber rings or a Perspex sheet. Some commodes incorporate a radiographic ruler for precise measurements when felt clinically necessary. Although the more sensitive seated position is preferable, proctography can be performed in the left-lateral position if a commode is unavailable or if the patient is incontinent

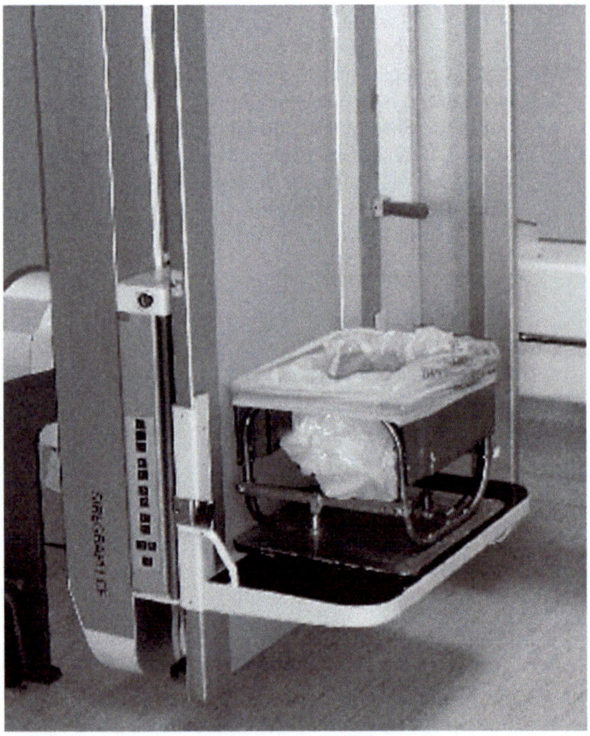

Fig. 4.1.1. The proctography commode placed on the footrest of the upright fluoroscopy table. Note the copper sheet immediately subadjacent to the seat, in order to balance radiographic contrast

(Poon et al. 1991), but it should be borne in mind that static values for pelvic floor position are higher (Jorge et al. 1994a). It may be helpful to shield the patient behind a portable screen, especially if the radiographic unit is remotely controlled, so that some privacy is afforded and embarrassment potentially avoided.

It is essential to obtain continuous or rapid recording of rectal evacuation, either by spot filming, cineradiography or videofluoroscopy. Although spot filming provides the best spatial resolution, the facility to replay the entire examination at any speed is an invaluable feature of video; this is also possible with modern digital systems, which also convey the lowest dose. Radiation dose has been a major and persistent concern, not least because many patients are young women in their childbearing years. However, because high spatial resolution is not a prerequisite for proctography, low-dose digital algorithms and added filtration may be applied without any significant diagnostic penalty (Hare et al. 2001). Intermittent imaging should also be employed to reduce the dose in patients whose evacuation is prolonged; there is no benefit to having multiple, identical images.

4.1.1.3 Normal Findings

Based on the findings in 56 asymptomatic patients, Mahieu defined five criteria for a normal examination: increased anorectal angulation, obliteration of the puborectal muscle impression, wide anal canal opening, total evacuation of contrast, and normal pelvic floor resistance (Mahieu et al. 1984). Several subsequent studies of asymptomatic volunteers have revealed a wide range of normal values, including some overlap with pathology, but the general consensus of what is normal agrees broadly with Mahieu's original description. There have been several studies of asymptomatic volunteers following Mahieu's description, with varying degrees of selection bias, sometimes unavoidable because of perceived problems with radiation dose. Others have even defined normality retrospectively in constipated patients who have a 'normal' proctogram, which is completely inappropriate. Probably the best study is by Shorvon and co-workers (1989) who examined 47 asymptomatic volunteers, most of whom were under 30 years old. Any proctographic examination can be considered in three stages: pre-evacuation, evacuation, and post-evacuation.

4.1.1.3.1 Pre-Evacuation

The patient should be initially imaged in the lateral position, which provides most information about anorectal configuration and pelvic floor position, and from which it is easiest to assess the degree of rectal emptying; a single lateral image at rest will suffice (Fig. 4.1.2a). The funnelled junction between the rectal ampulla and anal canal, the anorectal junction, is easy to appreciate at rest and for practical purposes defines the anatomical level of the posterior pelvic floor. The pubococcygeal line a line drawn between the inferior border of the symphysis pubis and the sacro-coccygeal junction, is generally believed to indicate the usual position of the pelvic floor. However, these bony landmarks may be difficult to identify with a limited field of view, and the inferior surface of the ischial tuberosities is often used instead. An even simpler approach is to use the top of the commode seat as a rough and ready estimate of pelvic floor position. The anorectal junction should be at or just above this plane: 0.4 cm above this level for women and 1.6 cm in men (Shorvon et al. 1989). The canal should also be tightly closed without any contrast leakage at rest.

The anorectal angle (ARA) is the angle subtended between the anal canal axis and the posterior aspect of the distal rectal ampulla. An alternative measurement uses the central rectal axis rather than the posterior rectal wall. The ARA is formed in part by the puborectalis muscle, which slings behind the anorectal junction and is thought to be important in maintaining continence because of the resultant acute angle formed between the rectal and anal axis, the 'flap-valve' theory of anal continence (Bartolo et al. 1986). Indeed, incontinent patients often have an obtuse ARA, and post-anal repair, an operation once commonly used to treat incontinence, aims to restore the ARA. However, although considerable attention has been devoted to this measurement, there is little practical evidence that it is worthwhile (especially since anal endosonography has superseded proctography as the radiological investigation of choice in incontinent patients); most investigators have abandoned it, not least because the normal range of values is very wide and there is considerable overlap with symptomatic patients (Shorvon et al. 1989). Nevertheless, as a broad guide the ARA should be approximately 90° at rest.

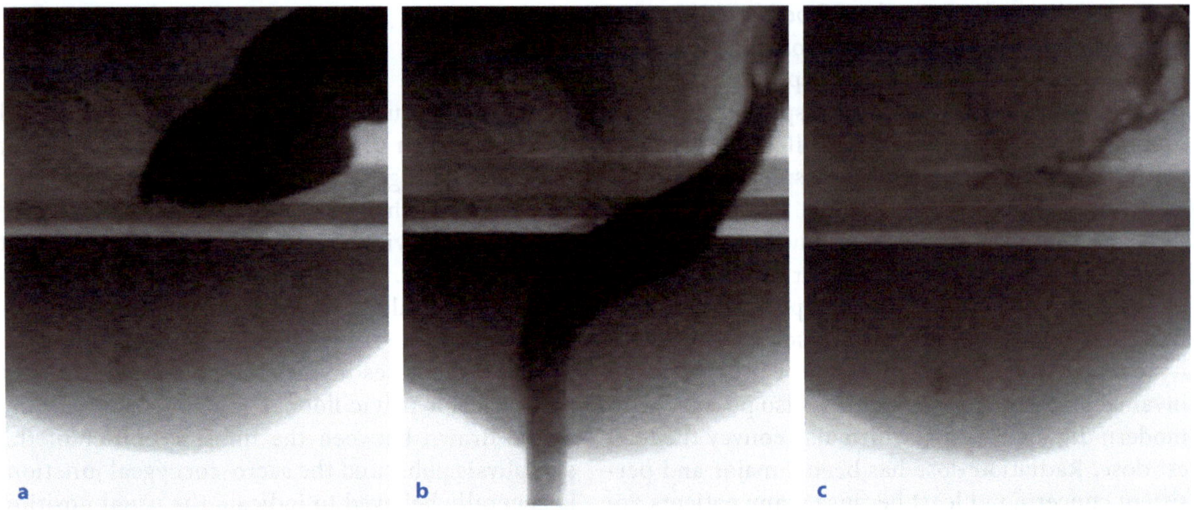

a b c

Fig. 4.1.2a–c. Normal evacuating proctogram. Asymptomatic volunteer. a Pre-evacuation phase. Resting rectal position and configuration are normal. The anal canal is tightly closed, and the anorectal junction is approximately at the level of the seat top. b Evacuation phase. The anorectal junction has descended, the anal canal has opened widely, and the anorectal angle has become more obtuse. The rectum empties smoothly and completely within 30 s. c Post-evacuation phase. The rectum is empty, the anal canal closed, and the anorectal junction has returned to its pre-evacuation position

Before rectal evacuation is attempted, many investigators advocate additional manoeuvres such as "squeeze" views to evaluate the strength of voluntary pelvic floor musculature, "cough" views to stress the continence mechanism, and "strain" views to assess pelvic floor descent. Although these seem reasonable things to do in the first instance, in practical terms there is little evidence that they discriminate enough between patients to be clinically useful. Ultimately, the authors believe that such manoeuvres merely add to procedural complexity. It is interesting to note that the ARA may paradoxically increase during strain manoeuvres in up to 30 per cent of normal subjects, reflecting pelvic floor contraction secondary to a desire to remain continent (Kelvin et al. 1994).

Lastly, when centring the pre-evacuation image it is important to allow for pelvic floor descent during subsequent evacuation. This may be considerable and can result in the rectum being displaced out of the radiographic field of view.

4.1.1.3.2 Evacuation

After the initial lateral resting view has been obtained, the patient is asked to evacuate their rectum as rapidly and completely as possible. In normal volunteers, evacuation is generally initiated quickly, and a substantial delay is positively associated with pelvic in-coordination and indicates functional disorder (Halligan et al. 1995a). Embarrassment may also cause delay. On evacuation the anorectal junction should descend in response to raised intraabdominal pressure; failure to descend represents inadequate effort, which may also be a sign of functional disorder (Halligan et al. 1995b). Once initiated, evacuation is rapid and complete in normal individuals; asymptomatic volunteers are able to void the majority of a 120-cc contrast enema within 30 s (Kamm et al. 1989). Prolonged evacuation usually indicates a functional abnormality and is occasionally associated with repetitive jerky pelvic floor movements. Pelvic floor descent (represented by inferior movement of the anorectal junction) should normally be no more than approximately 3.0 cm. The puborectal impression should flatten, and the ARA should become more obtuse. The anal canal should shorten and widen to allow evacuation (Fig. 4.1.2b). Generally, the rectal ampulla should empty smoothly and symmetrically, rather like a tube of toothpaste, although a wide variety of configurations are possible in normal individuals (Shorvon et al. 1989). Patients who need to use digital manoeuvres to aid rectal emptying, such as applying vaginal or posterior perineal pressure, should be instructed to do so, so that their effect may be evaluated.

4.1.1.3.3
Post-Evacuation

The examination generally finishes once evacuation is complete, or when it is clear that little or no evacuation is likely. After evacuation the anal canal closes, and the anorectal junction should ascend, returning to its pre-evacuation resting position (Fig. 4.1.2c). The ARA should also return to its pre-evacuation configuration. The rectum should be empty or nearly so. Occasionally, when the evacuation phase has raised the possibility of intussusception predominantly within the coronal plane (the rectal valves of Houston are best seen in this plane, for example), it may be worthwhile examining this further with the patient in the frontal position, which is also the best position to evaluate perineal hernias. The commode is simply turned around on the footrest and the subject asked to strain during fluoroscopy; there is usually enough residual barium to render the fold configuration visible (McGee and Bartram 1993). After the examination the collection bag can be simply lifted from the commode and disposed of, and the patient can visit the lavatory in order to void any residual barium and clean him or herself. The entire room time for the examination should be approximately 5 min or even less. The authors believe that evacuation proctography should be a rapid and simple technique, requiring much less effort from the staff and patient than a barium enema, for example.

4.1.1.3.4
Additional Manoeuvres

Extension of the basic technique of evacuation proctography is discussed below in Section 4.2, but, as a routine, the authors administer 100 cc oral barium suspension (100% weight/volume) diluted with 200 ml of water to which 10 ml of Gastrografin has been added. This is administered 30 min before proctography in order to facilitate diagnosis of enterocoeles. An alternative but less sensitive approach is to use a contrast-soaked gauze swab placed at the vaginal apex, or vaginal contrast gel; enterocoeles are then revealed by significant rectovaginal separation. However, tampons should not be used because of their propensity to splint the vagina and thus inhibit enterocoele formation (Archer et al. 1992).

4.1.1.3.5
Radiological Report

The radiological report should comment on rectal configuration at rest, the degree of pelvic floor descent during evacuation, the rate and completeness of evacuation, and the presence of any associated structural abnormality, such as a rectocoele, enterocoele, etc. In day-to-day clinical practice, formal measurement of various angles and distances is not required; an understanding of what is broadly normal and abnormal will suffice and will come with experience.

4.1.1.4
Alternative Approaches

It is worth noting that evacuation proctography can be performed using scintigraphic methods (Hutchinson et al. 1993). Although spatial resolution is relatively poor, impairing diagnosis of intussusception, for example, the technique provides very accurate assessments of the rate and degree of rectal emptying compared to conventional fluoroscopic methods, and radiation dose may be less than with some conventional systems. Recognising that the ability to evacuate is more important than the rectal configuration adopted to do so, some authors have employed a radioopaque rectal balloon instead of contrast (Preston et al. 1984), although such an approach will not reliably diagnose many structural abnormalities. Indeed, it has frequently been argued that the imaging component of the examination can be dispensed with altogether and a balloon (Barnes and Lennard-Jones 1985) or fluid used instead (Alstrup et al. 1997). Again, these methods will miss many morphological abnormalities, the significance of which remains controversial. Other investigators have performed proctography following intraperitoneal water-soluble contrast medium injection (Halligan and Bartram 1995), but this has not found general acceptance, possibly because it has been superceded by MR imaging. The next section discusses in detail some of the more common modifications made, whereby the basic proctographic examination is extended to include the middle and anterior pelvic floor. Ultimately, the level of information needed by the referring physician will largely define the radiological approach used.

4.1.2 Dynamic Cystoproctography

4.1.2.1 Introduction

The technique of evacuation proctography described above allows the practitioner to obtain information about rectal dynamics and configuration during attempted evacuation of barium paste. Those patients presenting specifically with disorders of evacuation are readily assessed by the technique (Chap. 6.1), which is quick, simple, and usually well tolerated. Limitations, however, include the relative inability to provide detailed information about the anterior and middle pelvic compartments.

Pelvic organ prolapse (a general term referring to any combination of organ descent, such as bladder, rectum, uterus, and bowel) is a very common condition–it is estimated that approximately one in nine women will ultimately need surgery for prolapse or stress incontinence (Olsen et al. 1997), with up to a third requiring repeated surgery due to recurrence. Consistent predisposing factors include vaginal delivery, advancing age, and increasing body-mass index, although chronic straining, previous hysterectomy, and abnormal connective tissue are all implicated (Jelovsek et al. 2007).

It is increasingly recognised that optimal corrective surgery requires a full appreciation of the dynamics of the whole pelvic floor, rather than relying on the traditional compartmentalised approach previously favoured by coloproctologists and uro-gynaecologists. Women who develop pelvic organ prolapse often have several concurrent symptoms–in a recent review combinations of bulge symptoms, urinary incontinence, urinary urgency or frequency, and faecal incontinence were all common (Ellerkmann et al. 2001). Physical examination is relatively successful at assessing pelvic organ prolapse, and clinical grading systems are well established (Bump et al. 1996). However, imaging techniques often reveal abnormalities that remain unsuspected during physical examination (Brubaker et al. 1993), and it is this that has been the foundation of their success.

A combined global approach to therapy for pelvic floor weakness is increasingly the norm (Chap. 5.1), and those imaging techniques providing a multicompartmental overview, notably dynamic cystoproctography (DCP) and functional MRI (Chap. 4.2), are of increasing importance. DCP differs from simple evacuation proctography in that additional radio-opaque contrast is administrated to allow visualisation of those pelvic organs predisposed to abnormal descent and prolapse, notably the bladder, vagina, and large and small bowel.

4.1.2.2 Technique

DCP essentially extends the basic technique adopted for evacuation proctography to provide a more complete assessment of the pelvic floor. True DCP as described by Kelvin and colleagues (1992) involves opacification of the bladder, vagina, and small bowel, although others advocate omitting bladder opacification (due to its relative invasive nature) and opacifying only the vagina and small bowel (so-called "extended proctography").

The timing and order of contrast administration prior to DCP is dependent on the preferred technique for the examination itself. A relatively simple approach is to opacify the bladder, vagina, and rectum concurrently and then to perform a single dynamic evacuatory study just as for simple proctography. Critics of this approach suggest it ignores the widely held concept of the "crowded pelvis" in which prolapsing organs must compete for space in the relatively small bony pelvic outlet. Thus, it is postulated that a large cystocoele may for example inhibit rectocoele formation (Fig. 4.1.3), and even hide a significant enterocoele by filling the distal pelvis and blocking small bowel descent. For this reason a staged approach to the examination may be preferable as described below, so that as many co-existing abnormalities as possible may be demonstrated at one sitting (Kelvin et al. 2000).

As for evacuation proctography, a careful and considered explanation of the procedure to the patient is essential. The basic equipment and commode are as detailed above (Sect. 41.2). Around 30 min prior to the examination proper, the patient is asked to drink positive oral contrast (e.g., barium suspension) to delineate the small bowel and so facilitate diagnosis of enterocoeles. For staged DCP, bladder filling is undertaken first. Using aseptic technique, the urinary balder is catheterised and around 50 ml of iodinated contrast instilled. Large volumes are usually not required for accurate diagnosis and may actually cause problems during subsequent bladder drainage. The patient then sits on the commode and

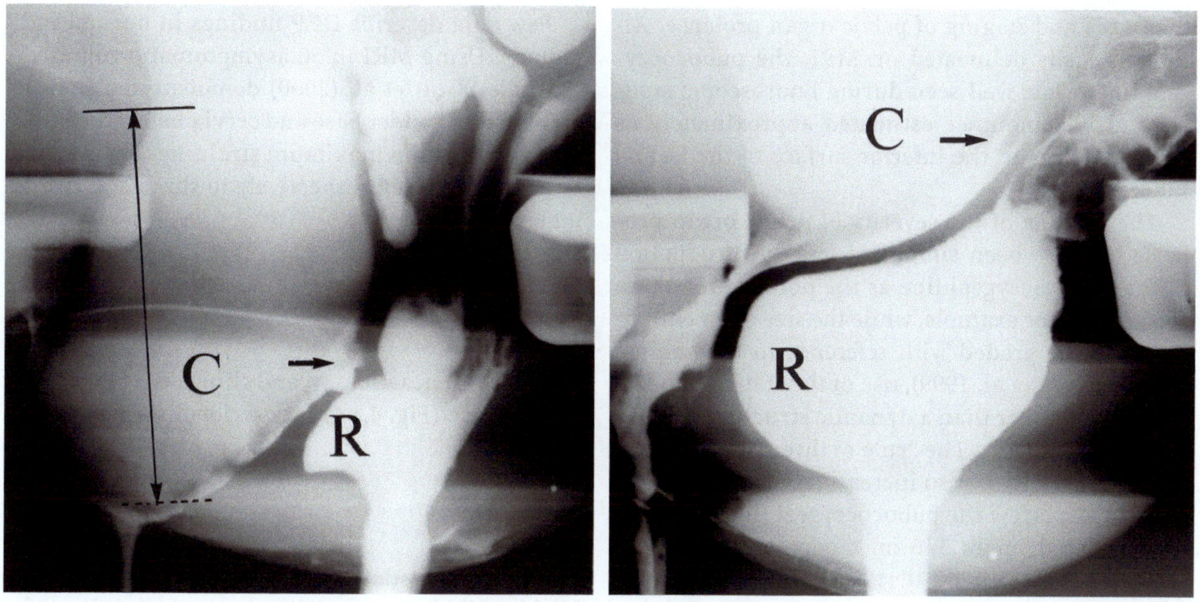

a b

Fig. 4.1.3a,b. Cystocoele minimizing size of rectocoele. **a** Cystoproctogram image taken during evacuation shows a very large cystocoele (*C*). The *uninterrupted line* represents the pubococcygeal line, the *dotted line* indicates the bladder base, and the *arrowed line* therefore indicates the depth of the cystocoele below the pubococcygeal line. There is a rectocoele (*R*), but its size is minimised by pressure from the large cystocoele. The *arrow* indicates the uppermost point of the vagina. **b** Six months later, following cystocoele repair, urethral suspension and sacrocolpopexy, the cystoproctogram was repeated. The cystocoele (*C*) is much smaller. The rectocoele (*R*) is now considerably larger as it is no longer compressed by the cystocoele. Note the elevation of the vaginal apex (*arrow*) as a result of sacrocolpopexy (reprinted with permission from Kelvin and Maglinte 1997)

resting and maximum strain images acquired to determine the presence of any cystocoele. The bladder is then drained and the catheter removed.

Opacification of the vagina is then performed via gentle syringe instillation of contrast (usually high viscosity barium). Use of a tampon is not recommended because of their propensity to splint the vagina and thus inhibit enterocoele formation (Archer et al. 1992). A small square of gauze may be placed over the introitus if contrast leaks persistently from the vagina (Ho et al. 1999). Finally, rectal opacification is achieved as described for evacuation proctography (Sect. 4.1.2).

Following organ opacification, the technique of DCP essentially mirrors that of simple evacuation proctography (Sect. 4.1.2). While some workers advocate the acquisition of resting and maximal contraction images prior to evacuation, others omit these for the reasons explained in sections above and simply acquire images of the rectal evacuatory phase. Finally, although not part of the authors' routine protocol, a strong argument can be made for allowing the patient to evacuate further in the privacy of the lavatory and then returning to the fluoroscopy suite for a final maximum straining image. Disadvantages of this final step are the additional time and staff effort required, but advantages include additional diagnostic information, for example, the unmasking of a cystocoele after rectocele emptying and the ability for the practitioner to assess if any anismus apparent during filming is actually an artefact due to embarrassment.

4.1.2.3 Normal Findings and Definition of Prolapse

Unfortunately, there is no standard adopted across all imaging modalities used in the assessment of the pelvic floor to define normality or indeed prolapse. Most workers, however, now reference dynamic pelvic floor movement to the pubococcygeal line, and this is the authors' preference. Even this line has various definitions [inferior border of the symphysis pubis to the sacro-coccygeal junction (Kelvin et al. 2000), symphysis pubis to the last coccygeal joint (Healy et al. 1997), etc.], although practically speaking such differences have little impact on the diagnosis and staging of pelvic organ prolapse. Although easily delineated on MRI, the pubococcygeal line is less well seen during fluoroscopic studies and is sometimes estimated approximately as corresponding to the inferior surface of the ischial tuberosities.

The grading of the severity of pelvic organ prolapse has also been simplified by the introduction of the pubococcygeal line as the point of reference (Fig. 4.1.3). For example, while the size of an enterocoele can be graded with reference to the vaginal apex (KELVIN et al. 1999), use of the static pubococcygeal line rather than a dynamic structure is likely to be more reliable. The "rule of threes" for grading prolapse severity is also increasingly used–prolapse of an organ below the pubococcygeal line by <3 cm is considered small, 3–6 cm moderate, and >6 cm large (LIENEMANN et al. 1997; GOH et al. 2000). However, it must be remembered that although use of a standard reference line for imaging investigations will facilitate a move toward standardisation between workers in the field, agreement with clinical grading of prolapse cannot be assumed (PANNU 2004). A line drawn through the long axis of the pubis approximates the location of the hymenal ring, the reference used for the clinical grading of prolapse, but even use of this line may not improve agreement between imaging and clinical evaluation (FAUCONNIER et al. 2007).

Few data describe DCP findings in normal individuals. Using MRI in 50 asymptomatic volunteers (25 male), GOH et al. (2000) demonstrated that descent of the bladder base and cervix below the pubococcygeal line on maximum straining was unusual, although was seen respectively in three and two females.

4.1.2.3.1 Rectocoele

The definition, aetiology, and clinical significance of a rectocoele (Fig. 4.1.4) is described in Chapter 6.1.

4.1.2.3.2 Cystocoele

A cystocoele is defined as abnormal decent of the bladder. Patients often present complaining of a feeling of anterior "fullness" or with stress incontinence. As the cystocoele progresses, patients may develop intermittent obstructed voiding, incomplete emptying, and hesitancy (JELOVSEK et al. 2007). On DCP a cystocoele is defined by descent of the bladder base (opacified by contrast) below the pubococcygeal line, although as noted above, this phenomenon may be seen in a small percentage of asymptomatic parous women. Even after emptying the bladder, a cystocoele may be inferred during the proctographic

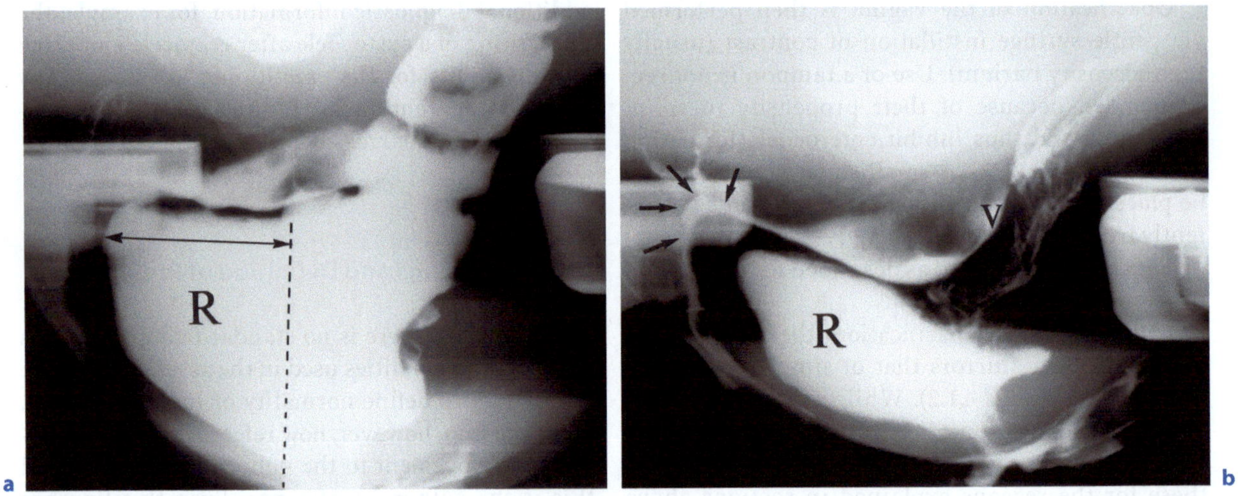

Fig. 4.1.4a,b. Large, symptomatic rectocoele. Patient with rectal discomfort and sensation of incomplete emptying after bowel movement. **a** During evacuation, a large outpouching arises from the anterior aspect of the lower rectum, indicating a large rectocoele (*R*). The depth of the rectocoele is measured by its maximal distance (*arrowed line*) from a line extended upwards from the anterior margin of the anal canal (*dotted line*). **b** Following evacuation, there is marked retention of contrast (barium trapping) within the rectocoele (*R*). Note the anterior displacement of the vagina (*arrows*) by the rectal protrusion (*V*=vaginal apex) (reprinted with permission from KELVIN and MAGLINTE 1997)

phase of the study by anterior indentation on the contrast-filled vagina. Indeed, as discussed above, the full extent of a cystocoele may only become apparent after the rectum has been emptied. Conversely, a large undrained cystocoele may prevent the formation of an enterocoele or rectocoele by occupying space in the pelvis (KELVIN and MAGLINTE 2003). Although depiction of urethral anatomy is superior using MRI (Chap. 4.2), information on motility can be inferred during DCP if the catheter is left in situ after bladder drainage.

4.1.2.3.3
Enterocoele and Sigmoidocoele

The rectogenital pouch (pouch of Douglas) is the most inferior aspect of the peritoneal cavity and usually terminates approximately at the level of the posterior vaginal fornix. Filling of this space with small bowel or sigmoid colon is termed an enterocoele (Figs. 4.1.5, 4.1.6) or sigmoidocoele (Fig. 4.1.7), respectively. The majority of women with enterocoeles have a prior history of vaginal delivery, and a significant proportion has also undergone hysterectomy, which leaves the pouch of Douglas exposed (HUDSON 1988). Unlike other forms of pelvic organ prolapse, clinical detection of enterocoeles is unreliable–in one study just 16% of proven enterocoeles were apparent on clinical examination (HOCK et al. 1993).

Enterocoeles are readily apparent during DCP because both the bowel and vagina are opacified. However, their demonstration may require repeated and prolonged straining (Fig. 4.1.6), and their formation may also be intermittent (HALLIGAN et al. 1996). There is good evidence that detection is improved by undertaking a repeat post-toilet straining image, and indeed up to 50% of enterocoeles may remain fluoroscopically undetected unless this manoeuvre is performed (Fig. 4.1.5) (KELVIN et al. 1999). In some patients, the enterocoele may be intravaginal, rather than entering the pouch of Douglas (Fig. 4.1.8). The clinical significance of an enterocoele is debated. It is now known, for example, that their presence does not cause obstructed defecation, but there is no doubt that they are associated with feelings of incomplete evacuation in some patients (HALLIGAN et al. 1996). Symptoms of pelvic pressure/dragging

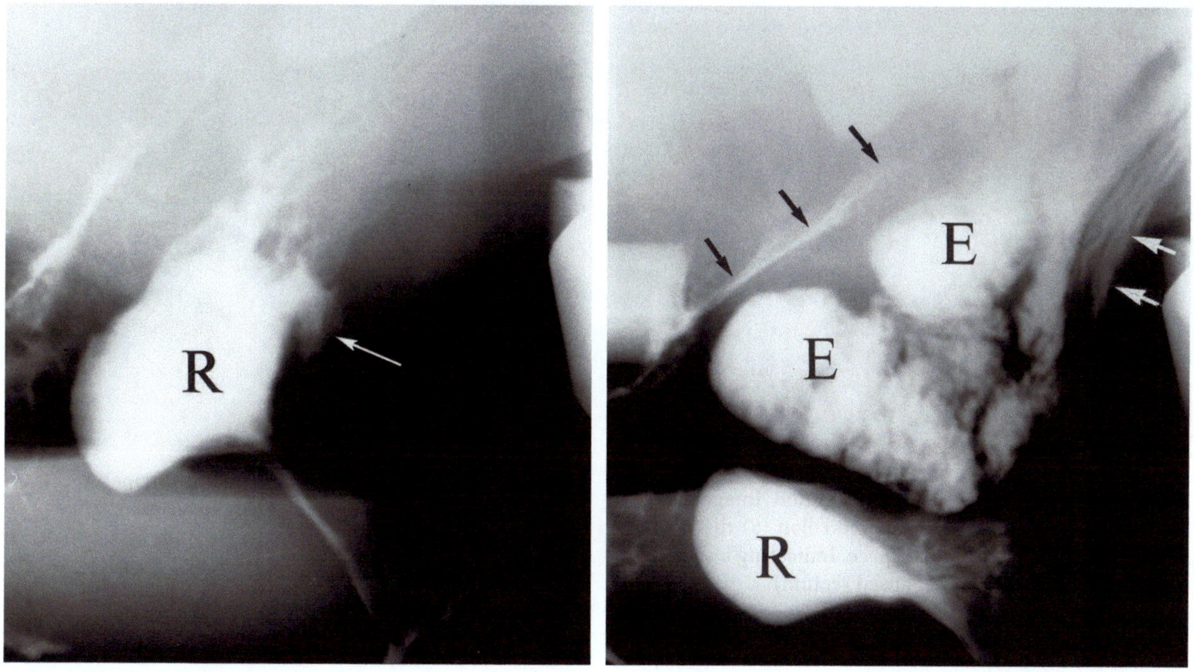

a b

Fig. 4.1.5a,b. Importance of post-toilet state for demonstration of enterocoele. **a** Post-evacuation image shows large rectocoele (*R*) with considerable barium trapping. Note also a posterior rectocoele (*arrow*) due to herniation through the levator ani. The rectovaginal space is widened, consistent with a peritoneocoele. **b** Following evacuation in the bathroom, the rectocoele (*R*) has almost completely emptied. The rectovaginal space is now filled by a large enterocoele (*E*) (reprinted with permission from KELVIN and MAGLINTE 1997)

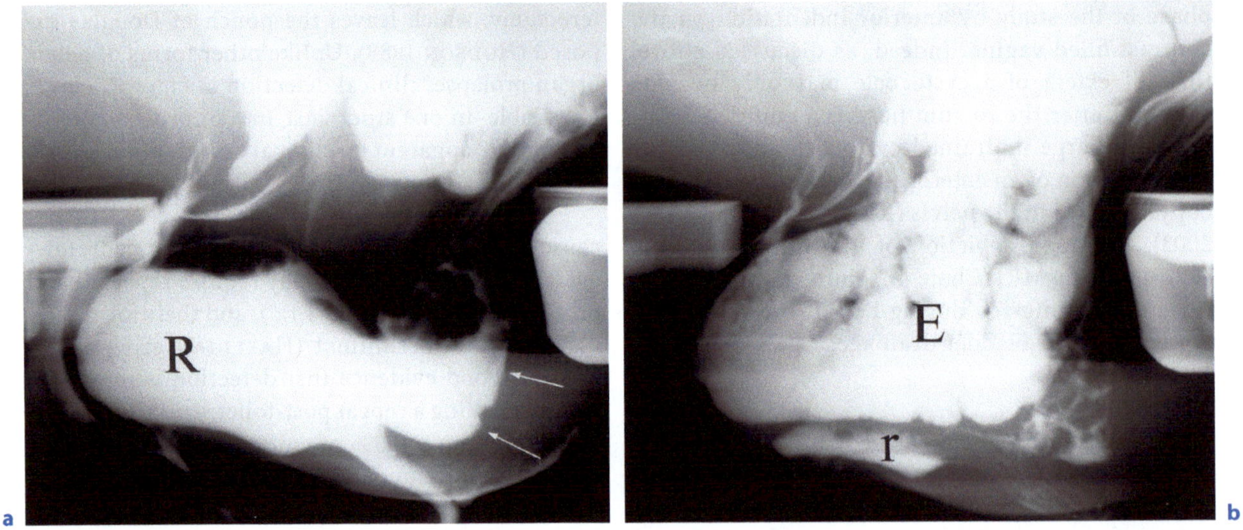

Fig. 4.1.6a,b. Enterocoele in rectovaginal space only visualised on straining maximally. **a** Post-evacuation image taken without straining shows no evidence of enterocoele. Note barium trapping in rectocoele (*R*). **b** On maximal straining, small bowel loops have descended between the vagina and collapsed upper rectum, indicating an enterocoele (*E*) in the rectovaginal space. Note descent of rectocoele (*r*) on straining (reprinted with permission from Kelvin and Maglinte 1997)

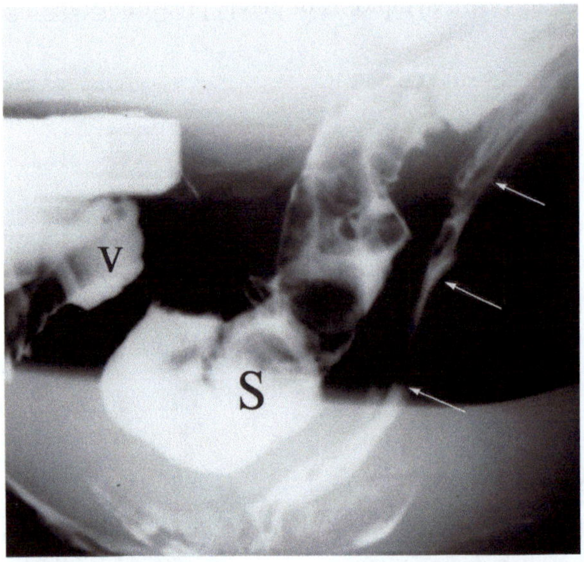

Fig. 4.1.7. Sigmoidocoele. Post-evacuation image demonstrates a stool-filled loop of sigmoid colon (*S*) that has descended into the rectovaginal space, indicating a sigmoidocoele (*V*=vagina, *arrows* collapsed rectum)

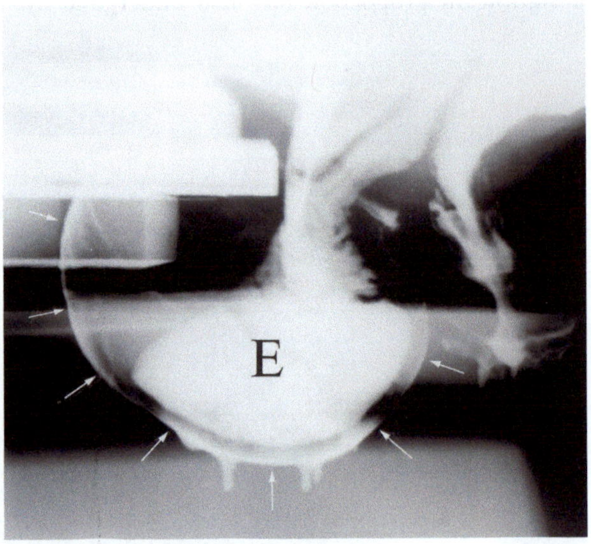

Fig. 4.1.8. Intravaginal enterocoele and competing cystocoele. Post-evacuation image shows external vaginal prolapse. The everted vagina is coated with contrast material (*arrows*). A large enterocoele (*E*) is present posteriorly within the prolapsed vagina, while the anterior half of the vagina is occupied by non-opacified cystocoele

and lower abdominal pain are often relieved by enterocoele repair (KELVIN and MAGLINTE 2003), and the presence of a significant enterocoele may indicate a trans-abdominal pelvic floor repair instead of a transvaginal approach. Detection is therefore an important role for pelvic floor imaging techniques.

Sigmoidocoeles are relatively unusual (around 5% of DCP examinations) (KELVIN 1999) and are likely underdiagnosed by DCP due to inadequate sigmoid opacification. However, clinical detection is also relatively poor, and it maybe MRI will prove superior to both clinical examination and DCP for diagnosis (Chap. 4.2). For uniformity of definition with other forms of pelvic organ prolapse, a sigmoidocoele may be defined as descent of the sigmoid below the pubococcygeal line (KELVIN and MAGLINTE 2003). However, others have proposed diagnosis is restricted to sigmoid decent by 4.5 cm below this reference line (FENNER 1996).

An association between sigmoidocoeles and constipation is well described (FENNER 1996), although which is the primary abnormality may sometimes be unclear. Stasis of faecal contents within a sigmoidocoele may lead to chronic straining (JORGE et al. 1994b), and resection can lead to dramatic relief of constipation in some patients (KELVIN and MAGLINTE 2003). It has been suggested that a large sigmoidocoele may physically obstruct defecation, the theory being the solid contents are more compressive compared to the "softer" consistency of an enterocoele (FENNER 1996).

4.1.2.3.4
Peritoneocoele

Positive contrast has been injected into the peritoneal cavity in order to investigate the configuration of the pelvic floor during rectal evaluation (HALLIGAN and BARTRAM 1995), a procedure known as "peritoneography" and necessary before MR imaging became widely available. To investigate proctographic widening of the rectovaginal space without an obvious enterocoele, Bremmer and colleagues (1997) used peritoneography to outline the distal peritoneal recess. In a study of 22 patients, 20 had a widened rectovaginal space due at least in part to a peritoneocoele (BREMMER et al. 1997), which is defined as decent of the rectouterine pouch below the upper third of the vagina, i.e., the pouch does not contain bowel (in which case it would be a simple enterocoele). Bremmer defined various subtypes of peritoneocoele, including rectal (located within a rectal intussusception), septal (descent into the recto-vaginal pouch), and vaginal (decent into the vagina). Peritoneocoeles may coexist with enterocoeles (up to 50%) (HALLIGAN et al. 1996), and their clinical import lies in the fact they probably predict enterocoele formation, thus indicating repair if prolapse surgery is undertaken (KELVIN et al. 2000). Although peritoneocoeles can be inferred from a widened rectovaginal space on DCP, they may be best visualised using MRI (Chap. 4.2).

4.1.2.3.5
Vaginal Vault Prolapse

Routine vaginal opacification during DCP usually permits reliable assessment of vault motility during maximum staining. Occasionally full vaginal prolapsed (Fig. 4.1.8) will be missed on DCP due to difficulties in identifying any residual vaginal contrast. However, such gross abnormality is of course readily apparent on clinical examination. Again for uniformity of definition, most workers consider vaginal prolapse as descent below the pubococcygeal line, regardless of the presence or not of the uterus. Vaginal prolapse rarely occurs in isolation and is usually associated with abnormal descent of other pelvic organs, notably an enterocoele.

Anterior displacement of the vagina on DCP may be secondary to rectocoele, enterocoele or large peritoneocoele, whilst posterior-inferior displacement is usually secondary to a cystocoele (KELVIN et al. 1999).

4.1.2.4
Comparison with Physical Examination

Correlation between physical examination findings and those on DCP have sometimes been disappointing. However, it must be remembered that both use different lines of reference–clinical examination uses the hymeneal ring and imaging the pubococcygeal line. When the mid-pubic line is used as the imaging line of reference, correlation with clinical findings is improved (PANNU et al. 2000). Furthermore, the ability of the patient to adequately strain is superior during evacuation as part of DCP than when lying semi-prone with a speculum in situ, and even the best trained finger cannot always correctly classify the full nature of a palpable bulge. Nevertheless, in a recent review, the role of imaging in the investigation of prolapse was described as "generally unnecessary"

(Jelovsek et al. 2007). This is despite the fact that enterocoeles and sigmoidocoeles are often clinically occult and revealed only by imaging. In one of the largest studies to date, Kelvin and colleagues (1999) retrospectively reviewed 170 DCP examinations. They found of 47 enterocoeles diagnosed on DCP, just 24 were detected clinically. Similarly, all 8 sigmoidocoeles and 27 cystocoeles were clinically occult. Importantly, even if early disease on DCP was excluded, clinical detection rates improved by just 1 to 2%, suggesting DCP was not "over-diagnosing" disease. Of note, however, 44 enterocoeles were detected clinically, but not seen radiologically. The authors questioned the use of clinical examination as the reference standard and pointed out even a surgical reference was an insufficient standard given the supine, anaesthetised state of the patient during the latter. The findings of Kelvin and colleagues have been replicated by other authors (Hock et al. 1993; Altringer et al. 1995), confirming the apparent inferiority of clinical examination. Furthermore it is increasingly clear that prolapse almost invariably involves multiple organs, often in all three pelvic compartments (Maglinte et al. 1997, 1999). Recent studies using MRI have confirmed a high prevalence of clinically occult prolapse in symptomatic women (Chap. 4.2), and pelvic floor imaging is increasingly used as clinicians begin to understand the importance of a holistic rather than compartmentalised approach to pelvic floor dysfunction (Kaufmann et al. 2001).

4.1.3 Summary

Evacuation proctography is a simple and rapid technique with which to assess the morphological and functional aspects of rectal evacuation. It is generally extremely well tolerated by patients, much more so than the barium enema, for example. The examination may be extended so that a global pelvic floor assessment is achieved, but this adds considerably to procedural complexity and is probably best reserved for urogynaecological practice, although the simple addition of oral barium to diagnose enterocoeles is worth considering. In day-to-day clinical practice, a formal measurement of various angles and distances is not required; an understanding of what is broadly normal and abnormal will suffice and will come with experience.

Acknowledgements

The authors would like to thank Dr. F. Kelvin for the original format of this chapter and providing Figures 4.1.3 to 4.1.8.

References

Alstrup N, Ronholt C, Chuangang F et al (1997) Viscous fluid expulsion in the evaluation of the constipated patient. Dis Colon Rectum 40:580–584

Altringer WE, Saclarides TJ, Dominguez JM et al (1995) Four-contrast defecography: pelvic "floor-oscopy." Dis Colon Rectum 38:695–699

Archer BD, Somers S, Stevenson GW (1992) Contrast medium gel for marking vaginal position during defecography. Radiology 182:278–279

Bannister JJ, Davison P, Timms JM et al (1987) Effect of stool size and consistency on rectal evacuation. Gut 28:1246–1250

Barnes PRH, Lennard-Jones JE (1985) Balloon expulsion from the rectum in constipation of different types. Gut 26:1049–1052

Bartolo DCC, Roe AM, Locke-Edmunds JC et al (1986) Flap valve theory of anorectal continence. Br J Surg 73:1012–1014

Bremmer S, Mellgren A, Holmstrom B et al (1997) Peritoneocele: visualization with defecography and peritoneography performed simultaneously. Radiology 202:373–377

Brubaker L, Retzky S, Smith C et al (1993) Pelvic floor evaluation with dynamic fluoroscopy. Obstet Gynecol 82:863–868

Bump RC, Mattiasson A, Bo K et al (1996) The standardization of terminology of female pelvic organ prolapse and pelvic floor dysfunction. Am J Obstet Gynecol 175:10–11

Ellerkmann RM, Cundiff GW, Melick CF et al (2001) Correlation of symptoms with location and severity of pelvic organ prolapse. Am J Obstet Gynecol 185:1332–1337

Fauconnier A, Zareski E, Abichedid J et al (2007) Dynamic magnetic resonance imaging for grading pelvic organ prolapse according to the international continence society classification: Which line should be used? Neurourol Urodyn 27:191–197

Fenner DE (1996) Diagnosis and assessment of sigmoidoceles. Am J Obstet Gynecol 175:1438–1442

Finlay IG (1988) Symposium: Proctography. Int J Colorect Dis 3:67–89

Goh V, Halligan S, Kaplan G et al (2000) Dynamic MR imaging of the pelvic floor in asymptomatic subjects. Am J Roentgenol 174:661–666

Halligan S, Bartram CI (1995) Evacuation proctography combined with positive contrast peritoneography to demonstrate pelvic floor hernias. Abdom Imaging 20:442–445

Halligan S, Bartram CI, Park HY et al (1995a) The proctographic features of anismus. Radiology 197:679–682

Halligan S, Thomas J, Bartram CI (1995b) Intrarectal pressures and balloon expulsion related to evacuation proctography. Gut 31:100–104

Halligan S, Bartram C, Hall C et al (1996) Enterocele revealed by simultaneous evacuation proctography and peritoneography: does "defecation block" exist? Am J Roentgenol 167:461–466

Hare C, Halligan S, Bartram CI et al (2001) Dose reduction in evacuation eroctography. Eur Radiol 11:432–434

Healy JC, Halligan S, Reznek RH et al (1997) Patterns of prolapse in women with symptoms of pelvic floor weakness: assessment with MR imaging. Radiology 203:77–81

Ho LM, Low VHS, Freed KS (1999) Vaginal opacification during defecography: utility of placing a folded gauze square at the introitus. Abdom Imaging 24:562–564

Hock D, Lombard R, Jehaes C et al (1993) Colpocystodefecography. Dis Colon Rectum 36:1015–1021

Hudson CN (1988) Female genital prolapse and pelvic floor deficiency. Int J Colorectal Dis 3:181–185

Hutchinson R, Mostafa AB, Grant EA et al (1993) Scintigraphic defecography: Quantitative and dynamic assessment of anorectal function. Dis Colon Rectum 36:1132–1138

Ikenberry S, Lappas JC, Hana MP et al (1996) Defecography in healthy subjects: comparison of three contrast media. Radiology 201:233–238

Jelovsek JE, Maher C, Barber MD (2007) Pelvic organ prolapse. Lancet 369:1027–1038

Jorge JMN, Ger GC, Gonzalez L et al (1994a) Patient position during cinedefecography. Dis Colon Rectum 37:927–931

Jorge JMN, Yang Y-K, Wexner SD (1994b) Incidence and clinical significance of sigmoidoceles as determined by a new classification system. Dis Colon Rectum 37:1112–1117

Kamm MA, Bartram CI, Lennard-Jones JE (1989) Rectodynamics–Quantifying rectal evacuation. Int J Colorect Dis 4:161–163

Kaufman HS, Buller JL, Thompson JR et al (2001) Dynamic pelvic magnetic resonance imaging and cystocolpoproctography alter surgical management of pelvic floor disorders. Disease Colon Rectum 44:1575–1583

Kelvin FM, Maglinte DDT (2000) Radiologic investigation of prolapse. J Pelv Surg 6:218–220

Kelvin FM, Maglinte DDT (2003) Dynamic evaluation of female pelvic organ prolapse by extended proctography. Radiol Clin N Am 41:395–407

Kelvin FM, Maglinte DDT, Hornback JA et al (1992) Pelvic prolapse: assessment with evacuation proctography (defecography). Radiology 184:547–551

Kelvin FM, Maglinte DDT, Benson JT et al (1994) Dynamic cystoproctography: a technique for assessing disorders of the pelvic floor in women. Am J Roentgenol 163:368–370

Kelvin FM, Hale DS, Maglinte DDT et al (1999) Female pelvic organ prolapse: diagnostic contribution of dynamic cystoproctography and comparison with physical examination. Am J Roentgenol 173:31–37

Kelvin FM, Maglinte DDT, Hale DS et al (2000) Female pelvic organ prolapse: a comparison of triphasic dynamic MR imaging and triphasic fluoroscopic cystocolpoproctography. Am J Roentgenol 174:8–88

Lienemann A, Anthuber C, Baron A et al (1997) Dynamic MR colpocystorectography assessing pelvic-floor descent. Eur Radiol 7:1309–1317

Maglinte DDT, Kelvin FM, Hale DS et al (1997) Dynamic cystoproctography: a unifying diagnostic approach to pelvic floor and anorectal dysfunction. Am J Roentgenol 169:759

Maglinte DDT, Kelvin FM, Fitzgerald K et al (1999) Association of compartment defects in pelvic floor dysfunction. Am J Roentgenol 172:439–444

Mahieu P, Pringot J, Bodart P (1984) Defecography: 1. Description of a new procedure and results in normal patients. Gastrointest Radiol 9:247–251

McGee SG, Bartram CI (1993) Intra-anal intussusception: diagnosis by posteroanterior stress proctography. Abdom Imaging 2:136–140

Olsen AL, Smith VJ, Bergstrom JO et al (1997) Epidemiology of surgically managed pelvic organ prolapse and urinary incontinence. Obstet Gynecol 89:501–506

Pannu HK (2004) MRI of pelvic organ prolapse. Eur Radiol 14:1456–1464

Pannu HK, Kaufman HS, Cundiff GW et al (2000) Dynamic MR imaging of pelvic organ prolapse: spectrum of abnormalities. Radiographics 20:1567–1582

Poon FW, Lauder JC, Finlay IG (1991) Technical report: Evacuating proctography–A simplified technique. Clin Radiol 44:113–116

Preston DM, Lennard-Jones JE, Thomas BM (1984) The balloon proctogram. Br J Surg 71:29–31

Shorvon PJ, McHugh S, Diamant NE et al (1989) Defecography in normal volunteers: results and implications. Gut 30:1737–1749

Wallden L (1952) Defecation block in cases of deep rectogenital pouch. A surgical, roentgenological and embryological study with special reference to morphological conditions. Acta Chir Scandinav (Suppl):165

Imaging Techniques

4.2 Dynamic MR Imaging of the Pelvic Floor

Joel G. Fletcher, Adil E. Bharucha, and Hassan Siddiki

CONTENTS

J. G. Fletcher, MD
Associate Professor of Radiology, Department of Radiology, Mayo Clinic, 200 First Street SW, Rochester, MN 55905, USA
A. E. Bharucha, MBBS, MD
Professor of Medicine, Clinical Enteric Neuroscience Translational and Epidemiological Research Program, Mayo Clinic, College of Medicine, 200 First Street SW, Rochester, MN 55905, USA
H. Siddiki, MD
Department of Radiology, Mayo Clinic, 200 First Street SW, Rochester, MN 55905, USA

4.2.1 Abstract-Role of MR in Evaluating Pelvic Floor Disorders

Over the last decade advances in commercial MR technology have facilitated the development and integration of dynamic MR imaging into the workup of patients with pelvic floor disorders. Dynamic MR imaging demonstrates movement of the pelvic floor and organs, providing functional information reflecting ligamentous or muscular injury, atrophy or dysfunction. Additionally, it has several advantages over conventional fluoroscopic cystoproctography. The intrinsic T2-weighted signal differences of the pelvic organs provide excellent visualization of the bladder, vagina, small bowel and rectum with minimal preparation, as well as direct visualization of the pelvic floor musculature. The use of cross-sectional imaging eliminates problems of superimposition, magnification and measurement at traditional fluoroscopy. The multiplanar capabilities of MR permit dynamic coronal and axial imaging unavailable using fluoroscopic methods. Because dynamic imaging of the pelvic floor is performed using time-efficient pulse sequences, it can be combined with high spatial resolution static (anatomic) imaging using endoluminal receiver coils, in order to permit a combined anatomic and functional assessment of defecatory disorders in a single setting.

4.2.2 Spectrum of MR Imaging for Pelvic Floor Disorders

In the early and mid 1990s, several investigators realized the potential of MR to identify pelvic visceral prolapse and abnormalities of pelvic floor shape (Christensen et al. 1995; Healy et al. 1997; Ozasa et al. 1992). The advent of fast imaging with steady-state precession (true FISP or FIESTA) and single-shot fast spin echo (SSFSE or HASTE) pulse sequences, which minimize motion artifacts, allowed acquisition of a single image every 1.2–2 s during pelvic floor motion with signal differences that adequately displayed pelvic floor organs and musculature (Lienemann et al. 1997; Busse et al. 2000; Gufler et al. 1999). In 1997 Lienemann et al. published results comparing dynamic MR colposyctorectography, traditional fluoroscopic colposyctorectography and clinical exam in 44 patients and 5 volunteers using sonographic gel in the rectum and vagina, and saline and thread in the bladder and urethra, respectively (Lienemann et al. 1997). They found that dynamic MR colposyctorectography performed with an equal or higher sensitivity than traditional fluoroscopy for prolapse at various sites, with MR being superior for the detection of enteroceles and uterine prolapse. While most radiologists performing dynamic MR have abandoned the instillation of contrast material within all pelvic structures except for the rectum, the findings recorded and methods in their study are largely followed today.

Static imaging of the pelvic floor is often performed in the same setting of dynamic MR imaging. Torso phased-array coils are generally used for dynamic imaging, but can also be used to visualize the shape and attachments of the levator plate, vagina and puborectalis (Strohbehn et al. 1996; Tunn et al. 1999; Hjartardottir et al. 1997). Additionally, experienced observers may be able to identify external anal sphincter atrophy using torso phased-array coils alone (Terra et al. 2006). Endoanal receiver coils additionally permit excellent visualization of tears or atrophy of the internal and external anal sphincters, as well as providing improved visualization of the urethra and vagina (Stoker and Rociu 1999; Hussain et al. 1995; Stoker et al. 2001). Endovaginal or endourethral receiver coils can also be used to provide optimal imaging of the urethra and its supporting ligaments (Tan et al. 1998; Macura 2006; Strohbehn et al. 1996). We routinely perform endoanal imaging to examine the sphincters, levator ani and puborectalis prior to dynamic MR imaging, with both static and dynamic imaging completed in about 45 min. Endoluminal imaging is generally performed prior to dynamic imaging owing to potential near-field artifacts caused by residual rectal or vaginal contrast.

4.2.3 Dynamic MR Proctography Technique

A variety of approaches to performing dynamic MR imaging of the pelvic floor have been advocated (Lienemann et al. 1997; Kelvin et al. 2000; Pannu et al. 2000; Comiter et al. 1999). Generally, most centers perform a three-phase examination consisting of (1) a squeeze maneuver to assess puborectalis contraction, (2) simulated defecation utilizing rectal contrast to examine for rectal abnormalities and pelvic organ prolapse and (3) post-defecation Valsalva imaging (i.e., a post-toilet phase) to maximize the detection of enteroceles and cystoceles.

4.2.3.1 Patient Instruction

Prior to imaging, patients are instructed in the maneuvers they will perform as part of the MR exam (i.e., squeeze, defecation and Valsalva). It is important to utilize easy-to-understand directions (e.g., "squeeze your anal muscles and pull your pelvic floor up;" "relax;" "bear down and expel all your rectal contents;" "bear down as hard as you can"). During the dynamic exam itself, patients are instructed to perform specific maneuvers prior to pulse sequence initiation and to initiate movement when they next hear the technologist's voice, so that image acquisition will begin at rest and proceed through the desired motion, and so that instructions can be heard above the noise of the magnet. Confirming that the patient has performed the right maneuver at the time of scan is important to assure acquiring the correct movement.

4.2.3.2 Patient Preparation and Positioning

No bowel preparation is required. The patient is gowned in a hospital robe with open access to the back and brought into the MR suite. A torso phased-array coil is placed directly on the MR table, covered by a sheet and plastic chucks directly over the location of the coil. During both endoanal and dynamic imaging, the patient is positioned such that the symphysis pubis is located in the middle of the torso phased array coil.

After endoanal imaging is performed, approximately 180 cc of ultrasound gel is inserted in the rectum for contrast. Several centers have reported improved pelvic descent when utilizing rectal gel, the expulsion of which can be used to gauge patient effort. To facilitate expulsion of rectal contrast, most investigators ask patients to flex their knees and place a large pillow under underneath them (Pannu et al. 2000).

4.2.3.3 MR Technique

Dynamic imaging is performed in a mid-sagittal plane during each maneuver. This plane should include (from anterior to posterior) the pubis, urethra, vagina, cervix (if present), anorectal junction and sacrococcygeal joint. Selection of this plane typically requires localizing axial scans or three-point localization techniques. For dynamic acquisition, we typically employ single-shot fast spin echo imaging with real-time image acquisition and reconstruction (Busse et al. 2000) so that we can insure patients have successfully performed each maneuver. Images are acquired every 1.2–1.4 s. Alternatively, sequential true-FISP imaging can be performed (Lienemann et al. 1997), with the selection between these pulse sequences likely depending upon the available MR equipment. Axial or coronal imaging can be performed across the pelvic floor during rest and straining, and is particularly helpful in discovering levator defects and hernias and their relationships to other pelvic organ prolapse.

The squeeze maneuver is performed to assess for puborectalis contraction and should be performed regardless of the appearance of the muscle. Dynamic imaging is then performed in a mid-sagittal plane, as described earlier. After two or three images are obtained at rest, the patient is asked to squeeze the anal muscles and contract the pelvic floor. The radiologist or technologist performing the exam should either see anterior and superior movement of the anorectal junction (as a result of puborectalis contraction) or insure that the patient properly understood the instructions and performed the maneuver (e.g., in the case of bilateral puborectalis injury or dysfunction).

Dynamic images are then acquired during simulated defecation in a similar manner. Images should be acquired until the patient expels all rectal contents or during multiple attempts. It should be realized that patients with puborectalis dysfunction and a minority of normal patients may be unable to expel any rectal contrast (Halligan et al. 1995; Bharucha et al. 2005). In such instances, the radiologist or technologist should insure that patient effort was maximal and that imaging findings of Valsalva are seen (clockwise rotation of the sacrum and ballooning of the abdominal wall musculature).

Dynamic post-defecation Valsalva images are performed after the patient has been excused to the restroom to complete rectal evacuation and empty the bladder. Emptying these structures maximizes detection of enteroceles and pelvic organ prolapse (Kelvin et al. 2000; Lienemann et al. 1997). Coronal images are also performed during Valsalva to detect eventration or hernias in the levator muscle and provide additional information regarding enteroceles, peritoneoceles or rectal prolapse (Pannu et al. 2000).

Additional maneuvers and problem-solving techniques can also be performed. Dynamic axial imaging of the levator plate can be helpful in evaluating pelvic organ prolapse by demonstrating pelvic organ descent not seen in a single mid-sagittal slice. Similarly, sagittal imaging during Valsalva can also be helpful in portraying the anatomy of enteroceles and levator ani hernias. While not required to measure vaginal descent, instillation of intra-vaginal contrast may be helpful when vaginal vault prolapse and eversion is present.

4.2.4 Exam Interpretation

Patients referred for dynamic imaging of the pelvic floor generally possess multiple abnormalities involving the anterior (bladder and urethra), middle (vagina and uterus) and posterior pelvic compartments (rectum and small bowel) (Maglinte et al. 1999). Abnormal descent and associated findings are described below for each organ. By convention the descent of pelvic organs and structures is measured from the pubococcygeal line, which is drawn from the inferior aspect of the pubis to the sacrococcygeal joint (Fig. 4.2.1). Descent of any particular structure/organ is measured along a perpendicular line from the pubococcygeal line to the structure. However, it must be noted that in most cases, studies that compare findings in properly selected asymptomatic controls to clinically confirmed cases are not available. In addition, the degree of movement seen is highly dependent on the degree of effort produced by the patient at the time of examination.

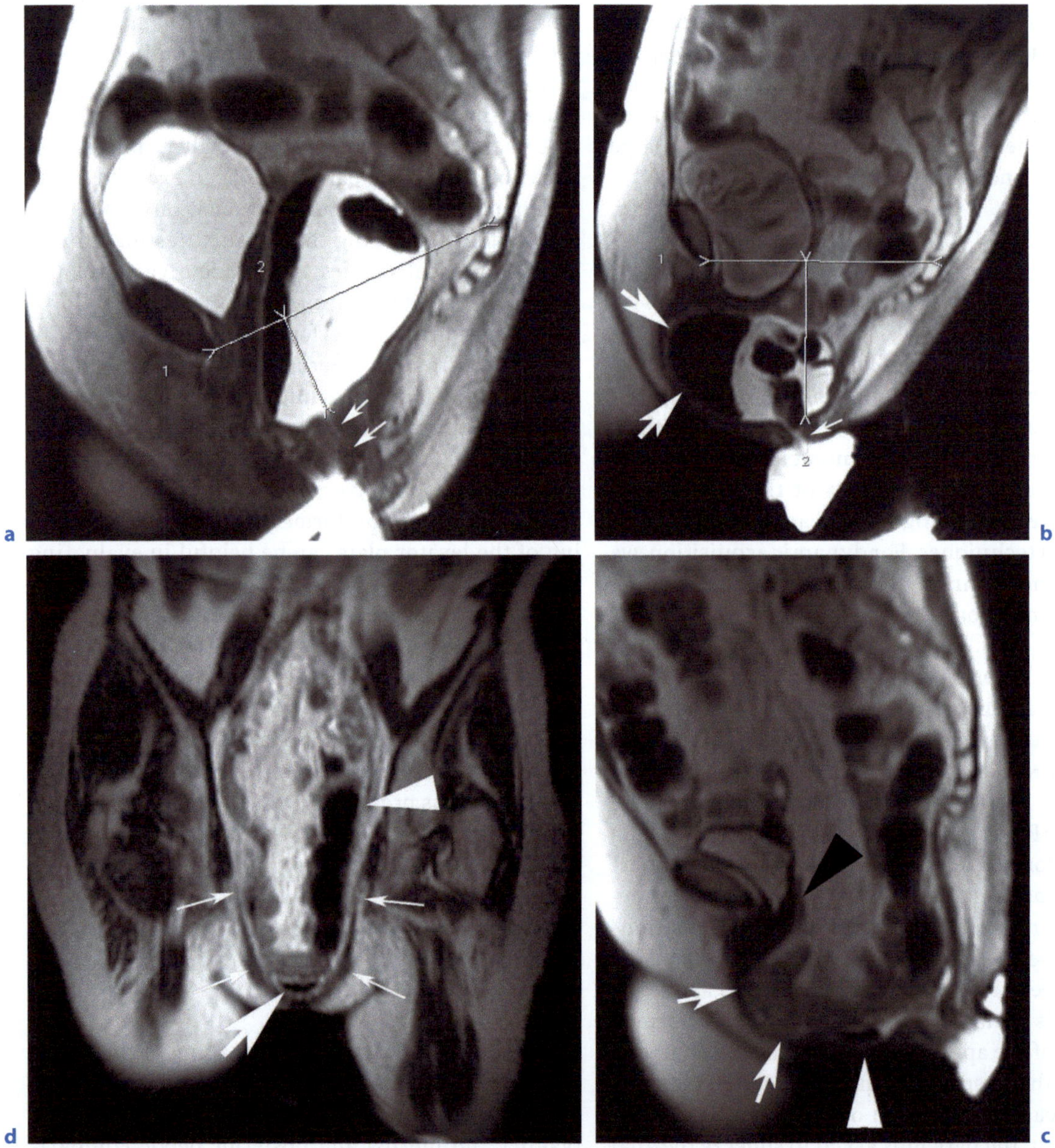

Fig. 4.2.1a–d. Dynamic MR proctography images in a patient with obstructive defecation at rest (**a**), during defecation (**b**), and during post-defecation Valsava (**c** and **d**). Descent is measured along a perpendicular drawn between the pubococcygeal line and the anorectal junction, and measures 4.2 at rest cm (**a**) and 9.1 cm during defecation (**b**). There is also a large 5-cm anterior rectocele during defecation (*large arrows*, **b**). Anal canal is denoted by *small arrows* (**a** and **b**). During post-defecation Valsalva imaging (after rectal and bladder emptying), a large enterocele (*small arrows*), along with decompressed rectocele (**c**, *arrowhead*). Coronal image shows that the enterocele contains sigmoid colon (**d**, *arrowhead*) in addition to small bowel loops

4.2.4.1 Bladder and Urethra

Stress urinary incontinence is related to intrinsic urethral sphincter deficiency and urethral hypermobility (Macura 2006), with the urethra and supporting ligaments best visualized at static MR with endoluminal receiver coils (Macura 2006) and hypermobility observed during dynamic imaging with Valsalva. Urethral hypermobility is demonstrated when the bladder base descends abnormally and the urethra rotates excessively. Funneling of the proximal urethra, or visualized filling of the proximal urethra, during rest or Valsalva is abnormal and associated with urinary incontinence, but can also be seen in some continent patients (Macura 2006). Many authors consider descent of the bladder base below the pubococcygeal line to be abnormal and to define the presence of a cystocele (Macura 2006; Kelvin et al. 2000; Pannu et al. 2000). However, some normal, continent patients demonstrate slight descent of the bladder base below the pubococcygeal line (Goh et al. 2000; Healy et al. 1997). Healy et al. found that the median descent of the bladder base with Valsalva in normal volunteers was 1.7 cm. Consequently, we utilize a cutoff of 2 cm below the pubococcygeal line to define a cystocele (Fig. 4.2.2), while others grade cystoceles as small when the distance between the pubococcygeal line and the bladder base is between 0 and 3 cm (Kelvin et al. 2000).

4.2.4.2 Vaginal, Uterus and Defects in Recto-Vaginal Fascia

The vaginal vault (in patients with hysterectomies) and cervicovaginal junction can be readily seen on mid-sagittal dynamic MR images (Fig. 4.2.2). It should be recognized that while many published series define vaginal vault or uterine prolapse as occurring when the vaginal vault or cervicovaginal junction descends below the pubococcygeal line (Lienemann et al. 1997), many asymptomatic patients will have mild descent of the vaginal vault to a point 3 cm or less below the pubococcygeal line (Healy et al. 1997), and such descent should be considered small (Kelvin et al. 2000). Moreover, even when the uterus descends more than 3 cm below the pubococcygeal line, the functional implications of its descent (i.e., whether or not it impedes rectal evacuation) should be described.

4.2.4.3 Puborectalis Function

The anorectal angle is drawn using tangents through the anal canal and along the posterior rectal wall (Shorvon et al. 1989; Bartram et al. 1988). Puborectalis function is evaluated by the changes in the anorectal angle during squeeze and defecation. Thus, the angle normally decreases, reflecting puborectalis contraction, during squeeze and increases, reflecting relaxation, during defecation. The utility of defecating proctography is limited by considerable inter-observer variability in anorectal angle measurements, which may be partly attributable to inter-observer variations in orientation of the rectal tangent, which may be drawn through the anterior, middle or posterior rectum (Barnett et al. 1999). However, inter-observer correlation for anorectal angle measurements by MR proctography can be excellent; based on the lowest 5th percentile in the group of asymptomatic control subjects, normal puborectalis contraction was defined by a reduction of the anorectal angle from rest to squeeze by 11° (Shorvon et al. 1989; Bharucha et al. 2005). During squeeze, the anorectal junction should move superiorly, and generally moves forward anteriorly, although this finding is variable in control subjects (Shorvon et al. 1989) (Fig. 4.2.3). Because variations in rectal contour also affect angle measurements even when electronic calipers are used, interpreting physicians should compare and insure that numeric measurements reflect their subjective impressions of puborectalis contraction.

During evacuation, the puborectalis normally relaxes, causing widening or an increase in the anorectal angle. Dynamic MR imaging reveals a smaller change in the anorectal angle, reflecting impaired puborectalis relaxation, during evacuation in patients with obstructed defecation compared to matched controls (Bharucha et al. 2005). Similar to barium proctography, the diagnosis of defecatory dysfunction should not be exclusively based on the anorectal angle change during evacuation because some asymptomatic subjects (17% in one study) may have an inadequate anorectal angle change during defecation, while some patients with clinical and manometric features of an evacuation disorder may have normal anorectal angle change during evacuation (Halligan et al. 1995; Bharucha et al. 2005). Thus, other findings (i.e., difficulty initiating evacuation, incomplete rectal evacuation, paradoxical puborectalis contraction as evidenced by increased puborectalis indentation and reduced perineal descent) should also be used to assess for disordered defecation. Indeed, there is increasing evidence for phenotypic heterogeneity in patients with defecatory disorders (Bharucha et al. 2005; Fletcher et al. 2003); for example, perineal decent may be normal, reduced or increased (Fig. 4.2.4) (Bharucha et al. 2005).

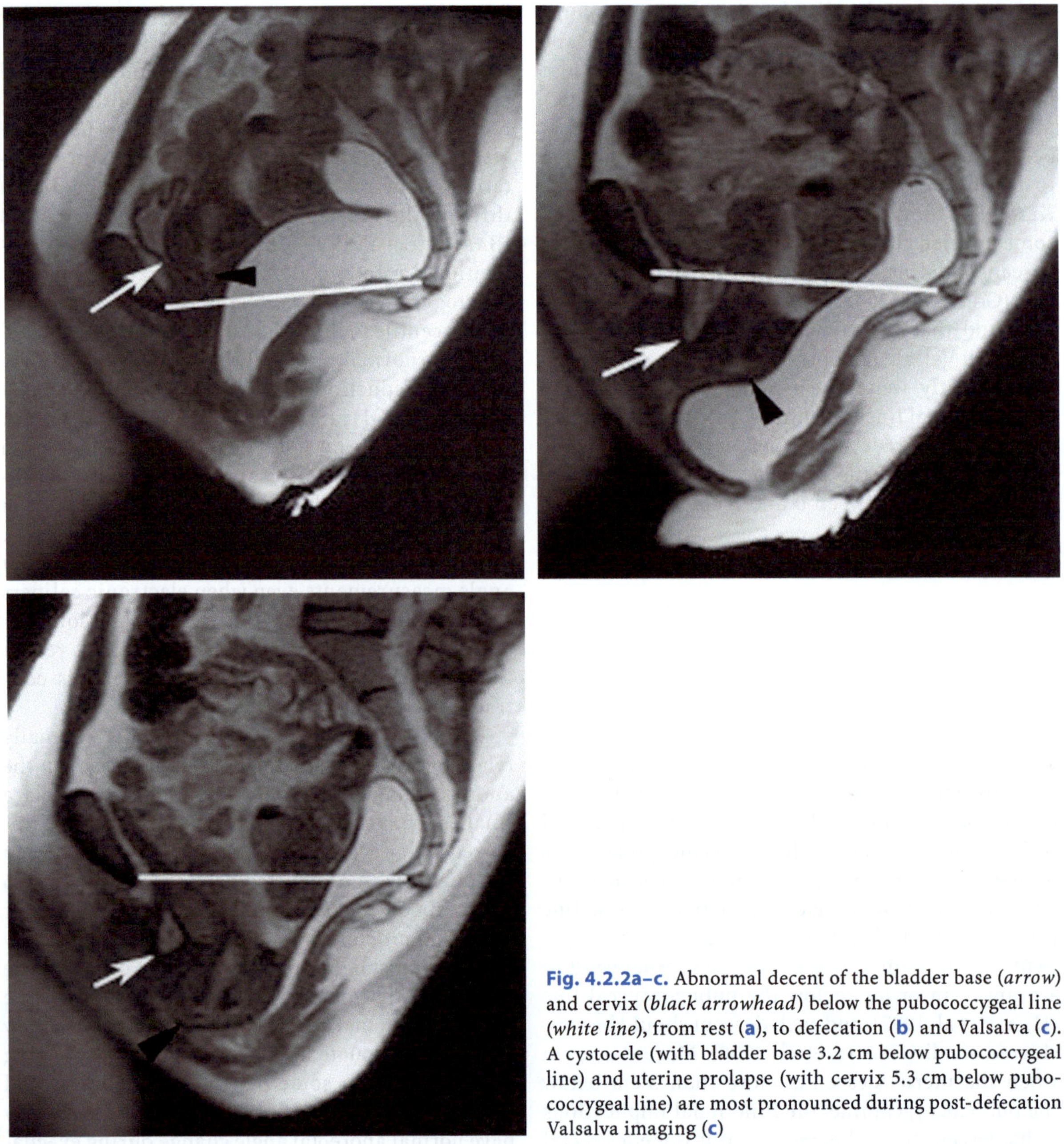

a b c

Fig. 4.2.2a–c. Abnormal decent of the bladder base (*arrow*) and cervix (*black arrowhead*) below the pubococcygeal line (*white line*), from rest (**a**), to defecation (**b**) and Valsalva (**c**). A cystocele (with bladder base 3.2 cm below pubococcygeal line) and uterine prolapse (with cervix 5.3 cm below pubococcygeal line) are most pronounced during post-defecation Valsalva imaging (**c**)

4.2.4.4 Rectal Abnormalities

Rectoceles are an outpouching of the (usually) anterior rectal wall, as measured from a line extended upward from the anal canal (Kelvin et al. 2000). Rectoceles less than 2 cm are considered to be clinically insignificant, particularly in older women. Rectoceles in excess of 4 cm are considered to be large (Kelvin et al. 2000). Conceptually, rectocoeles reflect "give-way" of the anterior rectal wall, often in the context of deficient support mechanisms (e.g., after a hysterectomy). It is important to recognize that rectocoeles are often secondary rather than

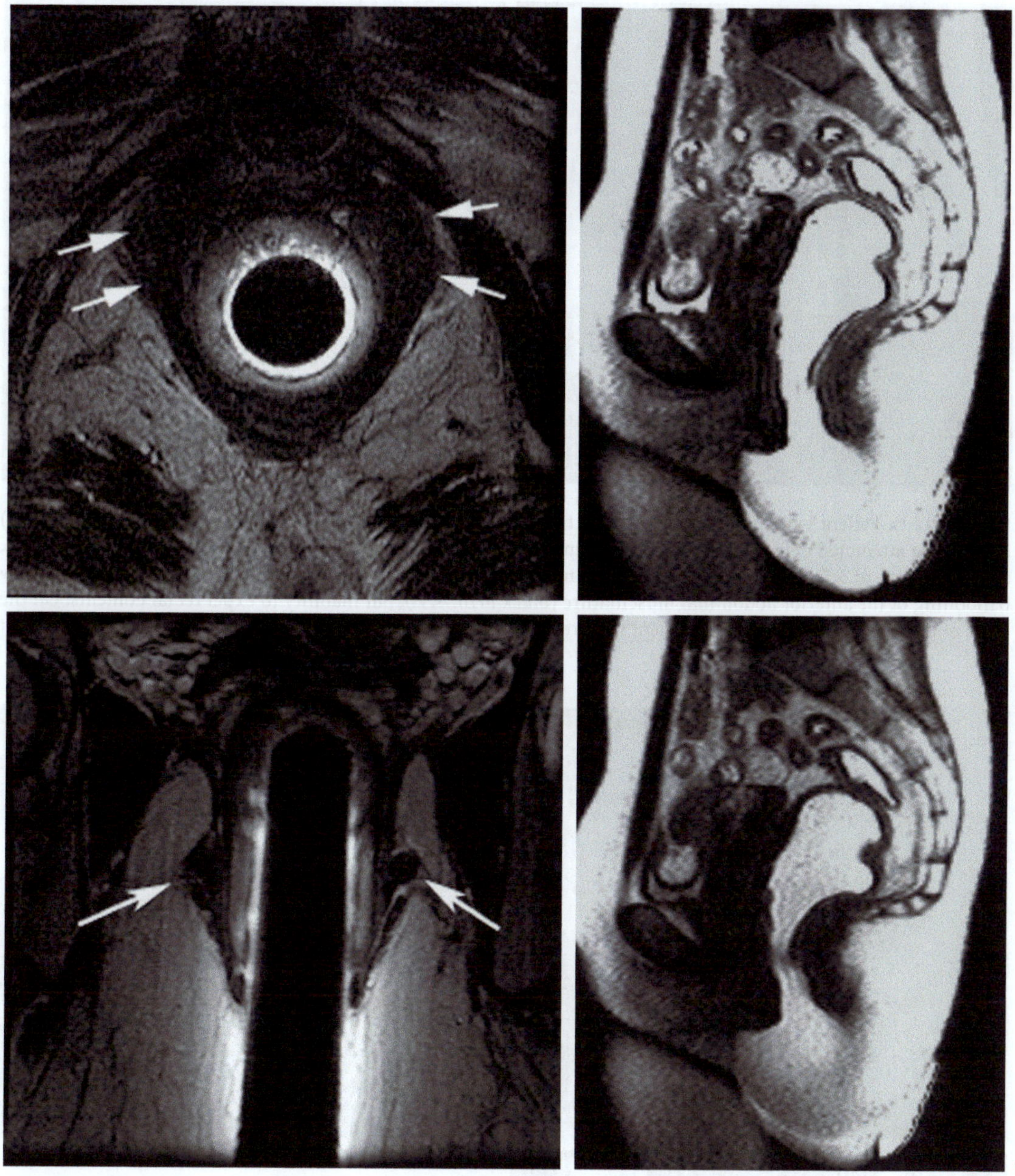

a c b d

Fig. 4.2.3a–d. Axial and coronal endoanal MR images (**a** and **b**, respectively) in an incontinent patient show normal-appearing puborectalis muscle and globally thickened internal anal sphincter (*arrows*, **a** and **b**). Dynamic MR images at rest (**c**) and squeeze (**d**) show a widely patulous anal canal and minimal puborectalis function, which correlated with reduced resting and squeeze pressures at manometry

primary abnormalities, i.e., they are caused by excessive straining in patients with impaired pelvic floor relaxation. Impaired emptying of a rectocele may contribute not only to symptoms of disordered defecation, but also to "passive" leakage (i.e., after defecation) in fecal incontinence. Rectocoele emptying should be assessed by images acquired after patients have had an opportunity to defecate on a toilet, perhaps on images acquired during a Valsalva maneuver (Greenberg et al. 2001). To describe rectal intussusception and prolapse at dynamic MR imaging, most subspecialists use grading systems developed at fluoroscopic proctography (Shorvon et al. 1989) (Fig. 4.2.5).

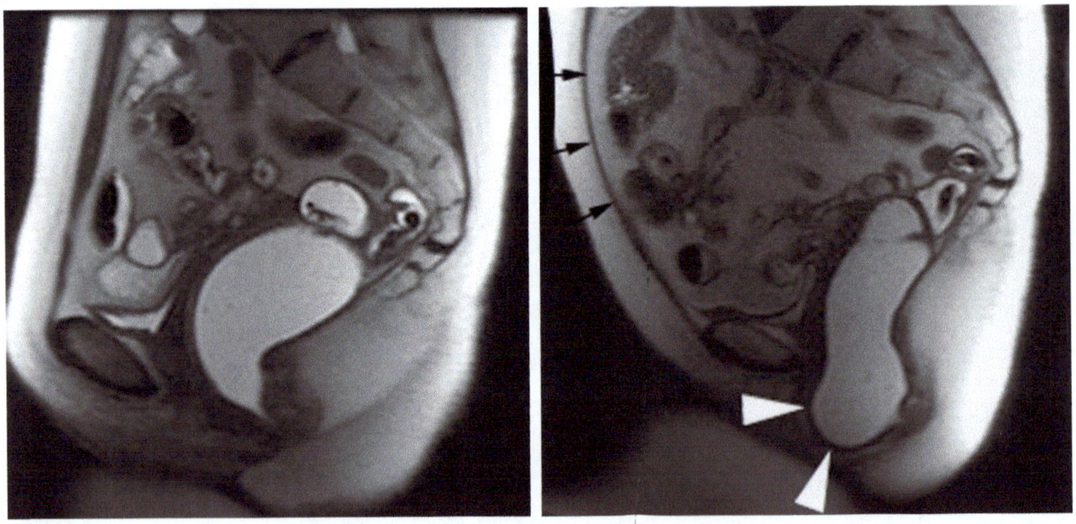

a b

Fig. 4.2.4a,b. Patient with symptoms of obstructive defecation, but negative balloon expulsion study at rest (**a**) and during attempted defecation (**b**). During attempted defecation, a broad-based anterior rectocele (*arrowheads*, **b**) and descent of 5.5 cm below pubococcygeal line is seen, with increased abdominal pressure demonstrated by ballooning of the anterior abdominal musculature (*black arrows*, **b**), but inability to expel rectal contents. On the basis of the MR and symptoms, the patient was treated with biofeedback with marked symptomatic improvement

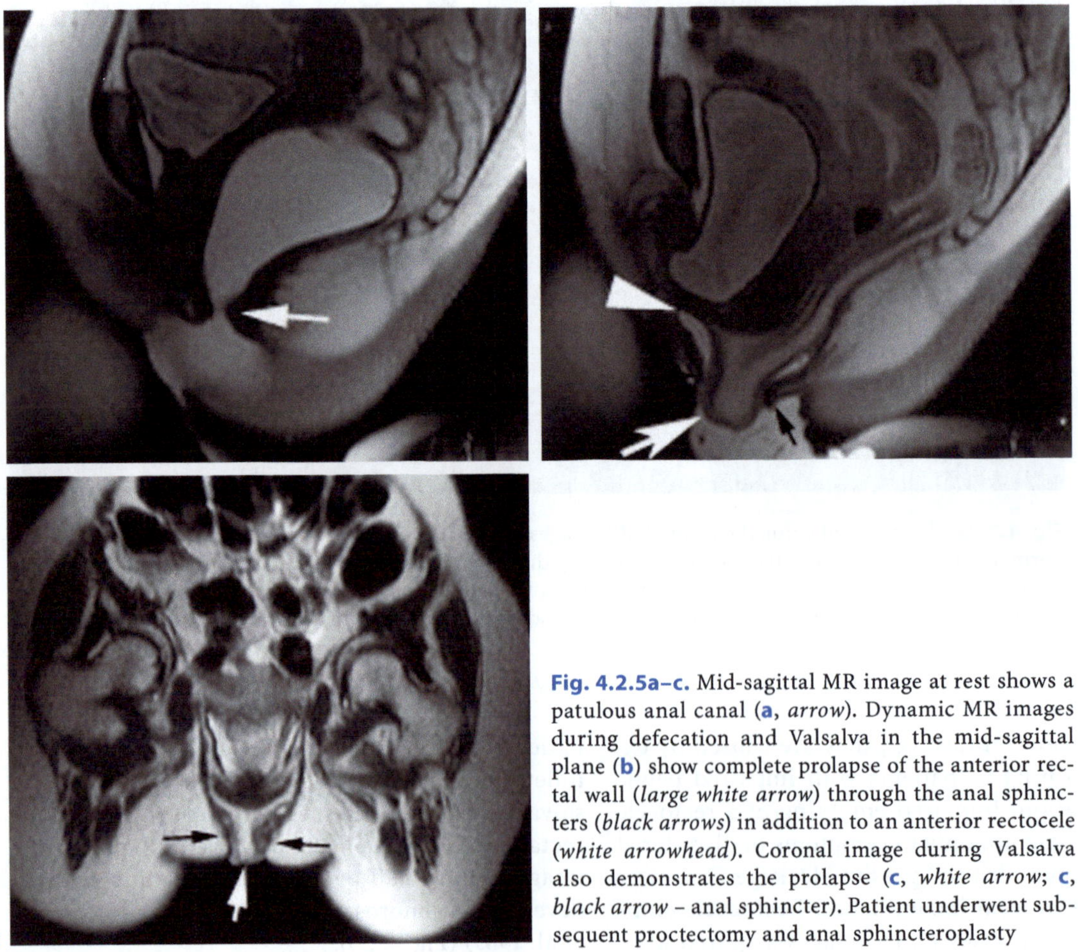

a b c

Fig. 4.2.5a–c. Mid-sagittal MR image at rest shows a patulous anal canal (**a**, *arrow*). Dynamic MR images during defecation and Valsalva in the mid-sagittal plane (**b**) show complete prolapse of the anterior rectal wall (*large white arrow*) through the anal sphincters (*black arrows*) in addition to an anterior rectocele (*white arrowhead*). Coronal image during Valsalva also demonstrates the prolapse (**c**, *white arrow*; **c**, *black arrow* – anal sphincter). Patient underwent subsequent proctectomy and anal sphincteroplasty

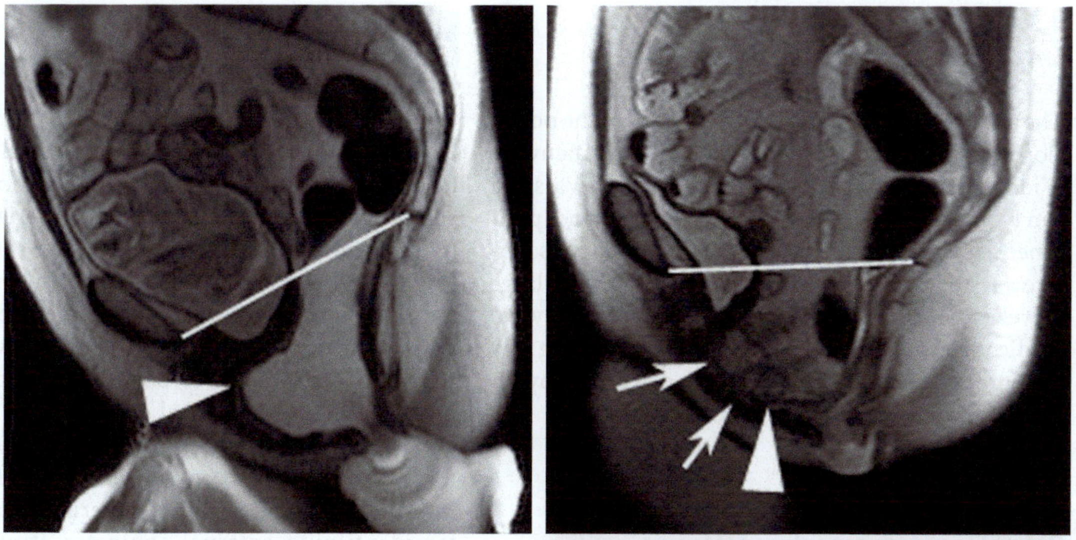

a b

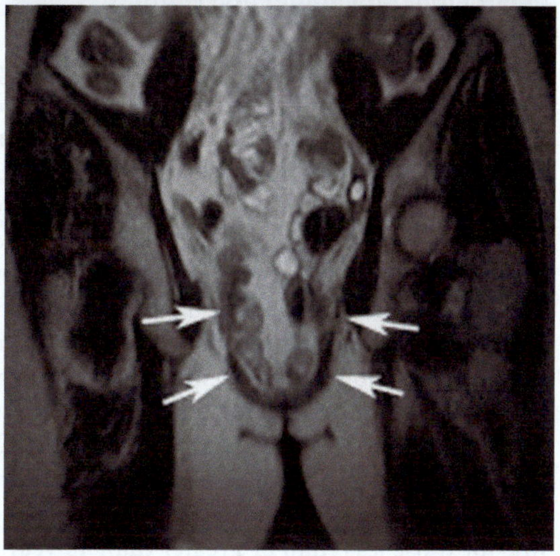

c

Fig. 4.2.6a–c. Dynamic MR imaging during defecation shows a 2.8-cm anterior rectocele (*arrowhead*, **a**) and decent of the anorectal junction to 6.7 cm below the pubococcygeal line, but no other findings. After rectal and bladder emptying, a large enterocele (*arrows*, **b** and **c**) is observed during Valsalva, in addition to the excessive descent and anterior rectocele seen previously (*arrowhead*, **b**)

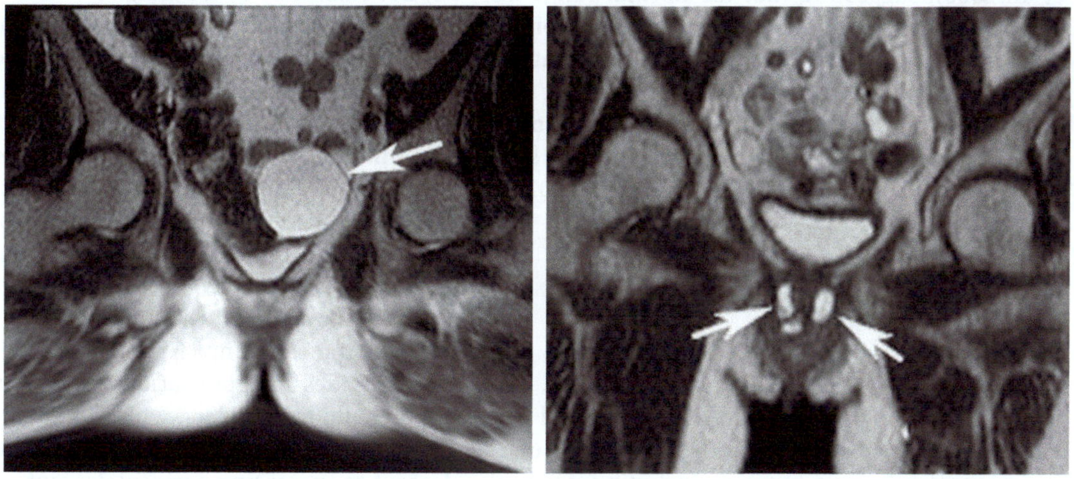

a b

Fig. 4.2.7a,b. A serous cystadenoma (**a**, *arrow*) and urethral diverticulm (**b**, *arrows*) in different patients, both of which were discovered incidentally at dynamic MR imaging in patients with pelvic floor disorders

4.2.4.5
Enteroceles and Peritoneoceles

The anterior rectum is normally opposed to the posterior vaginal wall throughout pelvic floor maneuvers. Widening of this space during defecation or Valsalva can be caused by descent of peritoneal fat alone (peritoneocele), peritoneal fat with small bowel loops (enterocele; Fig. 4.2.6) and/or peritoneal fat with large bowel (sigmoidocele or cecocele; Fig. 4.2.1). Several studies have suggested that dynamic MR imaging may be more sensitive than fluoroscopic defecography for detecting enteroceles (Lienemann et al. 1997).

4.2.4.6
Pelvic Floor Movement and Hernias

Movement of the anorectal junction during the squeeze maneuver has already been explained. Similar to anorectal angle measurement, various institutions have reported a variety of values for abnormal pelvic floor descent (measured between the pubococcygeal line and the anorectal junction at simulated defecation or Valsalva), largely owing to differences in technique and patient populations. Most radiologists employ a measurement of more than 2.5 cm below the pubococcygeal line at rest or greater than 3 cm of descent during maximum strain at MR for abnormal perineal descent (Goh et al. 2000). However, in asymptomatic subjects, anorectal descent to 4.6 and 5.5 cm below the pubococcygeal line for those less than or greater than 40 years old, respectively, has been observed at MR imaging (Fox et al. 2006), suggesting that the normal range for pelvic floor descent may be much higher than previously anticipated in the asymptomatic population. Coronal imaging during Valsalva at dynamic MR should also be used to detect hernias and eventrations in the levator ani muscle, which cannot be seen at traditional fluoroscopy (Kaufman et al. 2001).

4.2.4.7
Incidental Findings

HASTE and true-FISP imaging can, of course, display pelvic pathologies beyond the rectum and pelvic organ prolapse, most typically ovarian and uterine masses/pathology, but also including urethral diverticula, hydroureter, etc. (Comiter et al. 1999) (Fig. 4.2.7).

4.2.5
Patterns of Disease

Although imaging generally reveals distinct patterns in patients with fecal incontinence and defecatory disorders, there is some overlap because these conditions may coexist in the same patient (Fig. 4.2.8) (Bharucha et al. 2005). Anal sphincter and puborectalis injury (as manifested by tears, marked focal thickening or atrophy), which may be partly attributable to obstetric trauma, are frequently observed in fecal incontinence (Fig. 4.2.8 and 4.2.9) (Bharucha et al. 2005). While endoanal ultrasound and MRI are comparable for imaging the internal sphincter, MRI is superior to ultrasound for identifying external sphincter atrophy, which may be severe in up to one-fifth of incontinent patients and uncommon in asymptomatic controls (Bharucha et al. 2005; Terra et al. 2006). Anal sphincter injury is associated with sphincter weakness measured by manometry, i.e., reduced resting and squeeze pressures, reflecting internal and external sphincter weakness, respectively (Bharucha et al. 2005). Moreover, dynamic MR imaging often reveals a patulous anal canal, filled by rectal contrast, indicative of reduced anal resting pressure and diminished movement of the anorectal junction from rest to squeeze, indicative of impaired voluntary contraction (Fig. 4.2.9). Finally, anorectal structure and motion may appear normal, underscoring the contribution of other dysfunctions to fecal incontinence (e.g., diminished rectal capacity, altered rectal sensitivity and disordered bowel habits) not examined by imaging.

Patients with obstructive defecation may exhibit signs of pelvic floor dysynergia or paradoxical contraction of the external anal sphincter/puborectalis/pelvic floor while attempting to defecate (Fig. 4.2.4). Dynamic pelvic floor imaging can demonstrate a variety of findings in such patients, including reduced anorectal angle change during defecation (Bharucha et al. 2005) (Fig. 4.2.8), rectoceles and increased perineal descent in some patients (Bharucha et al. 2005), and bulging of the levator plate during straining (Healy et al. 1997). Indeed, MRI provides an appreciation of the natural history of pelvic floor disorders, which in some patients is characterized by a transition from reduced perineal descent to increasing perineal descent as the pelvic floor becomes weaker, perhaps in part due to excessive straining during defecation. The descending

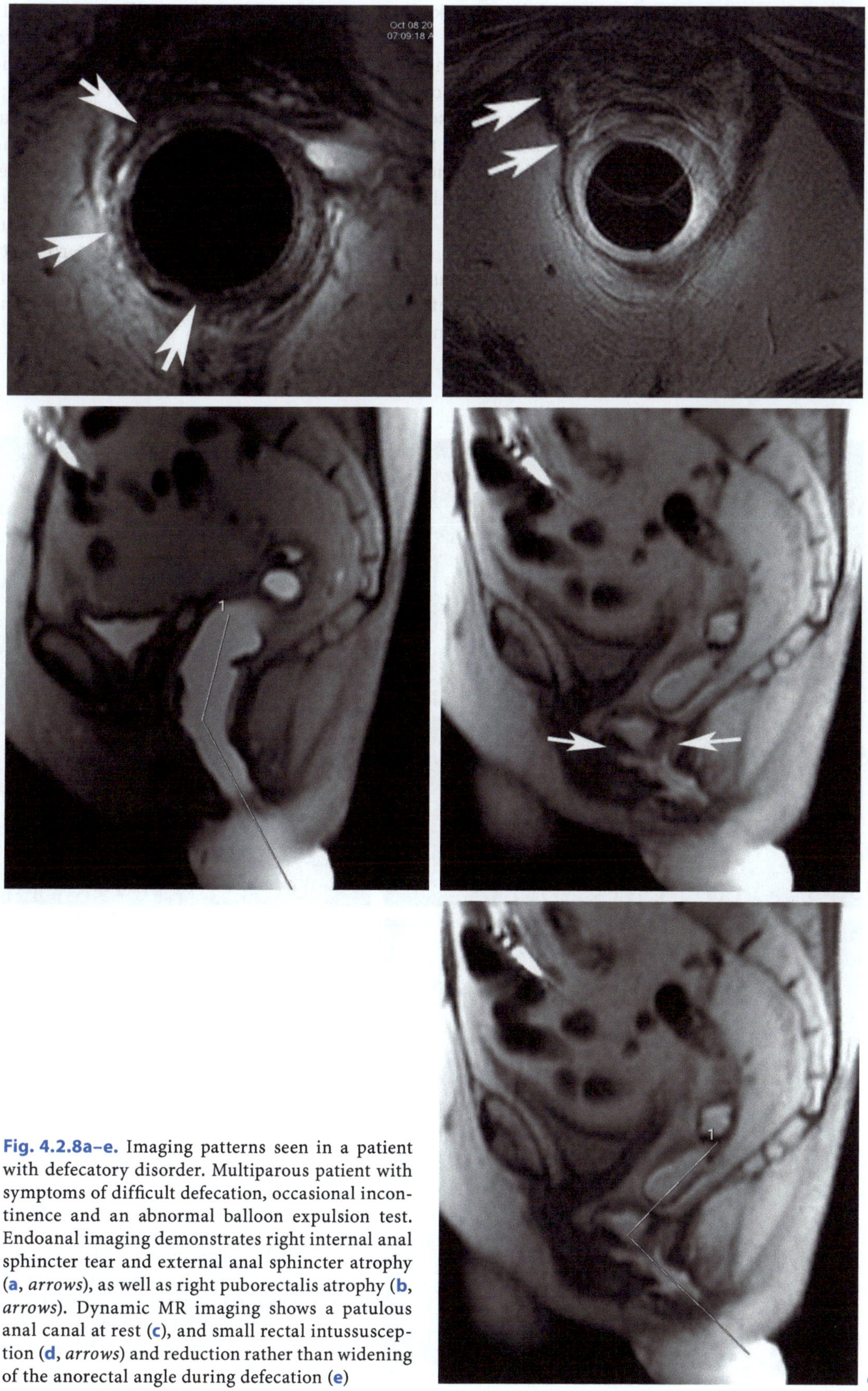

Fig. 4.2.8a–e. Imaging patterns seen in a patient with defecatory disorder. Multiparous patient with symptoms of difficult defecation, occasional incontinence and an abnormal balloon expulsion test. Endoanal imaging demonstrates right internal anal sphincter tear and external anal sphincter atrophy (**a**, *arrows*), as well as right puborectalis atrophy (**b**, *arrows*). Dynamic MR imaging shows a patulous anal canal at rest (**c**), and small rectal intussusception (**d**, *arrows*) and reduction rather than widening of the anorectal angle during defecation (**e**)

perineum syndrome is characterized by markedly abnormal perineal descent, which over time may cause a pudendal neuropathy, and lead to incontinence. In addition to impaired anorectal motion during defecation, defecatory disorders are also associated with impaired anorectal and pelvic floor motion during squeeze (i.e., when subjects contract their pelvic floor muscles), reflecting generalized pelvic floor dysfunction.

The role of imaging in anorectal disorders continues to evolve. While imaging findings are useful for understanding the pathophysiology of defecatory disorders and fecal incontinence, their impact on guiding management is unclear and a subject of debate, partly because there is a limited selection of therapeutic and particularly surgical options for these disorders (Bharucha 2006; Rao 2006; Wald 2006). For example, the role of anal sphincteroplasty in patients with anal sphincter defects presenting with fecal incontinence several decades after vaginal delivery is unclear, because although 85% of patients report improved continence in the short term after anal sphincteroplasty, full continence is maintained in only 28% at 40 months and in 11–14% at 60 months (Cheung and Wald 2004).

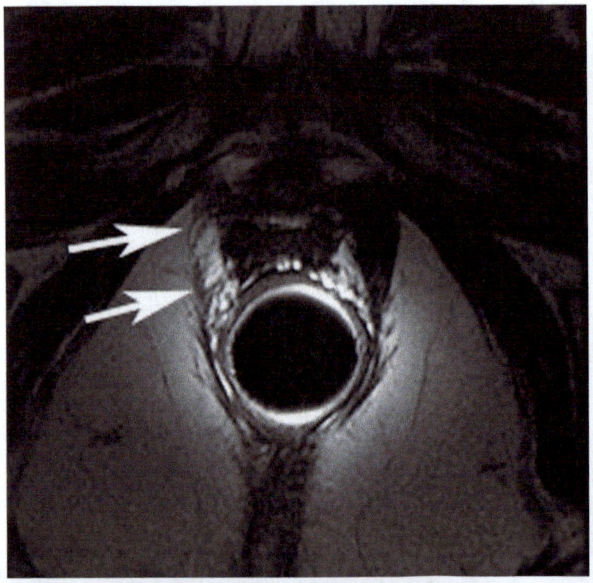
a

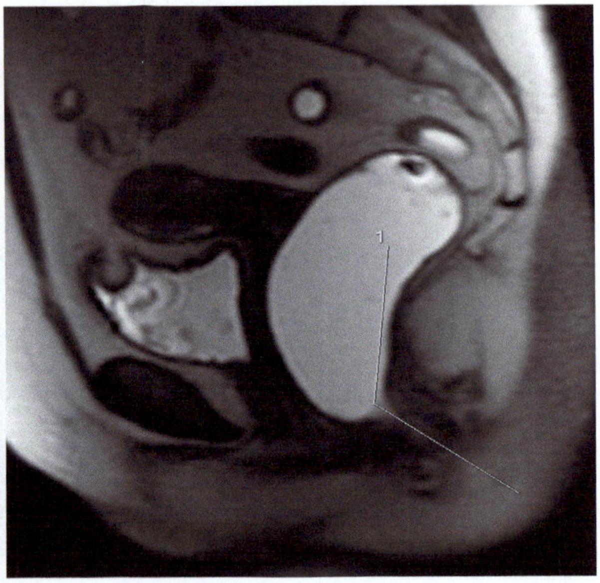
b

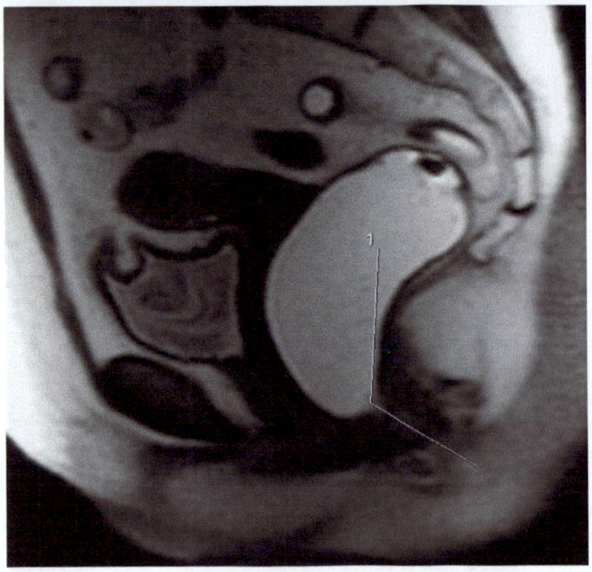
c

Fig. 4.2.9a–c. Imaging patterns in patients with fecal incontinence. Patient with symptoms of fecal incontinence had marked right puborectalis atrophy during static endoanal imaging (**a**, *arrows*). Dynamic imaging in the mid-sagittal planes demonstrated poor puborectalis function, with minimal lift of the anorectal junction and no change in the anorectal angle from rest (**b**, anorectal angle = 117) to squeeze (**c**, anorectal angle = 117)

In most patients, anal manometry and an abnormal balloon expulsion test suffice to confirm the diagnosis of an evacuation disorder. However, imaging is useful when routine diagnostic tests (e.g., anorectal manometry and rectal balloon expulsion) do not confirm the clinical suspicion of a rectal evacuation disorder, for example in patients who do not have florid perineal descent (i.e., perineal ballooning) on physical examination. A majority of these patients are typically diagnosed by abnormal balloon expulsion tests, but some are not, and these patients tend to have abnormal perineal descent at MR (Healy et al. 1997). Dynamic MRI also demonstrates generalized pelvic organ prolapse (e.g., cystocoele), which is associated with increased perineal descent and may require surgical correction. Finally, reviewing dynamic MR images with physicians provides patients with an improved appreciation of the disorder and management thereof. Finally, many patients present with mixed symptoms and imaging findings common to both fecal incontinence and obstructive defecation (Fig. 4.2.8).

4.2.6 Performance and Limitations of MR

Dynamic MR imaging is generally performed in the supine position, as opposed to the upright position used during fluoroscopic defecography. Several investigators have examined the potential impact of performing dynamic exams in the supine position. In general, variations in pelvic floor descent and pelvic organ prolapse are similarly observed at supine MR compared to upright MR or fluoroscopy (Lienemann et al. 1997; Kelvin et al. 2000; Fielding et al. 1998), although these findings have not been universal (Vanbeckevoort et al. 1999). Advantages of MR include increased visualization of the bladder, urethra and uterus without the time-consuming need for instillation of contrast in the anterior and middle pelvic compartments (Comiter et al. 1999), the potential for concomitant anatomic evaluation of the anal sphincters (Bharucha et al. 2005) and direct visualization of the pelvic floor and levator hernias (Kaufman et al. 2001).

The primary limitation of dynamic MR in the evaluation of pelvic floor disorders is temporal resolution and supine positioning. Subtle or transitory intussusception or prolapse may be missed or minimized under these imaging conditions (Kaufman et al. 2001). Moreover, in contrast to pelvic organ prolapse, rectal prolapse is better seen at fluoroscopy given the superimposition of the entire rectal lumen (as opposed to just a cross-section of it). If symptoms of prolapse are present and MR is negative, we typically recommend fluoroscopic defecography.

4.2.7 Conclusion

Defecation and continence are complex, multifactorial events for which a large variety of tests contribute to a holistic picture for any individual patient. Apart from detailed history and physical examination, patients typically undergo a variety of tests, which may include anorectal manometry, anatomic imaging of the anal sphincters (at MR or ultrasound), colonic motility testing, anal sphincter EMG and colonoscopy (to exclude structural lesions). Dynamic MR imaging of the pelvic floor has become a recognized adjunctive, problem-solving test in the evaluation of patients with defecatory disorders and is increasingly utilized in a routine fashion to affect management decisions (Hetzer et al. 2006). In the future we anticipate that MR imaging of the pelvic floor will continue evolve as a diagnostic tool in patients with defecatory disorders, providing additional functional information beyond pelvic floor movement and sphincter anatomy (Bharucha and Fletcher 2007). Moreover, functional information from dynamic MR will influence and inform the understanding the pathophysiology and unique disease subtypes in fecal incontinence and obstructive defecation (Bharucha et al. 2005; Deutekom et al. 2007).

References

Barnett JL, Hasler WL, Camilleri M (1999) American Gastroenterological Association medical position statement on anorectal testing techniques. American Gastroenterological Association. Gastroenterology 116:732–760

Bartram CI, Turnbull GK, Lennard-Jones JE (1988) Evacuation proctography: an investigation of rectal expulsion in 20 subjects without defecatory disturbance. Gastrointest Radiol 13:72–80

Bharucha AE (2006) Pro: Anorectal testing is useful in fecal incontinence. Am J Gastroenterol 101:2679–2681

Bharucha AE, Fletcher JG (2007) Recent advances in assessing anorectal structure and functions. Gastroenterology 133:1069–1074

Bharucha AE, Fletcher JG, Harper CM et al (2005) Relationship between symptoms and disordered continence mechanisms in women with idiopathic faecal incontinence. Gut 54:546–555

Bharucha AE, Fletcher JG, Seide B et al (2005) Phenotypic variation in functional disorders of defecation. Gastroenterology 128:1199–1210

Busse RF, Riederer SJ, Fletcher JG et al (2000) Interactive fast spin-echo imaging. Magn Reson Med 44:339–348

Cheung O, Wald A (2004) Review article: the management of pelvic floor disorders. Aliment Pharmacol Ther 19:481–495

Christensen LL, Djurhuus JC, Constantinou CE (1995) Imaging of pelvic floor contractions using MRI. Neurourol Urodyn 14:209–216

Comiter CV, Vasavada SP, Barbaric ZL et al (1999) Grading pelvic prolapse and pelvic floor relaxation using dynamic magnetic resonance imaging. Urology 54:454–457

Deutekom M, Dobben AC, Terra MP et al (2007) Clinical presentation of fecal incontinence and anorectal function: what is the relationship? Am J Gastroenterol 102:351–361

Fielding JR, Griffiths DJ, Versi E et al (1998) MR imaging of pelvic floor continence mechanisms in the supine and sitting positions. AJR Am J Roentgenol 171:1607–1610

Fletcher JG, Busse RF, Riederer SJ et al (2003) Magnetic resonance imaging of anatomic and dynamic defects of the pelvic floor in defecatory disorders. Am J Gastroenterol 98:399–411

Fox JC, Fletcher JG, Zinsmeister AR et al (2006) Effect of aging on anorectal and pelvic floor functions in females. Dis Colon Rectum 49:1726–1735

Goh V, Halligan S, Kaplan G et al (2000) Dynamic MR imaging of the pelvic floor in asymptomatic subjects. AJR Am J Roentgenol 174:661–666

Greenberg T, Kelvin FM, Maglinte DD (2001) Barium trapping in rectoceles: are we trapped by the wrong definition? Abdom Imaging 26:587–590

Gufler H, Laubenberger J, DeGregorio G et al (1999) Pelvic floor descent: dynamic MR imaging using a half-Fourier RARE sequence. J Magn Reson Imaging 9:378–383

Halligan S, Bartram CI, Park HJ et al (1995) Proctographic features of anismus. Radiology 197:679–682

Healy JC, Halligan S, Reznek RH et al (1997) Patterns of prolapse in women with symptoms of pelvic floor weakness: assessment with MR imaging. Radiology 203:77–81

Healy JC, Halligan S, Reznek RH et al (1997) Magnetic resonance imaging of the pelvic floor in patients with obstructed defaecation. Br J Surg 84:1555–1558

Hetzer FH, Andreisek G, Tsagari C et al (2006) MR defecography in patients with fecal incontinence: imaging findings and their effect on surgical management. Radiology 240:449–457

Hjartardottir S, Nilsson J, Petersen C et al (1997) The female pelvic floor: a dome – not a basin. Acta Obstet Gynecol Scand 76:567–571

Hussain SM, Stoker J, Lameris JS (1995) Anal sphincter complex: endoanal MR imaging of normal anatomy. Radiology 197:671–677

Kaufman HS, Buller JL, Thompson JR et al (2001) Dynamic pelvic magnetic resonance imaging and cystocolpoproctography alter surgical management of pelvic floor disorders. Dis Colon Rectum 44:1575–1583; discussion 1583–1584

Kelvin FM, Maglinte DD, Hale DS et al (2000) Female pelvic organ prolapse: a comparison of triphasic dynamic MR imaging and triphasic fluoroscopic cystocolpoproctography. AJR Am J Roentgenol 174:81–88

Lienemann A, Anthuber C, Baron A et al (1997) Dynamic MR colpocystorectography assessing pelvic-floor descent. Eur Radiol 7:1309–1317

Macura KJ GR, Bluemke DA (2006) MR imaging of the female urethra and supporting ligaments in assessment of urinary incontinence: spectrum of abnormalities. Radiographics 26:1135–1149

Maglinte DD, Kelvin FM, Fitzgerald K et al (1999) Association of compartment defects in pelvic floor dysfunction. AJR Am J Roentgenol 172:439–444

Ozasa H, Mori T, Togashi K (1992) Study of uterine prolapse by magnetic resonance imaging: topographical changes involving the levator ani muscle and the vagina. Gynecol Obstet Invest 34:43–48

Pannu HK, Kaufman HS, Cundiff GW et al (2000) Dynamic MR imaging of pelvic organ prolapse: spectrum of abnormalities. Radiographics 20:1567–1582

Rao SS (2006) A balancing view: Fecal incontinence: test or treat empirically-which strategy is best? Am J Gastroenterol 101:2683–2684

Shorvon PJ, McHugh S, Diamant NE et al (1989) Defecography in normal volunteers: results and implications. Gut 30:1737–1749

Stoker J, Rociu E (1999) Endoluminal MR imaging of diseases of the anus and rectum. Semin Ultrasound CT MR 20:47–55

Stoker J, Halligan S, Bartram CI (2001) Pelvic floor imaging. Radiology 218:621–641

Strohbehn K, Ellis JH, Strohbehn JA et al (1996) Magnetic resonance imaging of the levator ani with anatomic correlation. Obstet Gynecol 87:277–285

Strohbehn K, Quint LE, Prince MR et al (1996) Magnetic resonance imaging anatomy of the female urethra: a direct histologic comparison. Obstet Gynecol 88:750–756

Tan IL, Stoker J, Zwamborn AW et al (1998) Female pelvic floor: endovaginal MR imaging of normal anatomy. Radiology 206:777–783

Terra MP, Beets-Tan RG, van der Hulst VP et al (2006) MRI in evaluating atrophy of the external anal sphincter in patients with fecal incontinence. AJR Am J Roentgenol 187:991–999

Terra MP, Deutekom M, Beets-Tan RG et al (2006) Relationship between external anal sphincter atrophy at endoanal magnetic resonance imaging and clinical, functional, and anatomic characteristics in patients with fecal incontinence. Dis Colon Rectum 49:668–678

Tunn R, DeLancey JO, Howard D et al (1999) MR imaging of levator ani muscle recovery following vaginal delivery. Int Urogynecol J Pelvic Floor Dysfunct 10:300–307

Vanbeckevoort D, Van Hoe L, Oyen R et al (1999) Pelvic floor descent in females: comparative study of colpocystodefecography and dynamic fast MR imaging. J Magn Reson Imaging 9:373–377

Wald A (2006) Con: Anorectal manometry and imaging are not necessary in patients with fecal incontinence. Am J Gastroenterol 101:2681–2683

4.3 MRI of the Levator Ani Muscle

Wolfgang H. Umek and John O. L. DeLancey

CONTENTS

4.3.1 Introduction

One suggested rationale for using MR imaging to evaluate urinary incontinence and pelvic floor dysfunction derives from the observation that patients might present with symptoms isolated to one pelvic compartment, but may have concomitant defects in other compartments (Maglinte et al. 1999). Accurate diagnosis of coexisting abnormalities is essential in planning reconstructive pelvic floor and anti-incontinence surgery. Some authors have suggested that surgical failures result from the lack of thorough preoperative diagnosis and inadequate staging of pelvic floor dysfunction (Safir et al. 1999).

W. H. Umek, MD
Associate Professor, Department of Obstetrics and Gynecology, Medical University Vienna, Waehringer Guertel 18, 1090 Vienna, Austria
J. O. L. DeLancey, MD
Norman F. Miller Professor of Gynecology, L4000 Women's Hospital, University of Michigan, 1500 E. Medical Center Drive, Ann Arbor, MI 48109-0276, USA

Most diagnoses of pelvic floor prolapse are still made on detailed physical exam, but some studies have suggested the use of MRI in the diagnosis of pelvic floor dysfunction. This suggestion is based on the assumption that the pelvic exam has poor sensitivity and specificity in diagnosing certain forms of pelvic floor prolapse (Kelvin et al. 1997; 1999; Stovall et al. 2000). Whether or not this will improve surgical outcomes has not been investigated yet.

There is another reason for the increasing use of MR imaging in women with pelvic floor disorders: MR imaging can identify specific structural abnormalities that are associated with pelvic organ prolapse (DeLancey et al. 2007). Half of the women with prolapse have major morphologic defects in the levator ani muscles. Studies have reported a link between muscle impairment and operative failure after surgery for pelvic organ prolapse (Vakili et al. 2005).

A defective levator ani muscle is highly associated with pelvic floor dysfunction (Morgan et al. 2007; Shafik et al. 2003; Miller et al. 2004) and specifically pelvic organ prolapse where women with prolapse are shown to have a 40% lower force generated during a pelvic muscle contraction than women without prolapse (DeLancey et al. 2007). In addition, soft tissue imaging has clarified the cause of these defects.

Recent studies have identified vaginal birth as the source of levator ani muscle defects (DeLancey et al. 2003; Kearney et al. 2006; Dietz et al. 2005). There are also indications of neural damage during vaginal delivery (Allen et al. 1990). But the question of how much age-related changes, direct traumata to the muscle (avulsion, tearing), neurological damage, and secondary muscle atrophy contribute to levator ani defects is still not answered. A full understanding of the relationship between neural abnormalities and visible muscle defects is not yet available. This and several other questions about the relation of pelvic organ prolapse and the female pelvic floor are still unanswered, but the ability to objectively examine structural abnormalities in MR images is a promising development in understanding pelvic floor disorders. In the future, MR imaging may be used to detect these abnormalities so that different operative approaches can be used in women with high or low risk for operative failure.

4.3.2 MRI Appearance of the Normal Levator Ani Muscles

The term "pelvic floor" is generally used in two ways. In a broad sense, it refers to all structures that support and position the pelvic organs. These "pelvic floor" structures are: the perineal membrane, the levator ani muscles, and the connective tissue. In a restricted sense, "pelvic floor" refers to the group of muscles known collectively as levator ani muscles. We will use the term "levator ani" to describe these muscles and the term "pelvic floor" in its broader sense for the collection of supportive structures, recognizing that others use this term differently.

MR imaging has been used to study the normal female pelvic floor anatomy, the anatomy in symptomatic patients, and the anatomy of the aging female. The normal appearance of the levator ani muscle in asymptomatic, nulliparous women is well established. Side-by-side comparison of cadaver cross sections and corresponding MR images clarified the appearance of levator ani muscle anatomy (Strohbehn et al. 1996). Recent advances in MR imaging have enabled us to examine the levator ani muscles in detail in vivo in 2D (Margulies et al. 2006) and 3D images (Hoyte et al 2001).

There are five levator ani muscle subdivisions (Figs. 4.3.1 and 4.3.2):

1. the pubovisceral muscle with its components: pubovaginal, puboperineal, and puboanal muscle,
2. the puborectal muscle,
3. the iliococcygeus muscle.

The coccygeus muscle connects the coccyx to the ischial spine. Although the coccygeus muscle is contiguous with the levator ani muscle, it is generally considered separately and not included in the term "levator ani."

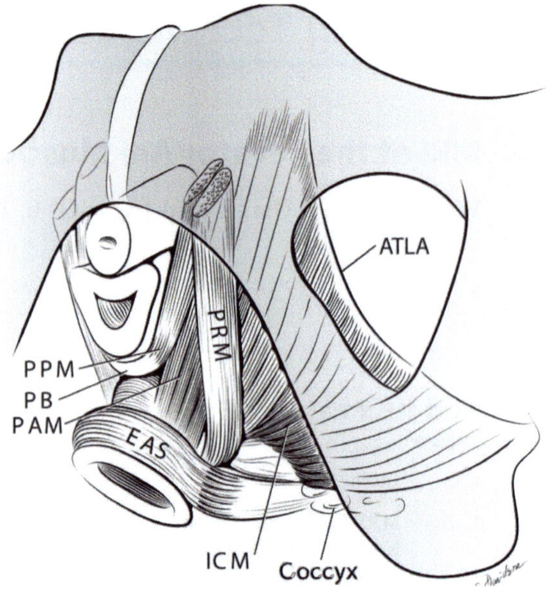

Fig. 4.3.1. Schematic view of the levator ani muscles seen from caudal left. Vulvar structures and perineal membrane have been removed showing: arcus tendineus levator ani behind the obturator foramen (*ATLA*), external anal sphincter (*EAS*), puboanal muscle (*PAM*), perineal body (*PB*) uniting the two ends of the puboperineal muscle (*PPM*), iliococcygeal muscle (*ICM*), and puborectal muscle (*PRM*). Note that the urethra and vagina have been cut just above the hymenal ring (from Kearney et al. 2004; © DeLancey 2003 with permission)

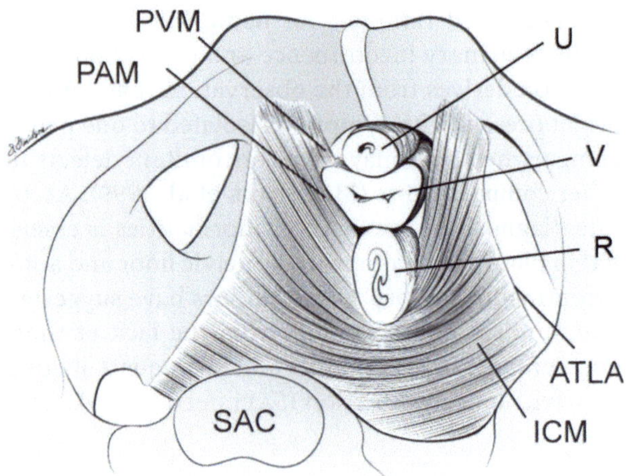

Fig. 4.3.2. The levator ani muscle seen from cranial right, looking over the sacral promontory (*SAC*) into the pelvis. The urethra (*U*), vagina (*V*), and rectum (*R*) have been cut just above the pelvic floor. Visible are: the pubovaginal muscle (*PVM*), puboanal muscle (*PAM*), arcus tendineus levator ani (*ATLA*), and iliococcygeal muscle (*ICM*) (from Kearney et al. 2004; © DeLancey 2003 with permission)

The puboviscerral muscle has previously been called the pubococcygeal muscle (Terminologia Anatomica 1998), but we favor Lawson's term "puboviscerral" (Lawson 1974), because it describes the origin and insertion accurately. A discussion of this topic was considered in depth in a recent article (Kearney et al. 2004). Our use of terminology is based on this analysis.

Each subdivision is defined by the muscle origin from and insertion to another structure. The suggested terms for these subdivisions, along with their origin/insertion points and their function, are listed in Table 43.1. The subdivisions of the levator ani muscle are visible on MRI scans, each with distinct morphology and characteristic features. Criteria for designation of a muscle subdivision on MRI are the clear and consistent visibility as a separate structure between adjacent structures. Additional visible characteristics are: fiber direction, and muscle origin and insertion.

Figure 4.3.3 shows a computer model of the levator ani subdivisions. This model helps to identify and understand the form, shape, and origin/insertion of each of the five levator ani subdivisions in Figures 4.3.4, 4.3.5, and 4.3.6.

4.3.2.1 Pubovisceral Muscle

The pubovisceral muscle arises from the pubic bone and passes beside the pelvic organs. It consists of subdivisions that originate from the pubic bone and insert to the perineal body (puboperineal part), to the vaginal wall (pubovaginal part), and to the anal canal and skin (puboanal part). The pubovisceral muscle elevates the perineal body, the vagina, and the anus.

In Figure 4.3.4, axial planes provide a clear view of the pubovisceral muscle and its subdivisions. The puboperineal, pubovaginal, and puboanal muscles originate together from the inner surface of the pubic bone (e.g., panels 0.0, +0.5) and course medial to the puborectal muscle next to the vagina. The pubovisceral subdivisions cannot be distinguished at their origin from the pubic bone, but the different insertion points can be distinguished. The attachment of the pubovaginal muscle to the right vaginal wall is seen in panel 0.0. The puboperineal muscle can be seen where it inserts into the perineal body (e.g., panels −2.0, −2.5). The puboanal muscle can be seen where it inserts into the intersphincteric space (e.g., panel +1.0).

Figure 4.3.5 shows the coronal plane in which the pubovisceral muscle lies perpendicular to the scan plane. The pubovaginal attachment is again identified as medial fusion of the muscle with the vaginal wall (e.g., panel −2.0). It is difficult to distinguish between the pubovisceral and the puborectal muscles in this orientation (e.g., panels −1.5 to −4.0) because muscle fibers are contiguous and without visible separation; pubovisceral and puborectal muscle are seen as a single body of muscle lateral to the vagina. Similarly, the subdivisions composing the pubovisceral muscle cannot be separated in the coronal MRI cross sections.

Table 4.3.1. Overview of the nomenclature and functional anatomy of the levator ani subdivisions (from Kearney 2004)

Terminologia Anatomica		Origin from	Insertion to	Function
Pubococcygeal muscle (we favour "pubovisceral")				
Subdivisions	Puboperineal muscle	Pubic bone	Perineal body	Elevates perineal body towards pubic bone
	Pubovaginal muscle	Pubic bone	Vaginal wall at the level of the mid-urethra	Elevates vagina towards pubic bone at the level of mid-urethra
	Puboanal muscle	Pubic bone	Intersphincteric groove between internal and external anal sphincter	Elevates the anus and its attached ano-derm towards the pubic bone
Puborectal muscle		Pubic bone	Forms sling dorsal to the rectum	Forms the anorectal angle and closes the urogenital hiatus
Iliococcygeal muscle		Tendinous arch of the levator ani	The two sides fuse in the iliococcygeal raphé	Spans the pelvic canal, forms a supportive diaphragm

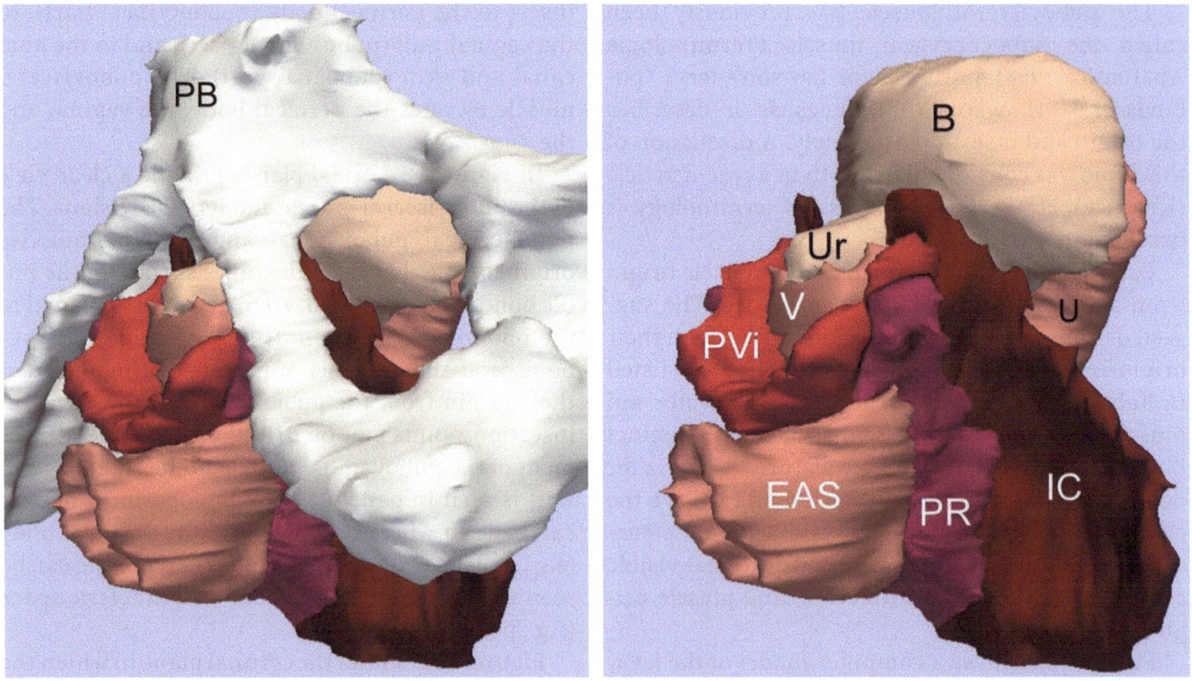

a b

Fig. 4.3.3. a Three-dimensional model of levator ani subdivisions including the pubic bone (*PB*) and pelvic viscera, left three-quarter view from caudal. This model was created by using the magnetic resonance images shown in Figures 4.3.4, 4.3.5 and 4.3.6. The pubovaginal, puboperineal, and puboanal muscles are all combined into a single structure: the pubovisceral muscle (*PVi*). **b** The same model without the pubic bone. *B*, bladder; *Ur*, urethra; *V*, vagina; *U*, uterus; *EAS*, external anal sphincter; *PR*, puborectal muscle; *IC*, iliococcygeus muscle (from Margulies et al. 2006; © DeLancey 2006 with permission)

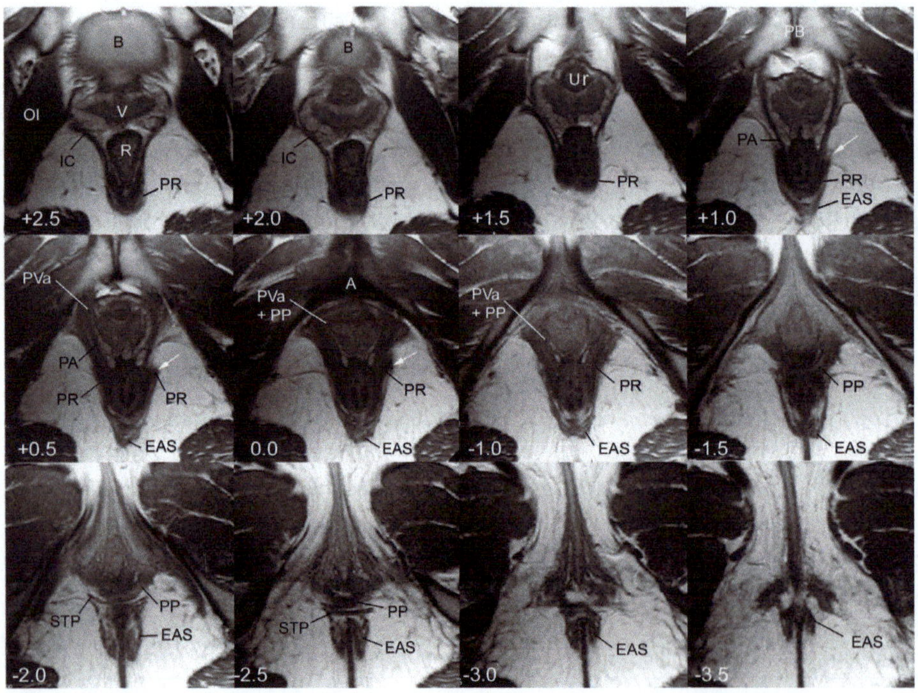

Fig. 4.3.4. Axial scan of a 25-year-old nullipara showing subdivisions of the levator ani muscle. Levels of single scan planes in centimeters relative to the arcuate pubic ligament (*A*) are indicated in *lower left corner* with positive numbers cranial to the ligament and negative numbers caudal. *B*, bladder; *V*, vagina; *R*, rectum; *PR*, puborectalis muscle; *OI*, obturator internus muscle; *IC*, iliococcygeal muscle; *Ur*, urethra; *EAS*, external anal sphincter; *PVa*, pubovaginal attachment; *PA*, puboanal muscle; *PP*, puboperineal muscle; *STP*, superficial transverse perineal muscle. *White arrows* indicate puborectal muscle progression (from Margulies et al. 2006; © DeLancey 2006 with permission)

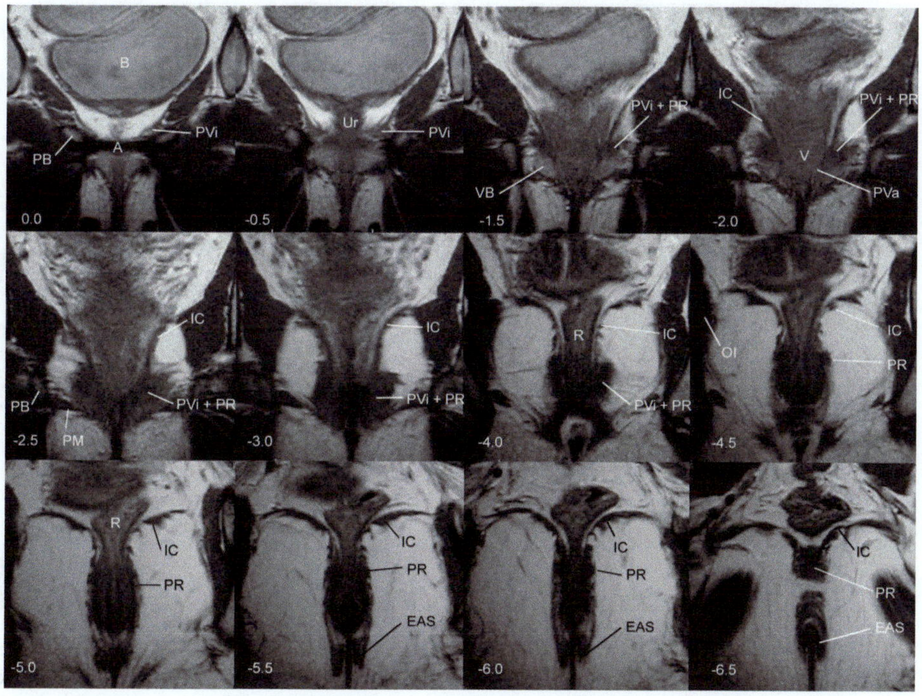

Fig.4.3.5. Coronal scans of the same subject depicted in Figs. 4.3.4 and 4.3.6. Levels of single scan planes in centimeters relative to the arcuate pubic ligament *A*) are indicated in the lower left corner with negative numbers dorsal to the ligament. Note that scans –1.0 and –3.5 have been omitted so that other scans could be included. *B*, bladder; *V*, vagina; *PB*, pubic bone; *PVi*, pubovisceral muscle; *VB*, vestibular bulb; *R*, rectum; *PR*, puborectalis muscle; *OI*, obturator internus muscle; *IC*, iliococcygeal muscle; *Ur*, urethra; *EAS*, external anal sphincter; *PVa*, pubovaginal attachment (from Margulies et al. 2006; © DeLancey 2006 with permission)

The sagittal plane (Fig. 4.3.6) offers the advantage of being parallel to the pubovisceral and puborectal muscle fiber directions, allowing the fiber direction to be seen. There is a clear view of the puboperineal portion, just cephalad to the perineal membrane (e.g., panels R1.5 to R0.5). The puboanal fibers can be seen as they course to the upper level of the external anal sphincter (e.g., panels R2.0, R1.5), but the pubovaginal attachment cannot be seen in this orientation.

4.3.2.2 Puborectal Muscle

The puborectal muscle originates from the dorsal aspect of the pelvic bone lateral to the pubovisceral muscle and courses lateral to it (Fig. 4.3.4). It forms a sling behind the rectum (e.g., panels +2.5 to –1.0) and is distinct from the pubovisceral muscle. The puborectal muscle helps create an angulation in the rectum, the ano-rectal angle, and is part of the anal continence mechanism. Puborectal and puboperineal muscles have fiber directions oblique to the axial scan plane. For this reason the entire muscle loop is not visible in any single axial slice alone. On coronal scans the bulk of the muscle can be identified lateral to the pubovisceral muscle (see Fig. 4.3.5, panels –1.5 to –6.5). On sagittal scans even fiber direction and the puborectal muscle bulk behind the anorectal junction are well visible (Fig. 4.3.6).

4.3.2.3 Iliococcygeus Muscle

The iliococcygeal muscle originates from the arcus tendineus levatoris ani, a condensation of obturator internus muscle fascia (Fig. 4.3.4, panels +2.5 and +2.0). In more cranial slices (not shown), it can be seen passing around the rectum above the fibers of the puborectal muscle. The iliococcygeal muscle forms a supportive diaphragm that spans the posterior part of the pelvis. It can be well visualized on sagittal scans with its wing-like configuration (Fig. 4.3.6, panels R2.5 through R1.0). The coronal plane is optimal for viewing the iliococcygeus in the dorsal parts of the pelvis (Fig. 4.3.5, panels –4.0 to –6.5). It originates laterally from the arcus tendineus levator ani over the obturator internus muscle and inserts to the iliococcygeal raphé in the midline. Here it interdigitates with the other side and connects with the superior surface of the sacrum and coccyx. The sagittal images show the shelf-like orientation of the iliococcygeus muscle, which is referred to as the "levator plate" (Fig. 4.3.6, panels R2.5 to R1.0).

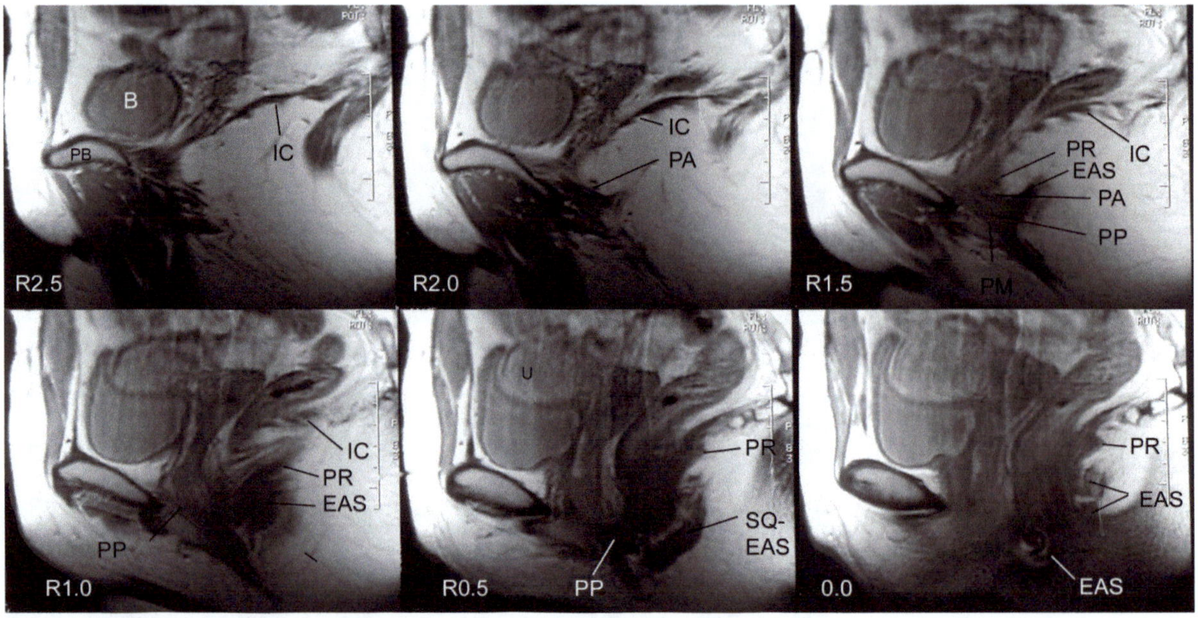

Fig. 4.3.6. Sagittal images of the right hemipelvis of the same subject depicted in Figures 4.3.4 and 4.3.5. Notations in the *lower left corner* of each panel indicate the distance of the scan plane in centimeters to the *right* of the midsagittal plane. *B*, bladder; *PB*; pubic bone; *IC*, iliococcygeal muscle; *PA*, puboanal muscle; *PR*, puborectal muscle; *EAS*, external anal sphincter; *PP*, puboperineal muscle; *PM*, perineal membrane; *SQ-EAS*, subcutaneous external anal sphincter (from Margulies et al. 2006; © DeLancey et al. 2006 with permission)

The levator ani muscle has a normal resting tone that closes the vagina in much the same way that the anal sphincters close the anal canal. There is a constant baseline activity that adjusts to the demands of increasing activity, for example, in the standing position when the loads on the muscle increase (Morgan et al. 2005). By holding the pelvic floor closed, the levator ani relieves the connective tissue supports from a portion of the load that they would otherwise need to carry. During voluntary pelvic muscle contractions, the levator musculature straightens and becomes more horizontal (Hjartardottir et al. 1997; Hugosson et al. 1991).

Each levator ani subdivision has its unique mechanical action. Injury to one component may have different mechanical effects than damage to another. For example, loss of the pubovaginal muscle would prevent elevation of the anterior vaginal wall (and urethra), while loss of the puborectal muscle would prevent kinking of the rectum in the postanal angle.

Like in other parts of the body, variation of muscle bulk can be observed on MRI (see Fig. 4.3.7). This is likely due to a combination of genetic factors and daily demands and exercise. The individual amount of muscle has implications for pelvic floor function and injury. A woman with a naturally bulky set of muscles may lose half of her muscle bulk due to injury or atrophy and still have the same amount of muscle as a woman with naturally delicate muscles. The consequences of these variations and damage remain to be determined.

4.3.3 Levator Ani Muscle and Pelvic Floor Dysfunction

Pelvic organ support is provided by the combined action of the levator ani muscles and the endopelvic fascia. The levator ani closes the urogenital hiatus. It creates a high pressure zone in the vagina (Guaderrama et al. 2005) similar to the high pressure zones created by the urethral and anal sphincter muscles. Together, the muscles and connective tissue must resist the downward forces that act on the pelvic floor by the superincumbent abdominal organs and the force from increases in abdominal

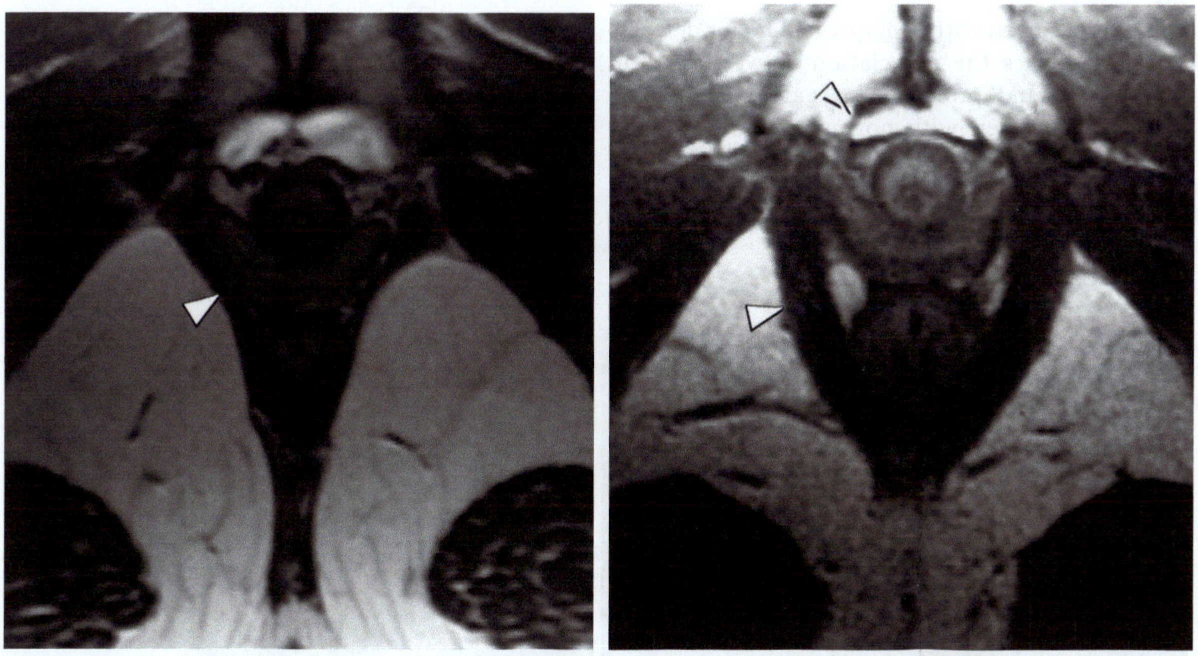

Fig. 4.3.7a,b. Variations in levator ani muscle thickness and configuration. Axial scans from two individuals are compared: **a** thin muscle (31-year-old nulliparous woman); **b** thicker muscle (36-year-old nulliparous woman). Note also that muscle is shaped like a "V" in **a** and more like a "U" in **b**. *Closed arrowhead*, right levator ani muscle; *open arrowhead*, insertion of arcus tendineus of fascia pelvis into pubic bone in **b** (from Tunn et al. 2003; © DeLancey 2003 with permission)

pressure during coughing, sneezing, or jumping. This normal load sharing between the adaptive action of the muscles and the energy-efficient action of static connective tissues is part of the load-bearing design of the pelvic floor (Morgan et al. 2005; Shafik et al. 2003).

When injury to one of these two components (muscles, connective tissue) occurs, the other must carry the increased demands placed on it. When the muscle is injured, the connective tissue is subjected to increased load (Chen et al. 2006). If the load exceeds the strength of the pelvic tissues, they may stretch or break, and prolapse may result. This forms a causal chain of events by which pelvic muscle injury may cause pelvic organ prolapse.

Levator ani damage was first reported in women with pelvic organ prolapse and described in detail in cadavers 100 years ago (Halban and Tandler 1907), and more recent work has demonstrated the importance of this observation (DeLancey et al. 2007).

In addition, there is accumulating evidence that surgery for pelvic organ prolapse has higher postoperative failure rates in women with levator ani muscle impairment. This has been assessed by biopsy (Hanzal et al. 1993) and muscle function testing (Vakili et al. 2005).

With the advent of modern imaging, we can directly see the pelvic floor muscles and their injuries. MRI can show us evidence of localized muscle injury (see Fig. 4.3.8) in an individual. It will be possible to better understand the relationship between injury to a specific part of the muscle and a certain female pelvic floor problem. Imaging has now demonstrated evidence of localized muscle loss, revealing a great variety of injury patterns in different women.

A simple scoring system to grade muscle defects has been shown to be reliable (Morgan et al. 2007). The scoring system uses grades: 0 = normal, 1 = mild defect (less than half of muscle bulk missing), 2 = moderate (more than half of muscle bulk missing), and 3 = severe (total or near total loss of muscle bulk). For examples, see Figure 4.3.9.

In a case-control study of 151 women with prolapse matched with 135 controls with normal pelvic organ support, it could be shown that women with prolapse are 3.4 times more likely to have a major levator ani defect than women with normal pelvic floor support (DeLancey et al. 2007). More than half of the women with prolapse had major defects. This establishes the association between levator impairment and prolapse. MILLER et al. (2004) studied 28 women with normal muscles and 17 women with complete bilateral loss of pubovisceral muscles. They found that women with intact muscles generated significantly higher urethral closure pressures than those without pubovisceral muscles (14 ± 11 versus 6 ± 9 cm H_2O). It should be emphasized, however, that this is not the only causal factor. The fact that 45% of women with prolapse do not have muscle injury clearly demonstrates that other factors, such as connective tissue strength and integrity, play a role as well.

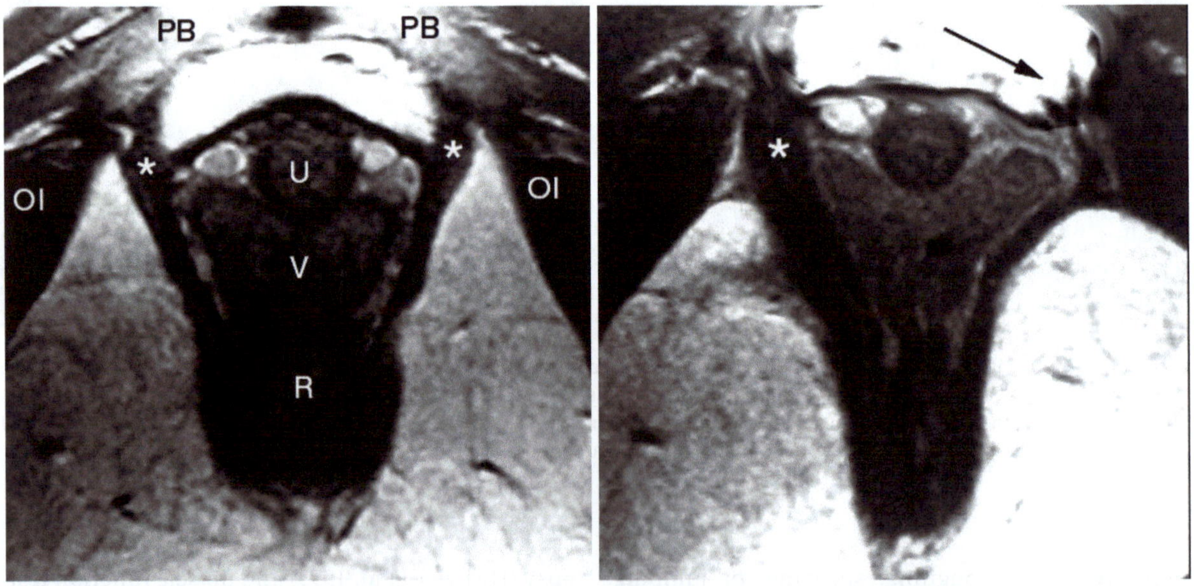

Fig. 4.3.8. Axial images at the level of the midurethra of two different women. Right panel showing a left-sided, unilateral pubovisceral muscle defect, left panel showing a normal pubovisceral muscle for comparison. Abbreviations: pubic bone (*PB*), obturator internus muscle (*OI*), pubovisceral insertion to the pubic bone (*asterisk*), location of missing pubovisceral insertion on the patient´s left side (*black arrow*), urethra (*U*), vagina (*V*), rectum (*R*), bladder (*B*) are shown (DELANCEY 2002 with permission)

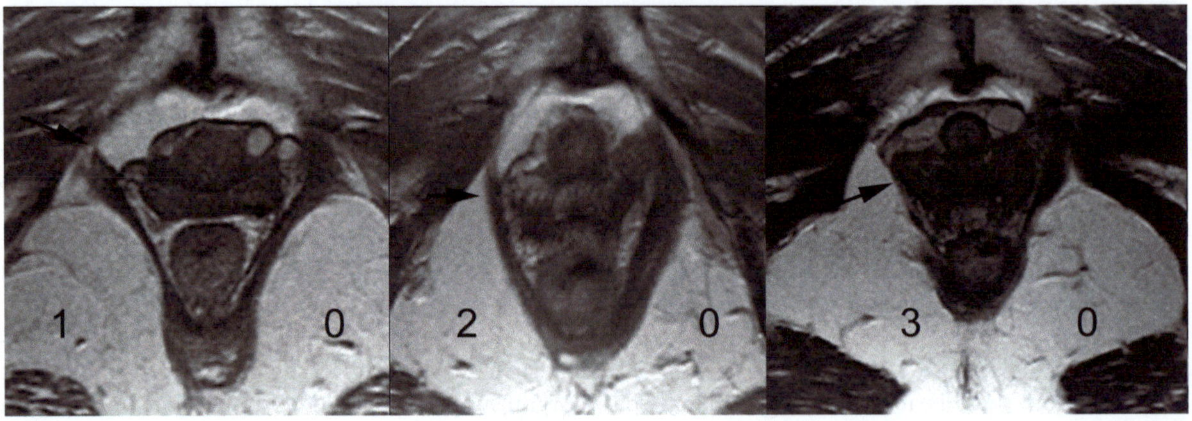

Fig. 4.3.9. Examples of grade 1, 2, and 3 unilateral defects in axial images. These were selected to illustrate degrees of defects in individuals with a normal contralateral pubovisceral muscle. The score for each side is indicated on the figure, and the *black arrows* indicate the location of the missing muscle (from DELANCEY et al. 2007; © DELANCEY 2006 with permission)

4.3.4 Pregnancy and Birth-Related Changes

Pregnancy and delivery both increase the likelihood that a woman will suffer from pelvic floor dysfunction (Mant et al. 1997; Rortveit et al. 2003). Vaginal birth has been identified as a cause of damage to the levator ani muscle (DeLancey et al. 2003). Soon after delivery the pelvic floor sags, and the urogenital hiatus is wider than normal (see Fig. 4.3.10).

Over the course of the first 6 months, post-partum muscle recovery results in resumption of the near-normal position in most women, and pelvic muscle strength also returns to normal (Sampselle et al. 1998). This corresponds to changes in muscle appearance following birth (see Fig. 4.3.11).

Recent studies using MRI have demonstrated that levator ani defects occur after vaginal delivery (Kearney et al. 2006). In a study of women after their first vaginal delivery, 32 of 160 (20%) had damage to the levator ani muscles (DeLancey et al. 2003). A nulliparous control group of 80 women was also studied, and none of these women had injuries. Twenty-nine of 32 visible levator ani injuries occurred in the pubovisceral muscle, and only 3 occurred in the iliococcygeal portion of the muscle. In a more recent study, Dietz and Lanzarone (2005) evaluated women before and after vaginal birth using 3D ultrasound and confirmed that these types of injury occur during vaginal delivery.

Among the women with injury to the pubovisceral muscle, the amount of muscle injury varies from one individual to another. Some of these injuries involve complete bilateral loss of pubovisceral muscle bulk (Fig. 4.3.12), while others may have only unilateral loss (Fig. 4.3.8). There is also variation in the amount of architectural distortion that occurs. Some individuals show major changes in the overall architecture, while others have intact spatial relationships.

It remains to be determined whether this represents the difference between a muscle rupture with subsequent distortion of muscle appearance or denervation that then results in loss of muscle without deformity. Recent computer models have suggested that some muscle damage during the second stage of labor may come from overstretching because those parts of the muscle that are stretched the most are those parts that are seen to be injured (Lien et al. 2004). Using a computer model of the levator ani muscle based on anatomy from a normal woman, the degree to which individual muscle bands are stretched could be studied (Fig. 4.3.13).

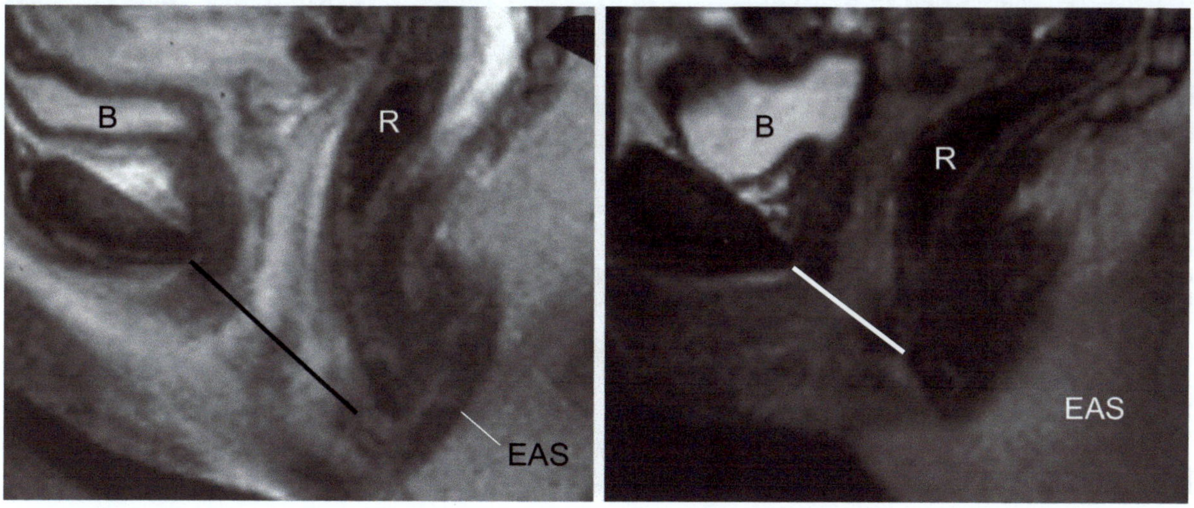

Fig. 4.3.10. T2-weighted sagittal sections of an 18-year-old woman, para2, 1 day (*left picture*) and 6 months (*right picture*) after spontaneous vaginal delivery. The external anal sphincter and perineal body that lies ventral to it are much lower in the 1st day after delivery compared with the anatomy 6 months later, and the urogenital hiatus is also larger (*line*) (from Tunn et al. 1999; © DeLancey 1999 with permission)

This analysis revealed that the muscle injured most often – the pubovisceral portion – was also the portion of the muscle that underwent the greatest degree of stretch. The second area of observed injury, the iliococcygeal muscle, was the second most stretched muscle. Furthermore, when the portion of the muscle at risk was identified in cross sections cut in the same orientation as axial MRI scans, the pattern of predicted injury matched the injury seen in MRI.

Birth-induced levator ani muscle injury may be accompanied by other types of injury that occurred during vaginal birth. A birth that was sufficiently difficult that it resulted in injury to the levator ani muscle may have also created injury to the connective tissue supports.

4.3.5 Conclusion

MR evaluation of the levator ani muscle is changing rapidly. The recent association of levator ani muscle damage and pelvic floor dysfunction has revealed the clinical importance of injury to this muscle. Identification of the injury mechanism provided important new knowledge about the pathophysiology of pelvic floor dysfunction. It is likely that the clinical course and treatment response of women who have levator ani muscle damage will be different from women with intact muscles. As this information becomes available, the need to know the muscle status to decide treatment will make levator ani muscle imaging a clinically important necessity.

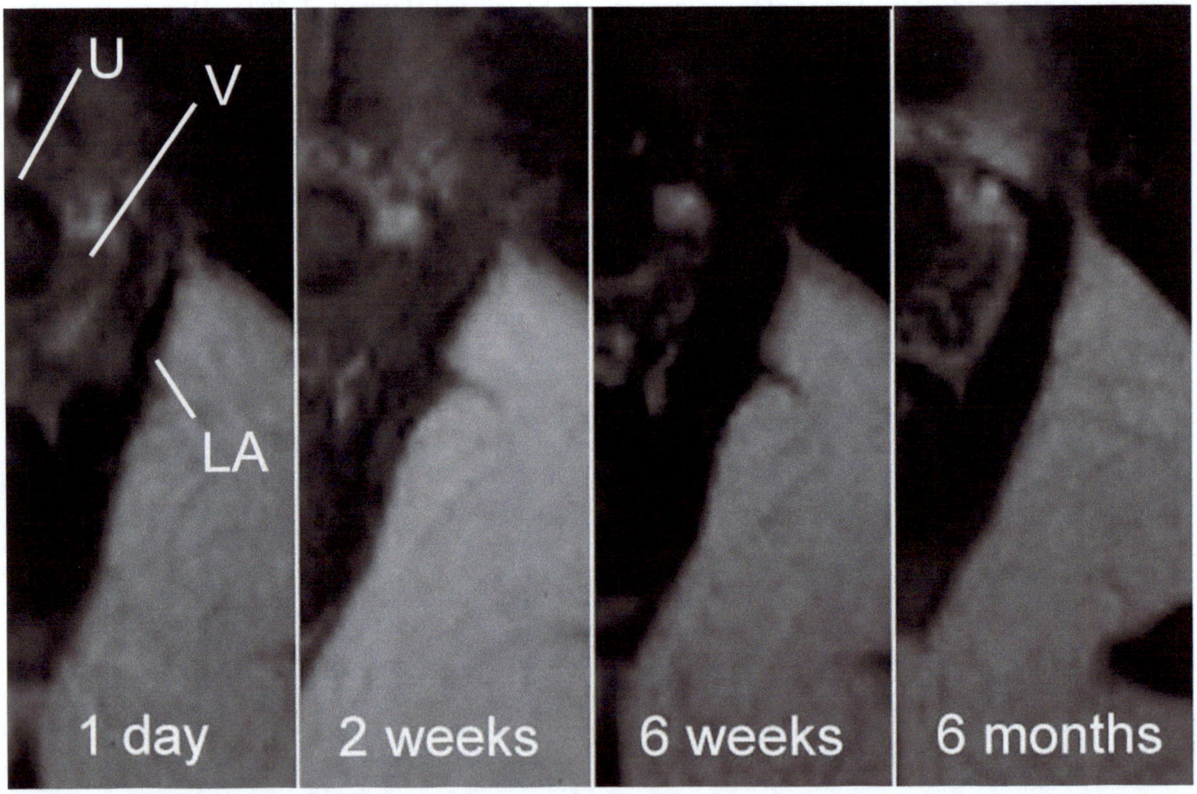

Fig. 4.3.11. Changes in muscle appearance following birth showing the left side of the pelvis at different time points after delivery. The urethra (*U*), vagina (*V*) and levator ani (*LA*) can be seen. Notice the increasing definition of the structures postpartum; especially the medial portion of the levator ani muscle adjacent to the vagina that is quite pale 1 day after delivery, but recovers its signal by 6 months (© DeLancey 1999 with permission)

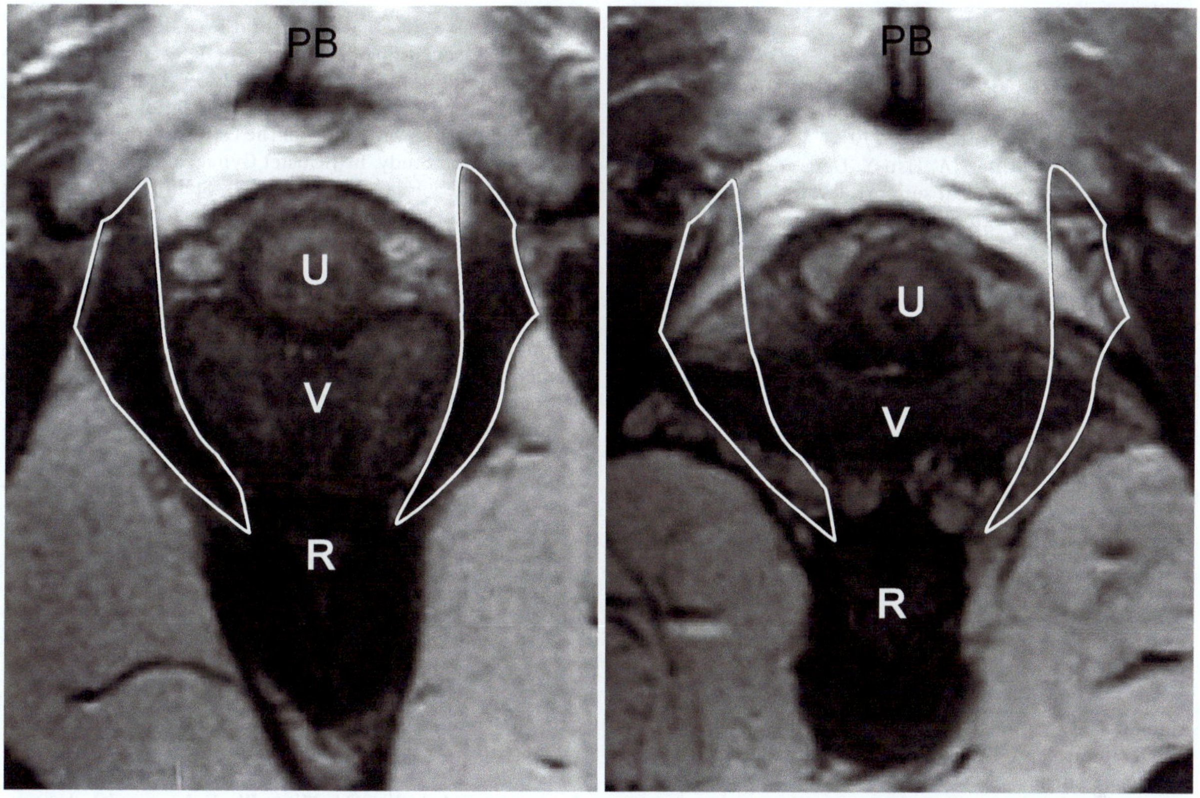

Fig. 4.3.12. Axial proton density MR on *left* shows normal pubococcygeal muscle with the muscle outlined at the level of the mid-urethra. On the *right* is a similar image from a woman with complete loss of the pubococcygeal muscle. Expected location of pubococcygeal muscles shown by *outline* (from DeLancey et al. 2005; © DeLancey 2005 with permission)

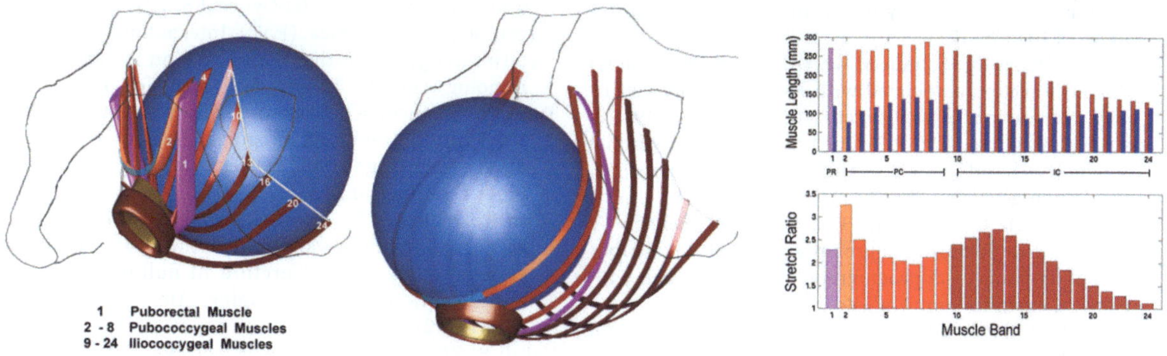

Fig. 4.3.13. *Left*, computer model of selected levator ani muscle bands before birth with muscle fibers numbered and the groups identified; the *middle figure* demonstrates muscle band lengthening present at the end of the second stage of labor; *right*, graphic representation of the original and final muscle (*top*) and the stretch ratio (*bottom*), indicating the degree to which each muscle band must lengthen to accommodate a normal-sized fetal head (from Lien et al. 2004; © Biomechanics Research Laboratory 2005 with permission)

References

Allen RE, Hosker GL, Smith AR, Warrell DW (1990) Pelvic floor damage and childbirth: a neurophysiological study. Br J Obstet Gynaecol 97:770–779

Chen L, Ashton-Miller JA, Hsu Y, DeLancey JO (2006) Interaction among apical support, levator ani impairment, and anterior vaginal wall prolapse. Obstet Gynecol 108:324–332

DeLancey JO (2005) The hidden epidemic of pelvic floor dysfunction: achievable goals for improved prevention and treatment. Am J Obstet Gynecol 192:1488–1495

DeLancey JO, Kearney R, Chou Q, Speights S, Binno S (2003) The appearance of levator ani muscle abnormalities in magnetic resonance images after vaginal delivery. Obstet Gynecol 101:46–53

DeLancey JO, Morgan DM, Fenner DE, Kearney R, Guire K, Miller JM, Hussain H, Umek W, Hsu Y, Ashton-Miller JA (2007) Comparison of levator ani muscle defects and function in women with and without pelvic organ prolapse. Obstet Gynecol 109:295–302

Dietz HP, Lanzarone V (2005) Levator trauma after vaginal delivery. Obstet Gynecol 106:707–712

Guaderrama NM, Nager CW, Liu J, Pretorius DH, Mittal RK (2005) The vaginal pressure profile. Neurourol Urodynam 24:243–247

Halban J, Tandler J (1907) Anatomie und Aetiologie der Genitalprolapse beim Weibe. Wilhelm Braumueller, Vienna, Leipzig

Hanzal E, Berger E, Koelbl H (1993) Levator ani muscle morphology and recurrent genuine stress incontinence. Obstet Gynecol 81:426–429

Hjartardottir S, Nilsson J, Petersen C. Lingtman G (1997) The female pelvic floor: a dome-not a basin. Acta Obstet Gynecol Scand 76:567–571

Hoyte L, Schierlitz L, Zou K, Flesh G, Fielding JR (2001) Two- and 3-dimensional MRI comparison of levator ani structure, volume, and integrity in women with stress incontinence and prolapse. Obstet Gynecol 185:11–19

Hugosson C, Jorulf H, Lingman G, Jacobsson B (1991) Morphology of the pelvic floor. Lancet 337:367

Kearney R, Sawhney R, DeLancey JO (2004) Levator ani muscle anatomy evaluated by origin-insertion pairs. Obstet Gynecol 104:168–173

Kearney R, Miller JM, Ashton-Miller JA, DeLancey JO (2006) Obstetric factors associated with levator ani muscle injury after vaginal birth. Obstet Gynecol 107:144–149

Kelvin FM, Maglinte DD (1997) Dynamic cystoproctography of female pelvic floor defects and their interrelationships. Am J Roentgenol 169:769–774

Kelvin FM, Hale OS, Maglinte DO, Patten BJ, Benson JT (1999) Female pelvic organ prolapse: diagnostic contribution of dynamic cystoproctograph and comparison with physical examination. Am J Roentgenol 173:31–37

Lawson JO (1974) Pelvic anatomy. I. Pelvic floor muscles. Ann R Coll Surg Engl 54:244–252

Lien KC, Mooney B, DeLancey JO, Ashton-Miller JA (2004) Levator ani muscle stretch induced by simulated vaginal birth. Obstet Gynecol 103:31–40

Maglinte DD, Kelvin FM, Fitzgerald K, Hale DS, Benson JT (1999) Association of compartment defects in pelvic floor dysfunction. Am J Roentgenol 172:439–444

Mant J, Painter R, Vessey M (1997) Epidemiology of genital prolapse: observations from the Oxford Family Planning Association Study. Br J Obstet Gynaecol 104:579–585

Margulies RU, Hsu Y, Kearney R, Stein T, Umek WH, DeLancey JO (2006) Appearance of the levator ani muscle subdivisions in magnetic resonance images. Obstet Gynecol 107:1064–1069

Miller JM, Umek WH, DeLancey JO, Ashton-Miller JA (2004) Can women without visible pubococcygeal muscle in MR images still increase urethral closure pressures? Am J Obstet Gynecol 191:171–175

Morgan DM, Kaur G, Hsu Y, Fenner D, Guire K, Miller J, Ashton-Miller JA, DeLancey JOL (2005) Does vaginal closure force differ in the supine and standing positions? Am J Obstet Gynecol 192:1722–1728

Morgan DM, Umek W, Stein T, Hsu Y, Guire K, DeLacney JOL (2007) Interrater reliability of assessing levator ani muscle defects with magnetic resonance images. Int Urogynecol J 18:773–778

Rortveit G, Daltveit AK, Hannestad YS, Hunskaar S; Norwegian EPINCONT Study (2003) Urinary incontinence after vaginal delivery or cesarean section. N Engl J Med 348:900–907

Safir MH, Gousse AE, Rovner ES, Ginsberg DA, Raz S (1999) Four defect repair of grade 4 cystocele. J Urol 16:587–594

Sampselle CM, Miller JM, Mims BL, DeLancey JO, Ashton-Miller JA, Antonakos CL (1998) Effect of pelvic muscle exercise on transient incontinence during pregnancy and after birth. Obstet Gynecol 91:406–412

Shafik A, Doss S, Asaad S (2003) Etiology of the resting myoelectric activity of the levator ani muscle: physioanatomic study with a new theory. World J Surg 27:309–314

Stovall DW (2000) Transvaginal ultrasound findings in women with chronic pelvic pain. Obstet Gynecol 95 (Suppl 1):S57

Strohbehn K, Ellis JH, Strohbehn JA, DeLancey JO (1996) Magnetic resonance imaging of the levator ani with anatomic correlation. Obstet Gynecol 87:277–285

Terminologia Anatomica (1998) International anatomical terminology/Federative Committee on Anatomical Terminology (FCAT). Theime, Stuttgart, New York

Tunn R, DeLancey JO, Howard D, Thorp JM, Ashton-Miller JA, Quint LE (1999) MR imaging of levator ani muscle recovery following vaginal delivery. Int Urogynecol J Pelvic Floor Dysfunct 10:300–307

Tunn R, DeLancey JO, Howard D, Ashton-Miller JA, Quint LE (2003) Anatomic variations in the levator ani muscle, endopelvic fascia, and urethra in nulliparas evaluated by magnetic resonance imaging. Am J Obstet Gynecol 188:116–121

Vakili B, Zheng YT, Loesch H, Echols KT, Franco N, Chesson RR (2005) Levator contraction strength and genital hiatus as risk factors for recurrent pelvic organ prolapse. Am J Obstet Gynecol 192:1592–1598

Imaging Techniques

4

4.4 Endoanal Ultrasound

Clive I. Bartram

CONTENTS

4.4.1 Introduction

Sonographic imaging of the anal sphincters poses several technical problems. The tissue layers are thin, and the acoustic impedance differences often minimal, requiring high anatomical resolution and good soft tissue differentiation to resolve. There is also the question of the anatomical plane the sphincters are examined in. As the sphincters are circular structures, ideally this would be axially through the sphincters. It is possible to obtain an angled axial image of the sphincters in women using a standard end-firing transducer placed on the perineum, but in men only imaging along the longitudinal axis of the sphincter is possible with a probe over the anus. Endoprobes have the advantage of imaging in the ideal anatomical plane, even although this will disturb the normal anatomy of the closed anus. Endoprobes for endoanal ultrasound need to be designed for axial imaging with high resolution, and currently only a few manufacturers have developed endoprobes for this work. One of the main contenders has been B-K Medical (Herlev, Denmark), and much of the developmental work has been accomplished using their systems. Other ultrasound manufacturers include Kretztechnik (Zipf, Austria), Hitachi [Hitachi Medical Systems Europe (Holding) AG, Zug, Switzerland] and Aloka (ALOKA Holding Europe AG, Zug, Switzerland).

The B-K Medical endoprobe type 1850 was designed for rectal scanning, to be inserted high into the rectum via a short sigmoidoscope. Acoustic contact with the rectal wall was achieved using a water-filled balloon. This could not be used in the anus as the balloon collapsed around the mechanically rotated transducer. The system was modified by replacing the balloon with a hard plastic cone (Law and Bartram 1989) that would not collapse around the rotating transducer and that had parallel walls to prevent anatomical deformity of the anus as the probe was moved within the canal. The width of the cone was minimised (17 mm) to reduce discomfort and stretching of the sphincters, and a 10 MHz crystal developed with near-field focussing for use in the anal canal. There is now a 3D probe, the 2050 with two crystals back to back, multifrequency 6–16 MHz, 900 radial lines and an axial resolution up to 0.2 mm and a lateral of 0.5 mm (Fig. 4.4.1).

C. I. Bartram, FRCS, FRCP, FRCR
Professor, Consultant Radiologist (retired), St Mark's Hospital, Princess Grace Hospital, Nottingham Place, London W1U 5NY, UK

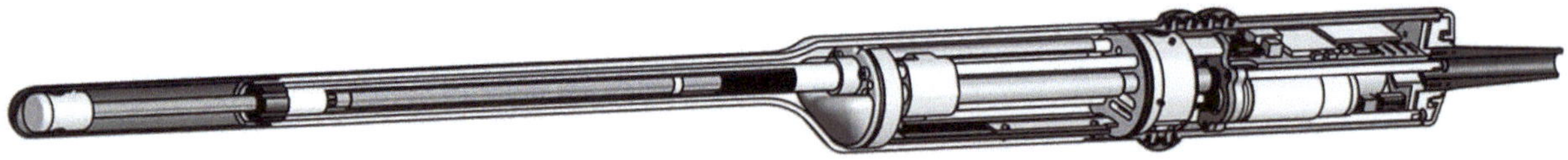

Fig. 4.4.1. Cut-away view of the B-K Medical 2050 3D probe. Courtesy of B-K Medical

4.4.2 Technique for Endoanal Ultrasonography

The standard B-K Medical endoprobe needed careful assembly to ensure there was no gas bubble within the plastic cone, but the new 2050 unit is sealed, requiring only a generous coating of ultrasound gel to the outside and inside of the protective sheath to ensure good acoustic contact.

The position in which the patient is examined is important. In men the left lateral is adequate, but in women either the prone or lithotomy position is preferred, as in the left lateral position the anus becomes deformed as the pelvic organs pull it over and symmetry of the anterior structures lost, which makes it more difficult to appreciate abnormalities in this important area (Frudinger et al. 1998).

The probe should be inserted until it is just into the rectum and then withdrawn and orientated so that anterior on the patient is uppermost on the image (Fig. 4.4.2). A series of images should be taken on withdrawal of the probe to record the appearances of the canal at all levels, with detailed scanning of any abnormality. The 2050 does not have to be moved, as the transducer moves within the probe. A complete dataset of the entire canal may be acquitted just by pressing a button. Patient movement must be restricted during acquisition. If the patient can hold their breath for the entire scan, this is ideal; otherwise they must breathe gently as respiration moves the pelvic floor, creating a misregistration artefact (Fig. 4.4.3).

4.4.3 Normal Anatomy

Muscle cells are of low reflectivity, and it is actually the complex connective tissue stroma around these, namely the endomysium, perimysium and epimysium, which create the series of parallel linear reflections typical of striated muscle. Reflectivity will also depend on the angle of the incidence ultrasound beam to the connective tissue planes, which may explain why the reflectivity varies in similar muscle structures, e.g. the puboanalis appears hyporeflective compared to the puborectalis as it runs in a different plane. The smooth muscle of the internal sphincter has a lower fibroelastic content, and presents as a well-defined ring of uniform low reflectivity (Bartram and Frudinger 1997).

The axial image is a composite of reflections from individual layers and interfaces between layers. Some layers, notably the internal sphincter, are sufficiently thick and of specific acoustic quality to be distinctive, but some are too thin, or of similar reflectivity, to be distinguished by their inherent acoustic properties. The interface reflections between different tissues planes then become important to allow recognition of the borders of some layers (Fig. 4.4.4).

The anus is fundamentally a four-layer structure (Fig. 4.4.5) that comprises from the inside outwards the:

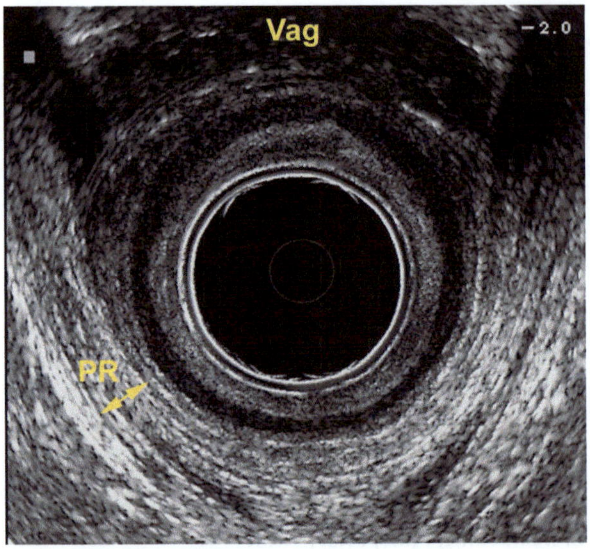

Fig. 4.4.2. Orientation of the probe in a female patient showing the "U" sling of the puborectalis (*PR*) with vagina anterior

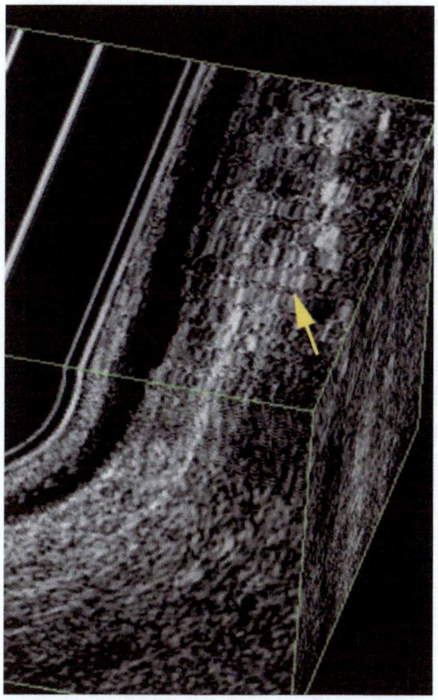

Fig. 4.4.3. Coronal plane view of 3D acquisition showing some linear misregistration (*arrow*) due to movement of the pelvic floor during respiration

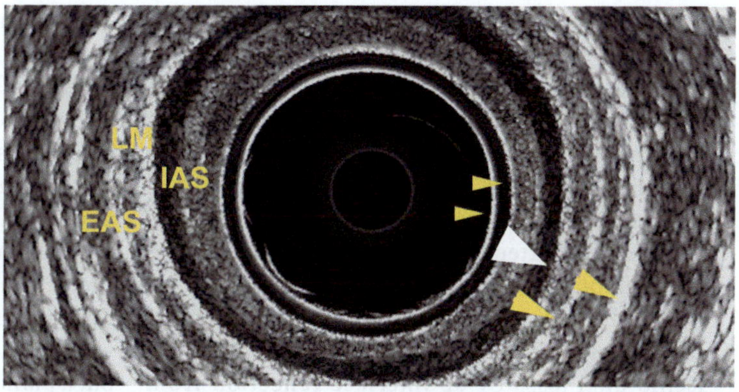

Fig. 4.4.4. Layer and interface reflections. Only the internal sphincter (*IAS*) may be identified by its inherent acoustic quality, whereas the longitudinal muscle (*LM*), external sphincter (*EAS*) and ischioanal fossa have comparable reflectivity and have to be distinguished by their interface reflections (*small yellow arrowheads* from cone; *large white interface* internal sphincter to longitudinal layer: *large yellow arrowheads* longitudinal layer to external sphincter and external sphincter to ischioanal fossa

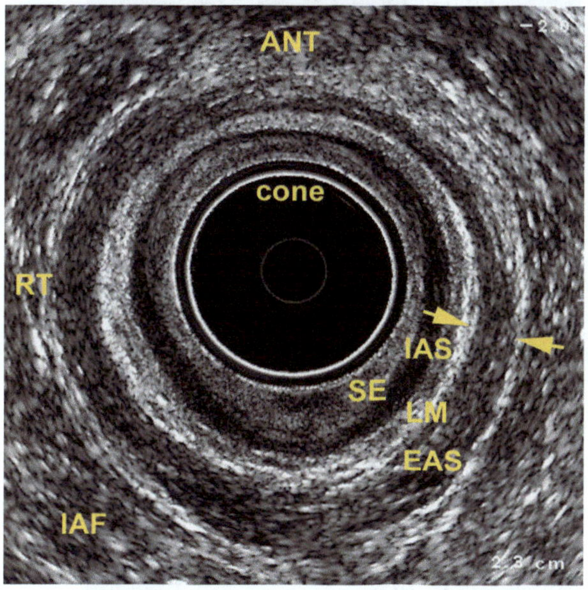

Fig. 4.4.5. Axial endosonographic image showing normal orientation with anterior uppermost (*ANT*) and right (*RT*) on the body right side. *IAF*=ischioanal fossa; *EAS*=external anal sphincter; *LM*=longitudinal layer; *IAS*=internal anal sphincter and *SE*=subepithelial tissues. *Two bright interface reflections* are seen from the cone with other interface reflections at fascial planes between the longitudinal layer/external sphincter and external sphincter/ischioanal fossa (*arrows*)

- Subepithelium – a moderately reflective layer. Thin low-reflective crescents of the muscularis submucosae ani may be visible in the upper canal. The dentate line is not discernible, but is situated approximately half way along the canal. Vascular channels may be seen at 6 and 12 o'clock, and are low-reflective tubular structures running longitudinally. The anal cushions are compressed by the probe and usually not visible unless haemorrhoidal.
- Internal anal sphincter – is a well-defined low-reflective ring about 2 mm thick. Usually symmetric in thickness, it is best measured at either 3 or 9. It may be slightly thicker just proximal to its termination, or more often at the cranial end. The termination is not always symmetric so that irregularity of the last mm or so should not be equated with a tear.
- Longitudinal layer – this is a complex layer comprising an extension of smooth muscle from the outer longitudinal layer of the rectum, striated muscle from the puboanalis and fibroelastic tissue from the endopelvic fascia (Fig. 4.4.6). Coronal views show how the two muscle layers fuse into the conjoined longitudinal muscle (Lunniss and Phillips 1992) that terminates in the mid canal with the fibroelastic component permeating through both sphincters into the ischioanal fossa and perianal skin, anchoring the anus into the pelvic floor (Fig. 4.4.7). Sub-adventitial fat on either side of this layer creates interface reflec-

tions, and the outer one, between the longitudinal layer and the external sphincter, may well represent the inter-sphincteric space that is the plane for surgical dissection between the sphincters.

- External anal sphincter – is considered to be in three parts: the deep part merges with the puborectalis dorsa-laterally, the superficial ends at the caudal extent of the internal sphincter, and the subcutaneous part curves inwards towards the anal margin (Fig. 4.4.8). The outer border of the external sphincter is demarcated from the ischio-anal fossa by an interface reflection from sub-adventitial fat (Fig. 4.4.4).

The junction of the anus to the striated muscles of the pelvic floor is complex. The puboanalis is an inner slip of the puborectalis that can be traced down into the longitudinal layer (Fig. 4.4.9). The fibre orientation is different so that it is seen as a low-reflective triangular structure immediately medial to the puborectalis (Fig. 44.10). The transverse perineii come in from both sides. In men these merge into the central point of the perineum with clear separation from the external sphincter (Fig. 44.11). In women they fuse into the external sphincter without a plane of dissection and are recognisable in 66% (Frudinger et al. 2002).

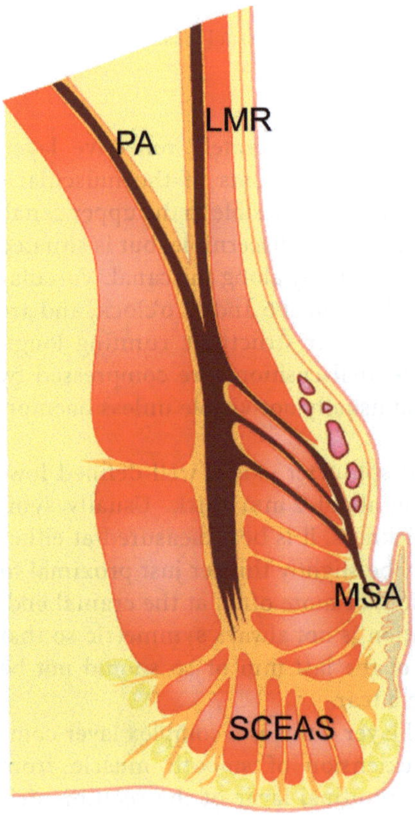

Fig. 4.4.6. The longitudinal muscle is a composite layer with smooth muscle from the longitudinal muscle of the rectum (*LMR*), striated from puboanalis (*PA*) and fibroelastic tissue from the endopelvic fascia. Slips from the longitudinal muscle run through the internal sphincter to the muscularis submucosae ani (*MSA*). Fibroelastic tissue also tracks through the subcutaneous external sphincter (*SCEAS*) to insert into the peri-anal skin

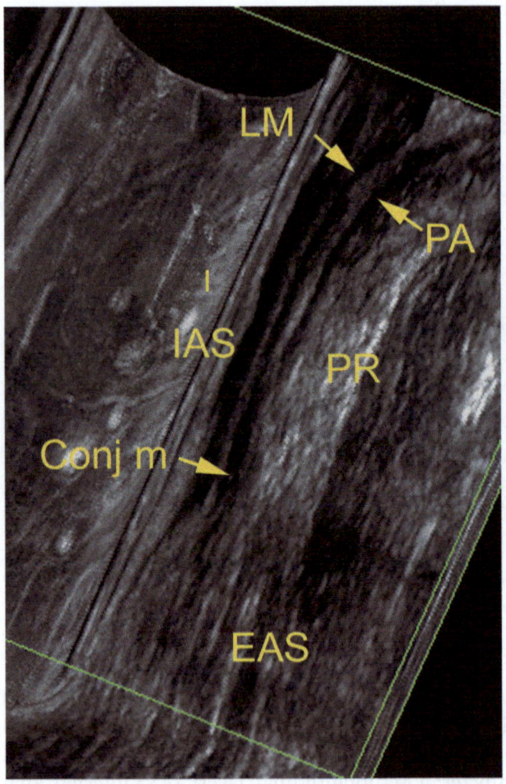

Fig. 4.4.7. Coronal image showing the longitudinal muscle from the rectum (*LM*) joining the puboanalis (*PA*) to form the conjoined longitudinal muscle (*Conj m*)

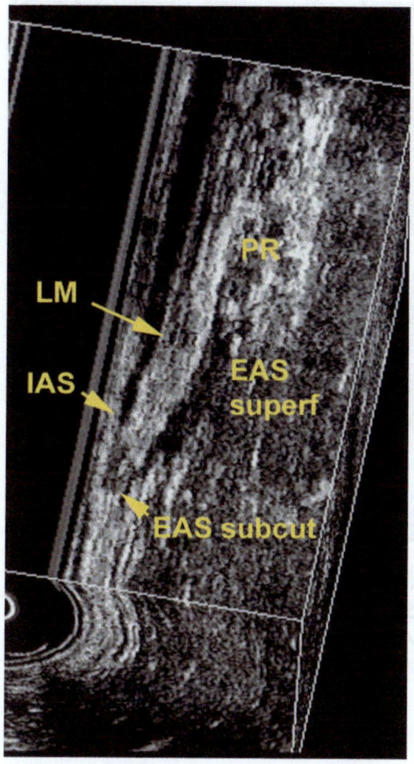

Fig. 4.4.8. Coronal image showing the typical hook-like appearance of the subcutaneous external anal sphincter

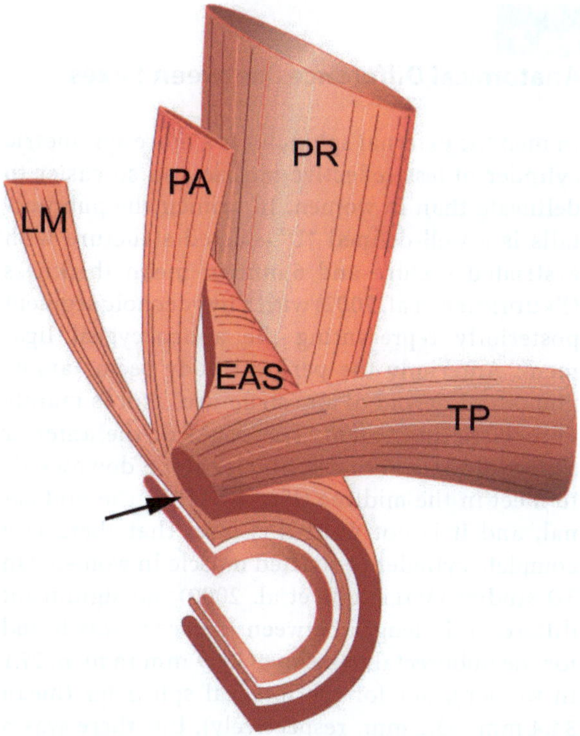

Fig. 4.4.9. The puboanalis (*PA*) rises from the medial border of the puborectalis (*PR*), joining the longitudinal muscle of the rectum (*LM*) to form the longitudinal layer (*arrow*). The transverse perineii is seen to fuse with the external anal sphincter

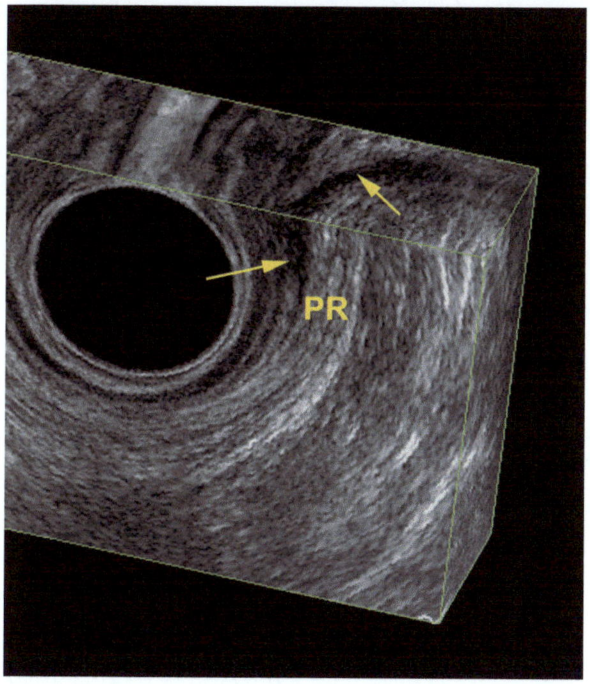

Fig. 4.4.10. The puboanalis (*arrows*) is a triangular low reflective segment medial to the puborectalis (*PR*)

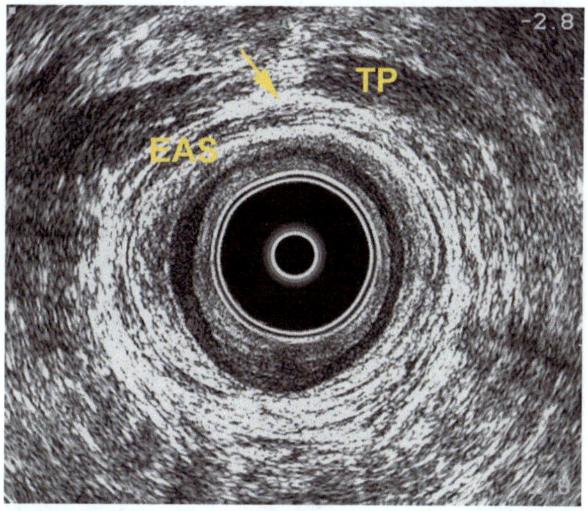

Fig. 4.4.11. The transverse perineii (*TP*) tend to be better defined in men and join the centre point of the perineum, creating a gap (*arrow*) between the transverse perineii and the external anal sphincter (*EAS*), whereas in women the transverse perineii fuse into the external sphincter directly

4.4.4 Anatomical Differences between Sexes

In men the external sphincter is a more symmetric cylinder of less reflective muscle and so easier to delineate than in women. In women the puborectalis is a well-defined "U"-shaped structure with a striated texture and 6 mm in mean thickness (Frudinger et al. 2002) with a hypoechoic segment posteriorly representing the anococcygeal ligament. Anteriorly the perineal body seems amorphous and devoid of any structure, as it is mainly fibroelastic in content. The edges of the anterior aspect of the external sphincter slope downwards to meet in the midline (Fig. 4.4.12) in the mid canal, and it is not until this level that there is a complete cylinder of striated muscle in women. On 3D studies (Williams et al. 2000), no significant difference in length between the sexes was found for the puborectalis (mean of 23.9 mm in men, 27.1 in women), nor for the internal sphincter (mean 34.4 mm, 33.2 mm, respectively), but there was a significant difference in the length of the external sphincter in all planes (anterior - 30.1:15.6; coronal - 31.6:19.5; posterior - 29.3:16.5, respectively). This confirms that the external sphincter is generally shorter, particularly anteriorly in women (Fig. 4.4.13), which is supported by endoanal MR studies (Rociu et al. 2000).

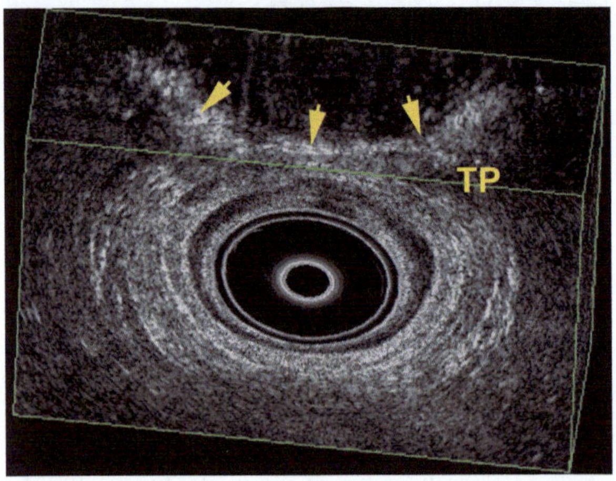

Fig. 4.4.12. A 3D view in a woman of the external sphincter sloping down to an intact anterior ring (*arrows*) with the transverse perineii (*TP*) fusing into this from each side

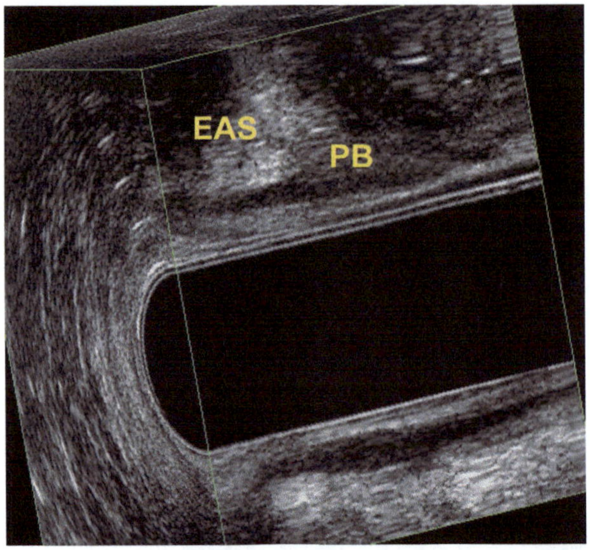

Fig. 4.4.13. Sagittal view of the moderately reflective external sphincter (*EAS*) caudal to the low reflective perineal body (*PB*), showing how this is shorter anteriorly in the female

4.4.5 Effects of Ageing

The internal anal sphincter is not constant in thickness. In neonates it is very thin (< 1 mm), measuring 1–2 mm in young adults, 2–3 mm in middle age and 3–4 mm in the elderly. A slight increase in reflectivity of the sphincter as it becomes thicker is also secondary to an increased connective tissue content. The external sphincter thins significantly in older nulliparous women, but the longitudinal layer, subepithelium or puborectalis was unchanged on endosonography (Frudinger et al. 2002), although the longitudinal layer has been shown to thin on endoanal MRI (Rociu et al. 2000). MR provides a more definitive measurement as it does not rely on interface reflections for measurement of some layers, which may explain these discrepancies.

4.4.6 Internal Anal Sphincter Abnormalities

The internal sphincter may show abnormalities of thickness or of loss of integrity. The sphincter may be either too thick or too thin for the patient's age. An abnormally thick sphincter (Fig. 4.4.14) may be

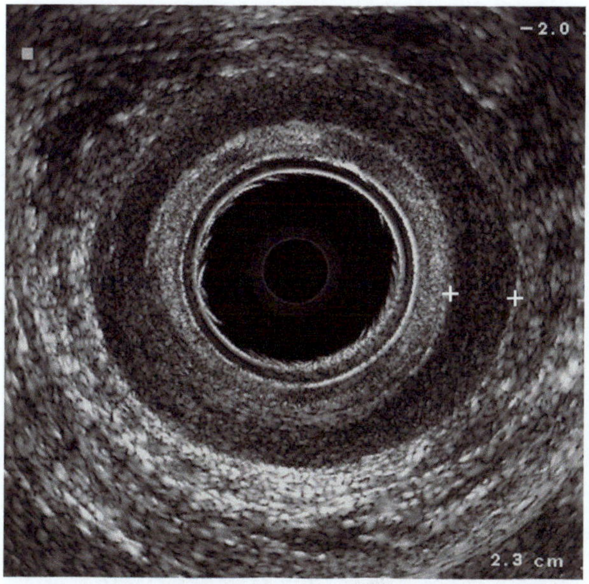

Fig. 4.4.14. A thick internal anal sphincter (4.3 mm between markers) in a 36-year-old woman with solitary rectal ulcer syndrome

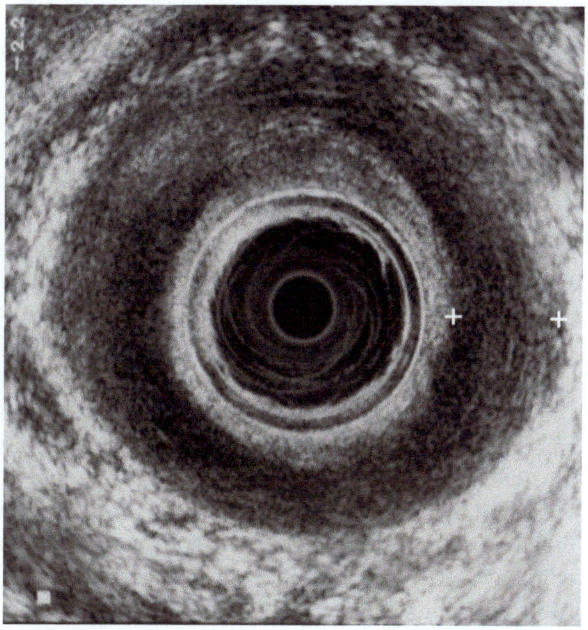

Fig. 4.4.15. Hereditary internal sphincter myopathy with a 7.6-mm internal sphincter thickness in a 76-year-old female with a long history of severe proctalgia fugax. Her mother had a similar history, and her daughter in her early 50s had just started having a similar pain

seen occasionally with uncomplicated constipation, but is invariably present in the solitary rectal ulcer syndrome with a 91% positive predictive value for high-grade rectal intussusception (Marshall et al. 2002) and is associated with intra-anal intussusception or rectal prolapse. A thick sphincter is an indication for evacuation proctography to exclude rectal prolapse if the diagnosis has not been made clinically. The internal sphincter and submucosa may become elliptical and thicker in the upper part of the canal (Dvorkin et al. 2004). The mechanism for this is uncertain and may just be secondary to mechanical stimulation from prolonged intussusception. Distension from a major rectal prolapse often damages the internal sphincter so that it becomes fragmented. A very rare condition is hereditary internal anal sphincter myopathy (Kamm et al. 1991), which produces a severe proctalgia fugax-type syndrome with gross thickening of the internal sphincter (Fig. 4.4.15). Proctalgia fugax is not uncommon, and in one series significant thickening of the internal anal sphincter was found in 30% (Gracia Solanas et al. 2005), so that endosonography may be used to determine which patients might be suitable for myectomy.

The internal sphincter should become thicker with age, but it is notable that in many patients with passive incontinence the internal sphincter is rather thin (Fig. 4.4.16). The cause of this is unknown, but

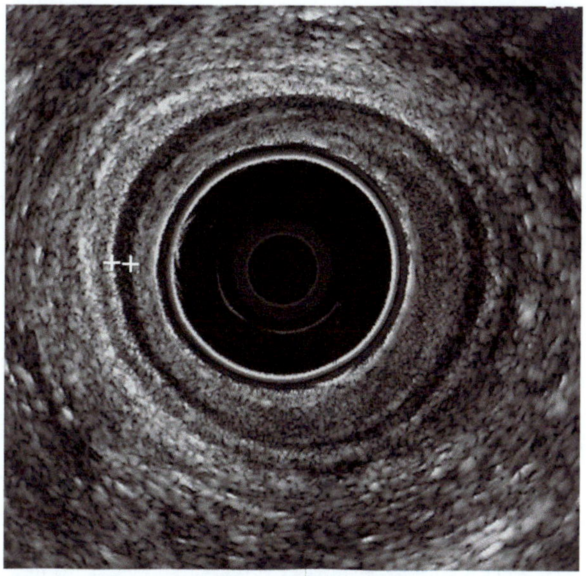

Fig. 4.4.16. A 70-year-old man with passive faecal incontinence. The sphincters are intact, but the internal sphincter is abnormally thin for this age, measuring 1.1 mm, indicative of internal sphincter degeneration

an internal sphincter of <2 mm thickness in a patient >50 years old is abnormal and may be called primary degeneration of the internal sphincter (Vaizey et al. 1997).

Lateral internal anal sphincterotomy was a common procedure prior to pharmacological treatments for anal fissure, but is now performed mainly for chronic unresponsive cases. The objective is to divide only the lower third of the internal sphincter. The cut ends spring apart, leaving a small gap that is easily visible on endosonography. If the entire internal sphincter is cut, the patient may not be totally incontinent, but will certainly have some degree of incontinence. Unfortunately this is easily done (Sultan et al. 1994a) (Fig. 4.4.17), suggesting the dentate line in women may not be a reliable reference point for the extent of sphincter division. In symptomatic patients who have been operated on, endosonography is useful to show how much, if any, of the internal sphincter has been divided, and to rule out any underlying sepsis. The coronal view may be used to calculate the percentage of sphincter divided (Fig. 4.4.18).

Abnormal dilatation of the anal canal for any reason or a stretch procedure may damage the internal sphincter. Stretch procedures are not performed as regularly as they were some years ago, but cases with sphincter disruption following this are still a relatively common finding (Fig. 4.4.19) and exhibit a range of changes from marked irregularity of the sphincter thickness, gross thinning of a segment, to fragmentation where only irregular isolated remnants of sphincter remain. Haemorrhoidectomy is also a cause of internal sphincter disruption, either from a stretch procedure being performed at the same time or from inadvertent division of part of the sphincter.

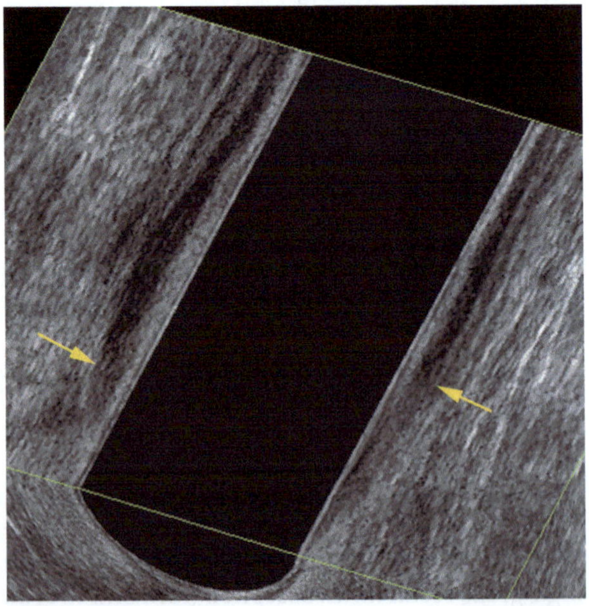

Fig. 4.4.18. Coronal view allows exact calculation of how much of the internal sphincter (*arrows*) has been divided

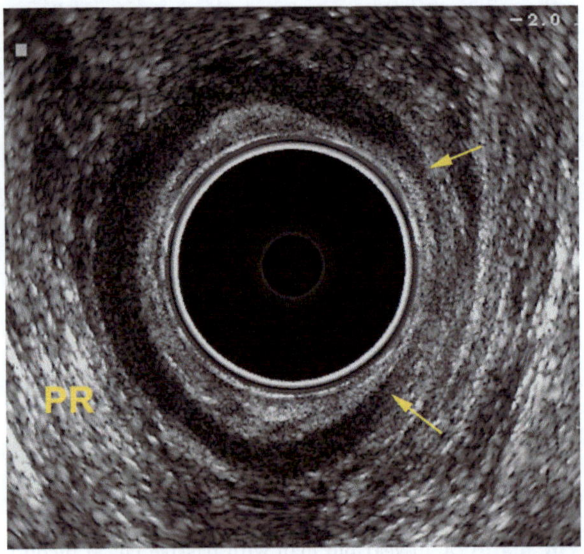

Fig. 4.4.17. Complete division of the internal anal sphincter with a defect (*arrows*) high in the canal at the level of the puborectalis (*PR*)

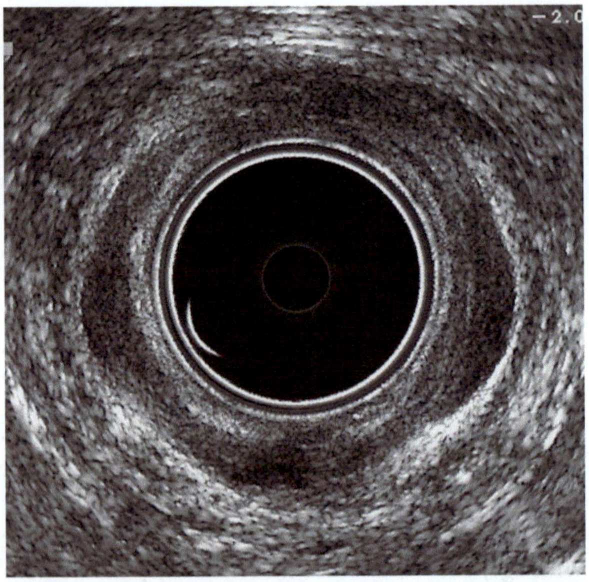

Fig. 4.4.19. Fragmentation of the internal anal sphincter following an anal stretch procedure

4.4.7 External Anal Sphincter Abnormalities

As with the internal anal sphincter, the external anal sphincter may be torn or abnormal in muscle fibre density. The latter is a complex issue, and one of the main indications for endoanal ultrasound is determining if the sphincter has been disrupted by childbirth. Direct trauma, from penetrating injuries or road traffic accidents, is quite rare by comparison (Fig. 4.4.20).

Tears from childbirth result either from overstretching, or possibly extension from an episiotomy, and may be complete or partial. The ruptured area heals with granulation tissue and fibrosis, forming a relatively homogeneous low-reflectivity segment within the external sphincter, usually involving other layers, particularly the longitudinal layer, and often the internal sphincter (Fig. 4.4.21).

Atrophy is undoubtedly the commonest abnormality, but unfortunately the most difficult to recognise on endosonography. The endocoil MRI criteria for external anal sphincter atrophy have been discussed elsewhere (Chap. 4.6). The reason that atrophy is difficult to diagnose relates to the histopathology of atrophy and how the outer border of the external sphincter is detected on sonography. Atrophy involves loss of muscle fibres with fat replacement diminishing the normal muscle to the subadventitial fat ratio to the extent that the acoustic interface on the outer border of the external sphincter will be lost, making a precise measurement of the thickness of the external sphincter impossible. The inability to recognise the outer border of the external sphincter may in itself be abnormal (Fig. 4.4.22), and coupled with a thin internal sphincter (<2 mm) gives a positive predictive value of 74% for atrophy (Williams et al. 2001b). As might be predicted, attempts to measure the external sphincter on 3D endosonography are not reliable for assessing atrophy (West et al. 2005). However, using a scoring system of mild, moderate and severe based on the clarity of the outer interface, the reflectivity pattern of the external sphincter and its length, good correlation with MR has been found (Cazemier et al. 2006). The texture of the external sphincter is therefore important. In women the normal subcutaneous part is hyper-reflective, with the deep and superficial parts more hypo-reflective with a striated pattern, whereas with atrophy the deep and superficial parts are amorphously hyper-reflective with loss of definition of the outer border. These sonographic changes all reflect the increased fat within the muscle layer, and therefore imply the presence of atrophy.

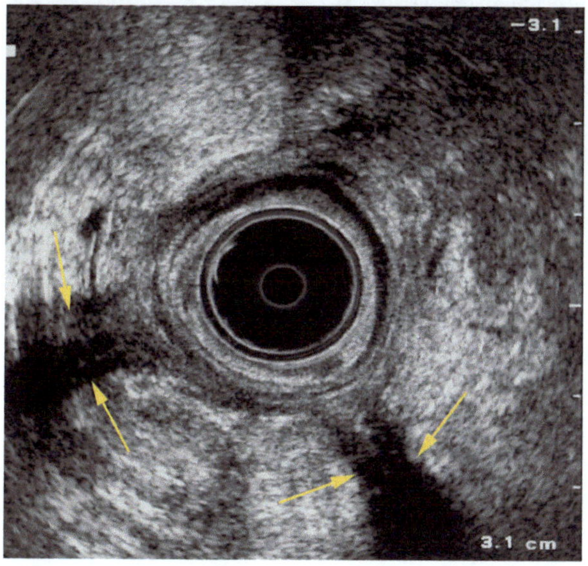

Fig. 4.4.20. Partial rupture of the sphincter with well-defined segmental scarring and acoustic shadowing (*arrows*) from this in a young boy who fell on a wooden stake

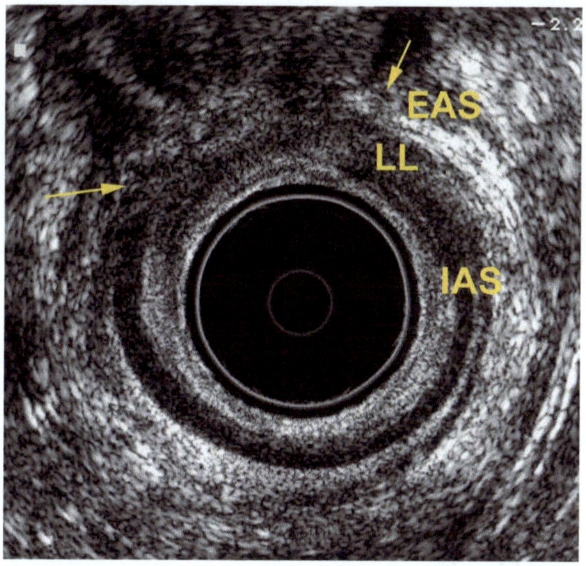

Fig. 4.4.21. Obstetric tears to the external sphincter (*EAS*), longitudinal layer (*LL*), and internal sphincter (*IAS*) between 10 and 1 o'clock

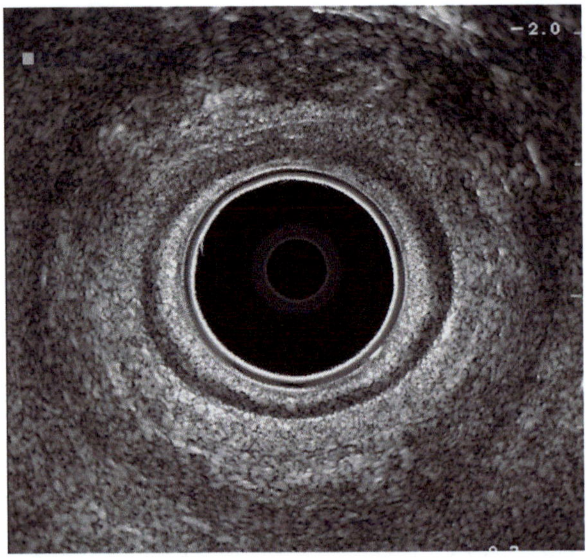

Fig. 4.4.22. External sphincter atrophy in a middle-aged woman with faecal incontinence. The sphincters are intact. The internal sphincter is thin (< 2 mm), but the interface between the longitudinal layer and the external sphincter as well as the outer border of the external sphincter is poorly defined, making it impossible to assess the thickness of the external sphincter

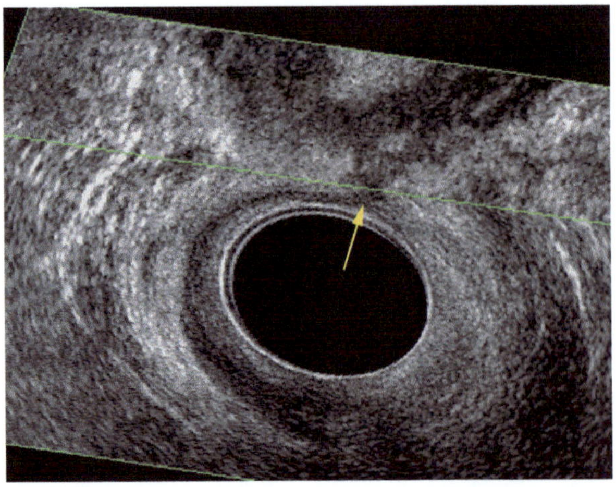

Fig. 4.4.23. Small anterior external sphincter tear 12-1 clearly visible on 3D imaging. Large obstetric tear between 10 and 2 o'clock (*arrows*) involving both the internal and external anal sphincters

4.4.8 Obstetric Trauma

Always examine in the prone (or lithotomy) position and assess the symmetry of the anal sphincters and perineal structures. Obstetric trauma affects only the anterior aspects of the sphincters, and disruption in the posterior half of the sphincters is due to some other cause. The extent of internal anal sphincter disruption usually matches that of the external sphincter. Internal sphincter tears do not occur without external sphincter damage. External sphincter continuity should be checked as the probe is slowly withdrawn, looking for the anterior parts coming together centrally to form a complete ring in the mid canal. If this is eccentric, it is a pointer for a tear. This may be confirmed on coronal imaging (Fig. 4.4.23). A tear should be mapped out in hours and longitudinal extent. Many involve just the upper part of the external sphincter, but may extend throughout its length. A complete tear of the perineum and sphincters results in a cloacal-type defect (Fig. 4.4.24).

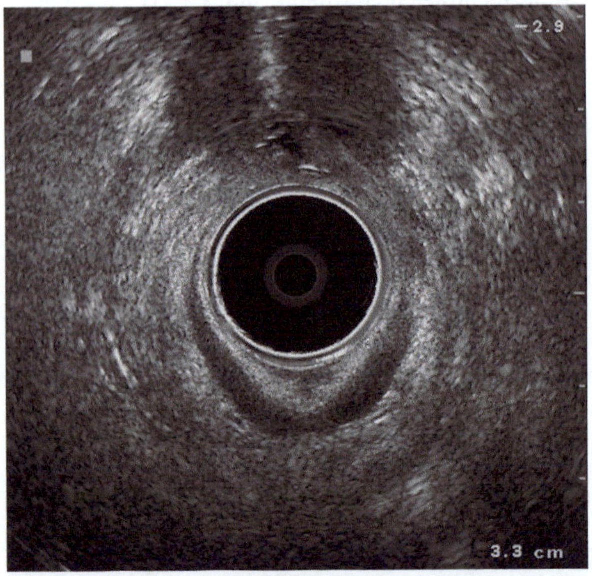

Fig. 4.4.24. Major obstetric tear with complete disruption of the perineum and only the posterior halves of the internal and external sphincters remaining, creating a cloacal defect

The reported incidence of obstetric trauma on endosonography varies from 11–35%, with an overall incidence of 26.9% from a meta-analysis (Oberwalder et al. 2003). This is very close to the incidence of 24.5% found on careful clinical examination immediately post partum by Andrews et al. (2006) who question the concept of "occult" tears, i.e. those found on endosonography when no tear has been reported clinically, suggesting that these are simply missed by current routine perineal inspection.

The differentiation of sphincteric from perineal tears may also be relevant. Tears of the transverse perineii and/or puboanalis are common, but do not affect sphincter pressures and may not therefore be functionally significant (Williams et al. 2001a).

Tears to the puboanalis create an area of low-reflective widening between the puborectalis and upper external sphincter that may be traced into the puboanalis (Fig. 4.4.25), whereas tears to the transverse perineii are just below the puborectalis and lateral to the external sphincter (Fig. 4.4.26). Tears may also involve the pelvic floor muscles, such as the puborectalis (Fig. 4.4.27), but these are more clearly visualised on MRI (Kearney et al. 2006).

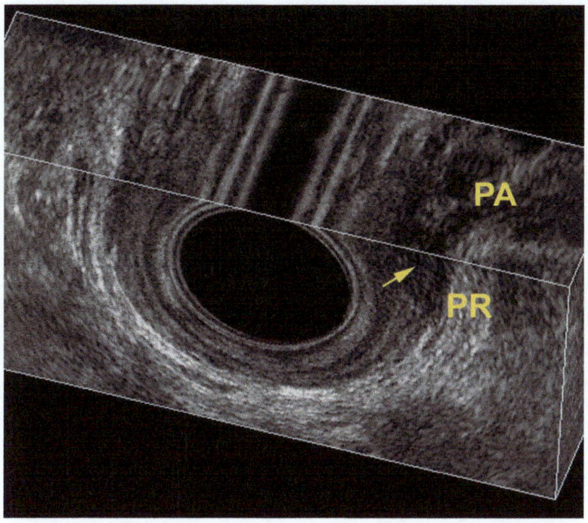

Fig. 4.4.25. Tear involving the left puboanalis (*PA*) with widening of the longitudinal layer (*arrow*) (compare to Fig. 4.4.10)

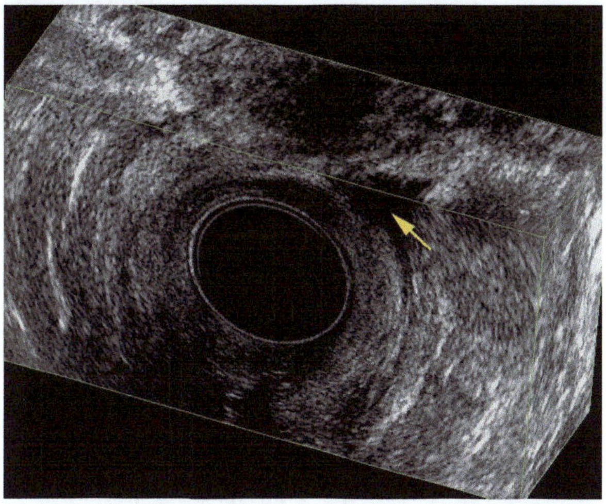

Fig. 4.4.26. Tear of the left transverse perineus (*arrow*) (compare to Figs. 4.4.11 and 4.4.12), lying caudal to the external sphincter ring. The right transverse perineus is intact

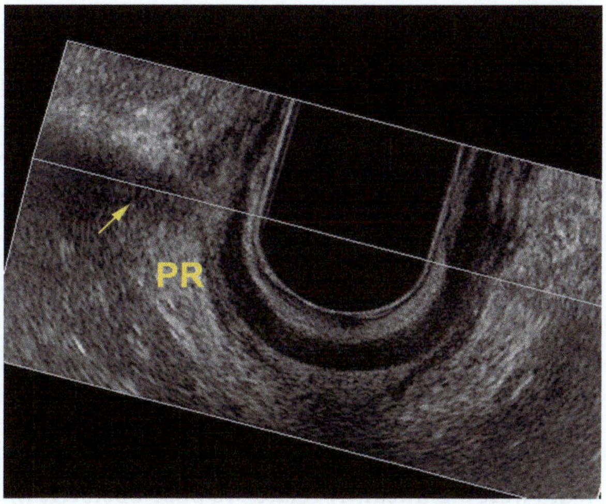

Fig. 4.4.27. Tear (*arrow*) of the right puborectalis (*PR*)

Caesarean section is not associated with any sphincter trauma. Damage is most frequent during the first delivery and with forceps assistance. There may be some permanent changes even when there is no tear. An initial study suggested thinning of the anterior external sphincter (Frudinger et al. 1999) and other layers. However, this was not a matched pre- and post-delivery study, and a later matched study (Williams et al. 2002) did not show any change in layer thickness. The only significant post-partum alteration was slight shortening of the external anal sphincter (21.7:20.5-mm post delivery) and increased angulation of the anterior segment (10:13.8° post delivery). Thinning of the perineal body has been noted in women with faecal incontinence post partum (Martinez Hernandez et al. 2003). This may be measured with endoanal examination using light digital contact with the inner perineum (Zetterstrom et al. 1998) to create a reverberation echo. A normal thickness of 12 ± 3 mm was found.

Third-degree tears, based on clinical detection, have an incidence of 0.6–9%. Endosonography after primary repair suggests that 90% have a persistent defect (Starck et al. 2006), which increases in size between 1 week and 3 months post repair, but thereafter remains unchanged. A relationship was found between larger defects, lower sphincter pressures and the higher risks of anal incontinence. In another study canal pressures were significantly lower with persistent combined defects compared to an intact sphincter after repair. Several studies have explored the relationship between the radial and longitudinal extent of sphincter tears and pressure changes. No difference in squeeze pressure has been found between partial or complete external sphincter tears, nor between < or >25% circumferential tears, but resting pressure was reduced in full-length external sphincter tears and with internal sphincter fragmentation (Voyvodic et al. 2003). However, in an incontinent group full-length external sphincter tears were associated with a lower squeeze pressure and internal sphincter defects with a lower resting pressure (Titi et al. 2007), and in another paper internal sphincter tears were significantly related to post-obstetric incontinence (Mahony et al. 2007). Tears and their size appear to have a significant relationship to symptoms (Damon et al. 2002).

4.4.9 Anismus, Rectocoele and Prolapse

The mechanism for anismus is thought to be paradoxical contraction of the pelvic floor during straining, and endosonography has been used with a linear probe to show that the puborectalis becomes shorter and thicker than controls during straining (Van Outryve et al. 2002), and on dynamic 3D that the angle between the puborectalis and the canal is significantly different also during straining (Murad-Regadas et al. 2007).

4.4.10 Endoanal Ultrasound in Relation to Other Techniques

Endocoil MR is discussed in detail in Chapter 4.6. When comparing these modalities, it is important to remember that experience is probably the most important factor in interpretation, although there are inherent differences that can tip the balance when looking for certain features. The internal sphincter is easier to see on endosonography, the external on MR as there is a clear distinction between muscle and fat. This also makes it easier to see major external sphincter tears on MR where there is fat replacement between the torn ends, and with experience it is easy to differentiate between scar tissue, which is homogeneous and more hypointensive compared to striated muscle on MRI. As one might expect, therefore several recent studies have found comparable performance for sphincter tears (Cazemier et al. 2006; Dobben et al. 2007; Pinta et al. 2004; West et al. 2005), with a preference for endosonography for the internal sphincter, but a definite advantage for MR in detecting external sphincter atrophy.

Endosonography is not the only method to image the anal sphincters, particularly in women where a transvaginal end-fire probe may be placed in the distal vagina/perineum and angled backwards to visualise the sphincters. This provides a unique view of the sphincter in its closed state. The anal cushions are seen (Fig. 4.4.28), and the subepithelial thickness may be measured. The internal sphincter is slightly thicker than on endoanal examination as it is not being stretched (Sultan et al. 1994b).

Good results have been reported for sphincter damage (Peschers et al. 1997; Stewart and Wilson 1999; Timor-Tritsch et al. 2005). Although one study suggested this was an unreliable method (Frudinger et al. 1997) for demonstrating sphincter tears, this may have reflected the type of probe used in this study. However, an inherent limitation remains with transvaginal/perineal ultrasound in orientating the probe to view the anal canal in right

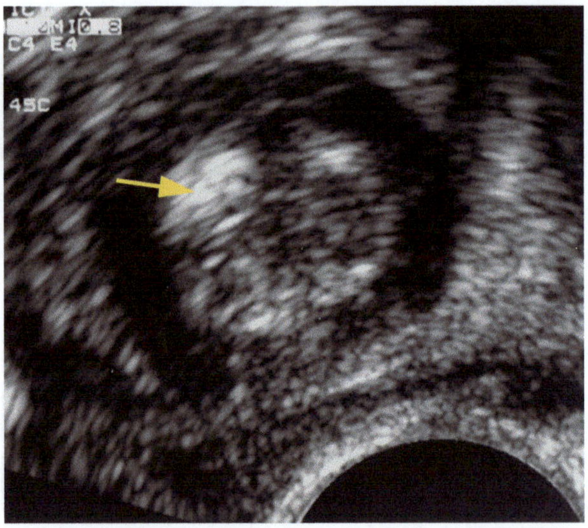

Fig. 4.4.28. Perineal ultrasound showing the anal cushions (*arrow*) in the closed canal, with a slightly thicker internal sphincter

angles throughout its length. In this respect, endoanal ultrasound remains the gold standard for detecting sphincter damage.

The pelvic floor may also be viewed by placing a probe on the perineum (see Chap. 4.5), and scanning in the sagittal and coronal planes with movement of the pelvic floor can be observed during straining and squeezing. The position of the puborectalis, bladder neck and anorectal angle may be measured. During straining, rectocoeles, cystocoeles and enterocoeles may be apparent and rectal intussusception imaged. Dynamic transperineal ultrasound has considerable potential as a simple, cheap and relatively non-invasive technique. Its relationship to other imaging methods and reliability await further assessment.

References

Andrews V, Sultan AH, Thakar R, Jones PW (2006) Occult anal sphincter injuries – myth or reality? Br J Obstet Gynaecol 113:195–200

Bartram CI, Frudinger A (1997) Handbook of anal endosonography. Wrightson Biomedical Publishing pp 21–42

Cazemier M, Terra MP, Stoker J et al (2006) Atrophy and defects detection of the external anal sphincter: comparison between three-dimensional anal endosonography and endoanal magnetic resonance imaging. Dis Colon Rectum 49:20–27

Damon H, Henry L, Barth X, Mion F (2002) Fecal incontinence in females with a past history of vaginal delivery: significance of anal sphincter defects detected by ultrasound. Dis Colon Rectum 45:1445–1450

Dobben AC, Terra MP, Slors JF et al (2007) External anal sphincter defects in patients with fecal incontinence: comparison of endoanal MR imaging and endoanal US. Radiology 242:463–471

Dvorkin LS, Chan CL, Knowles CH et al (2004) Anal sphincter morphology in patients with full-thickness rectal prolapse. Dis Colon Rectum 47:198–203

Frudinger A, Bartram CI, Kamm M (1997) Transvaginal versus anal endosonography for detecting damage to the anal sphincter. AJR Am J Roentgenol 168:1435–1438

Frudinger A, Bartram CI, Halligan S, Kamm M (1998) Examination techniques for endosonography of the anal canal. Abdom Imag 23:301–303

Frudinger, Halligan S, Bartram CI et al (1999) Changes in anal anatomy following vaginal delivery revealed by anal endosonography. Br J Obstet Gynaecol 106:233–237

Frudinger A, Halligan S, Bartram CI et al (2002) Female anal sphincter: age-related differences in asymptomatic volunteers with high-frequency endoanal US. Radiology 224:417–423

Gracia Solanas JA, Ramírez Rodríguez JM, Elía Guedea M et al (2005) Sequential treatment for proctalgia fugax. Mid-term follow-up. Rev Esp Enferm Dig 97:491–496

Kamm MA, Hoyle CH, Burleigh DE et al (1991) Hereditary internal anal sphincter myopathy causing proctalgia fugax and constipation. A newly identified condition. Gastroenterology 100:805–810

Kearney R, Miller JM, Ashton-Miller JA, DeLancey JO (2006) Obstetric factors associated with levator ani muscle injury after vaginal birth. Obstet Gynecol 107:144–149

Law PJ, Bartram CI (1989) Anal endosonography: technique and normal anatomy. Gastrointest Radiol 14:349–353

Lunniss PJ, Phillips RK (1992) Anatomy and function of the anal longitudinal muscle. Br J Surg 79:882–884

Mahony R, Behan M, Daly L et al (2007) Internal anal sphincter defect influences continence outcome following obstetric anal sphincter injury. Am J Obstet Gynecol 196:217–225

Marshall M, Halligan S, Fotheringham T et al (2002) Predictive value of internal anal sphincter thickness for diagnosis of rectal intussusception in patients with solitary rectal ulcer syndrome. Br J Surg 89:1281–1285

Martinez Hernandez Magro P, Villanueva Sáenz E, Jaime Zavala M et al (2003) Endoanal sonography in assessment of fecal incontinence following obstetric trauma. Ultrasound Obstet Gynecol 22:616–621

Murad-Regadas SM, Regadas FS, Rodrigues LV et al (2007) A novel procedure to assess anismus using three-dimensional dynamic anal ultrasonography. Colorectal Dis 9:159–165

Oberwalder M, Connor J, Wexner SD (2003) Meta-analysis to determine the incidence of obstetric anal sphincter damage. Br J Surg 90:1333–1337

Peschers UM, DeLancey JO, Fritsch H et al (1997) Cross-sectional imaging anatomy of the anal sphincters. Obstet Gynecol 90:839–844

Pinta T, Kylänpää ML, Luukkonen P et al (2004) Anal incontinence: diagnosis by endoanal US or endovaginal MRI. Eur Radiol 14:1472–1477

Rociu E, Stoker J, Eijkemans MJ, Laméris JS et al (2000) Normal anal sphincter anatomy and age- and sex-related variations at high-spatial-resolution endoanal MR imaging. Radiology 217:395–401

Starck M, Bohe M, Valentin L et al (2006) The extent of endosonographic anal sphincter defects after primary repair of obstetric sphincter tears increases over time and is related to anal incontinence. Ultrasound Obstet Gynecol 27:188–197

Stewart LK, Wilson SR (1999) Transvaginal sonography of the anal sphincter: reliable, or not? AJR Am J Roentgenol 173:179–185

Sultan AH, Kamm MA, Nicholls RJ, Bartram CI (1994a) Prospective study of the extent of internal anal sphincter division during lateral sphincterotomy. Dis Colon Rectum 37:1031–1033

Sultan AH, Loder PB, Bartram CI et al (1994b) Vaginal endosonography. New approach to image the undisturbed anal sphincter. Dis Colon Rectum 37:1296–1299

Timor-Tritsch IE, Monteagudo A, Smilen SW et al (2005) Simple ultrasound evaluation of the anal sphincter in female patients using a transvaginal transducer. Ultrasound Obstet Gynecol 25:177–183

Titi MA, Jenkins JT, Urie A, Molloy RG (2007) Correlation between anal manometry and endosonography in females with faecal incontinence. Colorectal Dis 10:131–137

Vaizey CJ, Kamm MA, Bartram CI (1997) Primary degeneration of the internal anal sphincter as a cause of passive faecal incontinence. Lancet 349:612–615

Van Outryve SM, Van Outryve MJ, De Winter BY, Pelckmans PA (2002) Is anorectal endosonography valuable in dyschesia? Gut 51:695–700

Voyvodic F, Rieger NA, Skinner S et al (2003) Endosonographic imaging of anal sphincter injury: does the size of the tear correlate with the degree of dysfunction? Dis Colon Rectum 46:735–741

West RL, Dwarkasing S, Briel JW et al (2005) Can three-dimensional endoanal ultrasonography detect external anal sphincter atrophy? A comparison with endoanal magnetic resonance imaging. Int J Colorectal Dis 20:328–333

Williams AB, Cheetham MJ, Bartram CI et al (2000) Gender differences in the longitudinal pressure profile of the anal canal related to anatomical structure as demonstrated on three-dimensional anal endosonography. Br J Surg 87:1674–1679

Williams AB, Bartram CI, Halligan S et al (2001a) Anal sphincter damage after vaginal delivery using three-dimensional endosonography. Obstet Gynecol 97:770–775

Williams AB, Bartram CI, Modhwadia D et al (2001b) Endocoil magnetic resonance imaging quantification of external anal sphincter atrophy. Br J Surg 88:853–859

Williams AB, Bartram CI, Halligan S et al (2002) Alteration of anal sphincter morphology following vaginal delivery revealed by multiplanar anal endosonography. Br J Obstet Gynaecol 109:942–946

Zetterstrom JP, Mellgren A, Madoff RD et al (1998) Perineal body measurement improves evaluation of anterior sphincter lesions during endoanal ultrasonography. Dis Colon Rectum 41:705–713

4.5 Pelvic Floor Ultrasound

Hans Peter Dietz

CONTENTS

4.5.1 Introduction

Physicians dealing with female pelvic organ prolapse, urinary and faecal incontinence and defecation disorders are slowly realising that clinical assessment alone is a very inadequate tool to assess pelvic floor function and anatomy. Our examination skills are limited, focusing on surface anatomy rather than true structural abnormalities, and recurrence after pelvic reconstructive surgery is common (DeLancey 2005).

While it may be possible to improve clinical assessment skills, this is unlikely to happen unless we allow imaging techniques to demonstrate what the actual problems are. To give just one example: the missing link between vaginal childbirth and prolapse – major levator trauma in the form of avulsion of the anteromedial aspects of the puborectalis muscle off the pelvic sidewall (Dietz and Lanzarone 2005; Kearney et al. 2006a) – is palpable, but palpation of levator trauma requires considerable skill and teaching (Dietz et al. 2005b; Kearney et al. 2006b; Dietz and Shek 2008), preferably with imaging confirmation. Certainly, diagnosis by imaging is a lot more reproducible than diagnosis by palpation, and much easier to teach. And suspected levator trauma or abnormal distensibility ('ballooning') is by no means the only reason to perform pelvic floor imaging (see Table 4.5.1).

Table 4.5.1. Indications for pelvic floor ultrasound

- Recurrent urinary tract infections
- Urgency, frequency, nocturia and/or urge urinary incontinence
- Stress urinary incontinence
- Insensible urine loss
- Bladder-related pain
- Persistent dysuria
- Symptoms of voiding dysfunction
- Symptoms of prolapse, i.e., the sensation of a lump or a dragging sensation.
- Symptoms of obstructed defecation such as straining at stool, chronic constipation, vaginal or perineal digitation and the sensation of incomplete bowel emptying
- Faecal incontinence
- Pelvic or vaginal pain after anti-incontinence or prolapse surgery
- Vaginal discharge or bleeding after anti-incontinence or prolapse surgery

H. P. Dietz, MD, PhD, FRANZCOG, DDU, CU
Associate Professor in Obstetrics and Gynaecology, Nepean Clinical School, University of Sydney, Nepean Hospital, Penrith NSW 2750, Australia

4.5.2 Equipment and Examination Technique

Basic requirements for translabial pelvic floor ultrasound include a B mode-capable 2D US system with cine loop function, a 3.5–6 Mhz curved array transducer and a videoprinter. A midsagittal view is obtained by placing a transducer (usually a curved array with frequencies between 3.5 and 8 MHz) on the perineum (see Fig. 4.5.1a), after covering the transducer with a glove, condom or thin plastic wrap. Recommendations for sterilisation of external transducers vary from one institution and country to another, ranging from alcoholic wipes to clean the transducer between patients (which the author considers sufficient) to an institutional requirement for sterilization.

Powdered gloves can markedly impair imaging quality due to reverberations and should be avoided. Imaging is usually performed in dorsal lithotomy, with the hips flexed and slightly abducted, or in the standing position. Requiring the patient to place her heels close to the buttocks will result in an improved pelvic tilt. Bladder filling should be specified; usually prior voiding is preferable. The presence of a full rectum may impair diagnostic accuracy and sometimes necessitates a repeat assessment after bowel emptying. Parting of the labia can improve image quality which generally is best in pregnancy and poorest in postmenopausal women with marked atrophy, most likely due to varying hydration of tissues. Vaginal scar tissue can also impair visibility, but obesity virtually never seems to be a problem.

The transducer can usually be placed firmly against the symphysis pubis without causing significant discomfort, unless there is marked atrophy. The resulting image includes the symphysis anteriorly, the urethra and bladder neck, the vagina, cervix, rectum and anal canal (see Fig. 4.5.1b). Posterior to the anorectal junction a hyperechogenic area indicates the central portion of the levator plate, i.e., the puborectalis muscle. The cul de sac may also be seen, filled with a small amount of fluid, echogenic fat or peristalsing small bowel. Parasagittal or transverse views may yield additional information, e.g. enabling assessment of the pubovisceral muscle and its insertion on the arcus tendineus of the levator ani, and for imaging of transobturator implants.

While there has been disagreement regarding image orientation in the midsagittal plane, the author prefers an orientation as on conventional transvaginal ultrasound (cranioventral aspects to the left, dorsocaudal to the right). The latter also seems more convenient when using 3D/4D systems. In Figure 4.5.2 one can see the standard representation of a 3D volume of the pelvic floor. The top left (a) represents the midsagittal plane, with the bottom left (c) being an axial plane slice, and the bottom right representing a rendered volume showing the levator hiatus (d).

The following paragraphs will describe the main clinical applications of the method in urogynecological imaging.

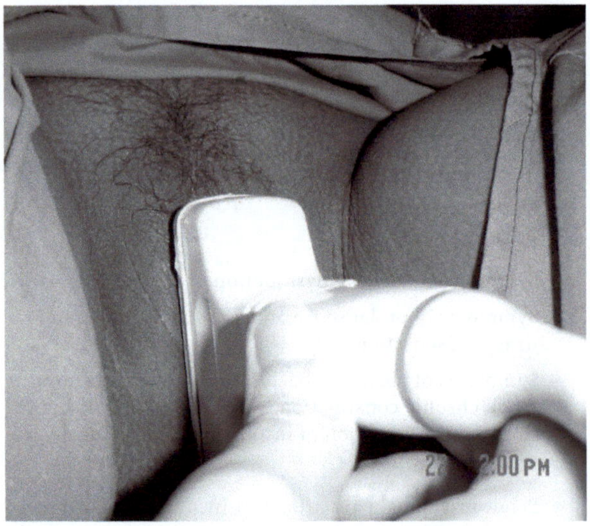
a

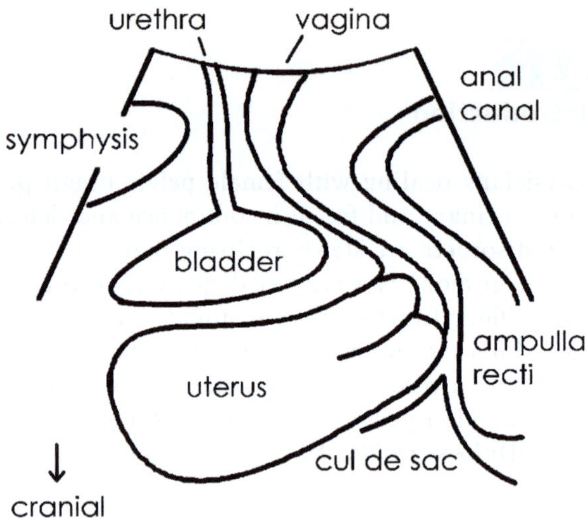

b

Fig. 4.5.1a,b. Transducer placement on the perineum (**a**) and schematic representation of imaging in the midsagittal plane. **a**, courtesy of Dr Nelinda Pangilinan, Manila; **b**, adapted from Ultrasound Obstet Gynecol 2004; 23:80–92, with permission

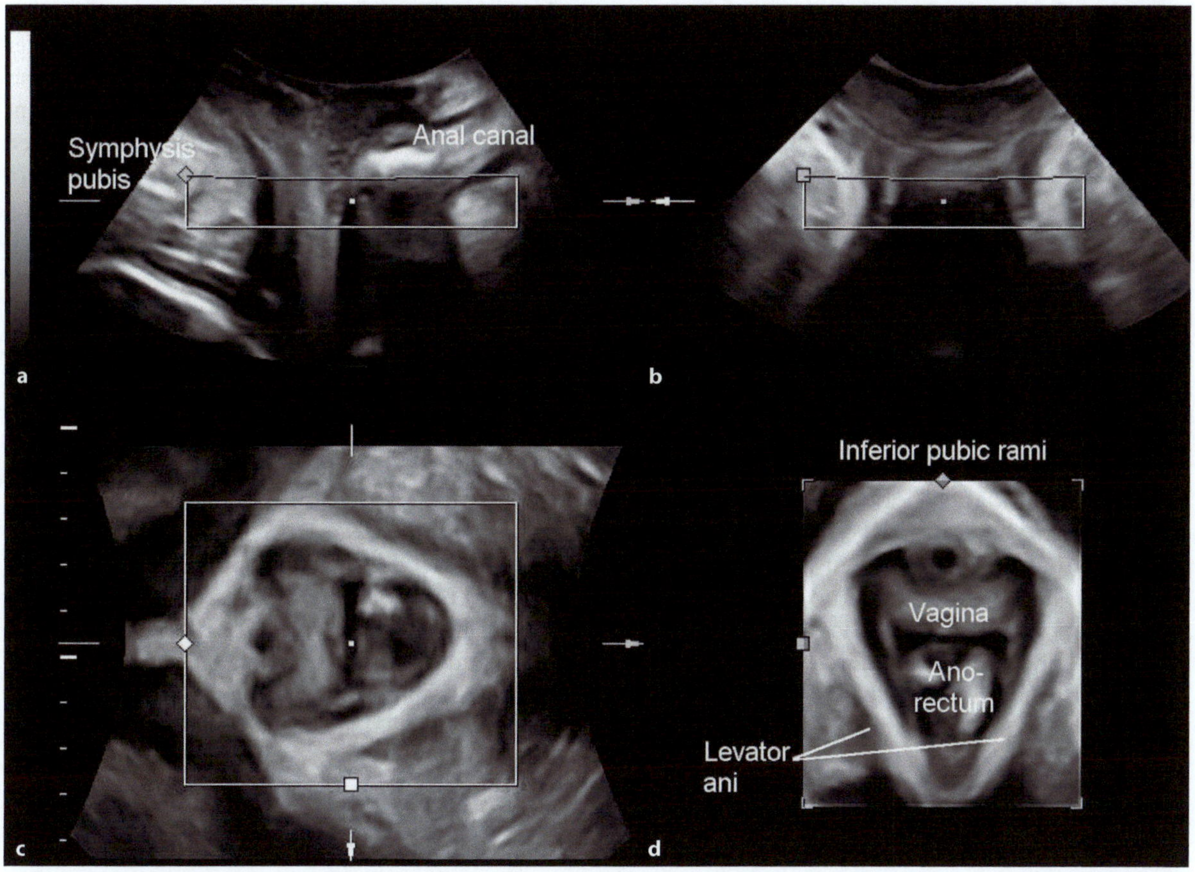

Fig. 4.5.2a–d. Standard acquisition screen of 3D pelvic floor ultrasound. The midsagittal plane is shown in (a), the coronal plane in (b), the axial plane in (c) and a rendered axial plane (i.e. a semitransparent representation of all pixels in the box seen in (a–c) in (d). From Ultrasound Bulletin 2007; 10: 17–23, with permission

4.5.3 Anterior Compartment

The original indication for pelvic floor ultrasound was (and still is) the assessment of bladder neck mobility and funnelling of the bladder neck, both of which are considered important in women with urinary incontinence. Figure 4.5.3 shows the standard orientation used to describe bladder neck mobility. The position of the bladder neck is determined relative to the inferoposterior margin of the symphysis pubis, and comparative studies have shown good correlations with radiological methods previously used for this purpose (for an overview see Dietz 2004a). The one remaining advantage of X-ray fluoroscopy may be the ease with which the voiding phase can be observed although some investigators have used specially constructed equipment to document voiding with ultrasound (Schaer et al. 1998).

4.5.3.1 Bladder Neck Position and Mobility

Bladder neck position and mobility can be assessed with a high degree of reliability. Points of reference are the central axis of the symphysis pubis (Schaer et al. 1995) or its inferoposterior margin (Dietz and Wilson 1998). The full bladder is less mobile (Dietz and Wilson 1999) and may prevent complete development of pelvic organ prolapse. It is essential to not exert undue pressure on the perineum so as to allow full development of pelvic organ descent. Measurements of bladder neck position are performed at rest and on maximal Valsalva, and the difference yields a numerical value for bladder neck descent. On Valsalva, the proximal urethra may be seen to rotate in a postero-inferior direction. The extent of rotation can be measured by comparing the angle of inclination between the proximal urethra and any other fixed axis. Some investigators measure the retrovesical angle (RVA or posterior urethrovesical angle PUV) between the proximal urethra and trigone; others determine the angle γ between the central axis of the symphysis pubis and a line from the inferior symphyseal margin to the bladder neck (Martan et al. 2001). The reproducibility of bladder neck descent seems good, with intraclass correlations of 0.75 or better, indicating 'excellent' agreement (Dietz et al. 2003).

There is no definition of 'normal' for bladder neck descent although cutoffs of 20 and 25 mm have been proposed to define hypermobility. Bladder filling, patient position and catheterization all have been shown to influence measurements (see Dietz 2004 for an overview), and it can occasionally be quite difficult to obtain an effective Valsalva manoeuvre, especially in nulliparous women who routinely co-activate the levator muscle (Oerno and Dietz 2007). Perhaps not surprisingly, publications to date have presented widely differing reference measurements in nulliparous women. While two recent series documented mean or median bladder neck descent of only 5.1 mm (Reed et al. 2002) and 5.3 mm (Brandt et al. 2000) in continent nulliparous women, another study on 39 continent nulliparous volunteers measured an average of 15 mm of bladder neck descent (Peschers et al. 2001). The author has obtained measurements of 1.2–40.2 mm (mean 17.3 mm) in a group of 106 stress continent nulligravid young women of 18–23 years of age (Dietz et al. 2004). It is likely that methodological differences account for the above discrepancies, with all known confounders tending to reduce descent.

The aetiology of increased bladder neck descent is likely to be multifactorial. The wide range of values obtained in young nulliparous women suggests a congenital component. Vaginal childbirth is probably the most significant environmental factor (Peschers et al. 1996; Dietz and Bennett 2003), with a long second stage of labour and vaginal operative delivery associated with increased postpartum descent. This association between increased bladder descent and vaginal parity is also evident in older women with symptoms of pelvic floor dysfunction (Dietz et al. 2002a).

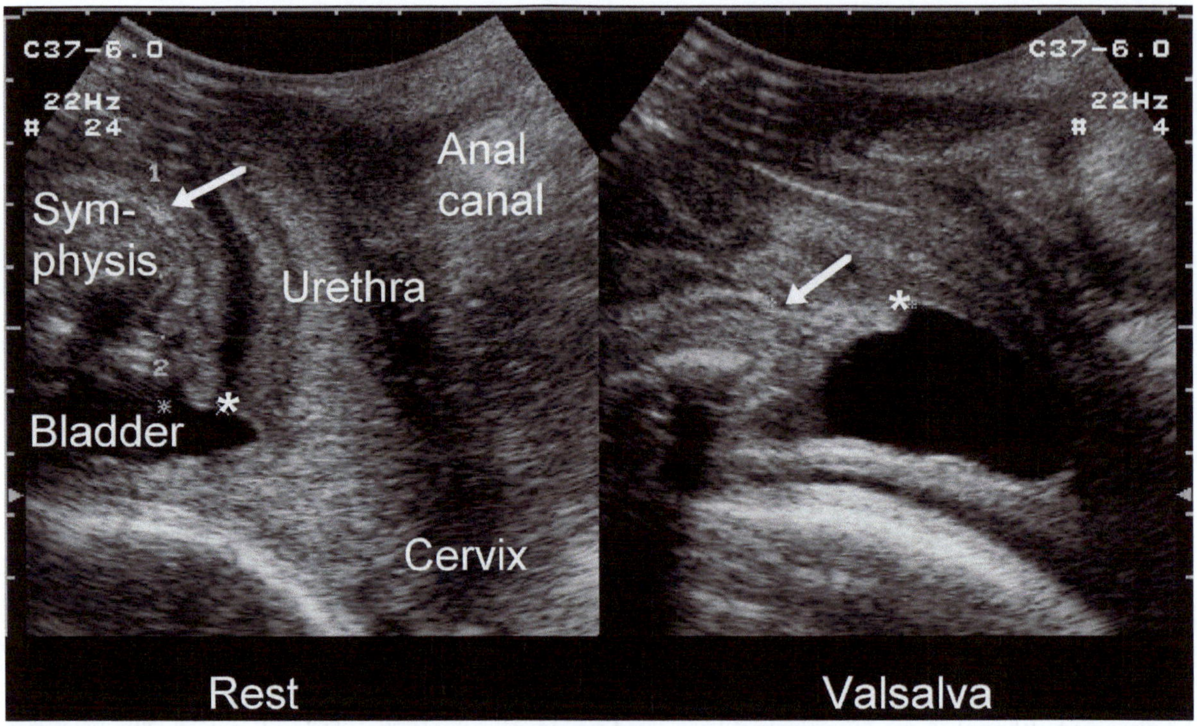

Fig. 4.5.3. Pelvic floor ultrasound, midsagittal plane. The image on the *left* is taken at rest; the one on the *right* is on maximal Valsalva. From Ultrasound Bulletin 2007; 10: 17–23, with permission

4.5.3.2
Funneling

In patients with stress incontinence, but also in asymptomatic women (SCHAER et al. 1999), funneling of the internal urethral meatus may be observed on Valsalva and sometimes even at rest. Funneling is often (but not necessarily) associated with leakage. Other indirect signs of urine leakage on B-mode realtime imaging are weak gray-scale echoes ('streaming') and the appearance of two linear ('specular') echoes defining the lumen of a fluid-filled urethra. However, funneling may also be observed in urge incontinence and can't be used to prove USI. Its anatomical basis is unclear. Marked funneling has been shown to be associated with poor urethral closure pressures (DIETZ and CLARKE 2001a; HUANG and YANG 2003).

4.5.3.3
Colour Doppler

Colour Doppler ultrasound can demonstrate urine leakage on Valsalva manoeuvre or coughing (DIETZ et al. 1999). Agreement between colour Doppler and fluoroscopy was high in a controlled group with indwelling catheters and identical bladder volumes (DIETZ and CLARKE 2001b). Both velocity and energy mapping were able to document leakage. CDV was slightly more likely to show a positive result, probably due to its better motion discrimination. Colour Doppler imaging may also facilitate the documentation of leak point pressures (MASATA et al. 2001). Whether this is in fact desired will depend on the clinician and his/her preferences, and one may well argue that urine leakage and leak point pressures can be determined much more easily.

4.5.3.4
Cystocele

Clinical examination is limited to grading anterior compartment prolapse, which we call 'cystocele'. In fact, imaging will identify a number of anatomical situations that are difficult, if not impossible, to distinguish clinically. There are at least two types of cystoceles with very different functional implications (see Fig. 4.5.4). A cystourethrocele is associated with above-average flow rates and urodynamic stress incontinence (top pair of images), while a cystocele with intact retrovesical angle (bottom pair of images) is generally associated with voiding dysfunction and a low likelihood of stress incontinence (DIETZ et al. 2002b). In addition, occasionally a protrusion of the anterior vaginal wall will turn out to be due to a urethral diverticulum (see Fig. 4.5.5 for a 3D representation of an unusual anterior urethral diverticulum), a Gartner duct cyst or an anterior enterocele, all likely to be missed on clinical examination. Urethral diverticulae are often overlooked for years in women with recurrent bladder infections and symptoms of frequency, urgency and pain or burning on voiding, until imaging is undertaken. Urethral structure and spatial relationships are much better appreciated in the axial plane (see Fig. 4.5.5), which is particularly useful in the differential diagnosis of Gartner cyst and urethral diverticulum.

4.5.3.5
Implants

Recently, synthetic suburethral slings have become very popular. Ultrasound can confirm the presence of such a sling, distinguish between transobturator and retropubic implants, especially when examining the axial plane (see Fig. 4.5.6), and may even allow an educated guess regarding the exact type and material of the tape (DIETZ et al. 2005b). As these implants are highly echogenic, ultrasound is superior to MR in identifying such meshes (SCHUETTOFF et al. 2006) and has helped elucidate their mode of action (DIETZ and WILSON 2004).

There is a worldwide trend towards implantation of permanent vaginal wall meshes, especially for recurrent prolapse, and complications such as failure and mesh erosion are not that uncommon. Polypropylene meshes such as the Prolift®, Perigee® and Apogee® are highly echogenic, and their visibility is limited only by persistent prolapse and transducer distance and alignment. Three-dimensional translabial ultrasound has demonstrated that the implanted mesh often 'shrinks', or more likely, does not remain as flat as it was on implantation (DIETZ et al. 2006a; TUNN et al. 2007; Shek et al. 2008a). Surgical technique seems to play a role here as fixation of mesh to underlying tissues results in a flatter, more even appearance. The position, extent and mobility of vaginal wall mesh can be determined, helping with the assessment of individual technique, and ultrasound may uncover complications such as dislodgment of anchoring arms (SHEK et al. 2007).

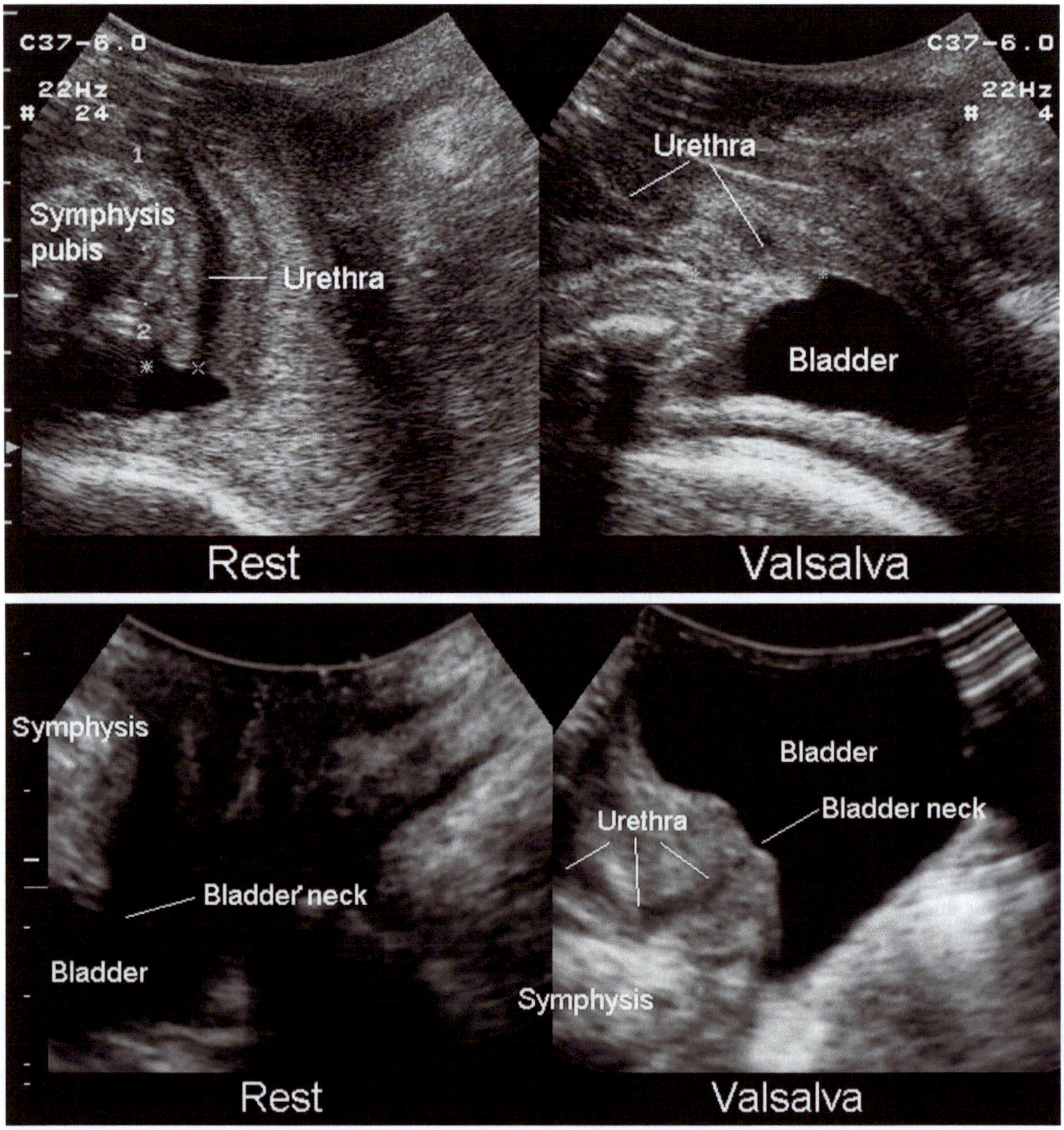

a b c d

Fig. 4.5.4a–d. The two main types of cystocele as imaged on maximal Valsalva in the midsagittal plane: **a,b** Cystourethrocele associated with urinary stress incontinence and good voiding function, and an 'isolated cystocele' (**c,d**) associated with prolapse and voiding dysfunction rather than stress incontinence. From Ultrasound Bulletin 2007; 10: 17–23, with permission

Clearly, translabial 4D ultrasound will be useful in determining functional outcome and location of implants, and will help in optimizing both implant design and surgical technique. Finally, most of the injectables used in anti-incontinence surgery are also highly echogenic and can be visualized as a hyperechoic donut shape surrounding the urethra.

4.5.3.6 Other Findings

Translabial ultrasound may detect foreign bodies or bladder tumours (Dietz 2004a; Tunn et al. 2003) and can be used to determine residual urine, using a formula originally developed for transvaginal ul-

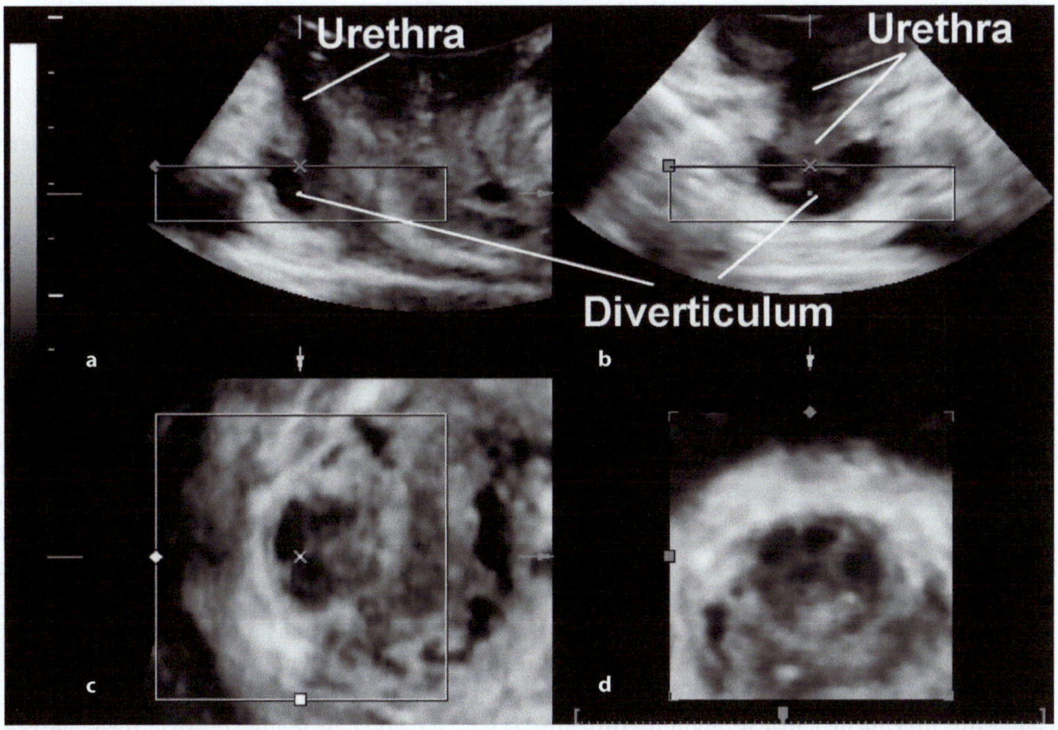

Fig. 4.5.5a–d. Anterior urethral diverticulum on 3D pelvic floor ultrasound. The orthogonal planes (**a–c**) clearly illustrate the location and extent of the diverticulum. From Ultrasound Bulletin 2007; 10: 17–23, with permission

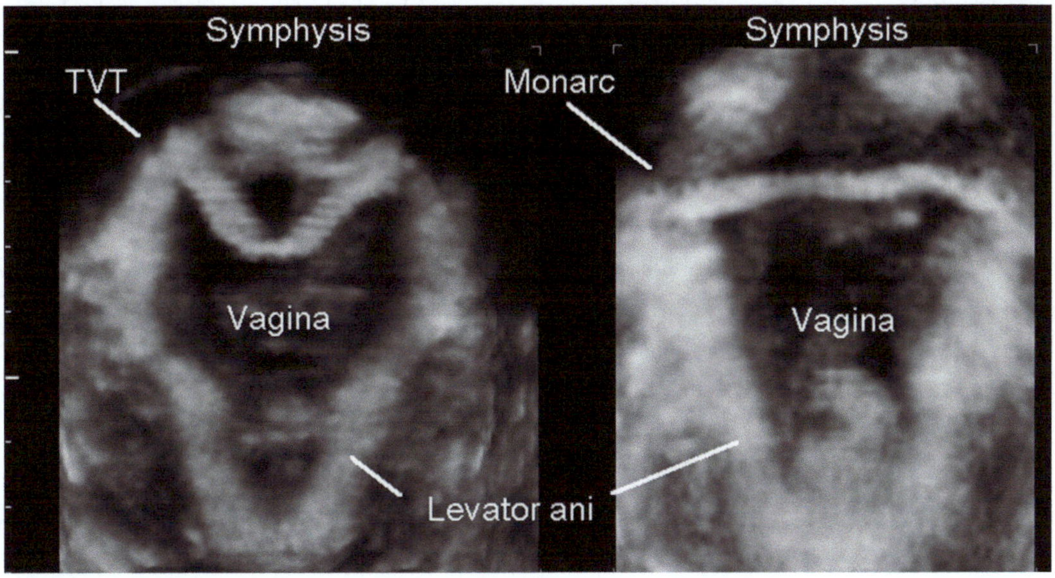

Fig. 4.5.6. Suburethral slings as seen on translabial ultrasound, axial plane. The TVT (*left*) is curving ventrally, while the Monarc arcs laterally towards the insertion of the levator ani muscle. From Ultrasound Bulletin 2007; 10: 17–23, with permission

trasound (Haylen et al. 1989). While detrusor wall thickness (DWT) has probably been overrated as a diagnostic tool in the context of detrusor overactivity (Yang and Huang 2003; Lekskulchai and Dietz 2008), increased DWT is associated with symptoms of the overactive bladder (Lekskulchai and Dietz 2008; Robinson et al. 2002), and may be a predictor of postoperative de novo urge incontinence and/or detrusor overactivity after anti-incontinence procedures (Robinson et al. 2005). As opposed to the situation in the male, DWT in women is not predictive of voiding dysfunction (Lekskulchai and Dietz 2006b).

4.5.4 Central Compartment

Tranbslabial ultrasound is somewhat less useful in the assessment of central compartment prolapse. Generally, uterine prolapse is obvious clinically, as is vaginal vault descent. Having said that, translabial ultrasound may graphically show the effect of an anteriorized cervix in women with an enlarged, retroverted uterus. This finding may help in explaining symptoms of voiding dysfunction and supporting surgical intervention in order to improve voiding in someone with a retroverted fibroid uterus. On the other hand, mild descent of an anteverted uterus may result in compression of the anorectum, explaining symptoms of obstructed defecation – a situation that is termed a 'colpocele' on defecation proctogram.

4.5.5 Posterior Compartment

It is in the posterior compartment where pelvic floor ultrasound is particulary useful. Clinically we diagnose 'rectocele', quite unaware that several different conditions can lead to prolapse of the posterior vaginal wall. A clinical second degree rectocele could be due to a true rectocele, i.e. a defect of the rectovaginal septum (most common, and associated with symptoms of prolapse, incomplete bowel emptying and straining at stool) (Dietz and Korda 2005), due to an abnormally distensible, intact rectovaginal septum (common and associated only with prolapse symptoms), a combined recto- enterocele (less common), an isolated enterocele (uncommon), or just a deficient perineum giving the impression of a 'bulge' (Dietz and Steensma 2005a). Occasionally a 'rectocele' turns out to be due to rectal intussusception, an early stage of rectal prolapse, where the wall of the rectum is inverted and enters the anal canal on Valsalva, propelled by an entorocele; see Figure 4.5.7 for a comparison of three of those conditions.

When a rectocele or rectal intussusception is identified on translabial imaging, one may want to provide the patient with visual biofeedback. Demonstrating that straining at stool is obviously counterproductive may help in modifying behaviour. Several studies have recently shown that ultrasound is much better tolerated than defecation proctography, and of course it is much cheaper. If there is a rectocele or a rectal intussusception/prolapse on ultrasound, this condition is very likely to be found on X-ray imaging (Perniola et al. 2008; Steensma

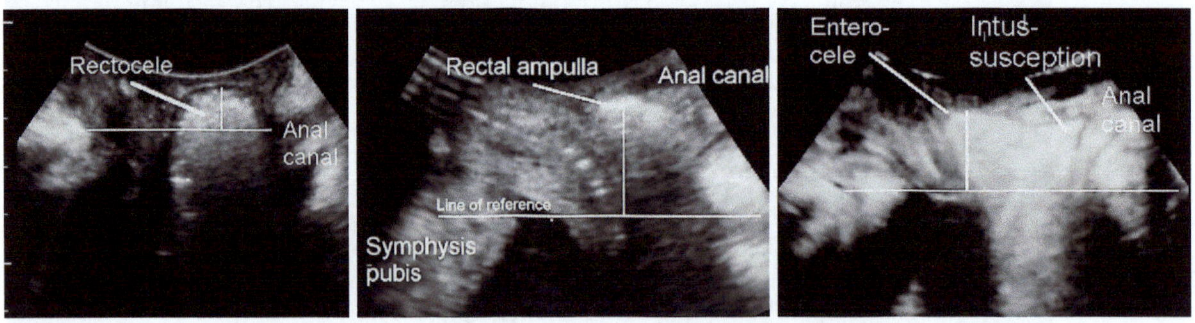

Fig. 4.5.7. The distinction between a 'true rectocele', i.e. a defect of the rectovaginal septum (shown by the *left image*), perineal hypermobility, i.e. descent of the rectal ampulla without fascial defect (*middle image*) and rectal intussusception (*right image*). All three conditions can manifest as a clinical 'rectocele' and are impossible to distinguish on examination

et al. 2007a; KONSTANTINOVIC et al. 2007). Consequently, it is likely that ultrasound will become an alternative to the radiological technique in the initial investigation of women with defecation disorders, avoiding ionizing radiation.

Assessment of the anal sphincter is the subject of Chapter 1 in this book and will receive full consideration there. The anal sphincter is generally imaged by endo-anal ultrasound. This method is firmly established as one of the cornerstones of a colorectal diagnostic workup for anal incontinence and beyond the scope of this review. Due to the limited availability of such probes in gynaecology, obstetricians and gynaecologists have taken to using high-frequency curved array or endovaginal probes placed exo-anally, i.e. transperineally, in the coronal rather than the midsagittal plane (PESCHERS et al. 1997; KLEINUBING et al. 2000; YAGEL and VALSKY 2006). There are advantages to this approach – not just from the point of view of the patient. Exo-anal imaging (see Fig. 45.8) reduces distortion of the anal canal and allows dynamic evaluation of the anal sphincter and mucosa at rest and on sphincter contraction, which seems to enhance the definition of muscular defects. However, resolutions are likely to be inferior (CORNELIA et al. 2002) to those obtained by endoanal ultrasound, and good comparative studies are still lacking.

4.5.6 The Axial Plane

The development of 3D/4D ultrasound has allowed us access to the axial plane, without the intrusiveness and distortion associated with an endovaginal or endoanal probe'. External imaging also has advantages when it comes to the observation of manoeuvres and of their effect on muscle and fascia. This is of major importance as most of the structures providing pelvic organ support are located lateral to the midline. A single volume obtained at rest with an acquisition angle of 70 degrees or higher will include the entire levator hiatus with symphysis pubis, urethra, paravaginal tissues, the vagina, anorectum and pubovisceral (puborectalis/pubococcygeus part of the levator ani) muscle from the pelvic sidewall in the area of the arcus tendineus of the levator ani (ATLA) to the posterior aspect of the anorectal junction. A Valsalva manœuvre however may result in lateral or posterior parts of the puborectalis being displaced outside the field of vision, especially in women with significant prolapse. For this reason higher acquisition angles of 80 or 85 degrees are preferable in pelvic floor imaging. For technical details on volume data acquisition see (DIETZ 2004b).

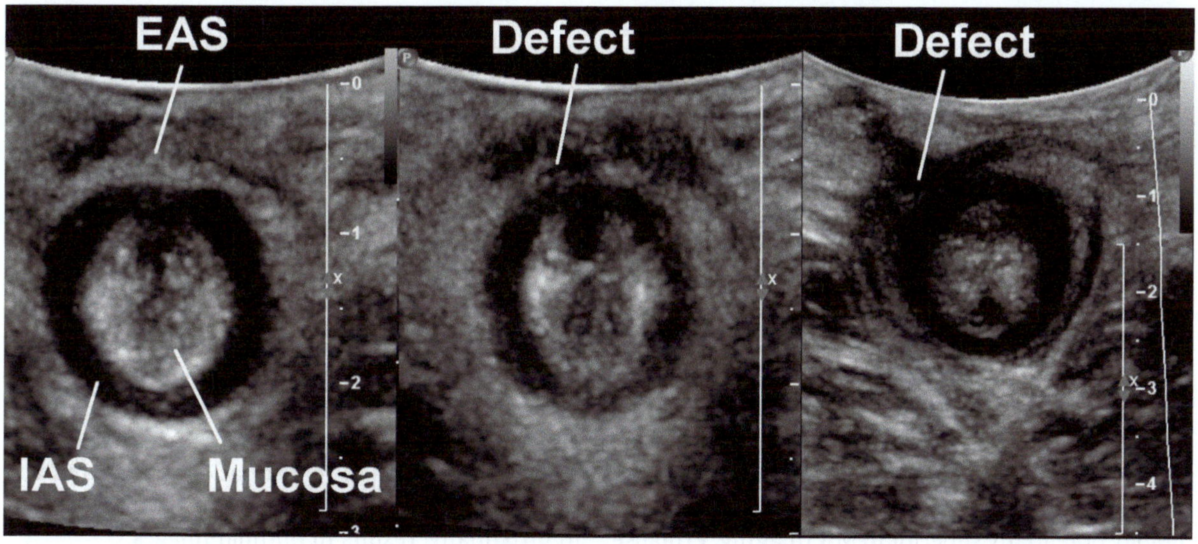

Fig. 4.5.8. Findings after repair of third degree tears. The image on the *left* shows an excellent repair with no discernible scarring of the external anal sphincter (*EAS*). The *central image* shows mild scarring in an asymptomatic patient. The *right* image illustrates a major residual defect that was palpable and associated with flatus incontinence. From: Pelvic Floor Ultrasound, 2007 Springer Verlag London, with permission

4.5.6.1 Display Modes

Figure 4.5.2 demonstrates the two basic display modes currently in use on 3D ultrasound systems. The multiplanar or orthogonal display mode shows cross-sectional planes through the volume in question. For pelvic floor imaging, this most conveniently means the midsagittal (top left), the coronal (top right) and the axial plane (bottom left). Imaging planes on 3D ultrasound can be varied in a completely arbitrary fashion in order to enhance the visibility of a given anatomical structure, either at the time of acquisition or offline at a later time. The levator ani for example usually requires an axial plane that is slightly tilted in a cranioventral to dorsocaudal direction.

The three orthogonal images are complemented by a 'rendered image', i.e. a semitransparent representation of all voxels in an arbitrarily definable 'region of interest'. The bottom right hand image in Figure 4.5.2 shows a standard rendered image of the levator hiatus, with the rendering direction set from caudally to cranially, which is the most appropriate for imaging the hiatus. The possibilities for post-processing are restricted only by the software used for this purpose.

4.5.6.2 Four-Dimensional Imaging

Four-dimensional imaging implies the real-time acquisition of volume ultrasound data, which can then be represented in orthogonal planes or rendered volumes. Many systems are now capable of storing cine loops of volumes, which is of major importance in pelvic floor imaging as it allows enhanced documentation of functional anatomy. Even on 2D single plane imaging, a static assessment at rest gives little information compared with the evaluation of manoeuvres such as a levator contraction and Valsalva. Their observation will allow assessment of levator function and delineate levator or fascial trauma more clearly.

The ability to perform a real-time 3D (or 4D) assessment of pelvic floor structures makes the technology potentially superior to MR imaging. Prolapse assessment by MR requires ultra-fast acquisition (Yang et al. 1991), which is of limited availability and will not allow optimal resolutions. Alternatively, some systems allow imaging of the sitting or erect patient, but again accessibility will be limited for the foreseeable future. The sheer physical characteristics of MRI systems make it much harder for the operator to ensure efficient manoeuvres as over 50% of all women will not perform a proper pelvic floor contraction when asked (Bo et al. 1988), and a Valsalva is often confounded by concomitant levator activation (Oerno and Dietz 2007). Observation of dynamic studies and interaction with the patient is needed until a satisfactory image is obtained, and this may be more conveniently done with ultrasound. Therefore, ultrasound has major potential advantages when it comes to describing prolapse, especially when associated with fascial or muscular defects, and in terms of defining functional anatomy. In addition, offline analysis packages allow distance, area and volume measurements in any user-defined plane (oblique or orthogonal), which is much superior to what is possible with DICOM viewer software on a standard set of single-plane MRI images.

4.5.6.3 Clinical Applications

At the moment, axial plane imaging is limited to the assessment of the levator ani muscle, occasionally extending to paraurethral tissues in patients with diverticulae or strictures. Translabial ultrasound has confirmed 60-year-old clinical data (Gainey 1943) and MRI studies (DeLancey et al. 2003) showing that major morphological abnormalities of levator structure and function are common in vaginally parous women (Dietz and Steensma 2006). Very recently it has been conclusively proven that such morphological abnormalities are due to vaginal delivery (Dietz and Lanzarone 2005; Dietz et al. 2007); see Figure 4.5.9 for a comparison of MR, ultrasound and clinical findings in one patient with unilateral levator avulsion. Such trauma can be documented on 2D ultrasound – either with a side-firing endocavitary probe (Athanasiou et al. 2007) or with a parasagittal probe orientation. However, the most convenient and reproducible approach is by using an abdominal 3D probe – the technology that is used to image a baby's face. Just as in that situation, a rendered volume, with the rendering direction set from distally to proximally, results in optimal images.

Major delivery-related levator trauma, affecting the inferomedial aspects of the pubovisceral muscle, clearly is part of the missing link between vaginal childbirth and prolapse. While there are

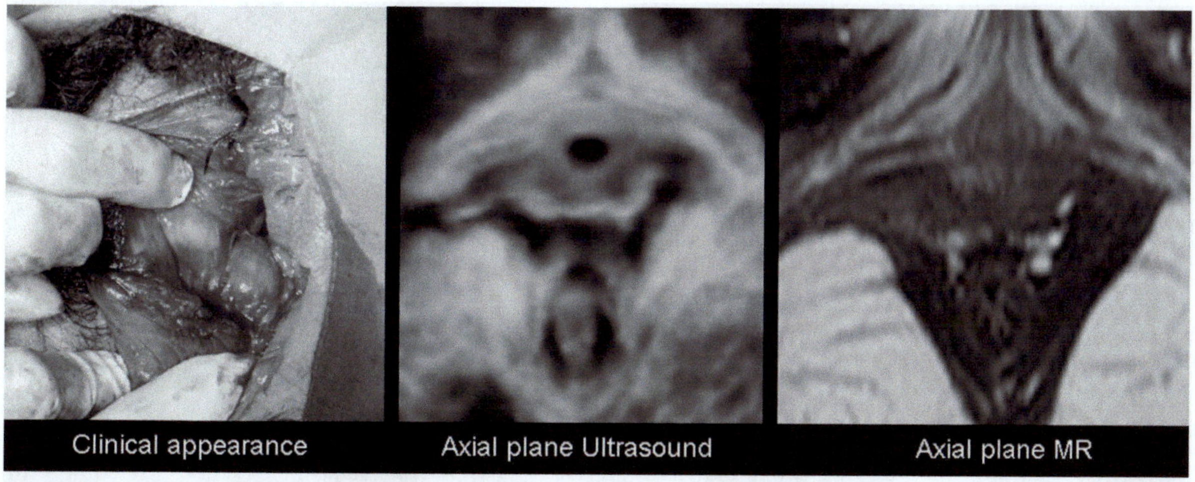

Fig. 4.5.9. Delivery-related levator trauma as seen on exploration of a large vaginal tear after vaginal delivery (*left*), as imaged on translabial 4D ultrasound (*middle*) and on MR (*right*). From Ultrasound Bulletin 2007; 10:17–23, with permission

other factors, probably including microtrauma or altered biomechanics of otherwise intact muscle, levator trauma seems to enlarge the hiatus (Dietz 2006) and results in anterior and central compartment prolapse (Dietz and Steensma 2006; Dietz and Simpson 2008). The larger the defect, the higher is the likelihood of prolapse (Dietz 2007), as quantified on multi-slice or tomographic ultrasound (see Fig. 4.5.10). Levator defects seem to be associated with cystocele recurrence after anterior repair (Adekanmi et al. 2005), in our population almost double the likelihood of significant prolapse (Dietz and Simpson 2008), and are associated with reduced contractile strength (Dietz and Shek 2008a; DeLancey et al. 2007). These defects are palpable, but palpation requires significant teaching (Kearney et al. 2006b; Dietz et al. 2006) and is clearly less repeatable ($\kappa = 0.41$) (Dietz and Shek 2008b) than identification by ultrasound (Cohen's kappa (κ) = 0.83 on analysis of whole volumes and $\kappa = 0.61$ for single slices in own data) (Dietz 2007; Weinstein et al. 2007a). There may be an increased prevalence of levator defects in women with anal sphincter defects, which is not really surprising given the overlap in risk factors (Weinstein et al. 2007b; Steensma et al. 2007b). Bilateral defects are more difficult to detect since there is no normal side to compare with, but they have a particularly severe impact on pelvic floor function and organ support (Dietz and Simpson 2008; Dietz and Shek 2008a).

Another factor only apparent on axial plane imaging is the degree of hiatal distension on Valsalva. Figure 4.5.11 gives an impression of the range of hiatal area measurements in patients attending a pelvic floor clinic. Measures of hiatal dimensions seem highly repeatable (Dietz et al. 2005c; Yang et al. 2006; Majida et al. 2006; Guaderrama et al. 2006; Kruger et al. 2007a) and correlate well with findings on magnetic resonance imaging (Kruger et al. 2007). Hiatal enlargement to over 25 cm^2 on Valsalva is defined as 'ballooning' on the basis of receiver operator characteristics statistics (Dietz et al. 2008) and normative data in young nulliparous women (Dietz et al. 2005c; Yang et al. 2006). The degree of distension is strongly associated with prolapse (Dietz and Steensma 2005b) and symptoms of prolapse (Dietz et al. 2008). It seems that ballooning is associated with prolapse recurrence after rectocele repair (Barry et al. 2006c), and the same probably holds true for other forms of prolapse surgery.

If delivery-related trauma and excessive distensibility of the levator are indeed risk factors for female pelvic organ prolapse and recurrence after reconstructive surgery, then of course we should know about it preoperatively and adjust our surgical approach accordingly. Some forms of prolapse are probably impossible to cure surgically unless one uses mesh implants such as the transobturator mesh shown in Figure 4.5.12. In future, we should aim to develop surgical methods that reduce the size and distensibility of the hiatus or reconnect the detached muscle in an attempt to prevent recurrence – and in 2008 this is no longer a hypothetical goal.

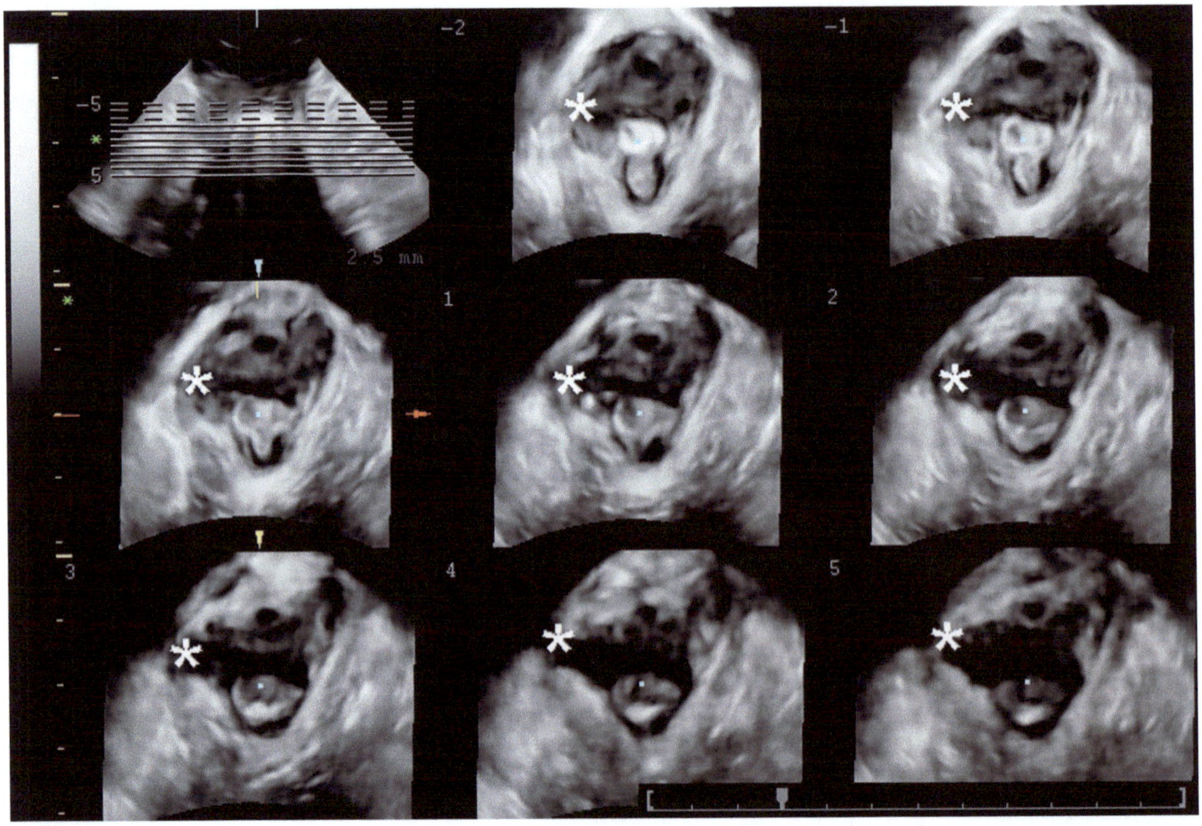

Fig. 4.5.10. Quantification of trauma on multislice/tomographic ultrasound imaging. There is a typical right-sided levator defect (indicated by * on the left hand side of the eight tomographic images) measuring about 2 cm in (dorsoventral) width and at least 1.75 cm in (craniocaudal) depth as it is apparent in all eight slices

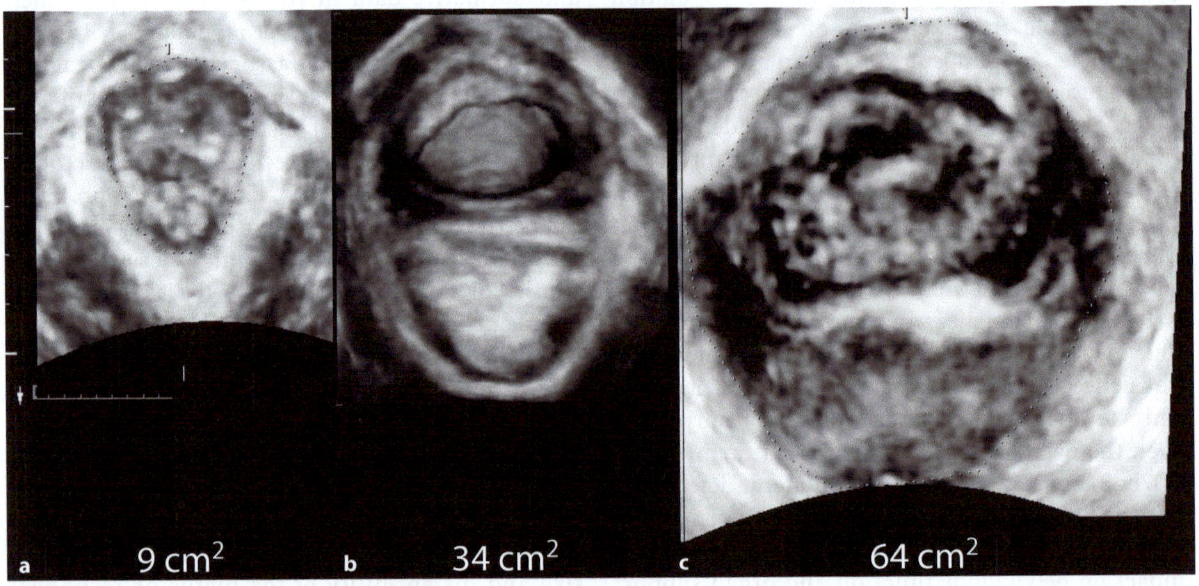

Fig. 4.5.11a–c. Hiatal area measurements (**a**, normal narrow hiatus at 9 cm^2; **b**, moderate ballooning in a parous patient at 34 cm^2; **c**, severe ballooning of 64 cm^2 in a patient with bilateral avulsion and three compartment prolapse) illustrating the range of findings that may be obtained in women with symptoms of lower urinary tract dysfunction

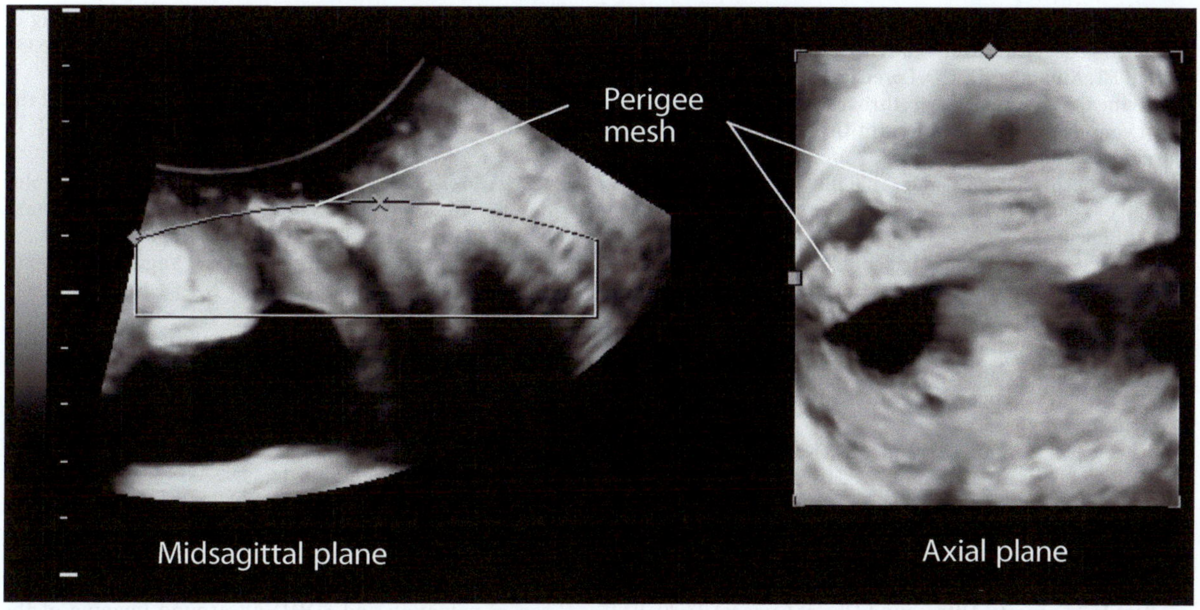

Fig. 4.5.12. 'Perigee' anterior vaginal wall mesh repair as imaged in the midsagittal plane (*left*) and a rendered volume in the axial plane (*right*). From Ultrasound Bulletin 2007; 10: 17–23, with permission

4.5.7 Conclusion

Even prior to the widespread introduction of 3D/4D imaging, pelvic floor ultrasound was a highly useful diagnostic tool for physicians dealing with pelvic floor disorders. As of 2008, this includes not just gynaecologists, urologists, urogynaecologists and radiologists, but also colorectal surgeons and gastroenterologists. Current trends, i.e. the near universal introduction of 4D ultrasound, new software options and increasing availability of training, will likely lead to more general acceptance of ultrasound as a standard diagnostic option in pelvic floor medicine. The issue of levator trauma, one of the most significant developments in clinical obstetrics since the introduction of foetal monitoring, will take pelvic floor ultrasound from a niche application into the mainstream and speed the convergence of clinical specialties dealing with pelvic floor disorders. The crucial issue, as always, is teaching and the provision of up-to-date resources, and it may still be another decade or two before this method truly becomes a fully accepted part of the diagnostic workup in women with pelvic floor disorders.

Further information may be obtained from the following website
http://web.mac.com/hpdietz1/iWeb/Site/Welcome.html
and the recently published 'Atlas of Pelvic Floor Ultrasound', Eds. HP Dietz, AB Steensma and L Hoyte, Springer Verlag London 2007.

References

Adekanmi OA, Freeman R, Puckett M, Jackson S (2005) Cystocele: Does anterior repair fail because we fail to correct the fascial defects? A clinical and radiological study. Int Urogynecol J 16:S73

Athanasiou S, Chaliha C, Toozs-Hobson P, Salvatore S, Khullar V, Cardozo L (2007) Direct imaging of the pelvic floor muscles using two-dimensional ultrasound: A comparison of women with urogenital prolapse versus controls. Br J Obstet Gynaecol 114:882–888

Barry C, Dietz H, Lim Y, Rane A (2006) A short-term independent audit of mesh repair for the treatment of rectocele in women, using 3-dimensional volume ultrasound: A pilot study. Aust NZ Continence J 12:94–99

Bo K, Larson S, Oseid S, Kvarstein B, Hagen R, Jorgensen J (1988) Knowledge about and ability to do correct pelvic

floor muscle exercises in women with urinary stress incontinence. Neurourol Urodyn 7:261–262
Brandt FT, Albuquerque CD, Lorenzato FR, Amaral FJ (2000) Perineal assessment of urethrovesical junction mobility in young continent females. Int Urogynecol J 11:18–22
Cornelia L, Stephan B, Michel B, Antoine W, Felix K (2002) Trans-perineal versus endo-anal ultrasound in the detection of anal sphincter tears. Eur J Obstet Gynecol Reproduct Biol 103:79–82
DeLancey JO (2005) The hidden epidemic of pelvic floor dysfunction: Achievable goals for improved prevention and treatment. Am J Obstet Gynecol 192:1488–1495
DeLancey JO, Kearney R, Chou Q, Speights S, Binno S (2003) The appearance of levator ani muscle abnormalities in magnetic resonance images after vaginal delivery. Obstet Gynecol 101:46–53
DeLancey JO, Morgan D, Fenner D, Kearney R, Guire K, Miller J, Hussain H, Umek W, Hsu Y, Ashton-Miller J (2007) Comparison of levator ani muscle defects and function in women with and without pelvic organ prolapse. Obstet Gynecol 109:295–302
Dietz HP (2004a) Ultrasound imaging of the pelvic floor: Part 1: 2d aspects. Ultrasound Obstet Gynecol 23:80–92
Dietz HP (2004b) Ultrasound imaging of the pelvic floor: 3d aspects. Ultrasound Obstet Gynecol 23:615–625
Dietz HP (2007) Quantification of major morphological abnormalities of the levator ani. Ultrasound Obstet Gynecol 29:329–334
Dietz HP, Wilson PD (1998) Anatomical assessment of the bladder outlet and proximal urethra using ultrasound and videocystourethrography. Int Urogynecol J 9:365–369
Dietz HP, Wilson PD (1999) The influence of bladder volume on the position and mobility of the urethrovesical junction. Int Urogynecol J 10:3–6
Dietz HP, Clarke B (2001a) The urethral pressure profile and ultrasound imaging of the lower urinary tract. Int Urogynecol J 12:38–41
Dietz HP, Clarke B (2001b) Translabial color doppler urodynamics. Int Urogynecol J 12:304–307
Dietz HP, Bennett MJ (2003) The effect of childbirth on pelvic organ mobility.[comment]. Obstet Gynecol 102:223–228
Dietz HP, Wilson PD (2004) The 'iris effect': How two-dimensional and three-dimensional ultrasound can help us understand anti-incontinence procedures. Ultrasound Obstet Gynecol 23:267–271
Dietz HP, Korda A (2005) Which bowel symptoms are most strongly associated with a true rectocele? Aust NZ J Obstet Gynaecol 45:505–508
Dietz HP, Lanzarone V (2005) Levator trauma after vaginal delivery. Obstet Gynecol 106:707–712
Dietz HP, Steensma AB (2005a) Posterior compartment prolapse on two- dimensional and three- dimensional pelvic floor ultrasound: The distinction between true rectocele, perineal hypermobility and enterocele. Ultrasound Obstet Gynecol 26:73–77
Dietz HP, Steensma AB (2005b) Dimensions of the levator hiatus in symptomatic women. Ultrasound Obstet Gynecol 26:369–370
Dietz HP, Steensma AB (2006) The prevalence of major abnormalities of the levator ani in urogynaecological patients. Br J Obstet Gynaecol 113:225–230
Dietz HP, Simpson J (2008) Levator trauma is associated with pelvic organ prolapse. Br J Obstet Gynecol, in print
Dietz HP, Shek C (2008a). Levator Avulsion and Grading of Pelvic Floor Muscle Strength. Int Urogynecol J 19:633–636
Dietz HP, Shek C (2008b) Validity and reproducibility of the digital detection of levator trauma. Int Urogynecol J; in print
Dietz HP, McKnoulty L, Clarke B (1999) Translabial color doppler for imaging in urogynecology: A preliminary report. Ultrasound Obstet Gynecol 14:144–147
Dietz HP, Clarke B, Vancaillie TG (2002a) Vaginal childbirth and bladder neck mobility. Aust NZ J Obstet Gynaecol 42:522–525
Dietz HP, Haylen BT, Vancaillie TG (2002b) Female pelvic organ prolapse and voiding function. Int Urogynecol J 13:284–288
Dietz HP, Eldridge A, Grace M, Clarke B (2003) Test-retest reliability of the ultrasound assessment of bladder neck mobility. Int Urogynecol J 14:S57–S58
Dietz HP, Eldridge A, Grace M, Clarke B (2004) Pelvic organ descent in young nulliparous women. Am J Obstet Gynecol 191:95–99
Dietz HP, Hyland G, Hay Smith E (2005a) A blinded comparison of palpation and 3D/4D ultrasound imaging of the pubovisceral muscle. Int Urogynecol J 16:S75
Dietz HP, Barry C, Lim YN, Rane A (2005b) Two-dimensional and three-dimensional ultrasound imaging of suburethral slings. Ultrasound Obstetr Gynecol 26:175–179
Dietz HP, Shek C, Clarke B (2005c) Biometry of the pubovisceral muscle and levator hiatus by three-dimensional pelvic floor ultrasound. Ultrasound Obstet Gynecol 25:580–585
Dietz HP, Hyland G, Hay-Smith J (2006) The assessment of levator trauma: A comparison between palpation and 4d pelvic floor ultrasound. Neurourol Urodyn 25:424–427
Dietz HP, Gillespie A, Phadke P (2007) Avulsion of the pubovisceral muscle associated with large vaginal tear after Normal Vaginal Delivery at term. A Case Report. Aust NZ J Obstet Gynecol 47:341–44
Dietz HP, Shek C, De Leon J, Steensma A (2008) Ballooning of the levator hiatus. Ultrasound Obstet Gynecol 31:676–680
Gainey HL (1943) Post-partum observation of pelvic tissue damage. Am J Obstet Gynecol 46:457–466
Guaderrama N, Liu J, Nager C, Pretorius D, Sheean G, Kassab G, Mittal R (2006) Evidence for the innervation of pelvic floor muscles by the pudendal nerve. Obstet Gynecol 106:774–781
Haylen BT, Frazer MI, Sutherst JR, West CR (1989) Transvaginal ultrasound in the assessment of bladder volumes in women. Preliminary report. Br J Urol 63:149–151
Huang WC, Yang JM (2003) Bladder neck funneling on ultrasound cystourethrography in primary stress urinary incontinence: A sign associated with urethral hypermobility and intrinsic sphincter deficiency. Urology 61:936–941
Kearney R, Miller J, Ashton-Miller J, Delancey J (2006a) Obstetric factors associated with levator ani muscle injury after vaginal birth. Obstet Gynecol 107:144–149
Kearney R, Miller JM, Delancey JO (2006b) Interrater reliability and physical examination of the pubovisceral portion of the levator ani muscle, validity comparisons using MR imaging. Neurourol Urodynamics 25:50–54

Kleinubing H Jr, Jannini JF, Malafaia O, Brenner S, Pinho TM (2000) Transperineal ultrasonography: New method to image the anorectal region. Dis Colon Rectum 43:1572–1574

Konstantinovic ML, Steensma AB, Domali E, Van Beckevoort D, Timmerman D, De Ridder D, Deprest J (2007) Correlation between 3D/4D translabial ultrasound and colpocystodefecography in diagnosis of posterior compartment prolapse. Ultrasound Obstet Gynecol 30:448

Kruger J, Heap X, Dietz HP (2007) A comparison of mri and ultrasound in the assessment of the levator hiatus. Ultrasound Obstet Gynecol 30:447

Kruger J, Heap S., Murphy B, Dietz HP (2008) Pelvic floor function in nulliparous women imaged using 3D Ultrasound and Magnetic Resonance Imaging. Obstet Gynecol 111:631–638

Lekskulchai O, Dietz HP (2006) Is detrusor hypertrophy in women associated with symptoms and signs of voiding dysfunction? ICS Annual Scientific Meeting

Lekskulchai O, Dietz HP (2008) Detrusor wall thickness as a test for detrusor overactivity in women. Ultrasound Obstet Gynaecol; in print

Majida M, Hoff Braekken I, Bo K, Umek W, Dietz HP, Ellstrom Engh M (2006) 3D and 4D ultrasound of the pelvic floor. An interobserver reliability study. Int Urogynecol J 17:S136–137

Martan A, Masata J, Halaska M, Voigt R (2001)Ultrasound imaging of the lower urinary system in women after burch colposuspension. Ultrasound Obstet Gynecol 17:58–64

Masata J, Martan A, Halaska M, Kasikova E, Otcenasek M, Voigt R (2001) Detection of valsalva leak point pressure with colour Doppler-new method for routine use. Neurourol Urodyn 20:494–496

Oerno A, Dietz HP (2007) Levator co-activation is a significant confounder of pelvic organ descent on valsalva maneuver. Ultrasound Obstet Gynecol 30:346–350

Perniola G, Dietz HP, Shek C, Chew S, Cartmill J, Chong C (2008). Defecation proctography and translabial ultrasound in the investigation of defecatory disorders. Ultrasound Obstet Gynecol 31:567–571

Peschers U, Schaer G, Anthuber C, DeLancey JO, Schuessler B (1996) Changes in vesical neck mobility following vaginal delivery. Obstet Gynecol 88:1001–1006

Peschers UM, DeLancey JO, Schaer GN, Schuessler B (1997) Exoanal ultrasound of the anal sphincter: Normal anatomy and sphincter defects. Br J Obstet Gynaecol 104:999–1003

Peschers UM, Fanger G, Schaer GN, Vodusek DB, DeLancey JO, Schuessler B (2001) Bladder neck mobility in continent nulliparous women. BJOG. 108:320–324

Reed H, Waterfield A, Freeman RM, Adekanmi OA (2002) Bladder neck mobility in continent nulliparous women: Normal references. Int Urogynecol J 13:S4

Robinson D, Anders K, Cardozo L, Bidmead J, Toozs-Hobson P, Khullar V (2002) Can ultrasound replace ambulatory urodynamics when investigating women with irritative urinary symptoms? BJOG: Int J Obstet Gynaecol 109:145–148

Robinson D, Khullar V, Cardozo L (2005) Can bladder wall thickness predict postoperative detrusor overactivity? Int Urogynecol J 16:S106

Schaer GN, Koechli OR, Schuessler B, Haller U (1995) Perineal ultrasound for evaluating the bladder neck in urinary stress incontinence. Obstet Gynecol 85:220–224

Schaer GN, Siegwart R, Perucchini D, DeLancey JO (1998) Examination of voiding in seated women using a remote-controlled ultrasound probe. Obstet Gynecol 91:297–301

Schaer GN, Perucchini D, Munz E, Peschers U, Koechli OR, DeLancey JO (1999) Sonographic evaluation of the bladder neck in continent and stress-incontinent women. Obstet Gynecol 93:412–416

Schuettoff S, Beyersdorff D, Gauruder- Burmester A, Tunn R (2006) Visibility of the polypropylene tape after tvt (tension-free vaginal tape) procedure in women with stress urinary incontinence – a comparison of introital ultrasound and mri in vitro and in patients. Ultrasound Obstet Gynecol 27:687–692

Shek C, Rane A, Goh JTW, Dietz HP (2007) Imaging of the perigee transobturator mesh and its effect on stress incontinence. Ultrasound Obstet Gynecol 30:446

Shek C, Dietz HP, Rane A, Balakrishnan S (2008). Transobturator mesh repair for large and recurrent cystocele. Ultrasound Obstet Gynecol; in print

Steensma AB, Oom DMJ, Burger CW, Schouten WR (2007a) Comparison of defecography and 3D/4D translabial ultrasound in patients with pelvic organ prolapse and/or evacuation disorders. Ultrasound Obstet Gynecol 30:447

Steensma AB, Schweitzer KJ, Burger CW, Schouten WR (2007b) Are anal sphincter injuries related to levator abnormalities? Ultrasound Obstet Gynecol 30:448

Tunn R, Petri E (2003) Introital and transvaginal ultrasound as the main tool in the assessment of urogenital and pelvic floor dysfunction: An imaging panel and practical approach. Ultrasound in Obstet Gynecol 22:205–213

Tunn R, Picot A, Marschke J, Gauruder-Burmester A (2007) Sonomorphological evaluation of polypropylene mesh implants after vaginal mesh repair in women with cystocele or rectocele. Ultrasound Obstet Gynecol 29:449–452

Weinstein MM, Pretorius D, Nager CW, Mittal R (2007a) Inter-rater reliability of pelvic floor muscle imaging abnormalities with 3D ultrasound. Ultrasound Obstet Gynecol 30:538

Weinstein MM, Pretorius D, Jung SY, Nager CW, Mittal R (2007b) Anatomic defects in the puborectalis muscle in women with fecal incontinence. Ultrasound Obstet Gynecol 30:637

Yagel S, Valsky DV (2006) Three-dimensional transperineal sonography for evaluation of the anal sphincter complex: Another dimension in understanding peripartum sphincter trauma. Ultrasound Obstet Gynecol 27:119–123

Yang A, Mostwin JL, Rosenshein NB, Zerhouni EA (1991) Pelvic floor descent in women: Dynamic evaluation with fast mr imaging and cinematic display. Radiology 179:25–33

Yang JM, Huang WC (2003) Bladder wall thickness on ultrasonographic cystourethrography: Affecting factors and their implications. J Ultrasound Med 22:777–782

Yang JM, Yang SH, Huang WC (2006) Biometry of the pubovisceral muscle and levator hiatus in nulliparous chinese women. Ultrsound Obstet Gynecol 26:710–716

Imaging Techniques

4.6 Endoanal Magnetic Resonance Imaging

Annette C. de Bruijne-Dobben and Jaap Stoker

CONTENTS

A. C. de Bruijne-Dobben, PhD
J. Stoker, MD, PhD
Department of Radiology, Academic Medical Center, University of Amsterdam, Meibergdreef 9, 1105 AZ Amsterdam, The Netherlands

4.6.1 Introduction

Disorders of the external and/or internal anal sphincter muscles are a major cause of fecal incontinence. External anal sphincter insufficiency is caused by a defect of the muscle or by damage to the pudendal nerve, resulting in atrophy of the external anal sphincter with subsequent weakness. Childbirth is the main cause of fecal incontinence in women. Both the muscle itself as well as the pudendal nerve can be damaged during delivery. The internal anal sphincter can also be damaged in combination with the external anal sphincter when a large rupture of the anal sphincter occurs. Isolated internal anal sphincter defects are mainly caused by anorectal surgery (anal sphincter trauma) (Kamm 1994).

Magnetic resonance imaging (MRI) with an endoluminal device has taken a prominent place in the evaluation of fecal incontinence. The high-resolution images obtained with endoanal MRI are very well suited for assessment of morphologic sphincter disorders (deSouza et al. 1996; Stoker et al. 1996). This has led to further insight into the pathogenesis of fecal incontinence.

4.6.2 Imaging Technique

4.6.2.1 Coil and Patient Preparation

There are some differences in the design and diameter of the endoluminal coils used for endoluminal imaging. In some institutions, a rectal coil with a balloon is used, but more optimal results are obtained with a dedicated anal coil without a balloon.

Cylindrical saddle geometry receiver coils, rectangular receive-only coils, as well as phased-array geometry coils are used (Stoker et al. 1999). With these coils high-spatial-resolution MR images can be obtained. The diameter of the coils available ranges from 7–17 mm, while the coil holder will add approximately 2 mm to the outer diameter. A larger diameter coil (e.g., 17 mm) can be recommended as this will result in a more uniform signal intensity of the anal sphincter muscles, while the diameter will not be a disadvantage in fecal-incontinent patients.

Patients need to be prepared carefully for the procedure. They first have to empty their bladder before the study in order to prevent discomfort from a distended bladder and consequent motion artifacts. The endoanal coil is covered with a condom and after application of a lubricant (we use ultrasound gel) inserted in the anal canal in a left lateral position. After positioning of the endoanal coil, the patient turns in a supine position, and supportive pads are used to stabilize the position of the endoanal coil. To reduce motion artifacts the patient is asked to fast for 4 h, and attention should be paid to patient comfort during the examination. Bowel relaxants (1 ml butylscopolamine bromide, Buscopan, 20 mg/ml, Boehringer Ingelheim, Germany – which is not approved in the USA – or 1 mg of glucagon hydrochloride, Glucagen, Bagsvaerd, Denmark) may be used to reduce bowel peristalsis. A bowel relaxant can be beneficial, but it is not scientifically proven. The patient should be informed not to squeeze the coil and to relax their anal sphincter and pelvic floor muscles.

Endoanal MRI is well tolerated by nearly all patients with fecal incontinence (Deutekom et al. 2006), although some patients refuse going into the magnet due to claustrophobia. Discomfort is comparable to that at endoanal ultrasound (US); however, the procedure is more time consuming (approximately 30 min versus 10 min room time).

4.6.2.2 Sequences and Protocol

The optimal imaging protocol for endoanal MRI in fecal-incontinent patients has not been established. T2-weighted sequences result in optimal contrast difference between the anal sphincters and the surrounding structures when relatively limited T2 weighting is used. The use of T1-weighted sequences without intravenous contrast medium is not beneficial (sphincters are hardly discernible), while the use of intravenous contrast medium has not been demonstrated to be superior to T2-weighted sequences.

The following T2-weighted fast spin-echo sequences are recommended for use at 1.5 T:TR 2,500–3,500 ms, TE 70–90 ms, echo train length 10, field of view 10 × 10 cm (axial) and 16 × 16 cm (coronal), imaging matrix 256 × 512, 3-mm slice thickness, 0.3-mm interslice gap, and two excitations. The TE is relatively short as this results in the most optimal demonstration of anal sphincter anatomy.

Axial images and coronal images are used with slice orientation perpendicular and parallel to the anal sphincter and endoanal coil to reduce partial volume effects. The axial or transverse plane is the most relevant and should be complemented by a coronal plane as the coronal plane reduces partial-volume effects and provides additional information on the extent of the disorder. The field of view encloses the whole anal sphincter, which indicates in the axial plane from at least one slice inferior to the sphincter to at least the anorectal verge cranially. The coronal plane encloses anteriorly the anovaginal septum in females and in males at least a part of the prostate. Posteriorly, the complete sphincter needs to be imaged. Endoanal MR studies can be performed on a MR machine with a field intensity of at least 0.5 T; most experience concerns 1.5 T. Although a higher image quality on 3 T compared to 1.5 T endoanal MRI can be expected, there is no literature yet to support this presumption.

4.6.3 Normal Anatomy, Variances, and Pitfalls

In the axial plane the anal sphincter surrounds the anal canal and is composed of several cylindrical layers. The innermost layer of the anal sphincter is the subepithelium that seals off the anal canal (anal cushions). The next layer is the cylindrical smooth muscle of the internal anal sphincter, supplied by autonomic nerves. The internal anal sphincter is approximately 2.9 mm thick on endoanal MRI (Rociu et al. 2000). The internal anal sphincter appears as a relatively hyperintense circular structure with a homogeneous uniform architecture (Fig. 4.6.1). In the coronal plane sometimes small horizontal lines can be identified, representing normal anatomy.

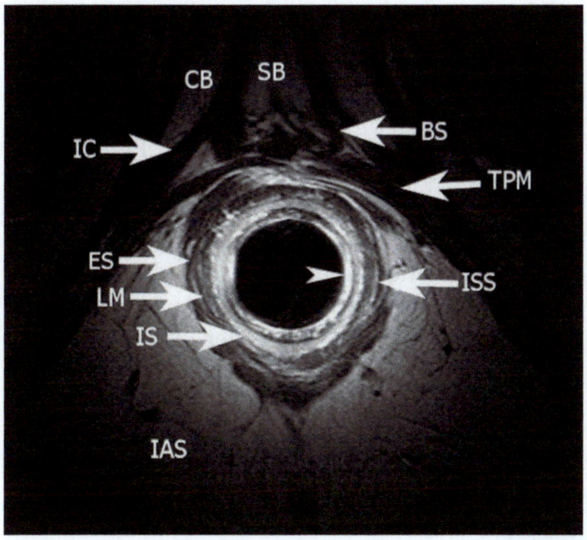

Fig. 4.6.1. Transverse endoanal T2-weighted fast spin-echo (2,500/70) MR image at the mid-anal canal shows normal anatomy in a 52-year-old man. The longitudinal muscle (*LM*) is clearly demonstrated within the intersphincteric space (*ISS*) between the internal (*IS*) and external (*ES*) anal sphincters. *Arrowhead* shows submucosa. *IAS* = ischioanal space, *CB* = cavernus body, *SB* = spongiose body, *IC* = ischiocavernous muscle, *TPM* = transverse perineal muscle, *BS* = bulbospongiosus muscle

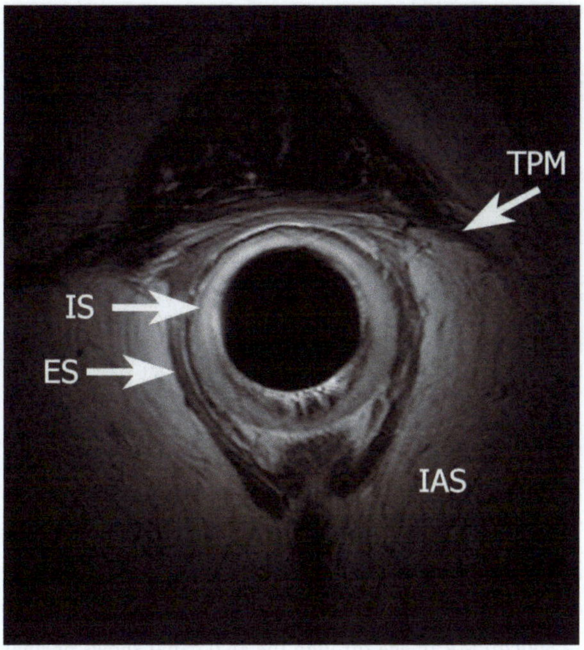

Fig. 4.6.2. Transverse endoanal T2-weighted fast spin-echo (2,500/70) MR image at the distal anal canal shows normal anatomy in a 56-year-old woman. The external anal sphincter (*ES*) is the hypointense outermost muscle; the internal anal sphincter (*IS*) is demonstrated as a hyperintense ring

The internal anal sphincter is the terminal continuation of the circular smooth muscle of the rectum and often separated from the longitudinal muscle. The longitudinal muscle layer is seen as a relatively hypointense layer within the hyperintense intersphincteric space (Fig. 4.6.1). The longitudinal layer is the fibromuscular continuation of the longitudinal muscular layer of the rectal wall.

The outermost layer comprises striated muscle with inferiorly the external anal sphincter and superiorly the puborectal muscle. The external anal sphincter is a muscle under voluntary control. The height of the external anal sphincter anteriorly is approximately 14 mm in women and 27 mm in men (Rociu et al. 2000). The thickness of the external anal sphincter is 4 mm on endoanal MRI. The external anal sphincter extends approximately 1 cm beyond the internal anal sphincter. The external anal sphincter is demonstrated as a clearly defined ring of hypointense signal intensity (Figs. 4.6.1, 4.6.2).

The puborectal muscle (also named the pubovisceral muscle) is part of the levator ani muscle, which also includes the levator plate at the anorectal junction. The puborectal muscle is a sling-like muscle and closely aligned to the deep part of the external anal sphincter. On endoanal MRI the puborectal muscle is approximately 28 mm high and 5.6 mm thick. Also, the puborectalis muscle and the levator ani muscle have a relatively hypointense signal intensity (Terra and Stoker 2006) (Fig. 4.6.3). The latter can be easily evaluated in the coronal plane (Fig. 4.6.3). The sphincter complex is embedded in the fat-containing ischioanal space, which is relatively hyperintense (Figs. 4.6.1, 4.6.2).

In the coronal plane (Fig. 4.6.3), the external anal sphincter has a characteristic "J" shape. Often a thin fat plane can be seen between the deep part and the puborectalis. Below this the superficial part is seen as a separate component. The subcutaneous part of the external anal sphincter curves around to form the bottom of the "J."

When starting the evaluation of the sphincter in the axial plane from the inferior, the lower edge of the external anal sphincter appears. At the caudal level the sphincter ring is not completely circular, but often shows discontinuity at the anterior and posterior side. Moving upwards to the mid-anal canal, the sphincter ring becomes completely circular, and both the inter-

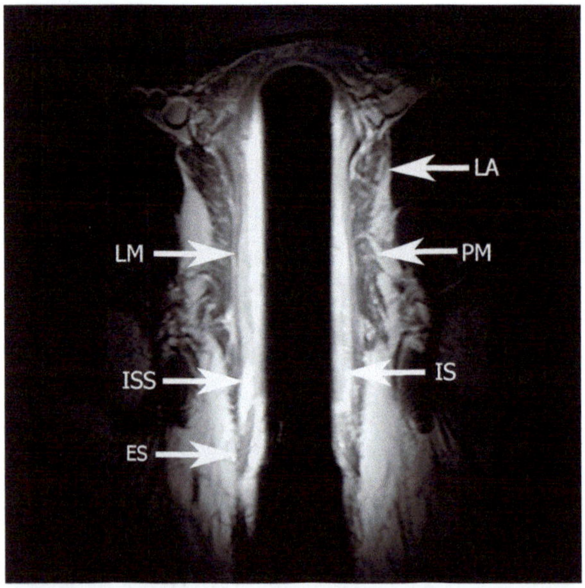

Fig. 4.6.3. Coronal endoanal T2-weighted fast spin-echo (2,500/70) MR image through the anal canal shows normal anatomy of the sphincter complex in a 52-year-old man with relatively hypointense external anal sphincter (*ES*), puborectal muscle (*PM*), and levator ani muscle (*LA*) and relatively hyperintense internal anal sphincter (*IS*). *LM* = longitudinal muscle, *ISS* = intersphincteric space

nal anal sphincter and longitudinal muscle appear. Since the signal intensity of either the longitudinal muscle or the external anal sphincter appears to be hypointense, they might be difficult to distinguish from each other when they are closely aligned. When moving upward to the proximal anal canal, the cranial part of the external anal sphincter is often fused with the puborectal muscle. At this level, the internal anal sphincter is still visible, but will disappear more proximally. The upper outer half of the anal sphincter is now sling-like (puborectal muscle).

The discontinuity of the sphincter edges at the lower level might easily be misinterpreted and diagnosed as a defect. On this level the lateral sides of the sphincter appear as symmetrically crescent-shaped. At the anterior side, discontinuity of the sphincter ring might be simulated by separation of the muscle groups with intermixing fibers inserting into the perineal body. This can be characterized by a cap-like morphology, which is a normal variant (Fig. 4.6.4). The external anal sphincter may appear to have a posterior defect as it is continuous at both sides with the anococcygeal ligament, which is also a normal variant (Fig. 4.6.5). Moving upward to the mid-anal canal, the external anal sphincter often will be seen to merge symmetrically posteriorly, reestablishing the sphincteric ring.

Sex-related differences should be taken into account. In women, the longitudinal muscle terminates just cranial to the external anal sphincter and contributes to the perineal body, whereas in men it extends to the caudal part of the external anal sphincter. The transverse perineal muscle also has a different relationship to the external anal sphincter. In women, the transverse perineal muscles fuse with the external anal sphincter, whereas in men they insert into the central point of the perineum (Figs. 4.6.1, 4.6.2).

4.6.4 Lesions of the Anal Sphincter

The most relevant lesions in the evaluation of fecal incontinence at endoanal MRI are disruption and volume anomalies of the internal and/or external anal sphincter. Disruption comprises sphincter defects and scar tissue; volume anomalies comprise sphincter thinning or thickening.

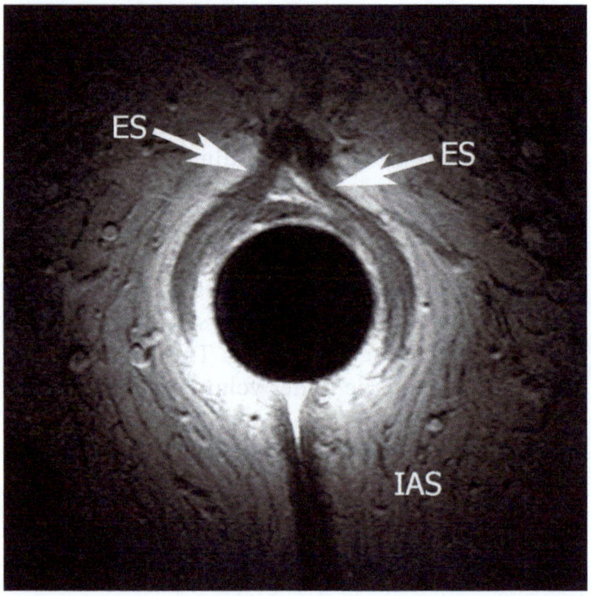

Fig. 4.6.4. Transverse endoanal T2-weighted fast spin-echo (2,500/70) MR image at the distal anal canal in a 77-year-old man shows normal anatomy of the external anal sphincter (*ES*). The ES anteriorly is demonstrated as a cap that might be interpreted as a defect since the muscle layer seems partly not continuous (*arrows*). *IAS* = ischioanal space

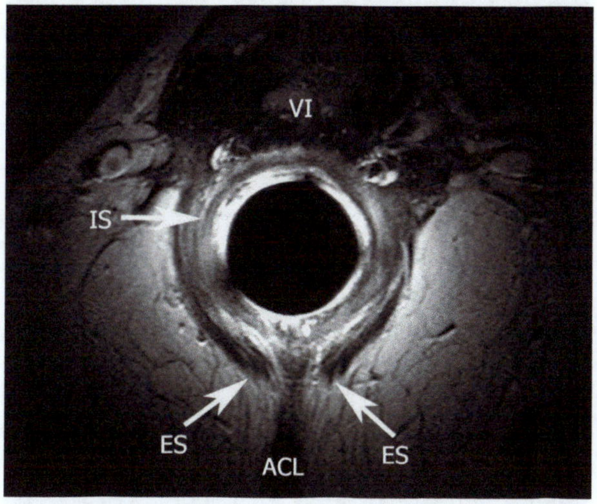

Fig. 4.6.5. Transverse endoanal T2-weighted fast spin-echo (2,500/70) MR image at the distal anal canal in a 57-year-old woman shows normal anatomy of the external anal sphincter (*ES*). The posterior part of the ES seems to discontinue at this level (*arrows*). This represents a normal variant and not a defect. The ES has posterior extension to the anococcygeal ligament at a higher level. At this level, the lower edge internal anal sphincter (*IS*) is visible and relatively hypointense at the anterior side due to scar tissue. *VI* = vaginal introitus, *ACL* = anococcygeal ligament

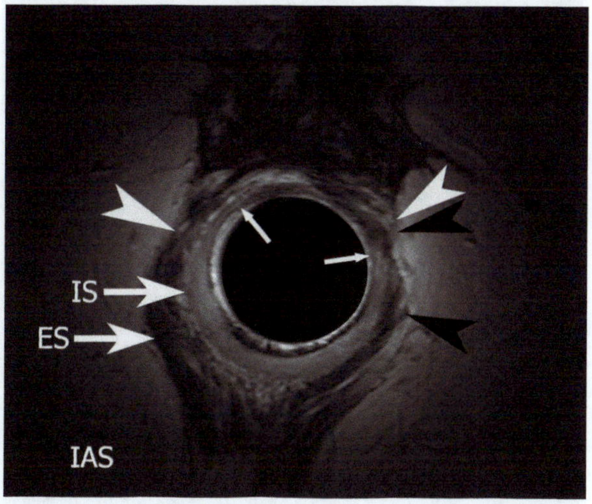

Fig. 4.6.6. Transverse endoanal T2-weighted fast spin-echo (2,500/70) MR image obtained from a 53-year-old fecal-incontinent woman after a complicated vaginal delivery (breech delivery and episiotomy) shows a defect of the external anal sphincter (*ES*) that is demonstrated by a discontinuity of the anterior outer sphincter ring (*black arrowheads*) and scar tissue (*white arrowheads*). Scar tissue anterior to the external anal sphincter is demonstrated as well as thinning and scar tissue of the anterior internal anal sphincter (*thin arrows*). *IS* = internal anal sphincter, *IAS* = ischioanal space

4.6.4.1 Scar Tissue and Defects

A defect of the anal sphincter at endoanal MRI is defined as a discontinuity of the muscle ring (anatomic defect) and/or is recognized by a hypointense deformation of the normal pattern of the muscle layer due to replacement of muscle cells by fibrous tissue (functional defect, scar tissue) (Rociu et al. 1999a).

Although with endoanal MRI a distinction can be made between an anal sphincter defect and scarring (Fig. 4.6.6), the importance of differentiation between these entities with respect to outcome has not been demonstrated yet. Secondary changes to the architecture of adjacent structures (longitudinal muscle, perianal fat) and involvement of both sphincters (Malouf et al. 2001) provide supportive evidence of a lesion.

4.6.4.1.1 Internal Anal Sphincter

Scarring of the internal anal sphincter is visible as mostly thinning of the internal anal sphincter combined with hypo-intense signal intensity of the internal anal sphincter. One should be aware that local thinning of the internal anal sphincter without changed signal intensity can be caused by compression by the endoanal coil.

Isolated internal anal sphincter defects are mostly due to prior anorectal surgery; obstetric trauma often causes a combined internal and external anal sphincter defect (Figs. 4.6.6, 4.6.7).

4.6.4.1.2 External Anal Sphincter

Scar tissue of the external anal sphincter can be subtle and may only comprise obliteration of the normal multilayered aspect of the external anal sphincter. Defects of the external anal sphincter can be isolated or may be accompanied by internal anal sphincter defects. Isolated external anal sphincter defects and combined internal and external anal sphincter defects have generally an obstetric origin. External anal sphincter defects can also be seen after surgery or other trauma. This may result in fragmentation of the whole sphincter. Defects following obstetric trauma are frequently located at the anterior part

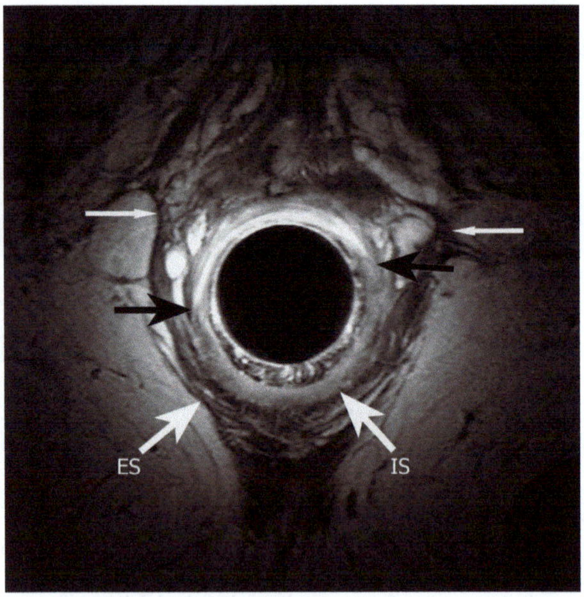

Fig. 4.6.7. Transverse endoanal T2-weighted fast spin-echo (2,500/70) MR image obtained from a 31-year-old woman after a complicated vaginal delivery (breech delivery, rupture) shows a defect (*thin arrows*) and scar tissue anterior to the external anal sphincter (*ES*) demonstrated by discontinuity of the sphincter ring, very low signal intensity, and disordered architecture. Also an anterior internal anal sphincter (*IS*) defect is depicted (*black arrows*), identifiable by the discontinuity of the anterior part of the internal anal sphincter and hyperintense fat interposing. Patient underwent anterior anal sphincter repair since she suffered from severe fecal incontinence

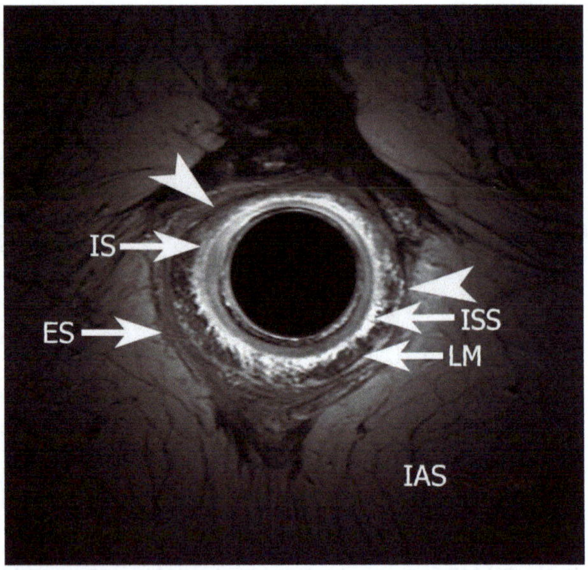

Fig. 4.6.8. Transverse endoanal T2-weighted fast spin-echo (2,500/70) MR image obtained from a 53-year-old fecal incontinent woman after a complicated vaginal delivery (long labor, assisted delivery, rupture) shows scar tissue of the external anal sphincter (*ES*) (*arrowheads*), which is demonstrated by a hypointense anterior outer sphincter ring that lacks the normal ES architecture (see posteriorly and see Figs. 4.6.1 and 4.6.2). Perineal scar tissue directly adjacent to the external anal sphincter. A thick longitudinal muscle (*LM*) is visible with a lesion at the anterior side of the ring. *IS* = internal anal sphincter, *IAS* = ischioanal space, *ISS* = intersphinteric space

of the anal sphincter complex (Fig. 4.6.8.) (Sultan et al. 1993; Kamm 1994). Continuity of the sphincter can be partially or completely destructed. Lesions cause an asymmetric disruption of the sphincter ring. Healing of defects is accompanied by the formation of granulation tissue, which leads to scar tissue which is of relatively low signal.

The extent and location of a defect can be indicated in hours (1–12 h) on a clock face using axial images and longitudinally in millimeters from the lower edge of the anal sphincter. When indicating defects in hours, one should be certain that the surgeon uses the same orientation. This potential pitfall can be prevented by indicating the location in segments, such as the left anterolateral.

Frank puborectal muscle lesions are relatively uncommon in fecal-incontinent patients. Defects of the puborectal muscle are primarily depicted in combination with internal and or external anal sphincter lesions. In addition, frank lesions of the levator ani plate present rarely in isolation in fecal-incontinent patients.

4.6.4.2 Atrophy

Generalized atrophy of the external anal sphincter, puborectal muscle, or levator ani muscle at endoanal MRI is characterized by thinning of the muscle fibers and/or fat replacement of muscle fibers by hyper-intense fat. Local atrophy represents local thinning or fatty degeneration of the external anal sphincter. Generalized atrophy of the internal anal sphincter is characterized by diffuse muscle thinning (muscle thickness less than 2 mm) (Rociu et al. 1999a).

4.6.4.2.1 Internal Anal Sphincter

Generally, the internal anal sphincter thickness in adults is considered to be normal when it ranges from 2 to 4 mm, irrespective of patient age. Abnormal thickening (> 4 mm) of the internal anal sphincter can be found in patients with solitary rectal ulcer syndrome and abnormally thinning (< 2 mm) in patients with idiopathic degeneration (Halligan et al. 1995; Vaizey et al. 1997). Atrophy of the internal anal sphincter is most easily appreciated at an axial image (Fig. 4.6.9).

4.6.4.2.2
External Anal Sphincter

In healthy subjects, the average thickness of the external anal sphincter at endoanal MRI is approximately 4 mm (Rociu et al. 2000). In contrast to external anal sphincter atrophy, pathological thickening of the external anal sphincter is seldom reported, and its clinical value is not well established. Atrophy of the external anal sphincter in fecal-incontinent patients is more often diagnosed in females ($p < 0.001$) and is associated with an impaired squeeze function (Terra et al. 2006a).

The coronal imaging plane is optimal for the evaluation of atrophy of the external anal sphincter (Fig. 4.6.10). When analyzing the volume of the external anal sphincter, it is important to bear in mind that women have a shorter external anal sphincter than men. On longitudinal images the lateral side of the external anal sphincter averages 27 mm in length in women and 28.6 mm in men, but the anterior aspect averages 14 mm in women compared to 27 mm in men. On mid-axial images, in young women (< 35 years) the external anal sphincter is thinner (4.32 mm average) than in young men (5.21 mm average) (Rociu et al. 2000).

Endoanal MRI is able to accurately depict generalized atrophy of the anal sphincter (Figs. 4.6.10, 4.6.11) and can differentiate between moderate (< 50% thinning of the external anal sphincter and/or replacement of external anal sphincter muscle by fat) and severe atrophy (≥ 50% thinning of the external anal sphincter and/or replacement of the external anal sphincter muscle by fat) (Briel et al. 2000; Terra et al. 2006a, 2006b). The internal anal sphincter thickness increases and the external anal sphincter thickness decreases with age (Rociu et al. 2000; Frudinger et al. 2002).

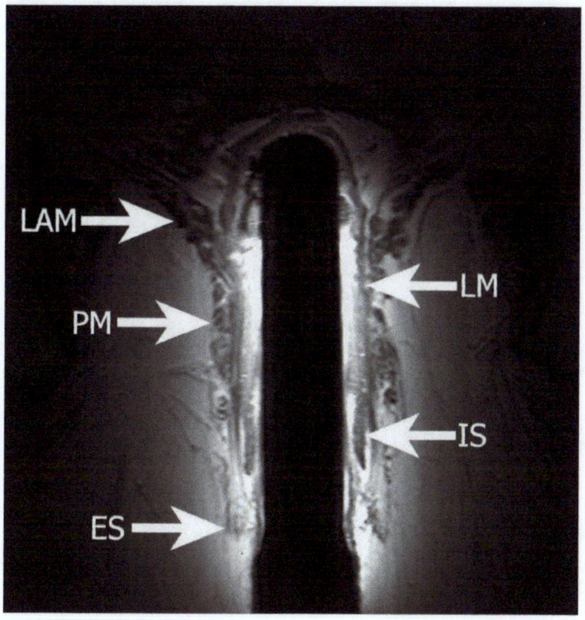

Fig. 4.6.10. Coronal endoanal T2-weighted fast spin-echo (2,500/70) MR image showing severe thinning of the external anal sphincter (*ES*) and diffuse replacement by fat in a 69-year-old fecal-incontinent woman with no risk factors for pudendal nerve damage in the past (compare to Fig. 4.6.3). The puborectal muscle and levator ani muscle are relatively spared. *IS* = internal anal sphincter, *IAS* = ischioanal space, *PM* = puborectal muscle, *LAM* = levator ani muscle, *LM* = longitudinal muscle

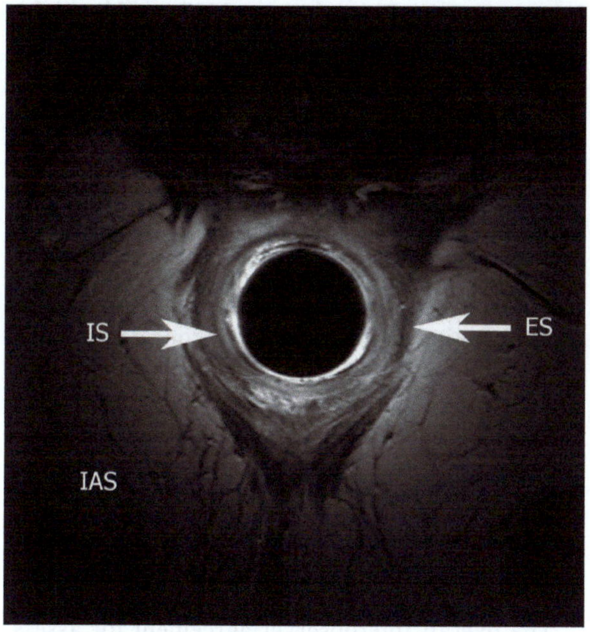

Fig. 4.6.9. Transverse endoanal T2-weighted fast spin-echo (2,500/70) MR image obtained from a 59-year-old fecal-incontinent woman after a complicated vaginal delivery (long labor, episiotomy, rupture) shows severe generalized atrophy of the internal anal sphincter (*IS*) demonstrated by a thin (less than 2 mm as measured on endoanal MRI) inner sphincter ring. *IAS* = ischioanal space

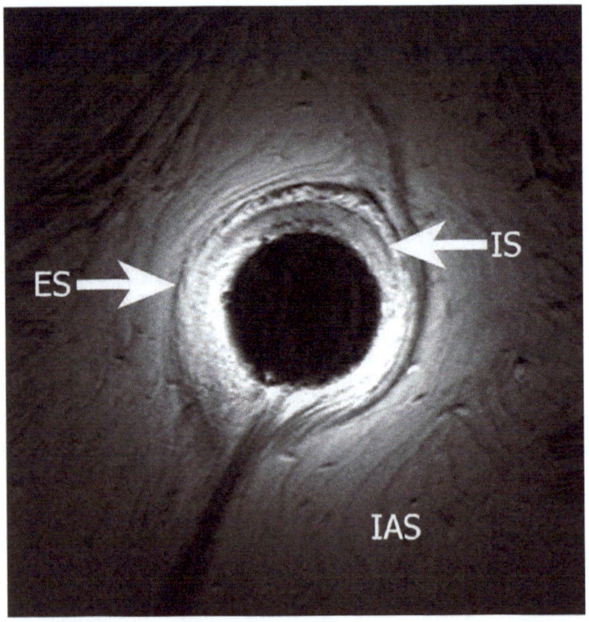

Fig. 4.6.11. Transverse endoanal T2-weighted fast spin-echo (2,500/70) MR image showing severe thinning of the external anal sphincter (*ES*) and diffuse replacement by fat in a 46-year-old man with fecal incontinence with a neurological disorder (spinal) in the past (compare to Figs. 4.6.1 and 4.6.2). At this level the anterior inferior edge of the internal anal sphincter (*IS*) is just visible

4.6.5 The Role of Endoanal MRI in the Diagnostic Workup

Continence is a complex function of multiple anatomic, physiologic, and psychological factors. A systematic evaluation of the patient should reveal the underlying pathophysiology, leading to appropriate therapy (Diamant et al. 1999). While anorectal physiology tests give insight in the (patho-) functional aspects of the anorectal region, imaging techniques are able to visualize the anatomy and pathology, such as defects, scar tissue, or atrophy, of the anal sphincter muscles. With digital rectal examination the presence or absence of an external anal sphincter defect can be assessed, and resting and squeeze pressure can be determined qualitatively. However, only major sphincter defects can be diagnosed accurately, and sphincter weaknesses are well, but not perfectly related to findings at manometry (Dobben et al. 2007a).

4.6.5.1 Comparison of Endoanal MRI versus Endoanal US

A comparison between endoanal MRI and endoanal ultrasound (US) in the depiction of sphincter lesions has been made in three studies. Malouf and colleagues (2000) performed a prospective study of 52 patients with an expert panel as reference standard. The expert panel was primarily familiar with endoanal US. They concluded that endoanal US and endoanal MRI are equivalent in diagnosing external anal sphincter injury. Complete agreement between endoanal MRI and endoanal US and the final diagnosis was found in 62%. The authors concluded that MRI is inferior in diagnosing internal anal sphincter injury.

A retrospective study performed by Rociu et al. (1999b) in 22 patients with surgery as reference standard emphasizes the precise description of the extent and structure of complex sphincter lesions and the superiority in clinical decision-making of endoanal MRI compared to endoanal US. Endoanal MRI findings showed better agreement with surgical results compared to findings at endoanal US for diagnosing lesions of the external anal sphincter (kappa value 0.85 versus 0.53) and of the internal anal sphincter (kappa value 0.64 versus 0.49). This is because MRI provides higher spatial resolution and better inherent image contrast for lesion characteristics. This group had a larger experience with endoanal MRI than with endoanal US.

A recent multi-center study (Dobben et al. 2007b) in 237 fecal-incontinent patients (214 women) evaluated the depiction of external anal sphincter defects with endoanal US and endoanal MRI. There was agreement between endoanal MRI and endoanal US in 146 patients (61%; $\kappa = 0.24$: fair agreement). Based on the imaging findings and other considerations, 36 patients had an anterior anal sphincter repair. There was no significant difference in the depiction of external anal sphincter defects between endoanal MRI and endoanal US ($P = 0.23$). Therefore, either technique can be considered as useful in the selection of patients as candidates for surgery (sensitivity and positive predictive value of endoanal MRI were 81% and 89%, respectively, versus 90% and 85% at endoanal US).

The overall interobserver agreement for assessment of sphincter integrity using endoanal MRI is strongest if the sphincters are either both intact or both disrupted (Malouf et al. 2001). For individual sphincters interobserver agreement for defects was fair (external anal sphincter) and moderate (internal anal sphincter). A study of 30 patients reported moderate to good interobserver agreement (Terra et al. 2005). Intraobserver agreement was fair to very good depending upon experience.

In summary, the present consensus in diagnosing disorders of the external anal sphincter is that endoanal US and endoanal MRI are equivalent. Even though internal anal sphincter disorders are adequately depicted at either endoanal US or endoanal MRI, there is still no consensus about the preferred technique of choice (Stoker et al. 2000; Malouf et al. 2000; Dobben et al. 2007b). The advantages of endoanal US are its availability and limited costs. Furthermore, endoanal US has been used for a longer period of time than MRI, resulting in more widespread experience with the endoanal US technique (Sultan et al 1994; Stoker et al. 2000; Bartram 2003). In contrast, endoanal MRI may allow for a clear visualization of the external anal sphincter as there is large contrast difference among the external anal sphincter muscle, its borders, and the surrounding fat. The accurate demonstration of the external anal sphincter facilitates the evaluation of external anal sphincter atrophy.

4.6.5.2 The Role of Endoanal MRI in Pre-Surgical Evaluation

In the selection of candidates for surgery, previous studies have shown that endoanal MRI is an accurate diagnostic technique in depicting external anal sphincter atrophy (deSouza et al 1995; Stoker et al. 1999; Briel et al. 1999; Rociu et al. 2000). A study by Briel et al. (1999) showed that external anal sphincter atrophy negatively affects continence after anterior anal sphincter repair. In this study 8 out of 20 consecutive female patients had external anal sphincter atrophy. Outcome was significantly better in those without external anal sphincter atrophy ($P = 0.004$).

In another study by Briel and colleagues (2001), endoanal MRI correctly identified sphincter morphology in 23 of 25 cases (92%). In detecting sphincter atrophy, endoanal MRI showed 89% sensitivity and 94% specificity. Microscopic histopathological investigation confirms findings of external anal sphincter atrophy revealed by endoanal MRI. Histologically, the external anal sphincter is considered to be atrophied when the striated muscle tissue exhibits diminished volume in association with replacement by fatty tissue (Briel et al. 2001; Williams et al. 2001).

A recent pilot study concerning the role of endoluminal imaging in the clinical outcome of anal sphincter repair of 30 patients (Dobben et al. 2007c) showed that baseline measurement of preserved external anal sphincter thickness at endoanal MRI correlated with a better outcome ($r = 0.42$; $P = 0.03$). As a consequence, preoperatively performed endoanal MRI might function as a potential predictor of surgical outcome. The role of endoanal MRI in selecting other surgical treatments has not been studied yet.

4.6.5.3 The Role of Endoanal MRI in Post-Surgical Evaluation

For postoperative assessment, the role of endoanal MRI has not been thoroughly investigated. In a pilot study by Dobben et al. (2007c), the authors found that patients with a visible anal sphincter overlap and less than 20% fat tissue at the level of overlap had a better outcome than patients with a non-visible, fatty sphincter overlap ($P = 0.037$). Although endoanal MRI could clearly depict the anal sphincter overlap (Fig. 4.6.12), the depiction of re-

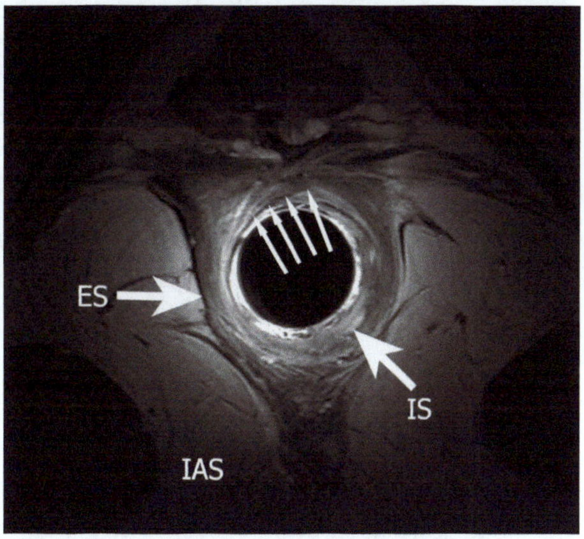

Fig. 4.6.12. Transverse endoanal T2-weighted fast spin-echo (2,500/70) MR image obtained from a 31-year-old woman (same patient as Fig. 4.6.7) after a complicated vaginal delivery (breech delivery, rupture). Patient underwent anterior anal sphincter repair. Overlap of the right anterior anal sphincter (*thin arrows*) over the left part is depicted. Much less disordered architecture is demonstrated as preoperatively (Fig. 4.6.7). The patient improved substantially

sidual external anal sphincter defects on endoanal MRI was insufficient. In contrast, the study showed that the depiction of residual external anal defect on endoanal US was effective. Surgical outcome was significantly worse in patients with a postoperatively depicted external anal sphincter defect at endoanal US compared to patients without an EAS defect ($P = 0.003$).

4.6.5.4
The Role of External Phased-Array MRI in Fecal Incontinence

Endoluminal techniques are primarily used at specialized centers as a dedicated device is necessary. In addition, the introduction of the endoluminal probe or coil leads to some discomfort. These two disadvantages of endoluminal techniques could be overcome with the use of external phased-array coils. External phased-array MRI has widespread use for imaging of pelvic diseases, but has not been used for sphincter visualization in patients with fecal incontinence. Although local spatial resolution is inferior to an endoluminal MRI, the detail acquired is adequate for appreciation of anal sphincter anatomy with subsequent sphincter measurements in normal individuals (Fig. 4.6.13) (Beets-Tan et al. 2001). A recent study in a cohort of fecal-incontinent patients showed that external phased-array MRI is comparable to endoanal MRI in the depiction of clinically relevant external ($P > 0.99$) and internal ($P > 0.99$) anal sphincter defects (Terra et al. 2005), providing that sufficient experience is available (Fig. 4.6.14). Either technique corresponded in 25/30 (83%) patients for the depiction of external anal sphincter defects and in 28/30 (93%) for the depiction of internal anal sphincter defects.

The depiction of atrophy by external phased-array MRI versus endoanal MRI has been evaluated in a comparative study in 30 patients with fecal incontinence (Terra et al. 2006b). The authors concluded that external phased-array MRI and endoanal MRI do not significantly differ in their ability to depict external anal sphincter atrophy ($P = 0.63$) with good agreement ($\kappa = 0.72$) when sufficient experience is available (Fig. 4.6.15).

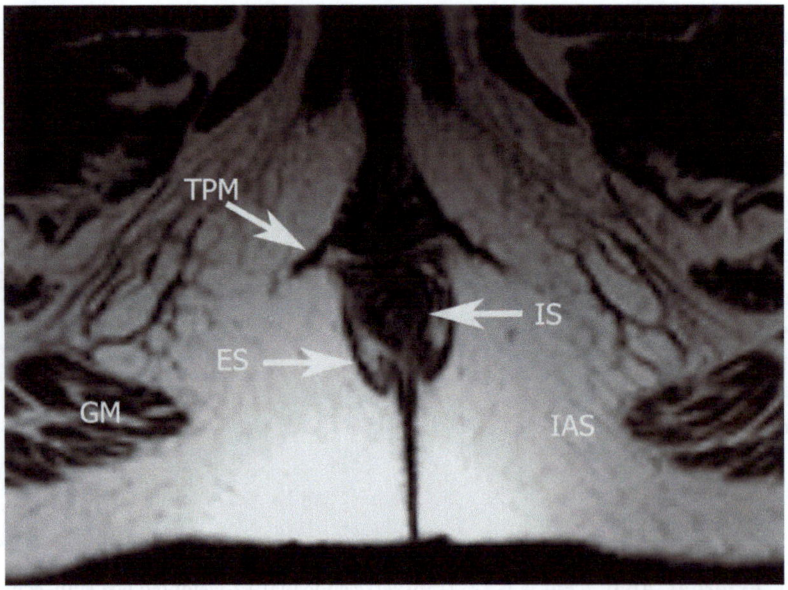

Fig. 4.6.13. Transverse T2-weighted fast spin-echo (2,500/70) external phased-array MR image shows the lower part of a normal external anal sphincter (*ES*) at the mid-distal anal canal in a 56-year-old woman. The external anal sphincter is demonstrated less with external phased-array MRI compared to endoanal MRI, but can be readily identified. The internal anal sphincter can be identified as a homogenous isointense to hypointense circular band surrounding the anal canal. *TPM* = transverse perineal muscle, *IAS* = ischioanal space, *GM* = gluteus muscle

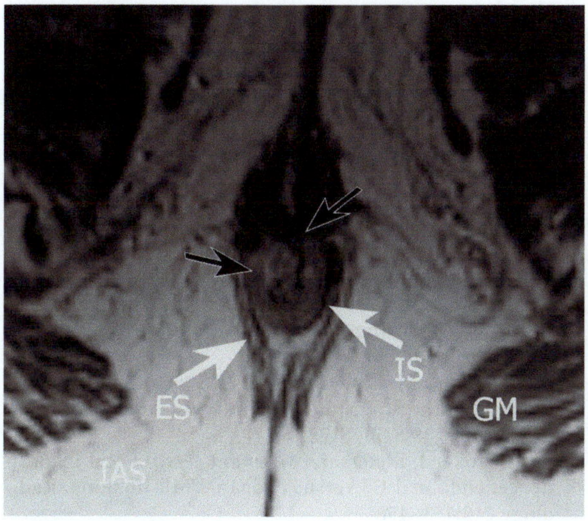

Fig. 4.6.14. Transverse T2-weighted fast spin-echo (2,500/70) external phased-array MR image obtained from a 42-year-old fecal-incontinent woman after a complicated vaginal delivery (long labor, assisted delivery, rupture). Scar tissue at the right anterior and anterior external anal sphincter. The anterior part of the internal anal sphincter is thinned and not well delineated. Note that scar tissue is more hypointense with distorted and asymmetric architecture. Moderate atrophy of the external anal sphincter. *IS* = lower part of the internal anal sphincter, *TPM* = transverse perineal muscle, *IAS* = ischioanal space, *GM* = gluteus muscle

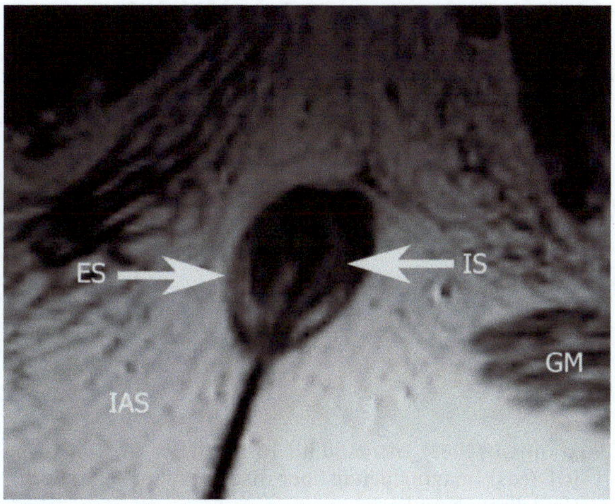

Fig. 4.6.15. Transverse endoanal T2-weighted fast spin-echo (2,500/70) MR image showing thinning of the external anal sphincter (*ES*) and diffuse replacement by fat in a 46-year-old man with fecal incontinence with a neurological disorder (spinal) in the past (same patient as Fig. 4.6.10). No generalized atrophy of the internal anal sphincter (*IS*) was depicted

4.6.5.5 Comparison of Endoanal MRI versus Three-Dimensional Endoanal US in the Depiction of Atrophy

With endoanal US, the presence of atrophy of the external anal sphincter can be evaluated to some extent. Recently, the evaluation of sphincter atrophy by three-dimensional (3D) endoanal US has been studied. In a study with 18 patients, 3D endoanal US and endoanal MRI showed no difference in the assessment of external anal sphincter atrophy ($P=0.25$), but there was a substantial difference in grading (Cazemier et al. 2006). Another study with 18 fecal-incontinent patients shows that correlation between the two imaging techniques for external anal sphincter thickness, length, and area was poor. In addition, correlation was also poor for external anal sphincter volume determined on 3D endoanal US and external anal sphincter thickness and area measured on endoanal MRI (West et al. 2005). This most likely can be attributed to the difficult delineation of the external anal sphincter at endoanal US. Fat replacement within the atrophied muscle causes loss of the normal muscle/fat interface border at the outer margin of the external anal sphincter. The outer border of the external anal sphincter is then not defined, and thickness cannot be accurately measured (Fuchsjäger and Maier 2003). The role of 3D endoanal US in the determination of sphincter atrophy has not been established yet. More research is needed with respect to this imaging technique.

4.6.6 Summary

For detection of internal and external defects, endoanal MRI is comparable to endoanal US. Given the widespread availability and experience with endoanal US and most likely lower costs, endoanal US can be used as the initial imaging technique. Endoanal MRI can be used as an alternative technique with comparable accuracy for sphincter defects. The major strength of endoanal MRI is in the detection of external anal sphincter atrophy, which is a predictor of poor outcome of anterior anal sphincter repair. Probably the best cost-benefit ratio can be obtained by having patients first undergo endoanal US, selecting patients as potential candidates for anterior anal repair. In potential candidates for surgery, endoanal MRI is preoperatively performed to study the presence of external anal sphincter atrophy. At the postoperative stage, it is presumably most efficient to perform only endoanal US when surgery has failed. The role of external phased-array MRI warrants further study.

References

Bartram CI (2003) Ultrasound. In: Bartram CI, DeLancey JOL (eds) Imaging pelvic floor disorders. Springer, Berlin Heidelberg New York

Beets-Tan RG, Morren GL, Beets GL et al (2001) Measurement of anal sphincter muscles: endoanal US, endoanal MR imaging, or phased-array MR imaging? A study with healthy volunteers. Radiology 220:81–89

Briel JW, Stoker J, Rociu E et al (1999) External anal sphincter atrophy on endoanal magnetic resonance imaging adversely affects continence after sphincteroplasty. Br J Surg 86:1322–1327

Briel JW, Zimmerman DD, Stoker J et al (2000) Relationship between sphincter morphology on endoanal MRI and histopathological aspects of the external anal sphincter. Int J Colorectal Dis 15:87–90

Cazemier M, Terra MP, Stoker J et al (2006) Atrophy and defects detection of the external anal sphincter: comparison between three-dimensional anal endosonography and endoanal magnetic resonance imaging. Dis Colon Rectum 49:20–27

deSouza NM, Puni R, Kmiot WA et al (1995) MRI of the anal sphincter. J Comput Assist Tomogr 19:745–751

deSouza NM, Hall AS, Puni R et al (1996) High resolution magnetic resonance imaging of the anal sphincter using a dedicated endoanal coil. Comparison of magnetic resonance imaging with surgical findings. Dis Colon Rectum 39:926–934

Deutekom M, Terra MP, Dijkgraaf MG et al (2006) Patients' perception of tests in the assessment of faecal incontinence. Br J Radiol 79:94–100

Diamant NE, Kamm MA, Wald A et al (1999) AGA technical review on anorectal testing techniques. Gastroenterology 116:735–760

Dobben AC, Terra MP, Deutekom M et al (2007a) Anal inspection and digital rectal examination compared to anorectal physiology tests and endoanal ultrasonography in evaluating fecal incontinence. Int J Colorectal Dis 22:783–790

Dobben AC, Terra MP, Slors JF et al (2007b) Comparison of endoanal magnetic resonance imaging and endoanal ultrasonography in the depiction of external anal sphincter defects in fecal incontinent patients. Radiology 242:463–471

Dobben AC, Terra MP, Deutekom M et al (2007c) The role of endoluminal imaging in clinical outcome of overlapping anterior anal sphincter repair in patients with fecal incontinence. AJR Am J Roentgenol 189:W70–77

Frudinger A, Halligan S, Bartram CI et al (2002) Female anal sphincter: Age-related differences in asymptomatic volunteers with high-frequency endoanal US. Radiology 224:417–423

Fuchsjäger MH, Maier AG (2003) Imaging fecal incontinence. Eur J Radiol 47:108–116

Halligan S, Sultan A, Rottenberg G et al (1995) Endosonography of the anal sphincters in solitary rectal ulcer syndrome. Int J Colorectal Dis 10:79–82

Kamm MA (1994) Obstetric damage and faecal incontinence. Lancet 344:730–733

Malouf AJ, Halligan S, Williams AB et al (2001) Prospective assessment of interobserver agreement for endoanal MRI in fecal incontinence. Abdom Imaging 26:76–78

Malouf AJ, Williams AB, Halligan S et al (2000) Prospective assessment of accuracy of endoanal MR imaging and endosonography in patients with fecal incontinence. AJR Am J Roentgenol 175:741–745

Rociu E, Stoker J, Zwamborn AW et al (1999a) Endoanal MR imaging of the anal sphincter in fecal incontinence. Radiographics 19:S171–S177

Rociu E, Stoker J, Eijkemans MJ et al (1999b) Fecal incontinence: endoanal US versus endoanal MR imaging. Radiology 212:453–458

Rociu E, Stoker J, Eijkemans MJ et al (2000) Normal anal sphincter anatomy and age- and sex-related variations at high-spatial-resolution endoanal MR imaging. Radiology 217:395–401

Stoker J, Hussain SM, van Kempen D et al (1996) Endoanal coil in MR imaging of anal fistulas. AJR Am J Roentgenol 166:360–362

Stoker J, Rociu E, Zwamborn AW et al (1999) Endoluminal MR imaging of the rectum and anus: technique, applications, and pitfalls. Radiographics 19:383–398

Stoker J, Rociu E, Wiersma TG et al (2000) Imaging of anorectal disease. Br J Surg 87:10–27

Sultan AH, Kamm MA, Hudson CN et al (1993) Anal-sphincter isruption during vaginal delivery. N Engl J Med 329:1905–1911

Sultan AH, Kamm MA, Talbot IC et al (1994) Anal endosonography for identifying external sphincter defects confirmed histologically. Br J Surg 81:463–465

Terra MP, Stoker J (2006) Fecal incontinence: Endoanal ultrasonography and MR imaging. In: Santoro GA, Di Falco G (eds) Benign anorectal diseases: diagnosis with endoanal and endorectal ultrasonography and new treatment options. Springer, Italy

Terra MP, Beets-Tan RG, van der Hulst VPM et al (2005) Evaluating anal sphincter defects in patients with fecal incontinence: Endoanal MR imaging versus external phased array MR imaging. Radiology 236:886–895

Terra MP, Deutekom M, Beets-Tan RG et al (2006a) External anal sphincter atrophy at endoanal MRI in patients with fecal incontinence. Dis Colon Rectum 49:1149–1159

Terra MP, Beets-Tan RG, van der Hulst VPM (2006b) MR imaging in evaluating atrophy of the external anal sphincter in patients with fecal incontinence. AJR Am J Roentgenol 187:991–999

Vaizey CJ, Kamm MA, Bartram CI (1997) Primary degeneration of the internal anal sphincter as a cause of passive faecal incontinence. Lancet 349:612–615

Williams AB, Bartram CI, Modhwadia D et al (2001) Endocoil magnetic resonance imaging quantification of external anal sphincter atrophy. Br J Surg 88:853–859

West RL, Dwarkasing S, Briel JW et al (2005) Can three-dimensional endoanal ultrasonography detect external anal sphincter atrophy? A comparison with endoanal magnetic resonance imaging. Int J Colorectal Dis 20:328–333

4.7 Urodynamics

Fadi Housami and Paul Abrams

CONTENTS

Abstract

Symptoms alone are not reliable in the evaluation of lower urinary tract dysfunction. Urodynamic investigations are used to assess the storage and voiding functions of the lower urinary tract. The patient symptoms are correlated to the urodynamics findings with the aim of providing a pathophysiological explanation and guiding clinical management. Urodynamics investigations encompass a variety of tests that are useful in clinical practice. Some are non-invasive and are routinely used in urology clinics, whilst others are more invasive and require specialist centres. Ultrasound imaging and video fluoroscopy form a significant part of these tests and provide live anatomical assessment of the lower urinary tract.

F. Housami, MD, MRCS
Clinical Research Registrar, Bristol Urological Institute, Southmead Hospital, Bristol BS10 5NB, UK
P. Abrams, MD, FRCS
Professor of Urology, Bristol Urological Institute, Southmead Hospital, Bristol BS10 5NB, UK

4.7.1 Functions of the Lower Urinary Tract

The urinary tract as a whole is responsible for the functions of urine production, storage and expulsion. The lower urinary tract is comprised by the bladder and urethra, which form a single unit that converts continuous urine production into intermittent micturition. Together they are responsible for the adequate low-pressure storage of urine and its efficient emptying at the appropriate time and place (Chapple and MacDiarmid 2000).

When considering the functions of the bladder and urethra, it is important to be clear on the functions of each during storage and voiding (Abrams 2006b). In normal storage the bladder remains relaxed and accommodates urine at low-pressure, while the urethral sphincter is contracted to prevent urine leakage. During normal voiding the urethral sphincter relaxes, while the bladder mounts a sustained contraction to expel urine out completely (Abrams 2006b). Once normal function is identified, it becomes easy to describe the principal forms of lower urinary tract dysfunction (Table 4.7.1) (Abrams 2006a).

Table 4.7.1. Lower urinary tract functions and dysfunctions (Abrams 2006a)

	Storage phase		Voiding phase	
	Normal	Abnormal	Normal	Abnormal
Bladder	Relaxed	Overactive	Contracted	Underactive
Urethra	Competent	Incompetent	Relaxed	Obstructive (functional or structural)

4.7.2 Lower Urinary Tract Symptoms

Evaluation of lower urinary tract dysfunction is based on a combination of full history, clinical examination, some laboratory tests and occasionally radiography, endoscopy or urodynamics (Chapple and MacDiarmid 2000). The various symptoms associated with lower urinary tract dysfunction (LUTD) have been classified by the International Continence Society (ICS) broadly into storage, voiding and post micturition symptoms (Table 4.7.2) (Abrams et al. 2002). All the terminology used in this chapter is ICS terminology, and clinicians are encouraged to learn and use the correct terminology to allow for clear communication between healthcare professionals (Abrams 2006b).

Unfortunately symptoms alone are not reliable in the evaluation of lower urinary tract dysfunction because there is considerable overlap among the symptoms for different urological conditions (Chapple and MacDiarmid 2000; Patel and Rickards 2005), and therefore further tests are usually necessary to identify different disorders.

Urodynamic investigations are objective tests of the storage and emptying functions of the bladder and urethra. When properly performed and accurately interpreted, they improve diagnostic capabilities and are useful in formulating treatment strategies and improving outcomes (Chapple and MacDiarmid 2000).

Table 4.7.2. Lower urinary tract symptoms (Abrams et al. 2002)

Function	Symptoms
Storage	• Urgency • Frequency • Nocturia • Urinary incontinence • Abnormal bladder sensation
Voiding	• Hesitancy • Straining • Slow or intermittent stream • Terminal dribble
Post micturition	• Post micturition dribble • Feeling of incomplete emptying

4.7.3 Urodynamic Investigations

The term urodynamics may encompass a variety of investigations of urinary tract function with varying complexity (see below) (Chapple and MacDiarmid 2000; Schafer et al. 2002). However, most practitioners use the term when referring to the assessment of bladder filling with cystometry and the assessment of bladder emptying with pressure-flow studies. Videourodynamics adds X-ray fluoroscopy, therefore combining both anatomical and functional assessments, which is useful as many of the functional symptoms are the consequence of a structural abnormality (Patel and Rickards 2005).

Urodynamic investigations include (Chapple and MacDiarmid 2000; Schafer et al. 2002):

- Frequency-volume charts
- Pad testing
- Uroflowmetry
- Cystometry
- Pressure-flow studies
- Videourodynamics
- Ambulatory urodynamics

- Urethral function studies
- Neuro-physiological investigation
- Upper tract urodynamics (Whitaker test)

4.7.3.1 Frequency-Volume Charts

The frequency-volume chart (FVC) is a useful tool in the assessment of storage and voiding symptoms. The patient measures the volumes voided and records the times and volumes over a period of 4–7 days. The chart provides an objective measure of the frequency of voiding as well as the urine output, which helps in identifying symptoms caused by increased urine output. The recording of incontinence episodes and use of pads gives the clinician more insight into the severity of symptoms. It is also useful as feedback on the effectiveness of treatment. The average volume voided is used as a guide to the filling volume in cystometry to prevent overfilling of the bladder.

Indications for a frequency-volume chart include:

- Baseline assessment of storage and voiding symptoms
- Objective feedback on the effectiveness of treatment
- Prior to filling cystometry to guide filling volume

4.7.3.2 Pad Testing

It is difficult to ascertain the severity of urinary incontinence objectively from clinical history as patients' bother of incontinence and use of pads varies greatly. The pad test is used as an objective measure of the amount of leakage caused by day-to-day activities. The patient wears a pre-weighed pad and performs various activities that would normally reproduce the patient symptoms; the pad's weight is measured and recorded at intervals. Due to possible weighing errors, sweating or vaginal discharge, an increase in pad weight of 1 g over 1 h is not considered as incontinence.

Indications for pad testing:

- Assessment of the presence and severity of incontinence
- Objective feedback on the effectiveness of treatment

4.7.3.3 Uroflowmetry with Ultrasound Estimation of Post-Void Residual

Urine flow studies investigate the voiding function of the lower urinary tract. Uroflowmetry involves a simple non-invasive technique (Abrams 2006b) where voiding is plotted as urine flow against time. The two main types of commercially available flowmeters are the gravimetric (measuring change in weight of urine collected against time) and rotating disk method (measuring the power requirement to keep a constant speed as urine falls on the disk) (Smith 1992).

The pattern of the flow plot is typically a smooth bell-shaped curve in a normal flow (Fig. 4.7.1a), while the flow curve is flattened in bladder outlet obstruction (Fig. 4.7.1b). It is important to identify artefacts that may modify the signal and result in misleading values from the flowmeter's automated analysis (Fig. 4.7.1c).

The main parameter obtained from uroflowmetry is the maximum flow rate (Q_{max}), which, as the name implies, is the highest flow rate reached for a given curve. Maximum flow is reached within the first third of the plot, and the higher the Q_{max}, the less likely it is for a patient to have bladder outlet obstruction. While 90% of patients with $Q_{max} < 10$ ml s^{-1} are obstructed, 35% of patients with a Q_{max} between 10 and 15 ml s^{-1} are not obstructed, and the low flow rate is due to detrusor underactivity (Abrams 2006b).

The results have to be interpreted within the context of a number of factors, including gender, age and voided volume. The voiding pattern has to be interpreted with caution if the voided volume is less than 150 ml. The results can be compared to published nomograms, such as the nomogram published by Siroky et al. (1979) and the Bristol nomogram.

In a normal flow the detrusor must elevate intravesical pressure enough to allow expulsion of urine past any resistance by the urethra. An abnormal flow indicates that some component in the lower urinary tract is abnormal (at least during voiding). Unfortunately, the converse is not always true; for example, a normal flow may still be seen in bladder outlet obstruction if this was produced by a stronger than normal detrusor contraction (Table 4.7.3) (Smith 1992). Furthermore, the test does not indicate the cause of the abnormality in most situations (Smith 1992), and a reduced Q_{max} despite a suitable voided volume does not differentiate between weak detrusor contractility and bladder outlet obstruction (Table 4.7.3). None-a

b

c

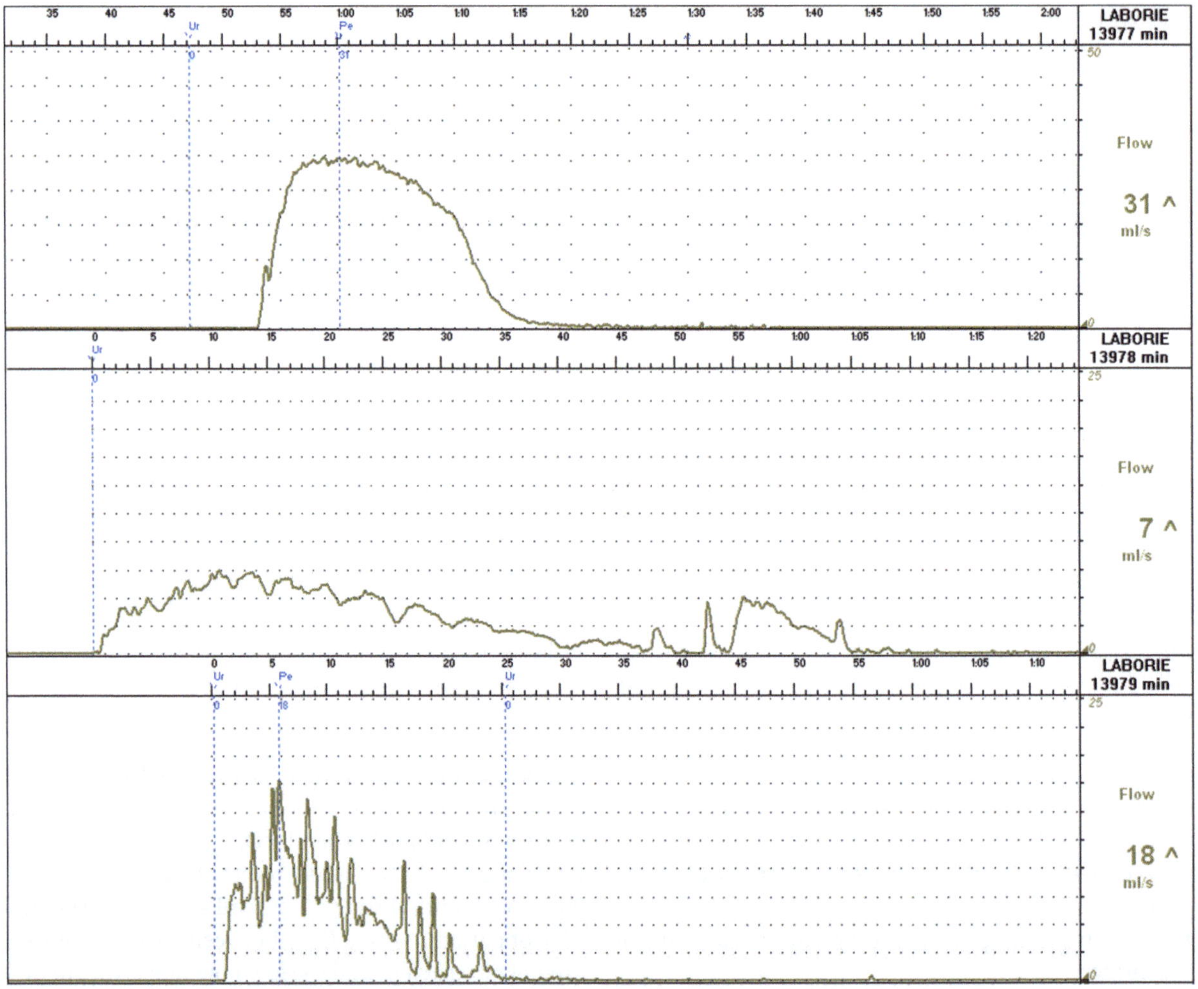

Fig. 4.7.1a–c. Uroflowmetry is a plot of urine flow rate against time. **a** The normal flow pattern is a bell-shaped curve with the maximum flow rate in the first third of the curve. **b** An elongated flow curve due to bladder outlet obstruction; note the prolonged flow with a reduced maximum flow rate. **c** Artefacts (spikes) due to patient movement and/or straining, which inaccurately increase the automated estimation of maximum flow rate (18 ml/s); the true maximum flow rate is closer to 12 ml/s

theless, uroflowmetry is very valuable in informing and directing further urodynamic investigations.

Uroflowmetry is combined with ultrasound of the bladder to provide further information on voiding function. The patient voids into a flowmeter, and the bladder is scanned soon after voiding to assess post-void residual volume (PVR). Bladder capacity can be calculated by adding PVR to the voided volume.

Indications of uroflowmetry include (Abrams 2006b; Smith 1992):

- Investigating voiding function
- Assessment of recurrent lower urinary tract infections
- Before and after pharmacological treatment of LUTS
- Before and after surgical procedures that modify the voiding function

Table 4.7.3. The relationship between lower urinary tract function and detrusor pressure and flow

Flow	Pressure	Obstruction	Contractility
Normal	Low	Unobstructed	Normal
Normal	Normal	Unobstructed	Normal
Normal	High	Obstructed	Strong
Low	High	Obstructed	Strong
Low	Normal	Equivocal	Equivocal
Low	Low	Unobstructed	Weak

4.7.3.4 Basic Urodynamics

There might be some variation in technique among urodynamics units, which may be due to the workload, expense or the experience of the staff. Nevertheless, the International Continence Society (ICS) has produced a guide to good urodynamic practice (Schafer et al. 2002).

Due to the various referral sources at our centre from urology, gynaecology, general practice and specialist nurses, it has been our practice to obtain full urological history prior to performing urodynamics. This allows the investigator to tailor the test to the patient's complaint.

Clinical examination is performed to elicit signs relevant to the patient's complaint. The patient's abdomen is examined for a palpable bladder, and neurological assessment of the lumbar and sacral roots, including perianal sensation and anal tone, is performed.

In men, digital rectal examination is performed in the left lateral position to assess prostate size and texture as patients with larger prostates respond better to 5-alpha reductase inhibitors. Pelvic floor strength could be assessed by asking the patient to squeeze around the examining finger; this is particularly important in those who present with incontinence.

In women, the patient is asked to cough while the urethral meatus is visualised in the supine position. This would demonstrate the sign of stress incontinence (Abrams et al. 2002). It is important to assess the oestrogenisation of the vaginal mucosa, which may play a significant part in urgency symptoms and bladder pain. The pelvic floor strength is assessed by asking the patient to tighten her pelvic floor during vaginal examination. Then the patient is asked to lie in a left lateral position to perform a speculum examination of the vagina using a Sims speculum to identify the presence of uterine/vault prolapse as well as anterior or posterior vaginal wall prolapse. The assessment of pelvic organ prolapse (POP) may be assessed using a POPQ assessment tool (Bump et al. 1996).

Remaining in a left lateral position, a rectal balloon catheter is inserted to measure abdominal pressure (p_{abd}), and then urethral catheters are inserted in supine position using aseptic technique. Any residual volume in the bladder is emptied via the urethral catheter, and the volume is recorded. Two separate urethral catheters may be used for bladder filling and measurement of vesical pressure (p_{ves}), or alternatively a biluminal catheter is used [the technique for inserting two catheters is described by Abrams (2006b)]. The activity of the detrusor muscle is assessed by measuring detrusor pressure (p_{det}), which is electronically calculated by the subtraction of p_{abd} from p_{ves} to remove the artefacts due to changes in abdominal pressure (Housami et al. 2007).

The ICS recommends that both abdominal and vesical pressures be zeroed to atmospheric pressure (Schafer et al. 2002) using the reference level of the upper symphysis pubis. Quality control of the pressures is achieved throughout the test by asking the patient to cough and noting equal spikes in pressure on both p_{ves} and p_{abd} lines.

The aim of urodynamics is to reproduce the patient's symptoms so that they could be related to synchronous urodynamics events, and some provocation may be necessary to elicit patient symptoms (Abrams 2006b). Asking the patient to cough or jog is used to elicit stress incontinence, and urgency may be provoked by the sound of running water. The test report should clearly indicate whether it was possible to reproduce the patient's symptoms (Abrams 2006b). A normal cystometrogram in a patient with LUTS should be considered normal only if the clinician is convinced that everything possible has been done to replicate the patient's symptoms (Smith 1992).

Filling cystometry describes the filling part of basic urodynamics where the pressure-volume relationship of the bladder is measured (Abrams 2006b; Chapple and MacDiarmid 2000). It is our practice to fill the bladder in a standing position in men and sitting position in women. A recent review of the literature concluded that performing filling cystometry in the supine position would miss a large proportion (33–100%) of detrusor overactivity (Al-Hayek et al. 2007). The bladder is filled with normal saline (contrast medium in videourodynamics) at room temperature with a controlled rate (usually 50 ml min^{-1}).

During bladder filling the patient is asked to report sensations of bladder filling, first desire to void, normal desire to void, strong desire to void and the presence of urgency. These should be annotated on the trace for future reference (Abrams et al. 2002).

The filling volume is usually guided by the patient's frequency-volume chart as well as the patient sensation at the time. The maximum cystometric capacity varies with age and gender, usually 400–600 ml in an adult male. Some patients have a reduced bladder capacity either due to early sensation of bladder filling or to poor bladder compliance (see below). In others the bladder capacity remains normal, but they fail to empty the bladder completely, leaving them with a reduced functional capacity.

Bladder compliance measures the relationship between the change in bladder volume and change in pressure using the equation:

$$\text{Compliance} = \Delta \text{ vol} / \Delta \text{ p} \quad (4.7.1)$$

Although the ICS has not defined a specific value for normal compliance, it is generally considered normal if it is greater than 40 ml cmH_2O^{-1} (Abrams 2006b).

During bladder filling, the bladder should remain relaxed despite provocation with little rise in pressure. Detrusor overactivity is a urodynamic observation characterised by an involuntary detrusor contraction that may be spontaneous or provoked (Abrams et al. 2002). This may also be associated with leakage (detrusor overactivity incontinence; Fig. 4.7.2). Detrusor overactivity is considered significant only if it replicates the patient's symptoms of urgency plus or minus urgency incontinence.

The normal urethra remains competent during storage and its incompetence causes urodynamic stress incontinence, which is demonstrated by involuntary leakage on increasing abdominal pressure (e.g., coughing) in the absence of detrusor contraction (Fig. 4.7.3) (Abrams et al. 2002). The abdominal leak point pressure is a crude measure of the ability of the bladder neck and urethral sphincter to maintain continence. It is the abdominal pressure at which leakage occurs when the patient is asked to do Valsalva manoeuvre with graduated increase in pressure (Chapple and MacDiarmid 2000). It is generally accepted that patients with intrinsic sphincter deficiency will leak at lower pressures (less than 60 cmH_2O) when compared to patients with stress incontinence due to reduced bladder neck support who leak at pressures more than 100 cmH_2O. The detrusor leak point pressure, on the other hand, is the detrusor pressure at which the leak occurs. It is used in the assessment of the risks to the upper tracts in patients with neuropathic disorders. In this group of patients the upper tracts are at higher risk of damage if the detrusor pressure rises to more than 30–40 cmH_2O during filling (Chapple and MacDiarmid 2000).

The voiding function is assessed with a pressure-flow study where synchronous measurements of vesical pressure, abdominal pressure and urine flow rate are taken. Prior to voiding, the bladder filling line is removed (to avoid an obstructive effect), while the pressure catheter is supported to remain in the bladder. After ensuring that the quality control of the pressures is satisfactory, the patient is asked to void into the flowmeter.

Pressure-flow studies allow for a physiological assessment of detrusor motor function as well as the resistance of the urethra during voiding. In normal voiding there is a sustained detrusor contraction with good continuous flow and complete emptying of the bladder (Fig. 4.7.4). Contraction of the detrusor muscle is reflected in a rise in both vesical and detrusor pressure (but not abdominal pressure) (Housami et al. 2007).

Much work has been done to try and identify men with bladder outlet obstruction from pressure-flow studies. The ICS developed a nomogram based on the previous work by (Abrams and Griffiths 1979) that groups voiding into obstructed, non-obstructed or equivocal obstruction. The maximum flow rate (Q_{max}) and detrusor pressure at maximum flow rate ($p_{detQmax}$) are used to calculate the bladder outlet obstruction index (BOOI) using the formula:

$$\text{BOOI} = p_{detQ_{max}} - 2\ Q_{max} \quad (4.7.2)$$

Patients are obstructed if the BOOI >40, equivocal if the BOOI is 20–40 and unobstructed if the BOOI <20 (Abrams 1999). The ICS also defined a bladder contractility index (BCI) based on work by (Schafer 1990) to assess the detrusor contractility during voiding.

$$\text{BCI} = p_{detQ_{max}} + 5\ Q_{max} \quad (4.7.3)$$

Using the above formula, strong contractility was defined as BCI >150, normal contractility BCI of 100–150 and weak contractility BCI <100 (Abrams 1999).

The quantification of obstruction and detrusor contractility is useful in predicting outcome and guiding further management. Patients with proven obstruction on pressure-flow studies have a high chance of success with TURP, while patients with weak detrusor contractility are at higher risk of retention following TURP (Abrams 2006b).

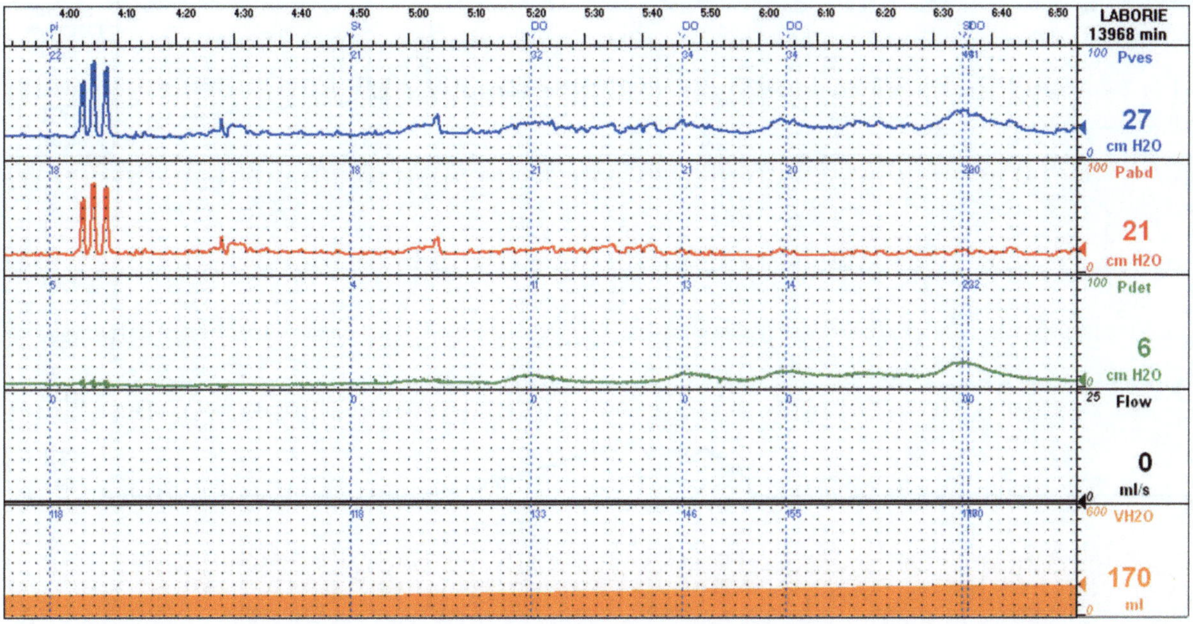

Fig. 4.7.2. Filling cystometry showing vesical pressure (*blue*), abdominal pressure (*red*) and detrusor pressure (*green*). The cough spikes on the *left* confirm a good trace quality (equal deflections on both vesical and abdominal lines). Note the waves in detrusor pressure (*green*) indicating detrusor overactivity (an abnormal finding), which is also marked on the trace as *DO*

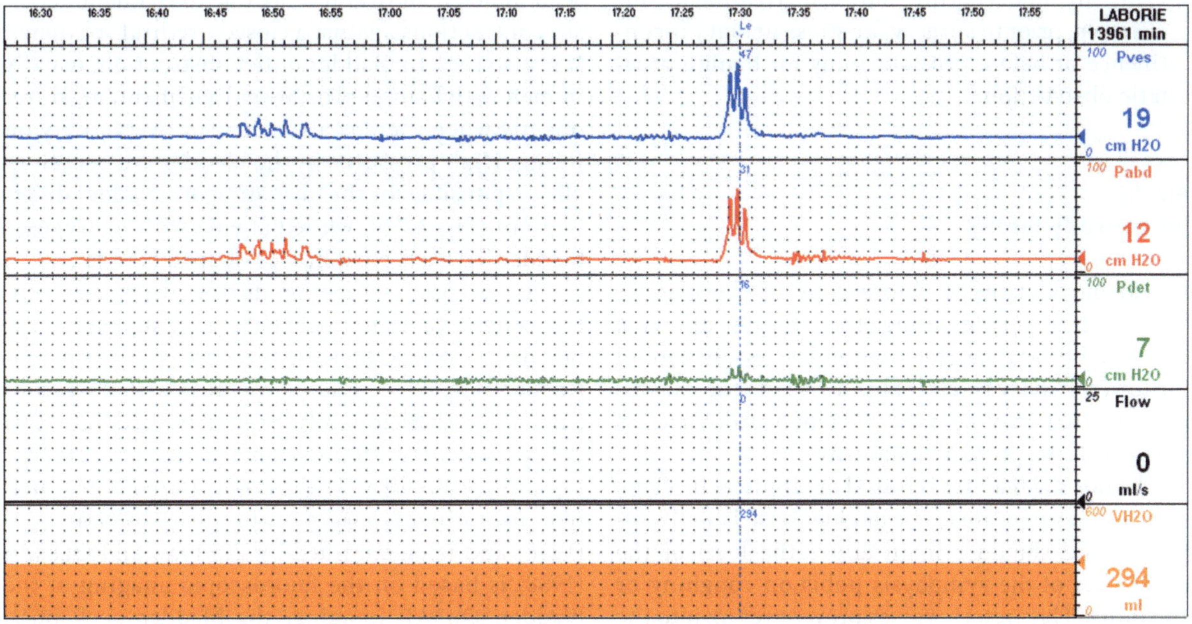

Fig. 4.7.3. Filling cystometry showing vesical pressure (*blue*), abdominal pressure (*red*) and detrusor pressure (*green*). Note the three consecutive coughs causing leakage marked on the trace as *Le*, whilst the detrusor pressure remains relatively flat. This is a typical example of urodynamic stress incontinence

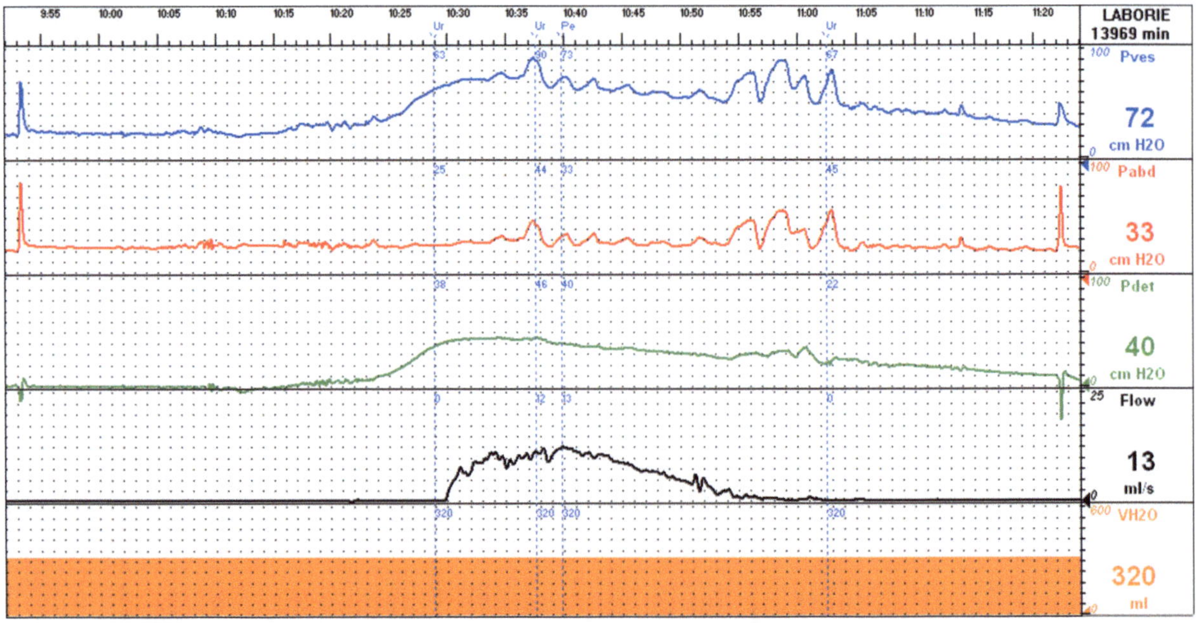

Fig. 4.7.4. Pressure-flow study during normal voiding showing vesical pressure (*blue*), abdominal pressure (*red*), detrusor pressure (*green*) and urine flow rate (*black*). The cough spikes on the *left* confirm a good trace quality (equal deflection on both vesical and abdominal lines). The patient has been given permission to void; note the sustained detrusor contraction during voiding with a corresponding urine flow

Indications for urodynamics include (Chapple and MacDiarmid 2000):

- Failure of medical management (e.g., persistent overactivity despite anti-muscarinics)
- Prior to undertaking surgical treatment, for example, prior to surgery for stress urinary incontinence or before prostatectomy for benign prostatic obstruction.

4.7.3.5 Videourodynamics

In videourodynamics, fluoroscopy of the bladder and urethra during filling and voiding allows a combined functional and anatomical assessment of the lower urinary tracts. Table 4.7.4 lists the various features that may be seen on video urodynamics along with the possible diagnosis.

The normal bladder is round or elliptical in shape with a smooth outline. The bladder base is well supported and should remain above the level of the lower part of the symphysis pubis on coughing or straining. The ureteric valves prevent reflux into the upper system during both filling and voiding. The urethral sphincter is closed during bladder filling, preventing any leakage, while it opens to allow voiding and contrast fills the urethra with a uniform calibre. At the end of voiding, there is no contrast remaining in the bladder.

Trabeculation of the bladder (Fig. 4.7.5) may be seen in detrusor overactivity due to frequent detrusor contractions against a closed urethral sphincter. It is also seen in bladder outlet obstruction, usually in men with benign prostate enlargement, most frequently when there is also detrusor overactivity on filling. High pressures in the bladder are occasionally responsible for the formation of a bladder diverticulum (Fig. 4.7.6), while patients with neurogenic bladder have a typical fir tree-shaped bladder.

Fluoroscopic screening during three consecutive coughs demonstrates the level of support to the bladder base as well as the presence of stress incontinence (Fig. 4.7.7). Causes of stress urinary incontinence have historically been classified into two groups, intrinsic sphincter deficiency and bladder neck hypermobility. The classification of stress urinary incontinence originally proposed by Green, Jr. (1968) and later modified by Blaivas and Olsson (1988) is based on the fluoroscopic imaging of the bladder. On AP imaging, the bladder neck position may be low (below the level of the upper third of symphysis pubis), signifying the loss of pelvic floor support (Chapple and MacDiarmid 2000).

Table 4.7.4. Normal and abnormal features on videourodynamics

	Video features	Possible diagnosis
1. Bladder shape	Round or elliptical shape	Normal
	Trabeculated	Detrusor overactivity with/without bladder outlet obstruction
	Fir tree shape	Neurogenic bladder
	Diverticulum	Detrusor overactivity with/without bladder outlet obstruction
	Low bladder	Reduced bladder support from pelvic floor muscle and endopelvic fascia and associated anterior vaginal wall prolapse
	Ureteric reflux	Recurrent UTIs
		Greater risk to upper tracts
		Neurogenic bladder
2. Bladder neck	Well supported	Normal
	Movement on coughing	Stress urinary incontinence
	Leakage on coughing	Stress urinary incontinence
3. Voiding features	Narrowing in urethra	Detrusor sphincter dyssynergia
		Benign prostatic obstruction
		Urethral stricture
	Ureteric reflux	Increased risk to upper tracts
	Residual urine	Recurrent UTIs
		Bladder outlet obstruction
		Weak detrusor contractility

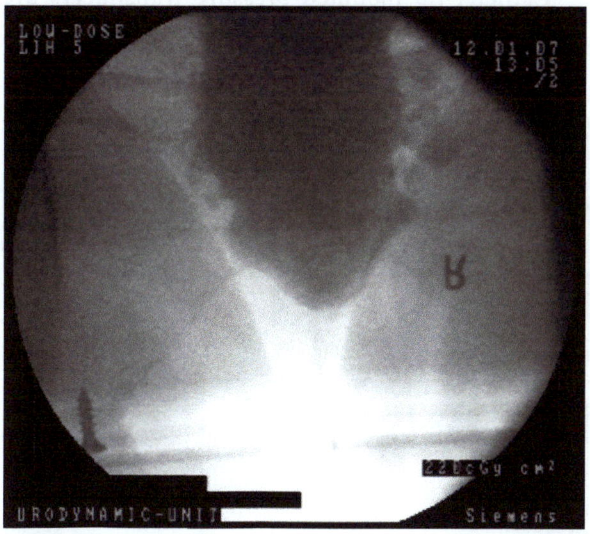

Fig. 4.7.5. Fluoroscopy of the bladder during filling showing trabeculation and marked sacculation of the bladder wall. Trabeculation is seen in patient with detrusor overactivity where the detrusor often contracts against a closed outlet

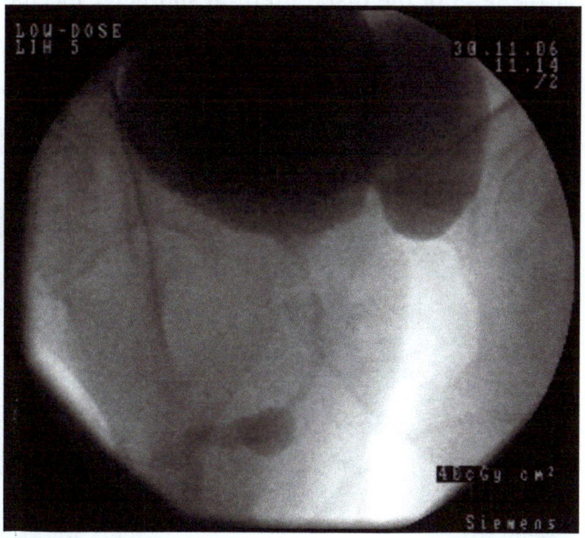

Fig. 4.7.6. Fluoroscopy of the bladder during voiding showing a large bladder diverticulum. The combination of focal detrusor wall weakness and high bladder pressure (usually against closed outlet) causes the formation of diverticuli. Large diverticuli could impair bladder function significantly; the diverticulum fills up during voiding and later refills the bladder, causing a post-void residual volume

When the urethra does not move, it is indicative of stress urinary incontinence due to intrinsic sphincter deficiency. Imaging in the transverse position may be used to differentiate between bladder neck and anterior vaginal wall prolapse (Chapple and MacDiarmid 2000).

Filtration of urine in the kidneys requires low pressure in the upper urinary tracts. It is, therefore, the function of the bladder to store urine in a low-pressure system and of the vesicoureteric valves to protect the upper tracts from the raised pressure during voiding. Vesicoureteric reflux (VUR) can be damaging to the kidneys and their function, especially in neurological patients who more frequently have high filling bladder pressures. On videourodynamics it is possible to identify VUR during filling or voiding (Fig. 4.7.8).

Fluoroscopy of the bladder and urethra during voiding allows a combined functional and anatomical assessment (Fig. 4.7.9), identifying the presence of ureteric reflux or the site of urethral obstruction. On voiding the bladder neck should open widely. If it remains closed despite high detrusor pressure, this is due to failure to relax (detrusor-bladder neck dyssynergia); a clue is trapping of urine in the proximal urethra (failure of retrograde emptying). Urethral overactivity occurs in neuropathic vesico-urethral dysfunction and is characterised by a narrowing at the level of the distal urethral sphincter mechanism.

Indications for videourodynamics include:

- Defining the site of bladder outlet obstruction (especially in younger men)
- Recurrent female stress incontinence after surgery
- Bladder neck position and support (usually females)
- Neurological disease likely to cause vesico-urethral dysfunction
- Surgical complications (e.g., post-prostatectomy incontinence)
- Children with abnormal voiding prior to invasive therapy
- Impaired renal function without intrinsic renal disease.

4.7.3.6 Ambulatory Urodynamics

The setting for routine urodynamics is rather artificial in terms of filling fluid, rate of filling and the environment around the patient. It is performed over a short time and in different circumstances to the patient's daily activities. Ambulatory urodynamics are used in situations where routine urodynamics fail to reproduce the patient's symptoms (Abrams 2006b).

Catheter-tip mounted pressure transducers are used, which are then connected to a small recording

a

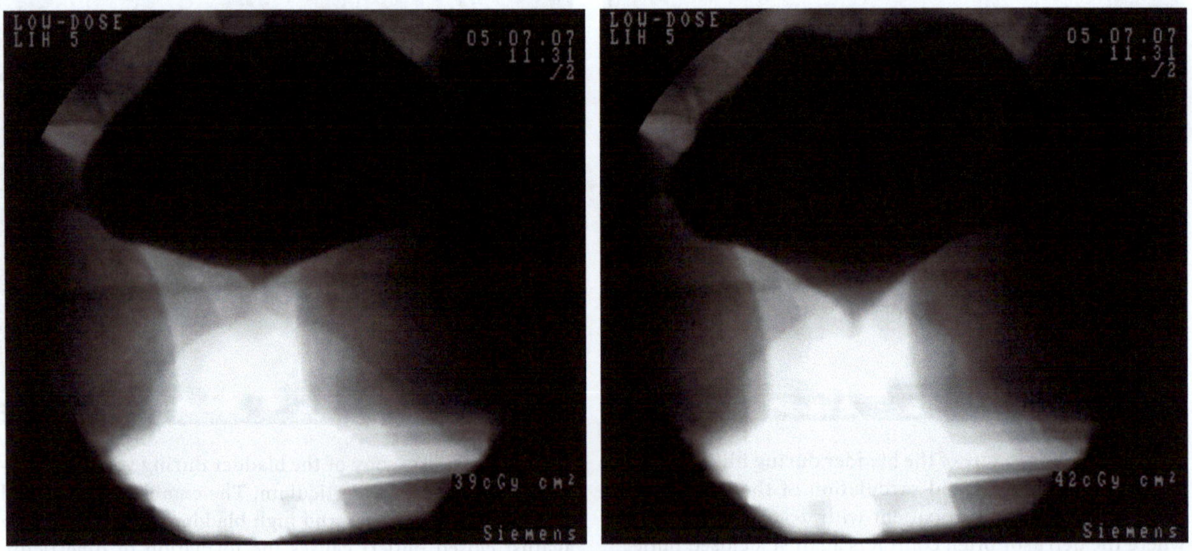

b

Fig. 4.7.7a,b. Fluoroscopy of the bladder during filling. The normal bladder neck is above the level of the symphysis pubis and should remain so during coughing. a In this patient the bladder neck beaks (opens slightly) and is behind the symphysis pubis at rest and (b) it descends with coughing, signifying reduced pelvic floor support

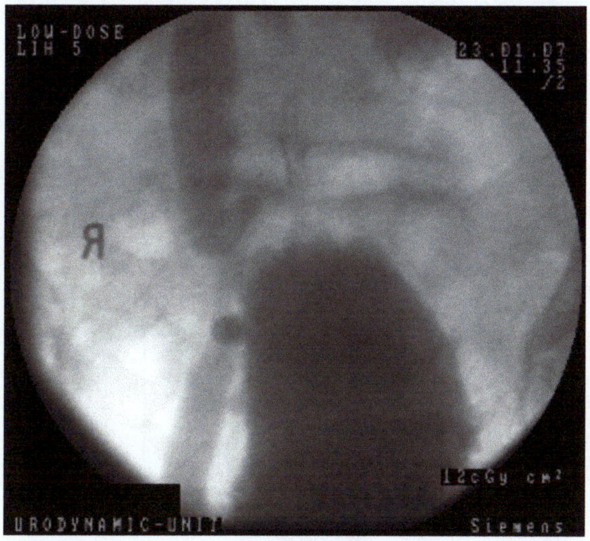

Fig. 4.7.8. Fluoroscopy of the upper part of the bladder during voiding showing right vesico-ureteric reflux. This is especially important in young patients as high pressure reflux puts the upper tracts at risk of kidney damage

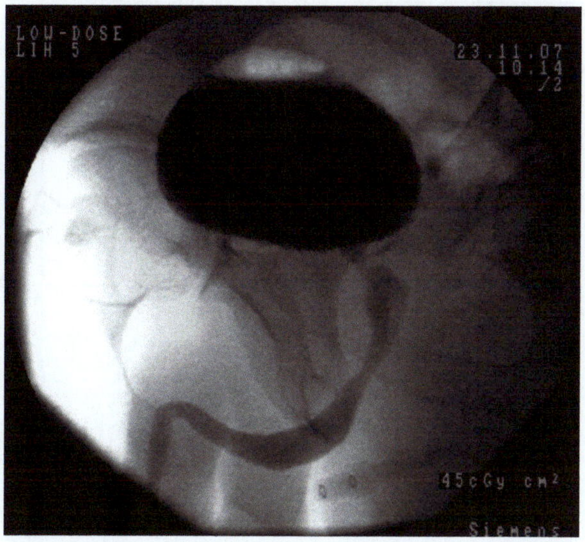

Fig. 4.7.9. Fluoroscopy of the bladder and urethra during normal voiding. The bladder and urethra are screened in 45° oblique view, which allows a better visualisation of the urethra. This provides an anatomical assessment of the urethra during voiding and allows for the localisation of obstructive lesions. It is also particularly useful in the assessment of urethral sphincter dysfunction

device for the patient to carry. The patient is asked to perform activities as close as possible to daily activities that are likely to provoke the symptoms; he/she is able to annotate the recording with the activities or events. These recordings can be correlated to the pressure changes when the recording is later reviewed.

As well as being closer to the patient's daily activities, ambulatory urodynamics differ in that the bladder is allowed to fill naturally over a longer period of time. It is possible to measure leakage by weighing the pads, and in some systems these have an electronic sensor to detect the timing and amount of leakage.

4.7.3.7 Urethral Function Tests

Normal urethral function requires a closed urethra during urine storage in order to maintain continence and for the urethra to relax and open completely when voiding is attempted. Measurement of urethral pressure, at rest, provides indirect data on its function.

The urethral pressure profile (UPP) is a plot of urethral pressure measurement along the length of the urethra. The typical UPP in females shows the maximum pressure at the mid-urethral point where the urethral sphincter is situated (Fig. 4.7.10). Edwards and Malvern (1974) suggested a formula of maximum urethral closure pressure to predict stress incontinence in females with an accuracy of 66%. The typical urethral pressure profile in a male demonstrates the pressure exerted by the prostate as well as the sphincter pressure (Fig. 4.7.11). Prostatic length, plateau height and prostatic area correlate with bladder outlet obstruction.

The urethral pressure profile is useful in the assessment of urethral sphincter function in females with symptoms of stress incontinence and in males with complications of surgery such as incontinence following TURP.

4.7.3.8 Neuro-Physiological Investigations

In the vast majority of patients, careful physical examination and detailed analysis urodynamic in-

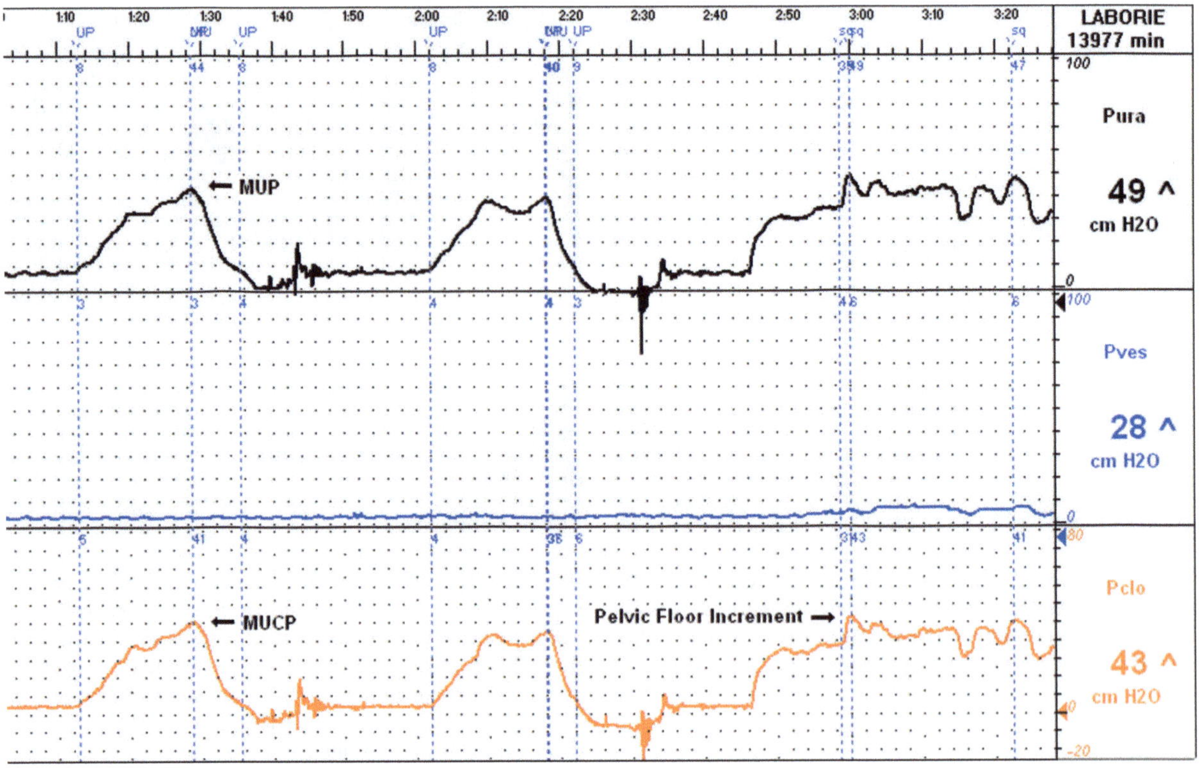

Fig. 4.7.10. Two urethral pressure profiles in a female; the urethral pressure is plotted along its length (from bladder to outside). The trace shows urethral pressure (*black*), vesical pressure (*blue*) and the urethral closure pressure (*orange*), which is calculated as the difference between urethral pressure and vesical pressure. The maximum urethral pressure (*MUP*) represents the urethral sphincter and may be used with the maximum urethral closure pressure (*MUCP*) by some clinicians to inform treatment decisions of stress incontinence. The pelvic floor increment (the increase in pressure above MUP with pelvic floor squeeze) represents the strength of the pelvic floor muscles

vestigations provide sufficient information to guide clinical management. However, in a small proportion of patients, neuro-physiological investigations provide useful information. The assessment of the urethral sphincter using surface or needle electromyography (EMG) allows for the study of the depolarisation of the striated muscle of the sphincter. Action potentials may be displayed on screen or played as sound waves. The tests require specific skills and therefore are only carried out in specialist centres. A high percentage of women with voiding difficulty have been shown to have abnormal sphincter activity as the cause of their symptoms (Fowler et al. 1988).

Indications for neuro-physiological investigations include:

- Neurogenic voiding dysfunction
- Women with voiding difficulty
- Children with dysfunctional voiding

4.7.3.9 Urodynamics of the Upper Tracts (Whitaker Test)

This is a functional pressure-flow assessment of the upper urinary tract and is indicated if other investigations have returned equivocal results (Chapple and MacDiarmid 2000). It is an invasive procedure that requires a nephrostomy to measure pressure in the renal pelvis, while bladder pressure is measured via a urethral catheter.

Dilute contrast is infused into the nephrostomy tube at 10 ml min^{-1} with simultaneous recording of the pressures. High pressures in the renal pelvis indicate ureteric obstruction, and fluoroscopy gives additional anatomical information (Chapple and MacDiarmid 2000).

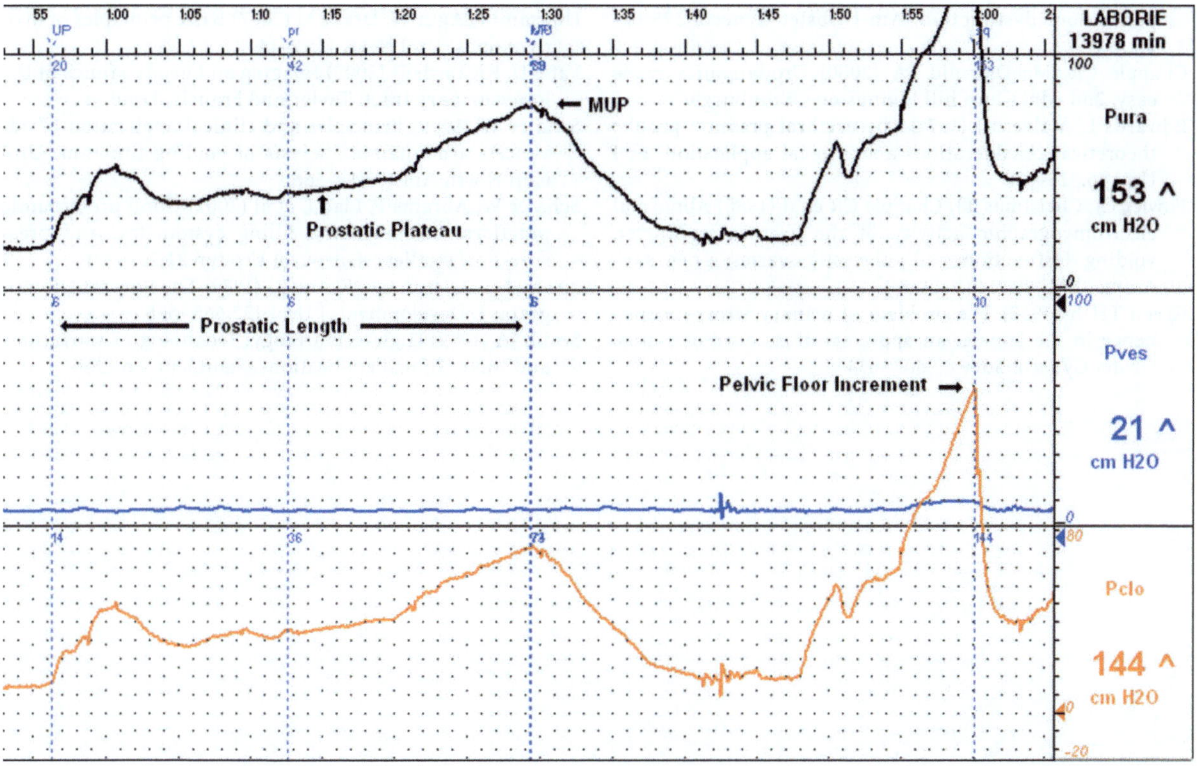

Fig. 4.7.11. Urethral pressure profile (*UPP*) plot in a male; the urethral pressure is plotted along its length (from bladder to outside). The trace shows urethral pressure (*black*), vesical pressure (*blue*) and the urethral closure pressure (*orange*), which is calculated as the difference between urethral pressure and vesical pressure. The male UPP starts with a prostatic rise in pressure to a prostatic plateau and then maximum urethral pressure (*MUP*) at the sphincter. The pelvic floor increment (the increase in pressure above MUP with pelvic floor squeeze) represents the strength of the pelvic floor muscles

Summary

Urodynamic investigations encompass a variety of tests investigating both storage and voiding functions of the lower urinary tract. Some of these are non-invasive and are used routinely in the assessment of lower urinary tract symptoms such as frequency-volume charts or uroflowmetry, whilst other tests such as neuro-physiological tests are reserved for a select group of patients. Interpretation of test results is dependent on the quality of the traces, and therefore quality control during the test is very important. Videourodynamics combines anatomical and functional assessments of the lower urinary tract, and it is especially useful in neurological disease or failure of surgical treatment. Clinicians are encouraged to follow the International Continence Society's guidance on good urodynamic practice.

References

Abrams P (1999) Bladder outlet obstruction index, bladder contractility index and bladder voiding efficiency: three simple indices to define bladder voiding function. BJU Int 84:14–15

Abrams P (2006a) A simple method for teaching about voiding disorders. BJU Int 98:463

Abrams P (2006b) Urodynamics, 3rd edn. Springer, London

Abrams PH, Griffiths DJ (1979) The assessment of prostatic obstruction from urodynamic measurements and from residual urine. Br J Urol 51:129–134

Abrams P, Cardozo L, Fall M et al (2002) The standardisation of terminology of lower urinary tract function: report from the Standardisation Sub-committee of the International Continence Society. Neurourol Urodyn 21:167–178

Al-Hayek S, Belal M, Abrams P (2008) Does the patient's position influence the detection of detrusor overactivity? Neurourol Urodyn 27:279–286

Blaivas JG, Olsson CA (1988) Stress incontinence: classification and surgical approach. J Urol 139:727–731

Bump RC, Mattiasson A, Bo K et al (1996) The standardization of terminology of female pelvic organ prolapse and

pelvic floor dysfunction. Am J Obstet Gynecol 175:10–17
Chapple CR, MacDiarmid SA (2000) Urodynamics made easy, 2nd edn. Churchill Livingstone, Edinburgh
Edwards L, Malvern J (1974) The urethral pressure profile: theoretical considerations and clinical application. Br J Urol 46:325–335
Fowler CJ, Christmas TJ, Chapple CR et al (1988) Abnormal electromyographic activity of the urethral sphincter, voiding dysfunction, and polycystic ovaries: a new syndrome? BMJ 297:1436–1438
Green TH Jr (1968) The problem of urinary stress incontinence in the female: an appraisal of its current status. Obstet Gynecol Surv 23:603–634
Housami F, Agur W, Drake M (2007) Basic principles of urodynamics. Urol News 11:12–14
Patel U, Rickards D (2005) Imaging and urodynamics of the lower urinary tract. Taylor and Francis, London
Schafer W (1990) Principles and clinical application of advanced urodynamic analysis of voiding function. Urol Clin North Am 17:553–566
Schafer W, Abrams P, Liao L et al (2002) Good urodynamic practices: uroflowmetry, filling cystometry, and pressure-flow studies. Neurourol Urodyn 21:261–274
Siroky MB, Olsson CA, Krane RJ (1979) The flow rate nomogram: I. Development. J Urol 122:665–668
Smith JA (1992) High tech urology: Technologic innovations and their clinical applications. Saunders, London

Imaging Techniques

4.8 Anorectal Physiology

Anton V. Emmanuel

CONTENTS

4.8.1 Introduction

Understanding the physiology of defaecation and continence requires an appreciation of the interplay among the anal sphincter, rectum and pelvic floor, which although anatomically simple is physiologically complex. Whilst gold standards to define function remain elusive, there are in routine use a number of techniques for studying the motor and sensory elements of anorectal physiology. Furthermore, recent studies have proposed a key role for rectal compliance and sensitivity in the pathogenesis of faecal incontinence and rectal evacuation disorders. This chapter focuses primarily on the rationale for, and the clinical value of, performing these tests with only brief detail of the methodology.

A. V. Emmanuel, MD, BSc, FRCP
Director of GI Physiology Unit, University College Hospital, 235 Euston Road, London NW1 2BU, UK

4.8.2 Clinical Features

The interpretation of anorectal physiology must take into account the impact of a patient's symptoms on the lifestyle and quality of life of that patient. An accurate history, which also encompasses an enquiry into relevant aetiological factors, remains the starting point of assessment. Symptom diaries and assessment questionnaires, completed prior to clinical examination, greatly assist this process by quantifying the extent, timing and social context of symptoms. However, questionnaires are only an adjunct to history taking. There is no existing symptom questionnaire that on its own addresses anorectal dysfunction comprehensively (Jorge and Wexner 1993; Vaizey et al. 1999). Recently, disease-specific quality-of-life instruments have been developed to complement this scored questionnaire data (Byrne et al. 2002; Voskiujl et al. 2004; Marquis et al. 2005). To date, the role of these instruments is mostly in the research setting.

Basic questioning in constipation should elicit a history of infrequent defaecation or evacuatory difficulty (or both). In a patient with incontinence, it is essential to differentiate between urge incontinence (loss of stool despite attempts to inhibit defaecation) and passive incontinence (loss of stool without patient awareness). Urge incontinence is usually associated with external anal sphincter dysfunction, whilst passive leakage reflects internal anal sphincter dysfunction (Engel et al. 1995). Nocturnal faecal incontinence suggests a neurological causation of symptoms. Anorectal physiology has a greater decision-assisting role in patients with incontinence compared to those with constipation, where it is important only in those with a lifelong history of constipation with no faecal soiling, as this raises the possibility of congenital disorders such as Hirschsprung's disease.

Physical examination may reveal a clue as to aetiology, such as a neurological or connective tissue disorder. Perineal examination may demonstrate soiling, or erythema and excoriation from chronic incontinence. Digital assessment may give an indication of anal tone, though this correlates poorly with clinical, manometric or histological assessment (Hallan et al. 1989; Sultan et al. 1994). If a patient is suspected of having an external rectal prolapse, this needs to be evaluated while the patient strains seated on a toilet. Rigid sigmoidoscopy is mandatory when there is any suspicion of organic disease. In both constipated and incontinent patients, digital examination is of value to detect faecal impaction.

4.8.3 Anorectal Manometry

Anal manometry determines the functional strength of the anal sphincter complex. The length of this complex is defined as the region where the resting pressure is >5 mmHg above rectal pressure. Traditionally a station pull-through method has been used to measure sphincter pressures, where a manometry catheter is inserted transanally into the rectum and pressure measurements recorded at 0.5-cm intervals as the catheter is withdrawn. The original manometry systems used air- or water-filled microballoons, and whilst they gave a pressure that equated to a summated "global" pressure, a major problem of poor reproducibility remained. Modern manometric methods use water-perfused systems or solid-state pressure transducers mounted on catheters. Such catheters typically carry between four to eight measuring ports (Fig. 4.8.1). Sphincter pressures are typically expressed as an average of the recordings from each transducer. The repeatability of this technique has been studied in small series with only moderate interobserver reproducibility demonstrated (Hallan et al. 1989; Rogers et al. 1989). A larger, more recent study (Nicholls et al. 2002) has shown that clinically accurate and reproducible results are obtained in up to 92% of patients. The limitations of solid-state catheters are that the sheer size (and expense) of the transducers limit the number of measurement ports that can be arranged radially. The water-perfused systems, being smaller, allow multiple measurement ports to be arranged radially and longitudinally along a catheter. A recent development is high-resolution anal manometry in which 16 measurement ports are available at one level, and it has been suggested that this may reduce the circumferential asymmetry that occurs with conventional four- or eight-channel manometry (Jones et al. 2007).

Whichever form of measurement is used, there are two primary measurements made with anorectal manometry – the resting and voluntary contraction anal sphincter pressures. Resting pressure correlates predominantly with internal anal sphincter tone, while contraction ("squeeze") pressure reflects predominantly external anal sphincter function (Engel et al. 1995). This implies that when making resting sphincter pressure measurements, the patient should be as relaxed as possible so as not to be contracting their external sphincter due to anxiety. Contraction pressure values are obtained by asking the patient to voluntarily squeeze their anal sphincter whilst the catheter is pulled through the anal canal. This can be assessed either as the average value obtained while the catheter is pulled rapidly through the canal or alternatively the average of multiple measurements made at discrete 0.5-cm "stations". Typical values for resting, internal sphincter pressure are between 50 and 65 mmHg, being slightly higher in men than women (Read et al. 1979; Loening-Baucke and Anuras 1984; McHugh and Diamant 1987; Nicholls et al. 2002). The range of normal values for contraction pressure is between 60 and 150 mmHg above resting sphincter pressure. Contraction pressures are consistently higher in men than women, and also tend to decline with age even in the absence of any pathology (Read et al. 1979; Loening-Baucke and Anuras 1984; McHugh and Diamant 1987; Nicholls et al. 2002).

Functional anal canal length is determined during the pull-through method, representing where anal sphincter pressure is greater than 5 mmHg above rectal pressure. There is seemingly a gender difference in this functional length, which in males is between 2.8 and 4.5 cm and in females is between 2.2 and 4.0 cm (Loening-Baucke and Anuras 1984; McHugh and Diamant 1987). An additional recording that is often made is of involuntary anal sphincter contraction pressure. The patient is asked to cough or in some other way to raise the intraabdominal pressure whilst concurrently recording the reflex increase in external sphincter contraction that occurs. This involuntary measure is held to reflect the maximal potential strength of the external sphincter and may be related to treatment outcome (Norton a 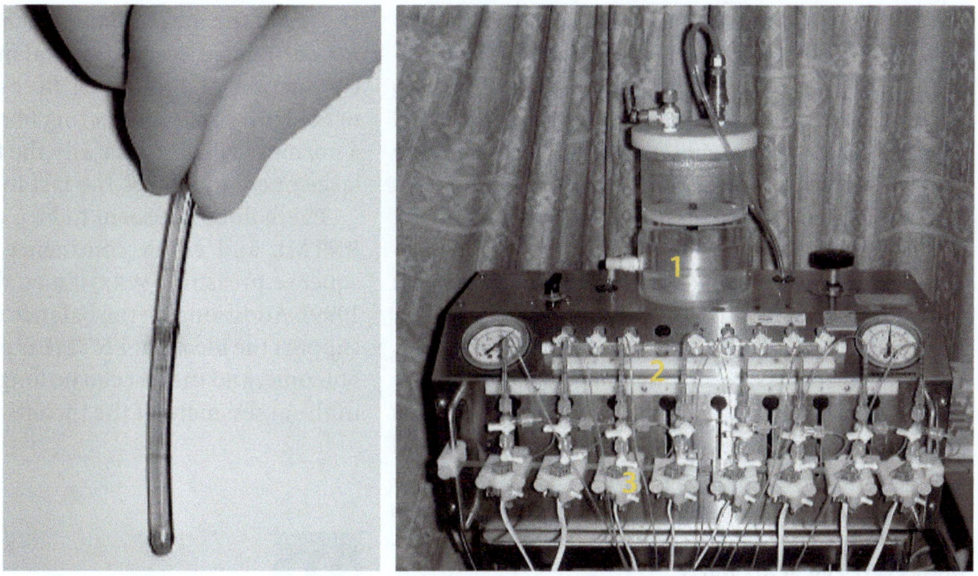

b

Fig. 4.8.1a,b. The eight radial catheter channels (**a**) are perfused with sterile water from (**b**) a pressurized reservoir (*1*) connected individually (*2*) to a capillary pressure transducer (*3*). Readings from each of these pressure transducers is sent to a PC for display and analysis

and Kamm 2002). An additional manometric measure that has been reported to reflect the fatigability of anal function is the duration of maximal squeeze pressure (Read et al. 1979; Marcello et al. 1998; Nicholls et al. 2002). These latter two measures, however, suffer from poor interobserver reproducibility, and their clinical value is as yet unproven.

One other clinically valuable manometric measure is confirming the presence of the rectoanal inhibitory reflex. This normal reflex is elicited by inflating a balloon in the rectum while simultaneously performing anal manometry. Absence of the reflex obviates the need for surgical histology in a patient with a history suggestive of Hirschsprung's disease (Tobon et al. 1968).

4.8.3.1 Vector Manometry

It is known that anal canal "pressures" are not radially symmetrical–in the proximal canal anterior quadrant pressures are lower, and in the distal canal posterior quadrant pressures are lower (Taylor et al. 1984). Vector manometry (vectometry) allows pressure profiling along the length of the anal canal to define this functional asymmetry. To date, however, there has been a disappointing absence of correlation between pressure asymmetry areas and defects on anal electromyography (see below) or endoanal ultrasound (Perry et al. 1990; Yang and Wexner 1994). Endoanal ultrasound remains the gold standard for identification of traumatic sphincter injury.

4.8.3.2 Anal Electromyography

Anal sphincter electromyography (EMG) provides information about the presence of sphincter defects and helps identify nerve injury. Measurement is performed by needle electrode (concentric or single-fibre), surface EMG pads or anal plugs. Concentric EMG samples the action potentials from up to 25 motor units, identifying areas of absent electrical activity representing either scarring or a frank defect in the muscle. Single-fibre EMG can be used to further define these areas of absent electrical activity, identifying denervated or reinnervated areas of muscle based on the patterns of reinnervation potentials. To avoid the discomfort of needle insertion, in recent years EMG studies have been performed using anal plugs, although the reproducibility of such measurements is undetermined. Surface EMG may be of benefit as part of biofeedback treatment in patients with constipation and incontinence.

Patients with incontinence have higher single-fibre density than controls, which is thought to reflect a neurogenic aetiology. However, there is no correlation between severity of symptoms and EMG changes (Bersma et al. 1992), and furthermore there is no validation of EMG changes in relation to histological evidence of denervation. Overall, the advent of anal endosonography has vastly improved the accuracy of quantification of sphincter injury (Sultan et al. 1994), and EMG is now of little value.

Recently, a surface EMG probe with 16 circumferential electrodes, recording motor units and their propagation around the external anal sphincter, has become available. The technique has been validated against needle EMG and used in patients with post-obstetric faecal incontinence, showing that there is correlation between EMG asymmetry and symptoms (Wietek et al. 2007).

4.8.3.3 Pudendal Nerve Latency Measurement

Kiff and Swash (1984) described a method to measure conduction in the pudendal nerve using a stimulating and recording electrode that is worn on a gloved finger (Fig. 4.8.2). A stimulus is applied (at the finger tip) to the pudendal nerve, and the latency until an external sphincter contraction occurs (recorded at the finger base) is measured. The normal value for this pudendal nerve terminal motor latency (PNTML) is 2±0.5 ms, increasing with age. However, the measurement technique is highly performer-related, and the actual measure reflects only conduction of the fastest fibres. Thus, a damaged nerve with some conducting fibres will still produce a normal PNTML; typically the fastest fibres are the large ones, which are the last to be damaged.

There does not seem to be a correlation between PNTML and either continence symptoms or anal squeeze pressure (Wexner et al. 1997; Fynes et al. 1999). Additionally, the balance of evidence does not support the idea that PNTML is predictive of surgical outcome, and the test can no longer be recommended in the assessment of the incontinent patient.

4.8.4 Anal Sensation

Anal sensation is served by specialized sensory endings in the anal mucosa and is important in maintenance of continence mechanisms (Miller et al. 1987; Sun et al. 1990). Reproducible thresholds for anal sensory perception can be obtained by passing a current between bipolar electrodes positioned in the anal canal (Rogers et al. 1989; Kamm and Lennard-Jones 1990). The normal value for anal electrosensation is 4.1±0.3 mA. The measure is an accurate reflection of denervation injury and has a role in predicting completeness of injury in spinal patients (Emmanuel et al. 2002).

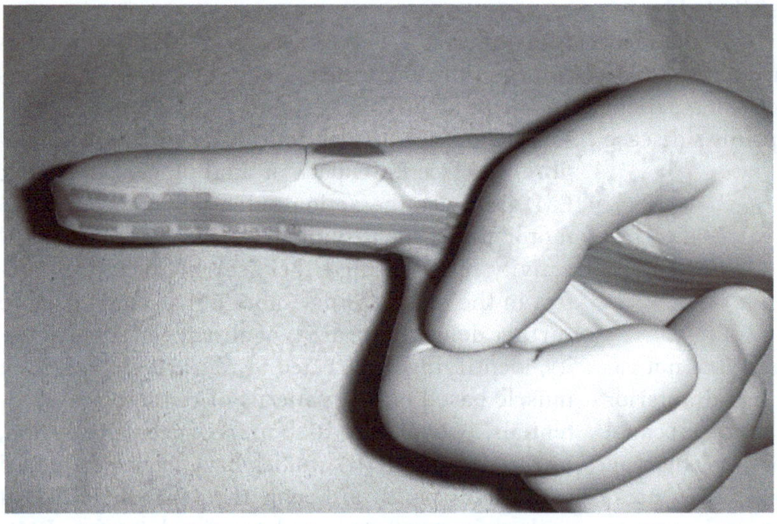
a

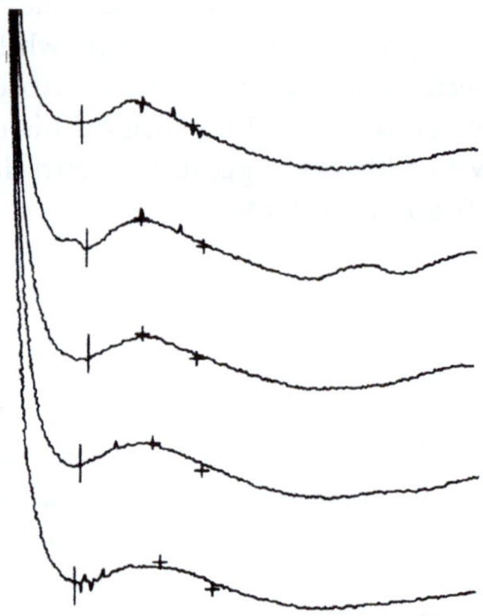
b

Fig. 4.8.2. a The St Mark's pudendal electrode for measuring pudendal nerve terminal motor latencies. The nerve is located by the tip of the ischial tuberosity. b The PNTML, measured in milliseconds, is the delay from the application of the stimulus to the onset of the external sphincter action potential

4.8.5 Rectal Sensation

Rectal sensitivity can be measured by either balloon distension or electrical stimulation. Balloon distension is performed by gradual inflation via a hand-held syringe of a balloon seated in the rectal ampulla. The patient is asked to report three separate feelings in succession: first ("threshold") sensation, feeling of urgency and finally maximal tolerable sensation. It is held that these sensations correlate to function of mucosal, muscular and serosal mechanoreceptors, respectively (Loening-Baucke and Anuras 1984; Caruana et al. 1991). The volumes obtained for these sensations depend on the type of balloon and the protocol for distension used, and to minimize the variability that this generates between different centres, it has been recommended that distension sensitivity is performed using a barostat. A barostat allows preset mechanical distension of an infinitely compliant balloon at fixed pressure, compensating for differences in rectal wall tension. Using a hand-held syringe and a party balloon, the normal range for threshold volume is 20–70 ml, for urge volume 35–120 ml and for maximum tolerated volume 100–260 ml (Nicholls et al. 2002). Heightened threshold volumes are found in patients with faecal incontinence, and these have been shown to normalize following successful biofeedback therapy (Miner et al. 1990).

Rectal electrical stimulation using a bipolar electrode as described for anal electrosensation is a more reproducible technique than balloon distension for measuring rectal sensation. This has proved a valuable technique for detecting hindgut denervation in patients with neurological disease (Emmanuel et al. 2002; Craggs et al. 2006).

4.8.6 Colonic Transit

Radio-opaque marker studies provide a useful measure of whole gut transit. A well-validated technique involves the ingestion of three geometrically different marker sets of 20 markers each on days 1, 2 and 3 with a plain film of the abdomen on day 6 (i.e. 120 h after the first ingestion later) when the remaining markers are counted. This in effect gives three transit studies for the one film and avoids the problem of clearing all the markers from a bowel motion early in the study if just one marker set was used (Hinton et al. 1969). The maximum number of markers that may be retained is less than four for the marker set given on day 1, less than six for the day-2 markers and less than 12 for the day-3 markers (Evans et al. 1992), and may be used to define slow colonic transit (Fig. 4.8.3). A modification of this is to give 20 markers for 3 days and then take

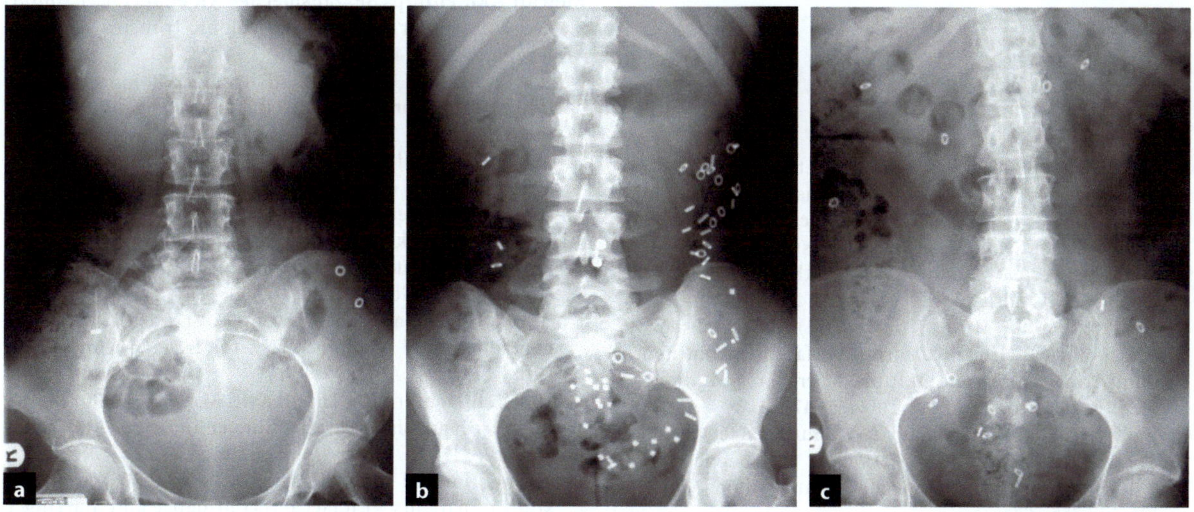

Fig. 4.8.3. **a** Normal transit with only three rings remaining (20 cubes given on day 1, 20 rods on day 2, 20 rings on day 3). **b** Slow colonic transit with 20 of each marker remaining. **c** Slow colonic transit on one of the marker sets only with all the cubes passed, 1 rod remaining, and 15 rings

a film on day 4. The number and distribution of markers may be used to calculate regional transit (Metcalf et al. 1987), although the significance of the concept of regional transit is uncertain. Scintigraphic assessment of colonic transit is the most accurate, but also the most complex, with no clear advantage over markers (van der Sijp et al. 1993).

4.8.7 Conclusion

Anorectal physiological techniques are of value in diagnosis and assessment of patients with incontinence and constipation, but must be interpreted in the context of a comprehensive clinical history and appropriate imaging. Anal manometry is of unequivocal value in defining the functional integrity of the anal sphincter muscles and in excluding Hirschsprung's disease. It complements the information obtained from endoanal ultrasound and helps in decision making prior to, and following, surgical repair. Endoanal ultrasound remains superior to anal vector manometry or electromyography in defining traumatic sphincter injury. Pudendal nerve latency measurement is not of value in assessing patients with faecal incontinence. Anorectal sensory testing is of value in identifying hindgut involvement in patients with neurological disease.

References

Bersma RJF, van Baren R, Koorevar M et al (1992) Anal endosonography: relationship with anal manometry and neurophysiologic tests. Dis Colon Rectum 35:944–949

Byrne CM, Pager CK, Rex J et al (2002) Assessment of quality of life in the treatment of patients with neuropathic fecal incontinence. Dis Colon Rectum 45:1431–1436

Caruana BJ, Wald A, Hinds JP et al (1991) Anorectal sensory and motor function in neurogenic faecal incontinence. Comparison between multiple sclerosis and diabetes mellitus. Gastroenterology 100:465–470

Craggs MD, Balasubramaniam AV, Chung EA et al (2006) Aberrant reflexes and function of the pelvic organs following spinal cord injury in man. Auton Neurosci 126-127:355–370

Emmanuel AV, Kamm MA, Middleton F (2002) Gut specific autonomic testing and bowel dysfunction in spinal cord injury. Gastroenterology 122 Supp 1:M1535

Engel AF, Kamm MA, Bartram CI et al (1995) Relationship of symptoms in faecal incontinence to specific sphincter abnormalities. Int J Colorectal Dis 10:152–155

Evans RC, Kamm MA, Hinton JM et al (1992) The normal range and a simple diagram for recording whole gut transit time. Int J Colorect Dis 7:15–17

Fynes MM, Donelly V, Behan M et al (1999) Effect of second vaginal delivery on anorectal physiology and faecal continence: a prospective study. Lancet 354:983–986

Hallan RI, Marzouk DE, Waldron DJ et al (1989) Comparison of digital and manometric assessment of anal sphincter function. Br Surg 76:973–975

Hinton JM, Lennard-Jones JE, Young AC (1969) A new method for studying gut transit times using radio-opapue markers. Gut 10:842–847

Jones MP, Post P, Crowell MD (2007) High-resolution manometry in the evaluation of anorectal disorders: a simultaneous comparison with water-perfused manometry. Am J Gastroenterol **102**:850–855

Jorge JM, Wexner SD (1993) Aetiology and management of faecal incontinence. Dis Colon Rectum 36:77–97

Kamm MA, Lennard-Jones JE (1990) Rectal mucosal electrosensory testing. Evidence for a sensory neuropathy in severe constipation. Dis Colon Rectum 33:419–423

Kiff ES, Swash M (1984) Slowed conduction in the pudendal nerves in idiopathic (neurogenic) faecal incontinence. Br J Surg 71:614–616

Loening-Baucke V, Anuras S (1984) Anorectal manometry in healthy elderly subjects. Am Geriatr Soc 32:636–639

Marquis P, De La Loge C, Dubois D et al (2005) Development and validation of the Patient Assessment of Constipation Quality of Life questionnaire. Scand J Gastroenterol 40:540–551

Marcello PW, Barrett BS, Coller JA et al (1998) Fatigue rate index as a new measurement of external sphincter function. Dis Colon Rectum 41:336–343

McHugh SM, Diamnt NE (1987) Effect of age, gender and parity on anal canal pressures: contribution of impaired anal sphincter function to faecal incontinence. Dig Dis Sci 32:726–736

Metcalf AM, Phillips SF, Zinsmeister AR et al (1987) Simplified assessment of segmental colonic transit. Gastroenterology 92:40–47

Miller R, Bartolo DCC, Roe AE et al (1988) Anal sensation and the continence mechanism. Dis Colon Rectum 31:433–438

Miner PB, Donnelly TC, Read NW (1990) Investigation of mode of action of action of biofeedback in treatment of faecal incontinence. Dig Dis Sci 35:1291–1298

Nicholls TJ, Solanki D, Emmanuel AV et al (2002) Inter-examiner reproducibility of anorectal motor and sensory function test. Gut 51, Supp II:A60

Norton C, Chelvanayagam S, Kamm MA (2002) Randomised controlled trial of biofeedback for faecal incontinence. Gut 51, Supp II:A61

Perry RE, Blatchford GJ, Christensen MA et al (1990) Manometric diagnosis of anal sphincter injuries. Am J Surg 159:112–117

Read NW, Harford WV, Schmulen AC et al (1979) A clinical study of patients with faecal incontinence and diarrhoea. Gastroenterology 76:747–756

Rogers J, Laurberg S, Misiewicz JJ et al (1989) Anorectal physiology validated: a repeatability study of the mo-

tor and sensory tests of anorectal function. Br J Surg 76:607–609
Sultan AH, Kamm MA, Talbot IC et al (1994) Anal endosonography for identifying external sphincter defects confirmed histologically. Br J Surg 81:463–465
Sun WM, Read NW, Prior A et al (1990) Sensory and motor responses to rectal distension vary according to rate and pattern of balloon inflation. Gastroenterology 99:1008–1015
Taylor BM, Beart RW Jr, Phillips SF (1984) Longitudinal and radial variations of pressure in the human anal sphincter. Gastroenterology 86:693–697
Tobon F, Reid NCRW, Talbert JL et al (1968) Nonsurgical test for the diagnosis of Hirschsprung's disease. New Engl J Med 278:188–194
Vaizey CJ, Carapet E, Cahill JA et al (1999) Prospective comparison of faecal incontinence grading systems. Gut 44:77–80
Voskuijl WP, van der Zaag-Loonen HJ, Ketel IJ et al (2004) Health related quality of life in disorders of defecation: the Defecation Disorder List. Arch Dis Child 89:1124-1127
van der Sijp JR, Kamm MA, Nightingale JM et al (1993) Radioisotope determination of regional colonic transit in severe constipation: comparison with radio opaque markers. Gut 34:402–408
Wexner SD (1997) Re: manometric tests of anorectal function in the management of defecation disorders. Am J Gastroenterol 92:1400
Wietek BM, Hinninghofen H, Jehle JC et al (2007) Asymmetric sphincter innervation is associated with fecal incontinence after anal sphincter trauma during childbirth. Neurourol Urodyn **26**:134–139
Yang Y, Wexner SD (1994) Anal pressure vectography is of no apparent benefit for sphincter evaluation. Int J Colorectal Dis 9:989–996

Urogenetical Dysfunction

5

5.1 Surgery and Clinical Imaging for Pelvic Organ Prolapse

Douglass S. Hale

CONTENTS

D. S. Hale, MD, FACOG, FACS
Director Female Pelvic Medicine & Reconstructive Surgery Fellowship, Associate Clinical Professor, Indiana University/Methodist Hospital, 1633 North Capitol Avenue, Suite 436, Indianapolis, IN 46202, USA

5.1.1 Introduction

The purpose of this chapter is to provide the radiologist interested in pelvic floor imaging with a surgical perspective of pelvic floor dysfunction. Although individual surgeons may have different reasons for requesting imaging studies, the basic question to be answered remains the same: the preoperative identification of all surgically treatable prolapse and pelvic floor dysfunction. It is estimated that 11.1% of women will undergo a single operation for pelvic floor dysfunction in their lifetime. Nearly 30% of these patients will require a second operation (Olsen et al. 1997). Projections over the next 30 years show the at-risk population will increase by 22%, but the demand for care will increase by 45%, reflecting a higher number of visits for patients as they age (Luber 2001). Improving the care of these patients has major implications for health-care systems.

To that end, preoperative identification of these conditions is critical to appropriate intervention. In the past, division of the pelvic floor into an anterior, middle, and posterior compartment has led to fragmentation of care. The anterior compartment with its urethra and bladder have been the realm of the urologist, the middle compartment containing the uterus and reproductive organs the domain of the gynecologist, and the posterior compartment with the small and large bowel belonged to the colorectal surgeon. These artificial divisions of the pelvis did not recognize the symbiotic relationship of these "compartments." Treatment of one compartment influences the structure and function of the others. Radiologic studies have helped clinicians recognize the interdependence of these compartments and the need to address them together in the treatment of pelvic disorders.

Advances in imaging techniques have evolved from studies involving single organs with their inherent limitations to more lengthy, but superior studies. Unfortunately, the best radiologic techniques for evaluating these conditions are time consuming, as they require individual filling and emptying of the organs along with various dynamic maneuvers. However, by combining the patient history, physical exam, and radiologic findings, the radiologist and the clinician can complement each other in the successful diagnosis and treatment of women with pelvic floor disorders.

5.1.2 Anatomy of Support

Care of women with these disorders begins with an understanding of the unique musculofascial system that supports the pelvic organs. No single ligament or muscle is responsible for supporting the pelvic organs. Rather a unique musculofascial system is in place that must work together for proper organ support. The levator ani muscles (puborectalis, pubococcygeus, iliococcygeus) provide an active platform of support for the pelvic organs, while a vast fascial connective tissue network suspends the organs on this platform. Damage to the levator ani muscles and pelvic nerves by childbirth, neurologic disease or injury, disuse atrophy, or various other conditions affecting neuromuscular integrity may lead to widening of the levator hiatus. As the hiatus widens, more stress is placed on the connective tissue network that holds the vaginal vault and pelvic organs in place. Eventually, this stress may lead to tearing or stretching of the supportive connective tissue. As the vaginal vault loses its support, the surrounding organs will begin to prolapse through the levator hiatus.

In place of true ligamentous support, the connective tissue of the pelvis is made up of varying degrees of collagen, elastin, smooth muscle, neural tissue, and vascular channels (Campbell 1950). The cardinal (Mackenrodt) ligaments and uterosacral ligaments form a continuous complex of support for the upper vagina and uterus. These should not be thought of as distinct, separate structures. The cardinal ligaments fan out to blend laterally with the parietal fascia of the pelvic sidewall muscles. The uterosacral ligaments are the postero-medial continuation of this complex, eventually joining the presacral fascia close to the sacroiliac joint. The importance of these structures for their role in support has been demonstrated in elegant yet simple cadaver studies (Mengert 1936). Working with these upper supports, a distinct fascial layer enveloping the vagina and serving as an independent support to the bladder and rectum has been described. Anteriorly this layer has been called the pubovesicocervical fascia, while posteriorly the term rectovaginal septum (Denovillier's fascia in the male) has been used. On the anterior vaginal wall, the pubovesicocervical fascia has been demonstrable grossly, but histologically has not been identified as a separate layer from the vaginal muscularis (Webber and Walters 1997). This fact may be explained by the blending of the uterosacral-cardinal connective tissue with vaginal muscularis; this is not a sharp clean attachment (Uhlenhuth and Nolley 1957). It is, therefore, important for both surgeons and radiologists involved in pelvic floor dysfunction to acknowledge that a distinct connective tissue layer separate from the anterior vaginal wall muscularis does not exist.

A similar controversy existed concerning the presence of a connective tissue layer supporting the posterior vaginal wall. In short, there is a rectovaginal septum distinct from the posterior vaginal muscularis. Problems in demonstrating the rectovaginal septum as a separate structure arise from its fusion with the caudal ½ to ⅓ of the vagina and its relatively short length (Milley and Nichols 1968). In a study of 44 women at laparoscopy, the mean length of the rectovaginal septum was found to be 2.1 cm, while the rectovaginal pouch extended 5.3 cm below the posterior vaginal apex (Kuhn and Hollyock 1982). The short length of the rectovaginal septum has been confirmed histologically and grossly in cadaver studies (DeLancey 1999). Therefore, the superior edge of the rectovaginal septum fuses with the muscularis of the posterior vaginal wall approximately 3 cm above the perineal body. Laterally, the rectovaginal septum fuses with the fascia of the levator ani muscles (Leffler et al. 2001). The perineal body is indirectly suspended to the sacrum by a series of connective tissue links involving the rectovaginal septum, the mid-vaginal muscularis, and the uterosacral ligaments.

To summarize, three different levels of support are recognized for the vagina (DeLancey 1992) (Fig. 5.1.1). The cardinal-uterosacral complex, which blends with the vaginal muscularis, supports the upper vagina and uterus. The mid vagina, level II support, is provided by the attachment of the vaginal muscularis to the arcus tendineus fascia pelvis and an intact vaginal muscularis. Level III support is the

Fig. 5.1.1. Three levels of vaginal connective tissue support: level I = uterosacral-cardinal complex; level II = arcus tendineus fascia pelvis; level III = perineal membrane and crura of levator muscles

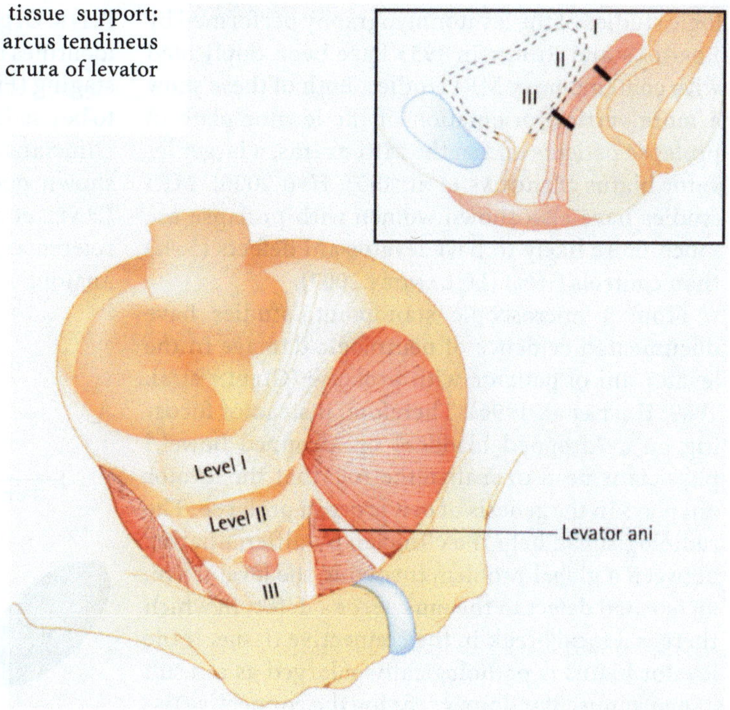

function of the rectovaginal septum and the perineal membrane. At all levels, the levator ani muscles have connective tissue extensions to aid with this support network (Zaccharin 1980). Not only do the well-recognized "ligamentous" supports of the urethra, vaginal vault, and lower uterine segment need to be intact, but also it appears the musculofascial tissue enveloping the vaginal epithelium must remain unbroken. As in all aspects of anatomy, variations do exist between patients, and this fact may help explain some of the pathogenesis of prolapse. Many surgeons correct breaks in the connective tissue support system at the time of surgery. MRI may have a role in identifying these connective tissue breaks that will then aid in the surgical planning. Understanding the anatomy and effectively communicating such imaging findings are paramount to the radiologists' interaction with the clinician.

5.1.3 Etiology of Prolapse

Pelvic organ prolapse (POP) has a multifactorial etiology. Vaginal parity, neuropathy, obesity, excessive Valsalva, connective tissue disorders, prior surgery, estrogen status, and advancing age are the most often cited risk factors (Smith et al. 1989; Gilpin et al. 1989; Norton et al. 1995; Davis 1996; Smith et al. 1990). Of these, vaginal parity and its associated neuropathy appear to play the biggest role. A 4- to 11-fold increase in prolapse is seen among vaginally parous women (Mant 1997).

Few epidemiological studies exist to follow the direct cause and progression of prolapse. As noted earlier, dysfunction of the levator ani muscle, whether from childbirth, neuropathy, or other factors, leads to an increased area between the levator ani muscles, i.e., the levator hiatus. Forces directed at the pelvic floor, namely Valsalva type maneuvers, further stress this situation by driving the organs through this hiatus. The connective tissue network begins to stretch and tear with resulting loss of support. Pelvic organ prolapse should not be thought of as the problem; rather it is the result of the problem, namely levator ani dysfunction. Reconstructed three-dimensional MRI comparison of the levator ani muscles has shown a marked difference in levator volume, shape, and integrity among asymptomatic patients, those with genuine stress incontinence, and those with prolapse, providing indirect evidence that levator ani dysfunction is intimately involved in the different clinical manifestations of pelvic floor dysfunction (Hoyte et al. 2001). The classic radiologic studies of the levator myography performed by Berglas and Rubin in 1953 have been duplicated with contemporary MRI studies. Both of these show a more vertical orientation of the levator plate in prolapse patients and in the MRI exams, a larger levator hiatus (Berglas et al. 1953; Hsu 2006). MRI studies have also shown women with prolapse are much more likely to have levator ani defects (56%) than controls (16%) (DeLancey 2007).

From a microscopic standpoint, studies have documented evidence of neurologic damage in the levator ani of patients with prolapse (Gilpin et al. 1989; Heit et al. 1996). Therefore, instead of focusing on a "dropped bladder" or "dropped bowel," physicians need to realize the role that the levator ani plays in the genesis of pelvic organ prolapse. The radiologist can help the clinician by differentiating between a global problem involving the levator ani, an isolated defect in the muscle, or a defect in which there is a focal break in the connective tissue. If the levator hiatus is pathologically enlarged as a result of neuromuscular damage, fixing the connective tissue break alone will not suffice. Without the support of the levator ani, the same stresses will be placed on the connective tissue, and prolapse will recur. Patients with a permanent, unrecoverable neuromuscular condition of the levator ani will often require graft placement to replace the damaged connective tissue. This graft material must be stronger than the native tissue and hold up better to the demands placed on the damaged pelvic floor. This global levator dysfunction may be diagnosed on MRI by levator ani ballooning, an enlarged levator hiatal area, or abnormal levator ani position and movement. This added knowledge can have a major impact on the surgical procedure chosen. Whether specific imaging findings will lead to specific surgeries for a given condition remains to be seen.

5.1.4 The Radiologist and the Clinician

A standardized pelvic organ prolapse grading system accepted by both radiologists and surgeons is the single most important factor slowing collaboration between radiologists and surgeons in the area of pelvic organ prolapse. The International Continence Society (ICS) has agreed on such a system for clinicians (Bump et al. 1996). Adopted in 1996, the Pelvic Organ Prolapse Quantification Exam (POPQ) identifies nine points for measurement and prolapse staging (Fig. 5.1.2). This allows a standardized exam to be used for follow-up, for communication between clinicians, and in scientific papers. The exam has shown good inter- and intra-observer correlation (Hall et al. 1996). The hymeneal ring serves as the reference point for most of these measurements, an anatomic landmark not readily visible during ra-

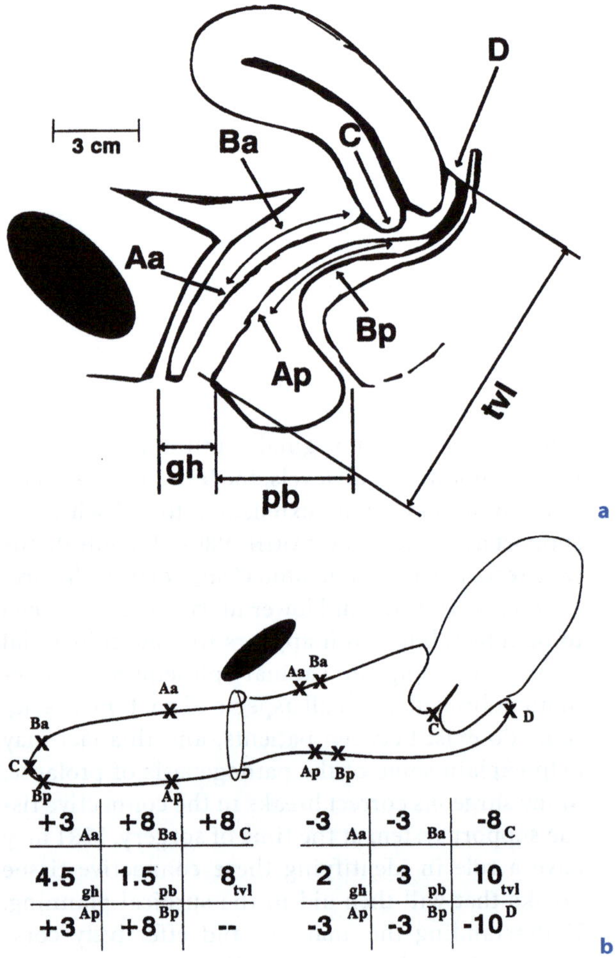

Fig. 5.1.2a,b. International Continence Society Pelvic Organ Prolapse grading system (Bump et al. 1996). **a** Nine points are measured in centimeters and recorded. The hymeneal ring serves as the reference point for most measurements. This diagram illustrates the measurements of the anterior vaginal wall (*Aa*, *Ba*), cuff or cervix (*C*), posterior fornix (*D*), posterior vaginal wall (*Ap*, *Bp*), total vaginal length (*TVL*), genital hiatus (*gh*), and perineal body (*pb*). **b** A total utero-vaginal vault eversion is juxtaposed with normal support. Where indicated, positive numbers represent tissue outside the hymeneal ring, while negative numbers represent tissue above the hymen. Overall and individual site staging can then be assigned based on these measurements

diologic studies. Attempts to identify a radiologic line that would allow direct comparisons with the ICS staging system have been frustrating. Several radiologic lines have been proposed, including the pubococcygeal line, the midpubic (hymeneal) line, the perineal line, the puborectal line, and the axial line (Comiter et al. 2001; Lieneman et al. 2004, Fauconnier et al. 2007) (Fig. 5.1.3). Unfortunately, despite good inter- and intra-observer reliability, no line has agreed with the clinical measurements in a meaningful way. In the most recent of these studies, the authors concluded that whatever line is chosen, the individual MRI measurements approximate very badly with the measurements performed at clinical examination. This fact poses the greatest challenge to meaningful communication between different disciplines.

Problems using the clinical ICS system involve using the hymen as a reference point. It is a mobile anatomic structure, particularly at the posterior forchette. The hymeneal line used radiologically tries to duplicate the clinical landmark, but it too showed poor agreement with the clinical exam (Fauconnier et al. 2007). Detachment of the perineal body from the rectovaginal septum cannot be appreciated by the current POPQ exam, but may be identified by MRI (Hsu 2006). Another problem is that the ICS system does not report on the highest level of support in cases where a hysterectomy has been performed. This information may influence the surgical approach. From the radiologic side, failure to understand the detailed anatomy of the pelvic floor has led to overstating prolapse. An example is the presence of an enterocele. Many radiologists diagnose an enterocele if there is any descent of small bowel posteriorly below the level of the vagina apex. However, the cul-de-sac depth in reported normal individuals may average over 5 cm (Kuhn and Hollyock 1982). The problem of over-diagnosing enteroceles on radiologic studies becomes evident. Further limitations are evident when one looks at the paucity of data regarding "normals." With the physical exam, ICS stage-II prolapse is a common finding in asymptomatic women. In one study, nearly 50% of 497 women seen for routine gynecologic care were asymptomatic and had ICS stage-II prolapse (Swift 2000). Radiologically, very few studies on normals have been performed, and most of these findings were obtained during an investigation of patients with prolapse. The overlap of normal subjects and symptomatic patients is considerable. Figure 51.4 shows an asymptomatic 19-year-old subject that by radiographic criteria has a moderate, contrast-retaining rectocele. Clearly, she does not require surgery. However, the same conclusion may not have been reached in a 60-year-old patient complaining of an evacuation disorder with similar radiologic findings. Rectoceles diagnosed radiologically may have no clinical symptoms. The complex, multifactorial etiology of bowel function makes reliance on one finding questionable. Nonetheless, a standardized staging system acceptable to both surgeons and radiologists is mandatory if further progress is to be made. If agreement cannot be reached on what constitutes prolapse and how it is measured, meaningful communication cannot take place.

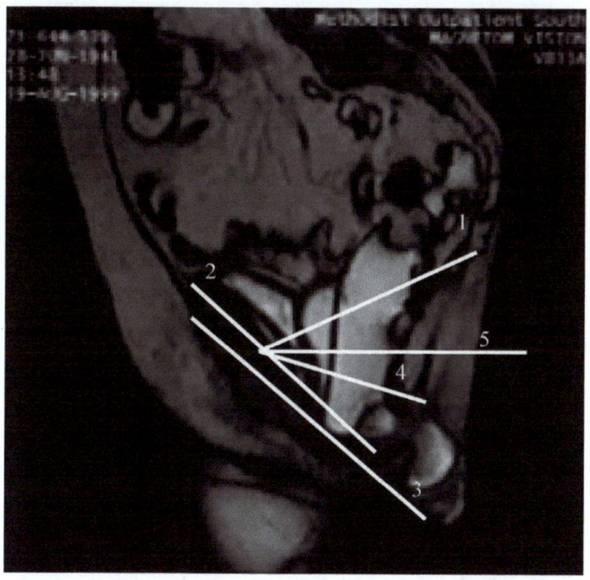

Fig. 5.1.3. Sagittal MRI showing the numerous lines proposed for radiologically measuring pelvic organ prolapse. Pubococcygeal line = *1*; midpubic (hymeneal) line = *2*; perineal line = *3*; puborectal line = *4*; axial line = *5*. None have shown agreement with the clinical ICS staging system

Historically, the gold standard for the presence or absence of prolapse has not been established. In general, radiographic studies have shown a higher degree of prolapse when compared to physical exam. This fact has been attributed to the complete relaxation of the levator ani muscles achieved during defecation on imaging studies, a condition rarely achieved during a physical exam. This relaxation allows for maximum distension of the urogenital hiatus, which in turn increases the extent of prolapse identified. As seen in Table 5.1.1, multiple comparative studies have shown that prolapse is more readily demonstrated on an imaging study than on physical exam. The discrepancy between the physical exam and im-

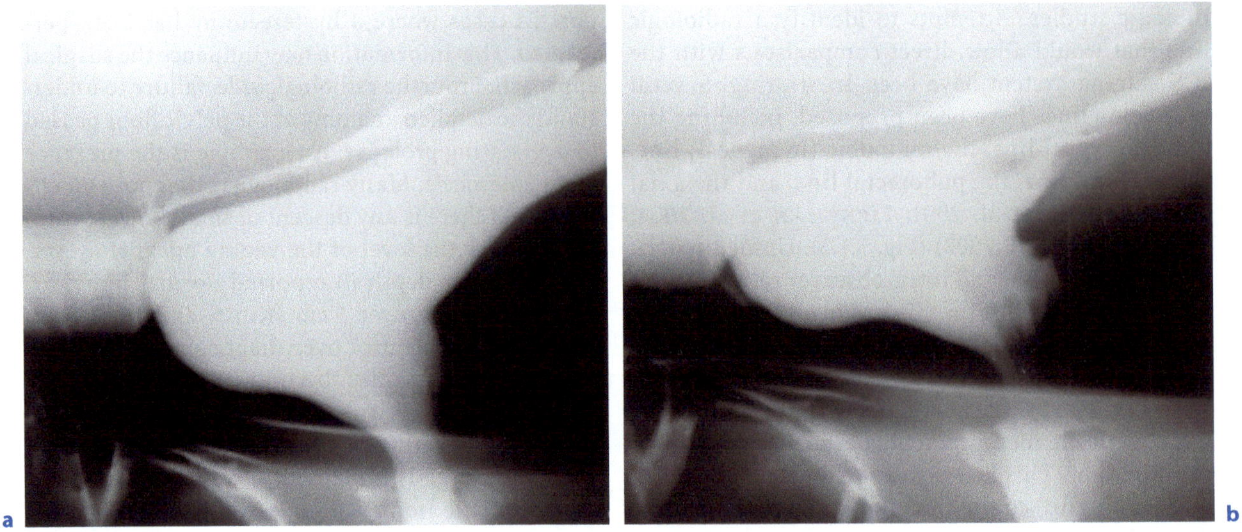

Fig. 5.1.4a,b. Moderate-sized rectocele during evacuation in a 19-year-old asymptomatic control. Following evacuation, contrast is retained in the same control. This demonstrates the difficulty in interpreting the clinical utility of these studies as an isolated finding

Table 5.1.1. Comparison of physical exam with fluoroscopy in detection of pelvic organ prolapse

Study	Rectocele			Enterocele			Cystocele		
	Found at DCP (n)	Found at PE		Found at DCP (n)	Found at PE		Found at DCP (n)	Found at PE	
		n	%		n	%		n	%
Hock et al. 1993	225	70	31	111	18	16	112	46	41
Altringer et al. 1995	46	24	52	33	16	48	44	32	73
Kelvin et al. 1999	155	119	77	47	24	51	159	132	83

aging studies may lead to a change in surgical planning. One study reported changing the initial surgical plan 41% of the time based on the results of the imaging study, while a second earlier study showed imaging changed the clinical diagnosis in 75% of their subjects (Kaufman et al. 2001; Altringer et al. 1995). Competition for the limited space within the urogenital hiatus is a major concern during both physical exam and imaging studies of the pelvis. The first organ to descend into the urogenital hiatus may prevent the descent of other organs. An unemptied cystocele may block descent of a rectocele or enterocele and therefore prevent its identification. Similarly, a large rectocele may prevent a cystocele or enterocele from being recognized (Fig. 5.1.5). Quickly performed imaging studies that do not systematically fill and empty the organs will miss the complete picture and add little to the physical exam. A triphasic technique has been proposed and seems to best address this issue. This systematic approach requires individual filling and emptying of the pelvic organs along with various dynamic maneuvers to help diagnose all organ prolapses (Kelvin et al. 2000). Although promising, sources of error including intra-observer error and week-to-week variation within a given subject have called triphasic MRI into question and need to be addressed (Morrena et al. 2005). In another example where imaging is helpful, a patient may have an obvious posterior wall defect by physical exam, which appears to be an enterocele. Imaging may diagnose this posterior wall defect to be a sigmoidocele. Sigmoidoceles are virtually never diagnosed by physical exam and can be present in up to 5% of patients with pelvic organ prolapse.

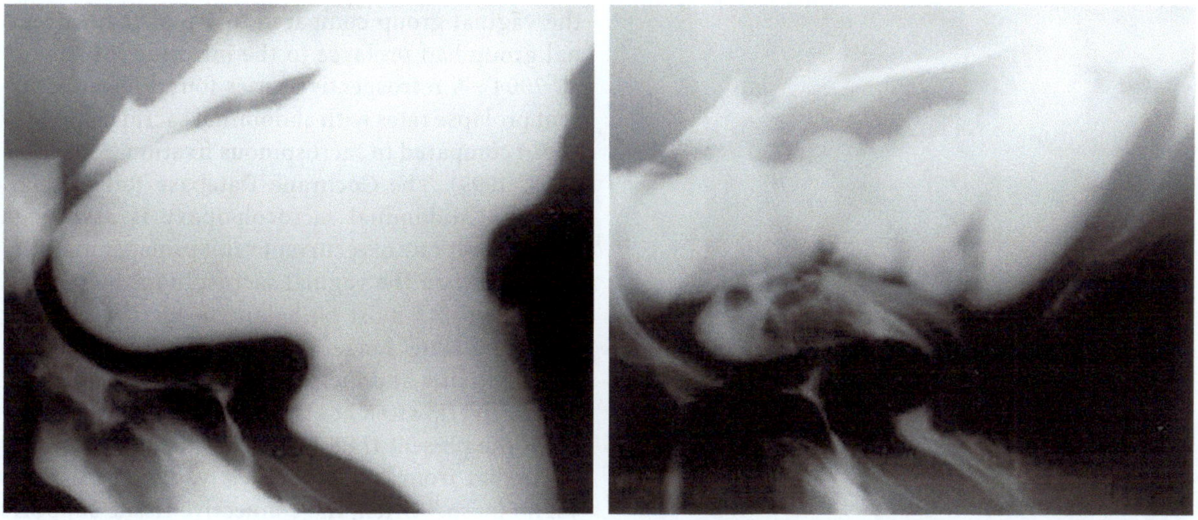

a b

Fig. 5.1.5a,b. An unemptied rectocele obscuring a large enterocele prior to complete rectal emptying. The same patient following complete contrast evacuation of the rectocele. A large enterocele is seen to descend into the urogenital hiatus, demonstrating competition for this limited space. Single-phase studies miss these coexisting prolapses, demonstrating the need for mutiphasic studies

Although some surgeons downplay the distinction between a sigmoidocele and enterocele and will not change their surgical approach, other surgeons will. These surgical changes may include a partial colectomy if a large sigmoidocele is associated with long-standing constipation (Jorge et al. 1994). In addition, detachment of the recto sigmoid from the presacral hollow with resulting prolapse may represent a different condition than a simple sigmoidocele alone. The former may need a rectopexy to reestablish rectosigmoid support rather than only cul-de-sac correction (Fig. 5.1.6). This represents a major change in surgical approach, one that is only made with the help of the radiologist. Some surgical experts argue that all prolapses can be identified at the time of surgery, and little is gained by extraneous preoperative radiologic studies. However, at the time of surgery the patient is asleep, unable to Valsalva, and usually in the dorsal lithotomy position. This is far from the ideal condition in which to identify prolapse and its extent.

For the clinician, different options exist when choosing an imaging study. Initial imaging studies of the pelvic floor were performed fluoroscopically. These have evolved into dynamic MRI studies and, in some research centers, reconstructed three-dimensional imaging. The individual study ordered will depend on the experience of the radiologist and the equipment available. The superior anatomic detail afforded by MRI would appear to make this the technique of choice. Other benefits of MRI are multiplanar views, detailed information about the levator ani muscle, patient comfort, and detection of other pelvic pathology as compared to fluoroscopic studies. Upright MRI allowing a more physiologic evacuation is available in only a few centers.

Cost may also be an issue. In a study of 22 patients having both MRI and fluoroscopy studies performed for constipation disorders, MRI was found to be ten times more expensive. In this small study there was no change in clinical management based on the results of one study compared to the other (Matsuoka et al. 2001). Pelvic floor imaging is not needed in every case of pelvic floor dysfunction. When the physical examination and patient complaints correlate, little may be gained by the imaging study. In complicated patients where the physical exam and patient complaints do not agree, an imaging study of the pelvic floor can be of diagnostic value and change surgical planning. As noted, the full extent of pelvic organ prolapse can only be appreciated when the levator ani completely relax. This relaxation only happens at times of evacuation, a condition not achieved during an office exam. As repeat surgeries are invariably more difficult and expose the patient to greater risk, care must be taken in planning the initial surgical repair. Although anatomic correction does not always lead to functional correction, the goal of pelvic surgery is to relieve patient symptoms and restore anatomy and function whenever possible.

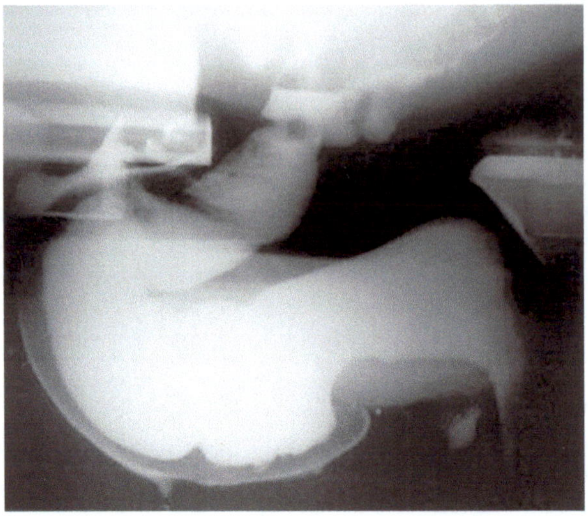

Fig. 5.1.6. Detachment of recto-sigmoid from presacral hollow. A rectopexy is required to restore normal support in addition to appropriate vaginal support

5.1.5 Surgical Approach

Details of each surgical procedure are beyond the scope of this chapter. However, information concerning basic understanding of the different surgeries available for prolapse should be helpful to radiologists. Many factors should be considered before selecting a route for reconstructive surgery. These factors include vaginal sexual function, concept of body image, a patient's medical condition, and possible fertility desires. Current surgical approaches include vaginal, abdominal, laparoscopic, or a combination of these routes. Adding to the complexity of deciding on which surgical approach to use is the issue of whether mesh is needed to perform the surgery or if native tissue should be used in these repairs. In general, biografts (allografts and xenografts) have shown inferior results when compared to synthetic grafts, but studies are limited. The experts who have published case series report a wide range of success rates with these varying techniques. Of course, the success rates of such expert surgeons may not apply universally. Three prospective studies have been published that randomized patients to either vaginal or abdominal routes for prolapse repair. Two found superior anatomic results with the sacral colpopexy (Benson et al. 1996; Lo and Wang 1998). The third found no statistical difference between the vaginal and abdominal procedures, although 17% of the vaginal group compared to 4% of the abdominal group had prolapse to the introitus (Maher et al. 2004). A retrospective series found lower recurrent prolapse rates with abdominal sacral colpopexy (19%) compared to sacrospinous fixation (33%) (Sze et al. 1999). The Cochrane Database Review concluded, "Abdominal sacrocolpopexy is associated with a lower rate of recurrent vault prolapse and dyspareunia than the vaginal sacrospinous colpopexy. These benefits must be balanced against a longer operating time, longer time to return to activities of daily living and increased cost of the abdominal approach" (Maher et al. 2007).

At the present time the debate focus has shifted somewhat from "abdominal vs. vaginal" to "mesh vs. no mesh." Often, the connective tissue supports are so damaged that attempting to repair them alone makes little sense. If the levator ani is a healthy, robust muscle capable of supporting the vagina and pelvic organs, surgical correction of breaks in the connective tissue may be appropriate. If the levator muscle cannot be rehabilitated by physical therapy, surgical support limited to the connective tissues may lead to the historically documented high recurrence rates. The desire to combine the success of the sacral colpopexy (mesh) with the benefits of a less invasive, vaginally approached surgery has led to proliferation of new prolapse repair "kits" using synthetic mesh. Widespread use of these kits before clinical trials have been conducted is of concern. Mesh can have significant complications, including but not limited to vaginal mesh exposure, erosion into surrounding organs, contracture, and pain. Many of these complications appear to be higher when vaginal incisions are used to place the mesh. Studies are ongoing to help make decisions about these new approaches, but at present few data exist. As the number of complications from mesh surgery rises, radiologists will be asked to assist in imaging these materials to better localize them prior to surgical removal.

In addition, there is also evidence that anterior vaginal wall dissection may lead to nerve damage involving the urethra and possibly also the bladder (Borirakchanyavat et al. 1997; Benson and McClellan 1993; Zivkovic et al. 1996; Ball et al. 1997). Experts believe that the most frequent offender is the anterior colporrhaphy, a procedure first described over 100 years ago that has changed little since that time (de Lamballe 1840). The exact relationship between this nerve damage and the clinical significance is debated.

Lastly, a laparoscopic or robotic approach may be useful in some patients (Su et al. 2007). Long-term efficacy studies of such approaches are lacking. If they are chosen, laparoscopic procedures should be performed as described for open cases. At the present time, relatively few surgeons have the skills required to attempt these repairs with the laparoscope. As further studies are carried out, answers to more of the "approach" questions will be found.

The following will discuss the different operations used for pelvic organ prolapse. Although divided into anterior, apical, and posterior wall procedures, the impact of one operation on another compartment cannot be emphasized enough. Just as important is the realization that rarely does one "defect" exist by itself. Our radiology colleagues who in one study showed 95% of prolapse patients had defects in all three compartments have demonstrated this (Maglinte et al. 1999).

5.1.6 The Anterior Vaginal Wall

A site-specific examination of the anterior vaginal wall focuses on the urethrovesical junction (UVJ), integrity of the lateral vaginal sulci, central vaginal wall defects, and lastly apical transverse defects (Richardson 1989) (Fig. 5.1.7). Patients with prolapse may also have co-existing or occult incontinence. A large prolapse may mask urinary incontinence by kinking of the urethra. In these cases, it has been suggested that the patients have the prolapse reduced and then have testing to uncover this occult incontinence. Preoperatively, occult incontinence is found with reduction testing in between 36–80% of patients with large prolapses (Bump et al. 1988). The importance of this was seen in a multicenter study of patients reporting no incontinence scheduled to undergo abdominal sacral colpopexy. Although not recognized as a repair for the anterior wall, the sacral colpopexy affects the anterior wall. Patients were randomized to receive a Burch (incontinence procedure) or no Burch in addition to their sacral colpopexy. The study was terminated at an interim analysis due to the high rate of symptoms of incontinence in the no-Burch group (44.1%) vs. the Burch group (23.8%) (Brubaker et al. 2006). The study concluded that in patients reporting no preoperative stress incontinence scheduled to undergo an abdominal sacral colpopexy, a Burch procedure significantly reduced the postoperative symptoms of stress incontinence. Whether the same conclusion can be reached for all prolapse surgeries is not known. In support procedures other than sacral colpopexy, selective support to the UVJ is encouraged in one form or another. This discussion needs to take place between the surgeon and the patient prior to surgery.

Historically, several terms have been used to describe cystoceles. Traction and displacement cystoceles are synonymous with paravaginal cystoceles, while pulsion or distension cystoceles are equivalent to central cystoceles (Pillai and Benson 1996). In a central cystocele, the apparent loss of contact between the vaginal epithelium and the muscularis leads to a smooth cystocele with no rugae. The bladder can be visualized herniating through the defect, separating the epithelium from the muscularis (Fig. 51.8). This contrasts a paravaginal cystocele where the central vaginal epithelium remains attached to the muscularis and rugae are maintained, but the lateral vaginal wall attachments to the arcus tendineus fascia pelvis are disrupted. This disruption almost always starts cephalad at the ischial spines and progresses distally (DeLancey 2002).

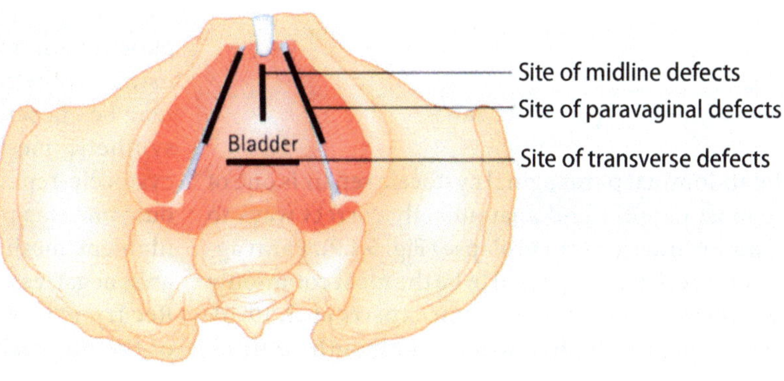

Fig. 5.1.7. Most common sites of anterior vaginal wall defects in the vaginal muscularis and connective tissue leading to cystocele: paravaginal, apical, central, and transverse

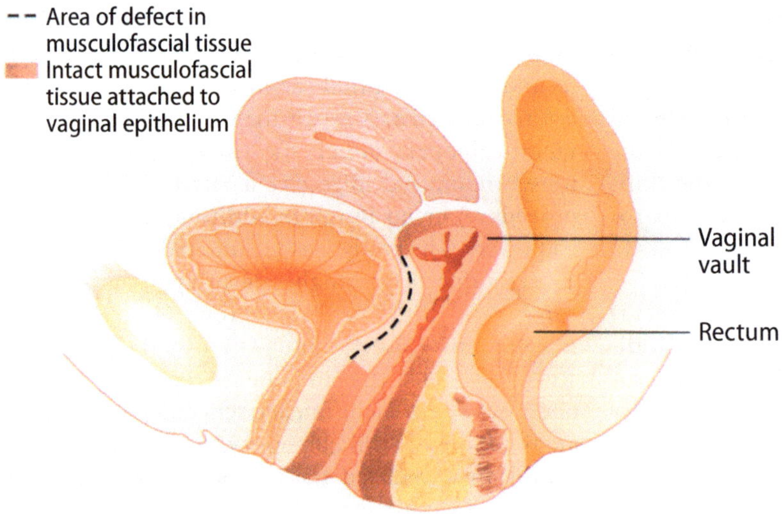

Fig. 5.1.8. Central cystocele: note the herniation of bladder through the muscularis separating the epithelium from the muscularis. No rugae will be seen on physical exam

Experts are realizing that anterior wall support is strongly linked to apical support and that the apex should be addressed in the majority of anterior wall repairs (Rooney et al. 2006; Summers et al. 2006). Identification of the musculofascial defects is essential to choosing the correct surgical approach. Use of the posterior blade of a speculum to isolate the anterior vaginal wall allows for these defects to be identified. The term urethrocele is used to denote loss of support of the distal anterior vaginal wall. It was previously thought that the support of the urethra was through a distinct structure called the pubourethral ligaments, making the distinction of an urethrocele more relevant. However, this support is in fact the termination of the arcus tendineus levator ani and the insertion of the puborectalis muscle. Therefore, the differentiation of an urethrocele and cystocele is merely the level where the support of the anterior vaginal wall is lost. The role of MRI in detecting these defects is evolving. To date, no prospective randomized studies exist comparing abdominal vs. vaginal surgical techniques for cystocele repair.

5.1.6.1 Paravaginal Cystocele Repair

The abdominal paravaginal cystocele repair is one of the most popular and anatomically correct ways to repair an anterior wall prolapse (Fig. 5.1.9). Paravaginal cystoceles are reported to be the most commonly encountered (White 1909; Richardson et al. 1976). Two series [n = 149, follow-up 6–48 months (Shull and Baden 1989) and n = 213, follow up 2–8 years (Richardson et al. 1981)] found 95% success rates for abdominal paravaginal repairs. Success was defined with respect to anterior wall support only. This has to be kept in mind as the latest data emphasize apical support in anterior wall prolapse (Rooney et al. 2006). A vaginal approach to repair paravaginal cystoceles has been described in several case series. One series of 56 women (follow-up ranging from 0.1–5.6 years, mean 1.6 years) showed 15 women (27%) had recurrent bladder support defects after surgery with 47% being either to or through the hymen. No defects were worse postoperatively (Shull et al. 1994). In another series of 100 women followed for a mean of 10.6 months, 22 had recurrent midline cystoceles, while 22 patients had persistent paravaginal cystoceles (Young et al. 2001).

5.1.6.2 Graft Placement

Experts may use an alternative to this procedure in a patient with multiple anterior wall defects. A repair using synthetic mesh, an allograft, or a xenograft may be chosen. A prospective, randomized trial of synthetic mesh versus anterior colporrhaphy for cystocele repair concluded that superior anatomic outcome was provided by use of a synthetic, monofilament mesh. This study illustrates the positives and negatives of using mesh in prolapse repairs. Recurrent prolapse at 12 months was found in 38.5% of the no-mesh group vs. 6.5% of the mesh group.

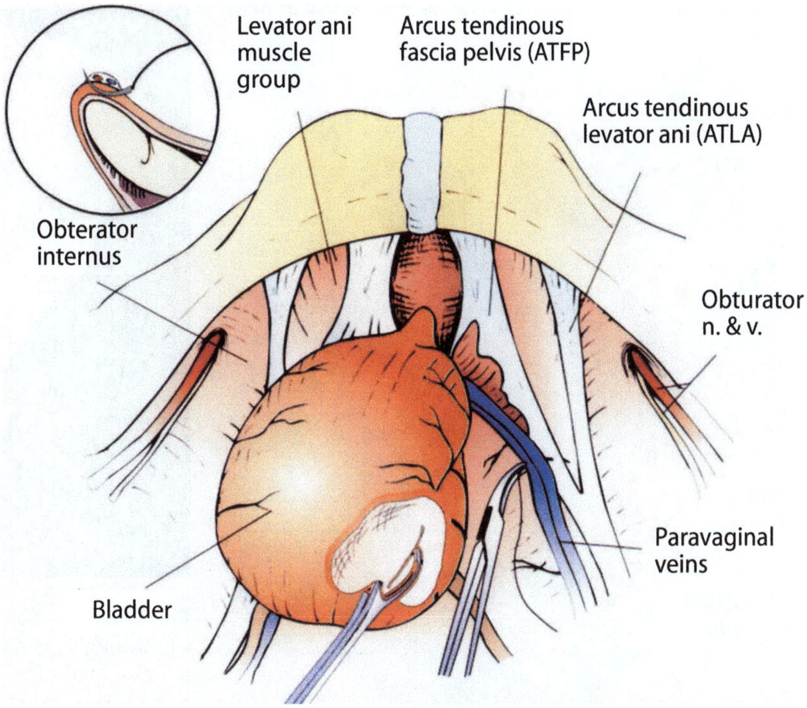

Fig. 5.1.9. Paravaginal cystocele repair: encircling the paravaginal veins with vaginal wall placement to the arcus tendineus fascia pelvis

However, stress incontinence was reported in only 10% of the no-mesh group compared to 23% of the mesh group (Hiltunen et al. 2007). The fact that structure does not equal function must be communicated with the patient prior to surgery. In general, grafts may be placed using suture fixation or placed in a tension-free manner. Using suture fixation, the graft is usually cut into a trapezoidal shape and strung like a hammock between the two arcus tendinei (Fig. 5.1.10). The superior edge of the graft is anchored to the apex of the vagina. The vaginal epithelium is then sutured to the graft, repairing the anterior vaginal wall defects (Word et al. 1992). As an alternative, tension-free graft placement can be used. Here, the body of the graft is attached to several long mesh arms that are placed though the obturator foramen lateral to the levator ani traversing through the ischiorectal fossa. The arms penetrate the levator ani proximally near the ischial spine and then distally by the ischiopubic ramus to enter the space of Retzius. The intent is to have the mesh lie against the arcus tendineus bilaterally held in place by the mesh arms and create a hammock for the bladder (Fig. 5.1.11). Outcome analyses for these techniques are limited and at this time are only case series.

5.1.6.3 Anterior Colporrhaphy

An anterior colporrhaphy is indicated for repair of central defects. The basic technique typically involves a midline vaginal incision with dissection laterally until adequate vaginal muscularis is identified. This muscularis is then plicated in the midline with one or several layers elevating the prolapsed bladder. A study randomized patients with anterior wall prolapse to one of three anterior colporrhaphy techniques: standard anterior colporrhaphy, standard repair plus polyglactin 910 mesh, or ultralateral anterior colporrhaphy. With a median follow-up of 23 months, there was no significant difference noted among techniques. Satisfactory or optimal results were obtained in 30% of anterior colporrhaphy patients, 42% of those with the added absorbable mesh, and 46% of the ultralateral patients (Weber et al. 2001). These numbers attest to the problem of using the patient's own tissue as the foundation of prolapse repair. The risk of damage to the urinary continence mechanism from nerve damage with anterior wall dissection should be considered before choosing this route of surgical correction.

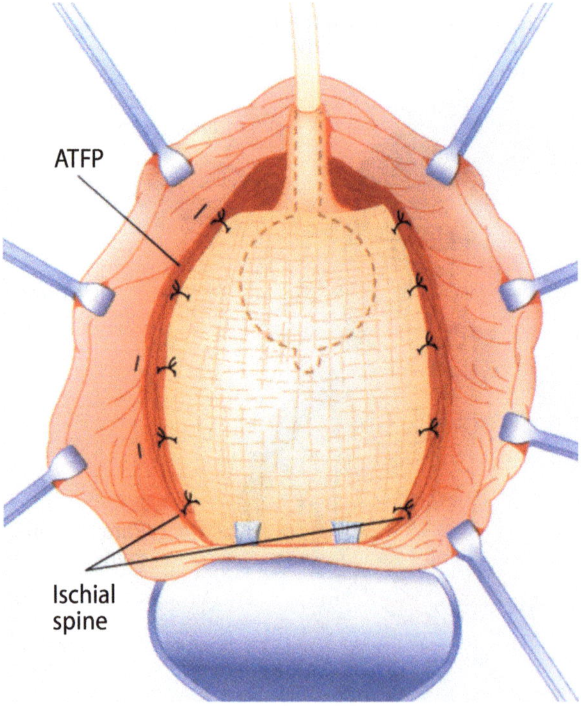

Fig. 5.1.10. Vaginal paravaginal repair using a graft to correct co-existing central and paravaginal defects. The superior edge of the fascia is sutured to the cuff and uterosacral ligaments. Bilaterally, the graft is anchored to the arcus tendineus

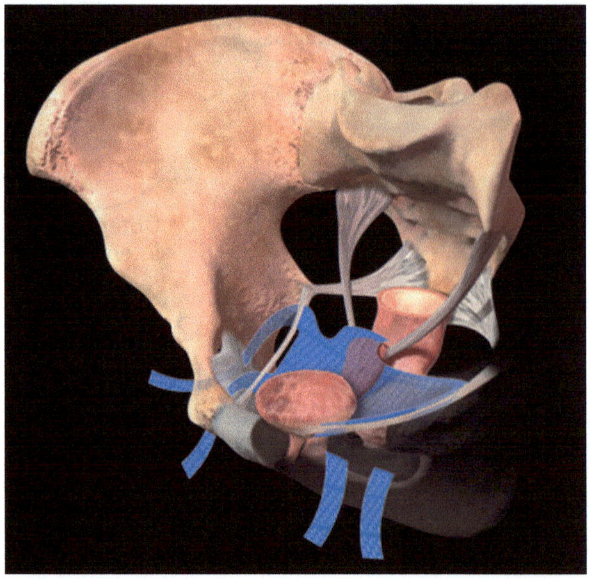

Fig. 5.1.11. Tension-free anterior wall graft with arms traveling through the obturator foramen penetrating the levator ani proximally by the ischial spine and distally by the insertion of the puborectalis. (©ETHICON, Inc.; reproduced with permission)

5.1.7 Surgery of the Vaginal Apex

Uterine preservation is an option for some women who desire future fertility or have other reasons for avoiding hysterectomy, but for most women with uterovaginal prolapse, hysterectomy is added to reconstructive efforts. With lesser degrees of apical prolapse (ICS stage 0–II), the uterosacral-cardinal ligament complex can be used to provide vault support through either an abdominal or vaginal approach. Often these ligaments will need shortening prior to being used, and ureteral location is essential before proceeding (Baden and Walker 1992a,b). After identification of these ligaments and possible shortening, the uterosacral complex is reattached to the musculofascial tissue of the anterior and posterior vaginal walls, and a culdoplasty is performed as needed. Consideration of these techniques should be given when performing any hysterectomy. For more severe apical prolapse, three surgical options exist: abdominal reconstruction, vaginal reconstruction, or obliterative surgery.

5.1.7.1 Abdominal Sacral Colpopexy or Colpoperineopexy

Abdominal sacral colpopexy is considered the gold standard operation for apical support (Maher et al. 2007; Nygard et al. 2004). The first techniques of sacral colpopexy described supporting the vaginal apex with a graft, either a synthetic mesh or autologous fascia (Timmons et al. 1992). Evolution of this technique has extended the support to the perineal body and deep into the vesicovaginal space (Cundiff et al. 1997; Fischer et al. 1997). This approach involves reinforcing the anterior and posterior vaginal wall with an allograft, xenograft, or synthetic mesh. The disadvantages of synthetic meshes include the potential of erosion or exposure in 3.4% of cases or an unnatural feel to the vaginal wall (Nygaard et al. 2004). The advantages of synthetic meshes are their strength, longevity, and in some the propensity to incite scar tissue formation, which may aid in pelvic support. Autologous fascia is an option, but is often impractical because such a large piece must be harvested. One series of ten patients had a 90% success rate (mean follow-up 26 months) with autologous fascia (Maloney et al. 1990). Allografts are generally not recommended due to a higher failure rate when compared to synthetic material (Culligan et al. 2005). Xenografts have been added to the pool of graft materials, but long-term studies are lacking.

The technique of abdominal sacral colpoperineopexy involves placement of a graft along the anterior and posterior vaginal walls. Posteriorly, the graft is extended along the entire length of the vagina wall to attach distally at the perineal body. At its caudal margin and laterally along the mid vagina, the posterior graft is attached to the fascia overlying the levator ani muscles just inferior to the ischial spine. This initial graft attachment uses a vaginal or laparoscopic approach. The remaining procedure is performed abdominally or laparoscopically. Over the proximal two thirds of the posterior wall, the graft is attached directly to the vaginal muscularis by spreading the graft as widely as possible. A stent placed vaginally aids in graft placement and also in dissection. Anteriorly, a second graft leaf is placed after dissecting into the vesicovaginal space. This also is spread as widely as possible on the anterior vaginal wall and sutured in place. By enveloping the vaginal vault in a graft, the integrity of the connective tissue network can be restored. Appropriate tension is applied, and the apices of the grafts are attached to the anterior longitudinal ligament of the spine over the S2–S3 levels (Fig. 5.1.12). The grafts are usually placed retroperitoneally to minimize bowel adhesions. Symmetrical placement of the graft over the vaginal wall is important to allow for equal distribution of forces. If a rectocele is not present, the approach may be completely abdominal or laparoscopic (Fig. 5.1.13). This requires that there is good support of the rectovaginal septum to the perineal body and that the upper edge of the rectovaginal septum is located high enough to be reached abdominally through the rectovaginal space. Often the perineal body is excessively mobile and, therefore, support should be extended to this level. Complications unique to this procedure include presacral hemorrhage and rare cases of osteomyelitis over the sacral site of graft attachment (Sutton et al. 1981; Weidner et al. 1997).

5.1.7.2 Sacrospinous Vault Suspension

Over the last 25 years the most common procedure performed for vaginal vault prolapse has been the vaginal sacrospinous vault suspension. Introduced into this country in 1971 (Randall and Nichols 1971), several clinical series have cited its success in providing apical support. Modified techniques utilizing iliococcygeus fascia, pubococcygeus fascia, or multiple points of vaginal fixation over the levator plate have been described. In a review of transvaginal repairs of vault prolapse, 1,062 patients pooled from 18 studies undergoing sacrospinous vault suspension and 322 patients (4 studies) treated with endopelvic

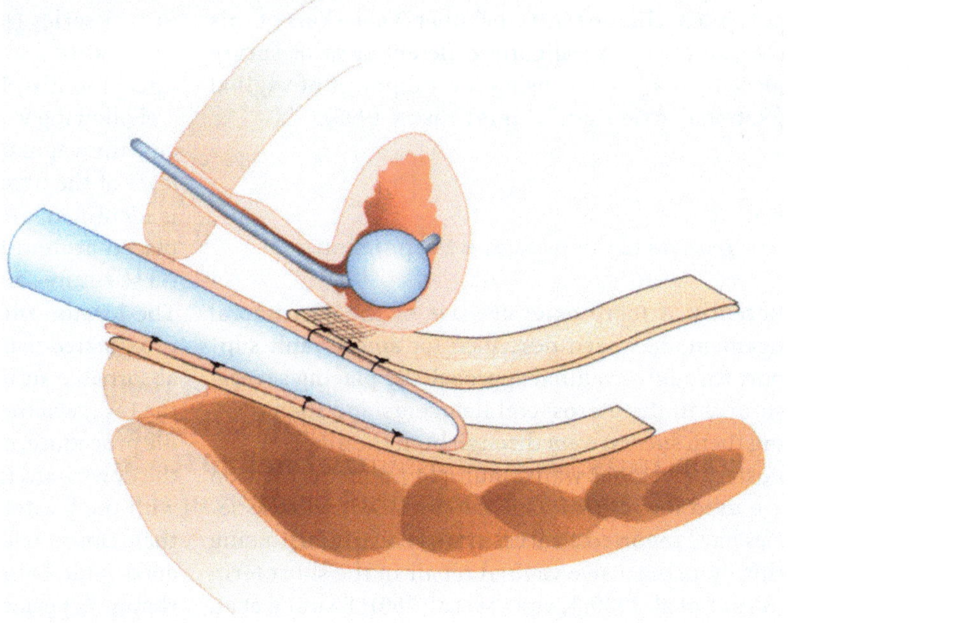

Fig. 5.1.12. Abdominal sacral colpoperineopexy, sagittal view. Anterior and posterior vaginal wall graft placement using a vaginal stent as a guide

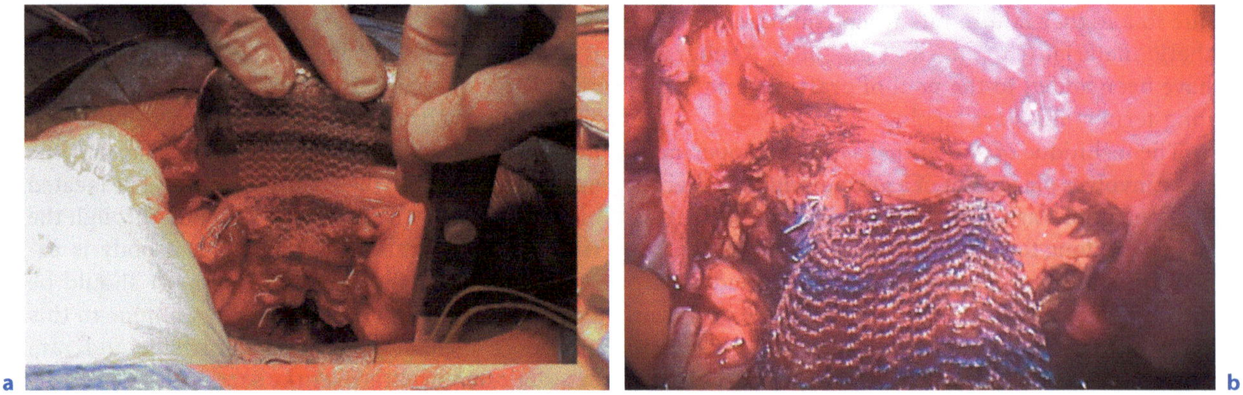

Fig. 5.1.13a,b. View looking at posterior wall graft extending down posterior vaginal wall into rectovaginal space using an open abdominal approach. View looking at posterior wall graft attached to perineal body extending into the rectovaginal space using a laparoscopic approach. The graft will be further attached along the whole posterior vaginal wall

vault suspension were available for follow-up. Recurrent prolapse occurred in 18% of the sacrospinous patients and 11% of the endopelvic fascial patients (Sze and Karram 1997). During this procedure, the right sacrospinous ligament and overlying coccygeus muscle are reached after vaginal dissection. Most often, two permanent sutures are placed 4 cm medial to the ischial spine into the sacrospinous ligament-coccygeus complex. Critical surrounding structures include the pudendal neurovascular bundle, inferior gluteal neurovascular bundle, and superiorly located lumbosacral plexus. The support sutures are then placed into the apical vaginal muscularis. This technique does deviate the vaginal axis to the right. Occasionally, a bilateral sacrospinous suspension is performed; however, there are no data to support one technique over the other. Variations of this procedure involve slightly different sites of suture placement as well as using several points of vaginal fixation (Peters and Christenson 1995).

5.1.7.3 Uterosacral Ligament Vault Suspension

Recently, a more extensive use of the uterosacral ligaments has been described for apical vault support through a vaginal approach. By placing several sutures in the uterosacral ligaments and then placing them successively through both the anterior and posterior vaginal walls, multiple points of fixation are used for vaginal vault support. Several case series have reported a success rate of nearly 90% using this more extensive vaginal repair in the short term (Shull et al. 2000; Karram et al. 2001; Barber et al. 2000). One case series reports an 84.7% success rate with 5 years of follow-up (Silva et al. 2006).

5.1.7.4 Obliterative Surgery

Utero-vaginal prolapse can be effectively treated with obliterative surgery. A LeFort colpocleisis, which does not remove the uterus, may be performed, although indications for this are becoming rare (Thompson 1992). It is usually reserved for a debilitated patient with minimal risk for endometrial cancer. An alternative approach combines total vaginal hysterectomy, if a uterus is present, with total colpocleisis. Excellent anatomic outcomes (97%) are reported in two series (n = 92, median follow-up 12 months, VonPechman et al. 2003 and n = 33, average follow-up 35 months, DeLancey and Morley 1997).

Following vaginal hysterectomy if a uterus is present, the vaginal epithelium is removed close to the level of the hymen. The apex of the prolapsing mass is identified, and successive purse string sutures are placed around the leading edge of the prolapse. As these sutures are tied, the enclosed tissue is reduced. The levator ani muscles are palpated and then approximated using a 0 or no. 1 permanent or delayed absorbable suture. Some support should be given to the UVJ, whether in the form of a Kelly plication, needle procedure, or pubovaginal sling to compensate for the downward traction that will be placed on the UVJ with the levator plication. The vaginal epithelium is then closed with a running suture, leaving a shortened vault, being at most 3 cm in length. A perineorrhaphy is performed to complete the procedure.

5.1.7.5 Uterine Preservation Procedures

Both vaginal and abdominal procedures exist to preserve the uterus in patients with symptomatic uterovaginal prolapse. These procedures are chosen for women who cannot tolerate the prolapse or pessary use and desire uterine preservation. In general, patients should be counseled to complete childbearing before reconstructive surgery is performed. If this is not acceptable, data from several small series exist. Pregnancy rates for potentially fertile patients ranged from 25%–67% (n = 168) in abdominally performed surgeries to 24%–67% (n=68) in vaginally performed surgeries. Term deliveries were 9%–50% and 5%–67%, respectively (Julian 1993; Chaudhuri 1979; Nassar 1967; Durfee 1966; Dastur et al. 1967; Kovac and Cruikshank 1993).

A wide range of operative techniques has been described. These include the use of graft material, uterosacral ligament fixation to the sacrospinous ligament, uterosacral ligament plication, the Manchester procedure, and round ligament suspension of the uterus (Nichols 1991; Shaw 1933; Thomas et al. 1995; Gilliam 1900). The lack of long-term studies makes makes it difficult to council patients on the long-term durability of these operations.

5.1.8 The Posterior Vaginal Wall

Defects of the posterior vaginal vault involve rectocele, enterocele, and sigmoidocele. Correction of the bulging may be attainable, but often the patient's symptoms are not relieved and in fact may be worsened (Kahn and Stanton 1997). Techniques of rectocele repair include traditional posterior colporrhaphy, defect repair, fascial replacement, rectal wall imbrication, and transanal repair.

5.1.8.1 Rectocele

Controversies remain regarding the symptoms and diagnosis of rectoceles. Symptoms linked to, but not diagnostic of rectocele, include incomplete rectal emptying, manual assisted defecation, rectal pressure, bleeding, pain, and constipation. Fluoroscopic and MRI studies have had their greatest impact in the diagnosis of posterior wall defects. There are no clear criteria that predict successful rectocele repair. Unfortunately, anatomic repair does not always lead to functional correction.

5.1.8.1.1 Posterior Colporrhaphy

The posterior colporrhaphy has its roots in the repair of perineal lacerations, dating back to the 16th century. The modern posterior colporrhaphy is linked to Simon in 1867 who coined the term still used today. Many modifications to this procedure have been made, but the basic procedure remains unchanged. The traditional posterior colporrhaphy plicates the musculofascial tissue (rectovaginal septum and vaginal muscularis) in the midline.

The posterior vaginal epithelium is opened in the midline and dissected laterally and superiorly. The thickened musculofascial tissue is plicated in the midline. Epithelial trimming is done only to remove redundant epithelium. Some experts recommend plication of the levator muscles between the vagina and rectum, while other experts avoid this as it can result in significant dyspareunia. Studies have reported the inability to have intercourse or severe dyspareunia in 30% of patients undergoing posterior repair (Jeffcoate 1959). In one study evaluating both subjective and objective outcomes, representative results for traditional rectocele repair were seen (Mellgren et al. 1995). Patients (n = 25) were evaluated with preoperative and postoperative questionnaires, physical exam, and defecography. Preoperatively, 96% suffered from constipation, while 48% used digital support for evacuation. All patients showed a rectocele by defecography, while 88% had a rectocele by physical exam. Surgical repair consisted of a posterior colporrhaphy with levator plication. Mean follow-up was 1 year. Constipation was eliminated in 52% of patients; an occasional complaint persisted in 32% and was frequent in 16%. No patients required digital maneuvers to aid in defecation following surgical correction. Defecography found that rectoceles were eliminated in 79% of patients. Physical exam detected rectoceles in only 4% of patients postoperatively. Nineteen percent of patients suffered from dyspareunia following repair. Subjective and objective improvement was achieved in approximately 80% of patients.

5.1.8.1.2 Defect Directed Repair of Rectocele

An alternative technique can be performed if a clear break in the rectovaginal septum is identified (RICHARDSON 1993). The defect repair is approached as in a traditional repair with a posterior midline incision just beneath the vaginal epithelium and continued with lateral dissection. With a finger placed rectally, the operator palpates the borders of the defect that is repaired using deep bites into the musculofascial tissue and rectovaginal septum with a long-lasting absorbable suture. Several case series report a range of anatomic cure from 82–100%, but persistent symptoms in many patients (PORTER et al. 1999; GLAVKIND and MADSEN 2000). Because of the anatomy of the rectovaginal septum, this repair only extends 3–4 cm along the posterior vaginal wall and is unable to treat higher rectoceles if used as an isolated procedure.

5.1.8.1.3 Graft Replacement

Replacement of fascia along the posterior wall has been described as part of the sacral colpoperineopexy. In the event that an isolated rectocele exists with poor musculofascial tissue, a graft may be attached to the perineal body, anchored to the levator ani muscles bilaterally and lastly placed to the uterosacral ligaments superiorly. Typically a graft 4×12 cm will be more than adequate. Each patient's graft is individualized based on their anatomy. Care is taken to not bridge the graft too tightly across the rectum (Fig. 5.1.14). Case series have reported success with both synthetic and biologic grafts for rectocele repair (KOHLI and MIKLOS 2003; GOH and DWYER 2001).

Only one prospective randomized study exists that compares the three major techniques for rectocele repair (PARAISO et al. 2006). In this study, 106 patients were randomized to traditional posterior colporrhaphy, defect repair, or defect repair with biograft overlay (FortaGen, Organogenesis, Inc., Canton, MA). At 1-year follow-up, anatomic failure defined as ICS stage II or greater was found in 14% of posterior colporrhaphy patients, 22% of defect repair patients, and 46% of defect repairs augmented with the biograft patients. In addition, postoperative worsening of colorectal or prolapse symptoms using QOL measures were found in 16% of posterior colporrhaphy patients, 12% of defect repair patients, and 21% of defect repair augmented with the biograft. This study questions the use of biologic grafts for rectocele repair, and although the majority of patients showed improvement in symptoms, a significant percentage actually had worsening of their symptoms.

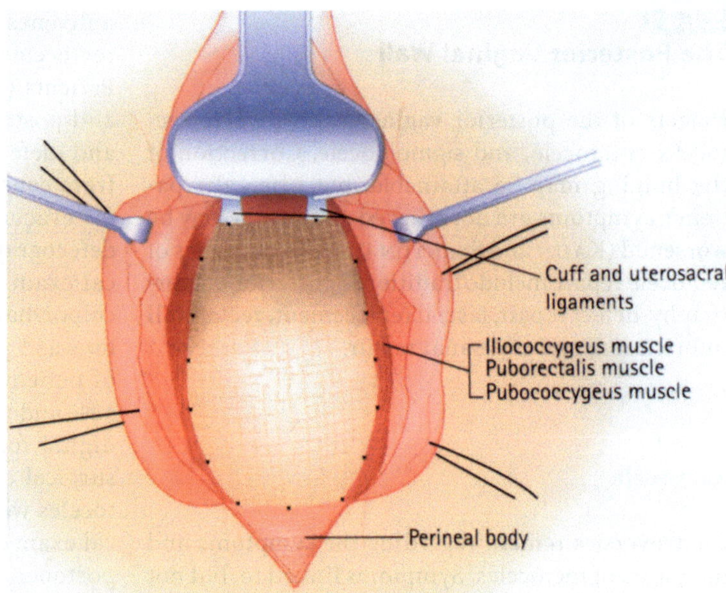

Fig. 5.1.14. Repair of rectocele using a posterior vaginal wall allograft or xenograft. Superiorly the graft is attached to the uterosacral ligament, laterally to the fascia of levator ani muscles, and inferiorly to the perineal body

5.1.8.1.4 Imbrication

Rectal wall imbrication can be approached either transvaginally or transrectally. In the transvaginal approach a midline posterior vaginal wall incision extending into the rectovaginal space is used (Benson 1992). Running interlocking sutures are placed in the rectal muscularis for the length of the rectocele. This results in the imbrication of the rectal wall narrowing the lumen. There are no published outcome studies of this technique with long-term follow-up. With the transrectal approach, the running interlocking suture is placed through the mucosa and submucosa. The incorporated tissue will undergo necrosis purportedly narrowing the rectal lumen and strengthening the muscularis layer. Outcome studies are also needed with the transrectal imbricating approach.

5.1.8.1.5 Transanal Repair

The transanal rectocele repair has been only rarely reported in the gynecologic literature, although its use by colorectal surgeons is well documented (Sullivan et al. 1968; Sehapayak 1985; Khubchandani et al. 1997; Karlbom et al. 1996; Janssen and van Dijke 1994). Rectal dilators are used to gain access to the rectum; long slightly curved clamps are placed along the rectal mucosa and redundant mucosa is pulled into the clamp. This mucosal excision is performed in one to three areas depending on the degree of redundancy. The musculofascial tissue and rectal muscularis are then reinforced with horizontal suturing. Several series of transanal repair with minor variations have been published with subjective improvement/cure rates ranging from 82% to 98% (Sehapayak 1985; Khubchandani et al. 1997). Transanal rectocele repair resulted in a postoperative fluoroscopic decrease in rectocele size, decrease in rectal area at rest, and increased rectal evacuation in 25 of 31 (81%) patients (Karlbom et al. 1996). In this study, a large rectal area at rest and use of enemas or bowel stimulants preoperatively was related to poor outcome. A second study using postoperative fluoroscopy also evaluated manometric measurements (Janssen and van Dijke 1994). Rectocele was eliminated objectively in 62%, while reduced in the remaining 38% (n=39). Subjectively at 1 year, an 87% improvement or cure rate was noted (n=76). No predictive defecographic parameters were identified. However, manometrically, a large first urge to defecate volume was a predictor of good clinical outcome. Lastly, the STARR procedure (stapled trans-anal rectal resection) has been reported with good anatomic and functional results (Boccasanta et al. 2004). This procedure requires further study before sound conclusions can be made.

However, with all these transanal repairs, it makes inherent sense that some rectoceles will not respond to vaginal wall operations alone as the rectal side of the rectocele may be intimately involved (Marks 1967). Some difference between the transvaginal approach used by gynecologists and the transanal approach used by colorectal surgeons may stem from different use of the term rectocele. In the gynecologic literature, it is associated with descent of the posterior vaginal wall through the introitus, while in the colorectal literature, it often denotes prolapse of the anal mucosa through the anus.

5.1.8.2 Enterocele

The cul-de-sac depth may have little bearing on the finding of an enterocele (Zaccharin 1977). Expert opinion suggesting a defect in the musculofascial layer of the posterior vaginal wall as being responsible for an enterocele has been challenged (Tulikangas et al. 2001). Although still debated, an enterocele is most likely the result of herniation of the small bowel through the posterior levator hiatus. In any repair to correct enterocele, the upper vaginal axis needs to be restored over the levator plate as part of the repair. The vaginal axis can be restored using an appropriate apical support technique. An alternative approach, thought seldom used today, involves suturing the posterior vaginal vault to the levator plate. Using this technique, the urogenital hiatus is shortened by a levator plication posterior to the rectum followed by vaginal fixation to the levator plate (Zaccharin 1985). No outcome measures are available for this technique.

More traditionally a Halban, Moschcowitz, or McCall type culdoplasty may be performed. The Halban or Moschcowitz approach requires sutures to be placed through only the peritoneal or serosal surfaces. Using the Halban technique, successive vertical sutures are placed down the serosal surface of the sigmoid colon, across the cul-de-sac, and along the posterior vaginal wall (Nichols et al. 1996). The sutures are placed 1 cm apart and no further lateral than 1 cm medial to the ureters. This prevents small bowel herniation between the sutures and avoids ureteral kinking. A Moschcowitz culdoplasty uses successive pursestring sutures to occlude the cul-de-sac (Moschcowitz 1912). Ureters are identified so as not to be pulled medially when the sutures are tied. These procedures do not rely upon the strength of this tissue, but rather provide apposition of peritoneal surfaces for scarification. With a vaginal approach, a McCall type culdoplasty can be used (McCall 1957). This approach requires identification of the uterosacral ligaments that are shortened and reattached to the vaginal apex.

Certain patients with apparent enteroceles may have sigmoidoceles. Of the patients undergoing defecography for pelvic floor defects, 4% (n = 234) were found to have sigmoidoceles. None were diagnosed by physical exam (Fenner 1996). Rarely, sigmoid resection may be indicated (Jorge et al. 1994).

Many patients with POP will have an enlarged vaginal introitus and reduced perineal body. Although experts agree that this procedure is frequently needed for a comprehensive reconstruction, the specific indications for the procedure remain vague. With significant perineal body decent, sacral fixation using the abdominal sacral colpoperineopexy is considered.

5.1.8.3 Prolapse Repair "Kits"

Several commercially available kits are available for prolapse repair. As discussed under the anterior wall, these kits usually involve long arms that extend from the body of the graft. These extension arms allow the graft to be held in place without the need for extensive suturing. Unique to these approaches is the use of the ischiorectal fossa. Anteriorly, a transobturator route is used to gain access to this space and secure the mesh in the space of Retzius (Fig. 5.1.15). Posteriorly, the ischiorectal fossa is approached though perianal incisions (Fig. 5.1.16a,b lateral and anterior view of Avaulta). The friction of the long arms helps secure the body of the graft. Initial short-term data show success of 95% at 6 months (Fatton 2007). High erosion rates have been reported in up to 12% of patients (Collinet 2007). These limited data show both promise and concern.

5.1.9 Conclusion

The collaboration between the radiologist and surgeon in the area of pelvic floor dysfunction continues to actively evolve. A unified language for grading dysfunction is frustratingly missing, and data concerning what is normal are needed. Radiologists need a thorough understanding of the supportive anatomy of the pelvis to aid in this communication. Clinicians need to recognize the value of imaging studies in helping to understand pelvic floor disorders. Physicians must also acknowledge the limitations of imaging remembering the multifactorial nature of pelvic floor disorders. Radiographic findings (and for that matter clinical findings) do not always correlate with patient symptoms, nor does structure equate to function. However, pelvic floor imaging can represent an unbiased high-quality assessment tool in the study of the pelvic floor and in surgical outcome studies. Working together, care for patients with these problems will continue to improve.

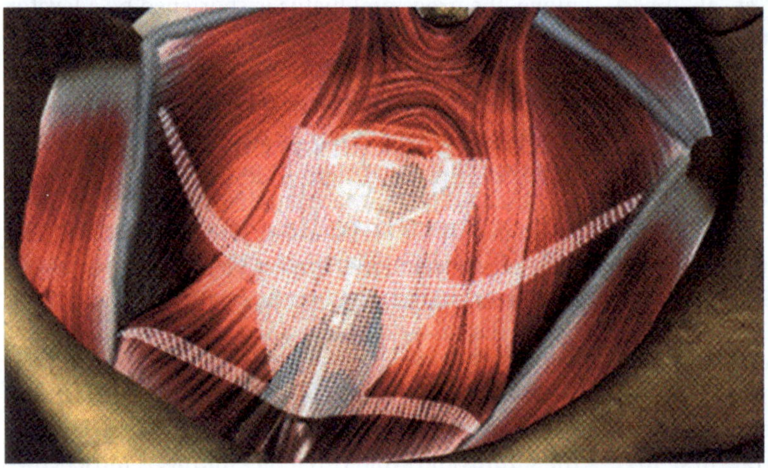

Fig. 5.1.15. Another example of a tension-free anterior wall graft repair extending from arcus tendineus fascia pelvis on each side bridging the levator hiatus. (Perigee®, AMS, Minnetonka, MN)

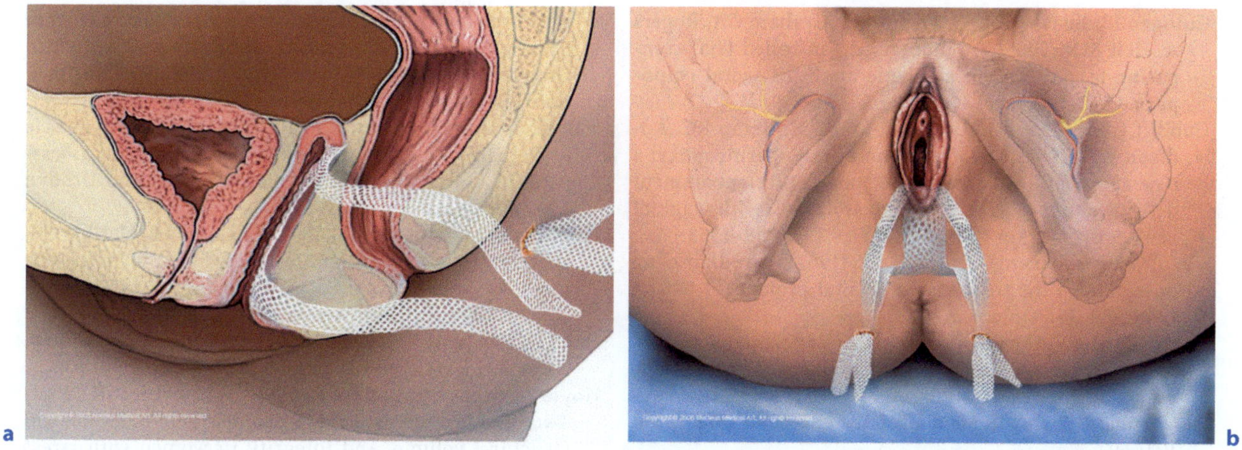

Fig. 5.1.16a,b. Example of a tension-free posterior wall graft with arms extending through the ischiorectal fossa, sagittal view. Example of the same mesh from an antero-posterior view

References

Altringer WE, Saclarides TJ, Dominguez JM, Brubaker LT, Smith CS (1995) Four-contrast defecography: pelvic "floor-oscopy." Dis Colon Rectum 38:695–699

Baden WF, Walker T (1992a) Abdominal approach to superior vaginal defects. In: Baden WF, Walker T (eds) Surgical repair of vaginal defects. JB Lippincott, Philadelphia, p 119

Baden WF, Walker T (1992b) Vaginal approach to superior vaginal defects. In: Baden WF, Walker T (eds) Surgical repair of vaginal defects. JB Lippincott, Philadelphia, p 161

Ball P Jr, Teichman JM, Sharkey FE, Rogenes VJ, Adrian EK Jr (1997) Terminal nerve distribution to the urethra and bladder neck: considerations in the management of stress urinary incontinence. J Urol 158:827–829

Barber MD, Visco AG, Weidner AC, Amundsen CL, Bump RC (2000) Bilateral uterosacral ligament vaginal vault suspension with site-specific endopelvic fascia defect repair for treatment of pelvic organ prolapse. Am J Obstet Gynecol 183:1402–1410

Benson JT (1992) Rectocele, descending perineal syndrome, enterocele. In: Benson JT (ed) Female pelvic floor disorders: Investigation and management. WW Norton, New York, p 384

Benson JT, McClellan E (1993) The effect of vaginal dissection on the pudendal nerve. Obstet Gynecol 82:387–389

Benson JT, Lucente V, McClellan E (1996) Vaginal versus abdominal reconstructive surgery for the treatment of pelvic support defects: a prospective randomized study with long-term outcome evaluation. Am J Obstet Gynecol 175:1418–1421

Berglas B, Rubin IC (1953) Study of the supportive structures of the uterus by levator myography. Surg Gynecol Obstet 97:677–692

Boccasanta P, Venturi M, Salamina G, Cesana BM, Bernasconi F, Roviaro G (2004) New trends in the surgical treatment of outlet obstruction: clinical and functional results of two novel transanal stapled techniques from a randomised controlled trial. Int J Colorectal Dis 19:359–369

Borirakchanyavat S, Aboseif SR, Carroll PR, Tanagho EA, Lue TF (1997) Continence mechanism of the isolated female urethra: an anatomical study of the intrapelvic somatic nerves. J Urol 158:822–826

Brubaker L, Cundiff G, Fine P, Nygaard I, Richter H, Visco A, Zyczynski H, Brown MB, Weber A (2003) A randomized trial of colpopexy and urinary reduction efforts (CARE): design and methods. Control Clin Trials 24:629–642

Bump RC, Fantl JA, Hurt WG (1988) The mechanism of urinary continence in women with severe uterovaginal prolapse: results of barrier studies. Obstet Gynecol 72:291–295

Bump RC, Hurt WG, Theofrastous JP, Addison WA, Fantl JA, Wyman JF, McClish DK (1996a) Randomized prospective comparison of needle colposuspension versus endopelvic fascia plication for potential stress incontinence prophylaxis in women undergoing vaginal reconstruction for stage III or IV pelvic organ prolapse. The Continence Program for Women Research Group. Am J Obstet Gynecol 175:326–333

Bump RC, Mattiasson A, Bo K, Brubaker LP, DeLancey JO, Klarskov P, Shull BL, Smith AR (1996b) The standardization of terminology of female pelvic organ prolapse and pelvic floor dysfunction. Am J Obstet Gynecol 175:10–17

Campbell RM (1950) The anatomy and histology of the sacrouterine ligaments. Am J Obstet Gynecol 59:1–12

Chaudhuri SK (1979) The place of sling operations in treating genital prolapse in young women. Int J Gynaecol Obstet 16:314–320

Collinet P, Belot F, Debodinance P, Ha DE, Lucot JP, Cosson M (2006) Transvaginal mesh technique for pelvic organ prolapse repair: mesh exposure management and risk factors. Int Urogynecol J Pelvic Floor Dysfunct 17:315–320

Comiter CV, Vasavada SP, Barbaric ZL, Gousse AE, Raz S (1999) Grading pelvic prolapse and pelvic floor relaxation using dynamic magnetic resonance imaging. Urology 54:454–457

Culligan PJ, Blackwell L, Goldsmith LJ, Graham CA, Rogers A, Heit MH (2005) A randomized controlled trial comparing fascia lata and synthetic mesh for sacral colpopexy. Obstet Gynecol 106:29–37

Cundiff GW, Harris RL, Coates K, Low VH, Bump RC, Addison WA (1997) Abdominal sacral colpoperineopexy: a new approach for correction of posterior compartment defects and perineal descent associated with vaginal vault prolapse. Am J Obstet Gynecol 177:1345–1353

Dastur B, Gurubaxani G, Palnitkar SS (1967) Shirodkar sling operation in the treatment of genital prolapse. J Obstet Gynaecol Br Commonw 74:125–128

Davis GD (1996) Uterine prolapse after laparoscopic uterosacral transection in nulliparous airborne trainees. A report of three cases. J Reprod Med 41:279–282

De Lamballe J (1840) Mem de l'Acad Roy De Med., vol VIII:697

DeLancey JO (1992) Anatomic aspects of vaginal eversion after hysterectomy. Am J Obstet Gynecol 166:1717–1724

DeLancey JO (1999) Structural anatomy of the posterior pelvic compartment as it relates to rectocele. Am J Obstet Gynecol 180:815–823

DeLancey JO (2002) Fascial and muscular abnormalities in women with urethral hypermobility and anterior vaginal wall prolapse. Am J Obstet Gynecol 187:93–98

DeLancey JO, Morley GW (1997) Total colpocleisis for vaginal eversion. Am J Obstet Gynecol 176:1228–1232

DeLancey JO, Morgan DM, Fenner DE, KearneyR, Guire K, Miller JM, HussainH, Umek W, HsuY, Ashton-Miller JA (2007) Comparison of levator ani muscle defects and function in women with and without pelvic organ prolapse. Obstet Gynecol 109:295–302

Durfee RB (1966) Suspension operations for treatment of pelvic organ prolapse. Clin Obstet Gynecol 9:1047–1061

Fatton B, Amblard J, Debodinance P, Cosson M, Jacquetin B (2007) Transvaginal repair of genital prolapse: preliminary results of a new tension-free vaginal mesh (Prolift technique) – a case series multicentric study. Int Urogynecol J Pelvic Floor Dysfunct 18:743–752

Fauconnier A, Zareski E, Abichedid J, Bader G, Falissard B, Fritel X (2008) Dynamic magnetic resonance imaging for grading pelvic organ prolapse according to the international continence society classification: Which line should be used? Neurourol Urodyn 27:191–197

Fenner DE (1996) Diagnosis and assessment of sigmoidoceles: Am J Obstet Gynecol 175:1438–1441

Fischer JR, Hale DS, Benson JT et al (1997) Combined rectocele repair and abdominal sacralcolpopexy. A new method for repair of Denonvillier's fascia. Presented at the AUGS 18th Annual Scientific Meeting, Tucson, Arizona

Gilliam DT (1900) Round-ligament ventrosuspension of the uterus: A new method. Am J Obst 52:1028

Gilpin SA, Gosling JA, Smith AR, Warrell DW (1989) The pathogenesis of genitourinary prolapse and stress incontinence of urine. A histological and histochemical study. Br J Obstet Gynaecol 96:15–23

Glavkind K, Madsen H (2000) A prospective study of the discrete fascial defect rectocele repair. Acta Obstet Gynecol Scand 79:145–147

Goh J, Dwyer P (2001) Effectiveness and safety of polypropylene mesh in vagina prolapse surgery. Urogynecol J 12:S90

Hall AF, Theofrastous JP, Cundiff GW, Harris RL, Hamilton LF, Swift SE, Bump RC (1996) Interobserver and intraobserver reliability of the proposed International Continence Society, Society of Gynecologic Surgeons, and American Urogynecologic Society Pelvic Organ Prolapse Classification System. Am J Obstet Gynecol 175:1467–1470

Heit M, Benson JT, Russell B, et al. (1996) Levator ani muscle in woman with genitourinary prolapse: Indirect assessment of muscle by histopathology. Neurol and Urodyn 15:17–29

Hiltunen R, Nieminen K, Takala T, Heiskanen E, Merikari M, Niemi K, Heinonen PK (2007) Low-weight polypropylene mesh for anterior vaginal wall prolapse: a randomized controlled trial. Obstet Gynecol 110:455–462

Hock D, Lombard R, Jehaes C, et al. (1993) Colpocystodefecography. Dis Colon Rectum 36:1015–1021

Hoyte L, Schierlitz L, Zou K, Flesh G, Fielding JR (2001) Two- and 3-dimensional MRI comparison of levator ani structure, volume, and integrity in women with stress incontinence and prolapse. Am J Obstet Gynecol 185:11–19

Hsu Y, Summers A, Hussain HK, Guire KE, DeLancey JO (2006) Levator plate angle in women with pelvic organ prolapse compared to women with normal support using dynamic MR imaging. Am J Obstet Gynecol 194:1427–1433

Janssen LW, van Dijke CF (1994) Selection criteria for anterior rectal wall repair in symptomatic rectocele and anterior rectal wall prolapse. Dis Colon Rectum 37:1100–1107

Jeffcoate TN (1959) Posterior colpoperineorrhaphy. Am J Obstet Gynecol 77:490–502

Jorge JM, Yang YK, Wexner SD (1994) Incidence and clinical significance of sigmoidoceles as determined by a new classification system. Dis Colon Rectum 37:1112–1117

Julian TM (1993) Response to Kovac SR, Cruikshank SH. Successful pregnancies and vaginal deliveries after sacrospinous uterosacral fixation in 5 of 19 patients. Am J Obstet Gynecol 168:1778–1786

Kahn MA, Stanton SL (1997) Posterior colporrhaphy: its effects on bowel and sexual function. Br J Obstet Gynaecol 104:82–86

Karlbom U, Graf W, Nilsson S, Pahlman L (1996) Does surgical repair of a rectocele improve rectal emptying? Dis Colon Rectum 39:1296–1302

Karram M, Goldwasser S, Kleeman S, Steele A, Vassallo B, Walsh P (2001) High uterosacral vaginal vault suspension with fascial reconstruction for vaginal repair of enterocele and vaginal vault prolapse. Am J Obstet Gynecol 185:1339–1342

Kaufman HS, Buller JL, Thompson JR, Pannu HK, DeMeester SL, Genadry RR, Bluemke DA, Jones B, Rychcik JL, Cundiff GW (2001) Dynamic pelvic magnetic resonance imaging and cystocolpoproctography alter surgical management of pelvic floor disorders. Dis Colon Rectum 44:1575–1583

Kelvin FM, Maglinte DD (2003) Dynamic evaluation of female pelvic organ prolapse by extended proctography. Radiol Clin North Am 41:395–407

Kelvin FM, Maglinte DD, Hornback JA, Benson JT (1992) Pelvic prolapse: assessment with evacuation proctography (defecography). Radiology 184:547–551

Kelvin FM, Hale DS, Maglinte DD, Patten BJ, Benson JT (1999) Female pelvic organ prolapse: diagnostic contribution of dynamic cystoproctography and comparison with physical examination. AJR Am J Roentgenol 173:31–37

Kelvin FM, Maglinte DD, Hale DS, Benson JT (2000) Female pelvic organ prolapse: a comparison of triphasic dynamic MR imaging and triphasic fluoroscopic cystocolpoproctography. AJR Am J Roentgenol 174:81–88

Khubchandani IT, Clancy JP III, Rosen L, Riether RD, Stasik JJ Jr (1997) Endorectal repair of rectocele revisited. Br J Surg 84:89–91

Kohli N, Miklos J (2003) Dermal graft augmented rectocele repair. Int Urogynecol J 14:146–149

Kovac SR, Cruikshank SH (1993) Successful pregnancies and vaginal deliveries after sacrospinous uterosacral fixation in 5 of 19 patients. Am J Obstet Gynecol 168:1778–1783

Kuhn RJ, Hollyock VE (1982) Observations on the anatomy of the rectovaginal pouch and septum. Obstet Gynecol 59:445–447

Leffler KS, Thompson JR, Cundiff GW, Buller JL, Burrows LJ, Schon Ybarra MA (2001) Attachment of the rectovaginal septum to the pelvic sidewall. Am J Obstet Gynecol 85:41–43

Lienemann A, Sprenger D, Janssen U, Grosch E, Pellengahr C, Anthuber C (2004) Assessment of pelvic organ descent by use of functional cine-MRI: which reference line should be used? Neurourol Urodyn 23:33–37

Lo T, Wang AC (1998) Abdominal colposacropexy and sacrospinous ligament suspension for severe uterovaginal prolapse: A comparison. J Gynecol Surg 14:59–64

Luber KM, Boero S, Choe JY (2001) The demographics of pelvic floor disorders: current observations and future projections. Am J Obstet Gynecol 184:1496–1501

Maglinte DD, Kelvin F M, Fitzgerald K, Hale DS, Benson JT (1999) Association of compartment defects in pelvic floor dysfunction. AJR Am J Roentgenol 172:439–444

Maher CF, Qatawneh AM, Dwyer PL, Carey MP, Cornish A, Schluter PJ (2004) Abdominal sacral colpopexy or vaginal sacrospinous colpopexy for vaginal vault prolapse: a prospective randomized study. Am J Obstet Gynecol 190:20–26

Maher C, Baessler K, Glazener CM, Adams EJ, Hagen S (2007) Surgical management of pelvic organ prolapse in women. Cochrane Database Syst Rev:CD004014

Maloney JC, Dunton CJ, Smith K (1990) Repair of vaginal vault prolapse with abdominal sacropexy. J Reprod Med 35:6–10

Mant J, Painter R, Vessey M (1997) Epidemiology of genital prolapse: observations from the Oxford Family Planning Association Study. Br J Obstet Gynaecol 104:579–585

Marks MM (1967) The rectal side of the rectocele. Dis Colon Rectum 10:387–388

Matsuoka H, Wexner SD, Desai MB, Nakamura T, Nogueras JJ, Weiss EG, Adami C, Billotti VL (2001) A comparison between dynamic pelvic magnetic resonance imaging and videoproctography in patients with constipation. Dis Colon Rectum 44:571–576

McCall ML (1957) Posterior culdeplasty; surgical correction of enterocele during vaginal hysterectomy; a preliminary report. Obstet.Gynecol 10:595–602

Mellgren A, Anzen B, Nilsson BY, Johansson C, Dolk A, Gillgren P, Bremmer S, Holmstrom B (1995) Results of rectocele repair. A prospective study. Dis Colon Rectum 38:7–13

Mengert WF. Mechanics of uterine support and position. Am J Obstet Gynecol 1936:775–782

Milley PS, Nichols DH (1968) A correlative investigation of the human rectovaginal septum. Anat Rec 163:443–452

Morrena GL, Balasingamb AG, Wells JE (2005) Triphasic MRI of pelvic organ descent: sources of measurement error. Eur J Radiol 54:276–283

Moschcowitz AV (1912). The pathogenesis, anatomy and cure of prolapse of the rectum. Surg Gynecol Obstet 15:7

Nassar GF (1967) Modified Williams-Richardson operation for uterine prolapse. Obstet Gynecol 30:233–237

Nichols DH (1991) Fertility retention in the patient with genital prolapse. Am J Obstet Gynecol 164:1155–1158

Nichols DH, Randall CL (1996) Enterocele. In: Nichols DH, Randall CL (eds) Vaginal surgery, 4th edn. Williams and Wilkins, Baltimore, p 348

Norton PA, Baker JE, Sharp HC, Warenski JC (1995) Genitourinary prolapse and joint hypermobility in women. Obstet Gynecol 85:225–228

Nygaard IE, McCreery R, Brubaker L, Connolly A, Cundiff G, Weber AM, Zyczynski H (2004) Abdominal sacrocolpopexy: a comprehensive review. Obstet Gynecol 104:805–823

Olsen AL, Smith VJ, Bergstrom JO, Colling JC, Clark AL (1997) Epidemiology of surgically managed pelvic organ prolapse and urinary incontinence. Obstet Gynecol 89:501–506

Paraiso MF, Barber MD, Muir TW, Walters MD (2006) Rectocele repair: a randomized trial of three surgical techniques including graft augmentation. Am J Obstet Gynecol 195:1762–1771

Peters WA III, Christenson ML (1995) Fixation of the vaginal apex to the coccygeus fascia during repair of vaginal vault eversion with enterocele. Am J Obstet Gynecol 172:1894–1900

Pillai A, Benson JT (1996) Cystocele. In: Brubaker LT, Saclarides TJ (eds) The female pelvic floor: Disorders of function and support.FA Davis Company, Philadelphia, p 269

Porter WE, Steele A, Walsh P, Kohli N, Karram MM (1999) The anatomic and functional outcomes of defect-specific rectocele repairs. Am J Obstet Gynecol 181:1353–1358

Randall CL, Nichols DH (1971) Surgical treatment of vaginal inversion. Obstet Gynecol 38:327–332

Richardson AC, Lyon JB, Williams NL (1976) A new look at pelvic relaxation. Am J Obstet Gynecol 126:568–573

Richardson AC, Edmonds PB, Williams NL (1981) Treatment of stress urinary incontinence due to paravaginal fascial defect. Obstet.Gynecol 57:357–362

Richardson AC (1989) Pelvic support defects in women (urethrocele, cystocele, uterine prolapse, enterocele and rectocele). In: Skandalakis J, Gray S, Mansberger A Jr, Colborn G, Skandalakis L (eds) Hernia: Surgical anatomy and technique. McGraw-Hill, New York, pp 238–263

Richardson AC (1993) The rectovaginal septum revisited: Its relationship to rectocele and its importance in rectocele repair. In: Pitkin RM, Scot JR, DeLancey JOL (eds) Clinical obstetrics and gynecology, vol 36. JB Lippincott Co, Philadelphia, p 977

Rooney K, Kenton K, Mueller ER, FitzGerald MP, Brubaker L (2006) Advanced anterior vaginal wall prolapse is highly correlated with apical prolapse. Am J Obstet Gynecol 95:837–1840

Sehapayak S (1985) Transrectal repair of rectocele: an extended armamentarium of colorectal surgeons. A report of 355 cases. Dis Colon Rectum 28:422–433

Shaw WF (1933) The treatment of prolapses uteri, with special reference to the Manchester operation of colporrhaphy. Am J Obstet Gynecol 26:667
Shull BL, Baden WF (1989) A six-year experience with paravaginal defect repair for stress urinary incontinence. Am J Obstet Gynecol 160:1432–1439
Shull BL, Benn SJ, Kuehl TJ (1994) Surgical management of prolapse of the anterior vaginal segment: an analysis of support defects, operative morbidity, and anatomic outcome. Am J Obstet Gynecol 171:1429–1436
Shull BL, Bachofen C, Coates KW, Kuehl TJ (2000) A transvaginal approach to repair of apical and other associated sites of pelvic organ prolapse with uterosacral ligaments. Am J Obstet Gynecol 183:1365–1373
Silva WA, Pauls RN, Segal JL, Rooney CM, Kleeman SD, Karram MM (2006) Uterosacral ligament vault suspension: 5-year outcomes. Obstet Gynecol 108:255–263
Smith AR, Hosker GL, Warrell DW (1989) The role of partial denervation of the pelvic floor in the aetiology of genitourinary prolapse and stress incontinence of urine. A neurophysiological study. Br J Obstet Gynaecol 96:24–28
Smith P, Heimer G, Norgren A, Ulmsten U (1990) Steroid hormone receptors in pelvic muscles and ligaments in women. Gynecol Obstet Invest 30:27–30
Su KC, Mutone MF, Terry CL, Hale DS (2007) Abdominovaginal sacral colpoperineopexy: patient perceptions, anatomical outcomes, and graft erosions. Int Urogynecol J Pelvic Floor Dysfunct 18:503–511
Sullivan ES, Leaverton GH, Hardwick CE (1968) Transrectal perineal repair: an adjunct to improved function after anorectal surgery. Dis Colon Rectum 11:106–114
Summers A, Winkel LA, Hussain HK, DeLancey JO (2006) The relationship between anterior and apical compartment support. Am J Obstet Gynecol 194:1438–1443
Sutton GP, Addison WA, Livengood CH III, Hammond CB (1981) Life-threatening hemorrhage complicating sacral colpopexy. Am J Obstet Gynecol 140:836–837
Swift SE (2000) The distribution of pelvic organ support in a population of female subjects seen for routine gynecologic health care. Am J Obstet Gynecol 183:277–285
Sze EH, Karram MM (1997) Transvaginal repair of vault prolapse: a review. Obstet Gynecol 89:466–475
Sze EH, Kohli N, Miklos JR, Roat T, Karram MM (1999) A retrospective comparison of abdominal sacrocolpopexy with Burch colposuspension versus sacrospinous fixation with transvaginal needle suspension for the management of vaginal vault prolapse and coexisting stress incontinence. Int Urogynecol J Pelvic Floor Dysfunct 10:390–393
Thomas AG, Brodman ML, Dottino PR, Bodian C, Friedman F Jr, Bogursky E (1995) Manchester procedure vs. vaginal hysterectomy for uterine prolapse. A comparison. J Reprod Med 40:299–304
Thompson JD (1992) Malposition of the uterus. In: Thompson JD, Rock JA (eds) TeLinde's operative gynecology, 7th edn. JB Lippincott Co, Philadelphia, pp 846–849
Timmons MC, Addison WA, Addison SB, Cavenar MG (1992) Abdominal sacral colpopexy in 163 women with posthysterectomy vaginal vault prolapse and enterocele. Evolution of operative techniques. J Reprod Med 37:323–327
Tulikangas PK, Walters MD, Brainard JA, Weber AM (2001) Enterocele: is there a histologic defect? Obstet Gynecol 98:634–637
Uhlenhuth E, Nolleyg GW (1957) Vaginal fascia, a myth. Obstet Gynecol 10:349–358
von Pechmann WS, Mutone M, Fyffe J, Hale DS (2003) Total colpocleisis with high levator plication for the treatment of advanced pelvic organ prolapse. Am J Obstet Gynecol 189:121–126
Weber AM, Walters MD (1997) Anterior vaginal prolapse: review of anatomy and techniques of surgical repair. Obstet Gynecol 89:311–318
Weber AM, Walters MD, Piedmonte MR, Ballard LA (2001) Anterior colporrhaphy: a randomized trial of three surgical techniques. Am J Obstet Gynecol 185:1299–1304
Weidner AC, Cundiff GW, Harris RL, Addison WA (1997) Sacral osteomyelitis: an unusual complication of abdominal sacral colpopexy. Obstet Gynecol 90:689–691
White GR (1909) Cystocele. A radical cure by suturing lateral sulci of vagina to white line of pelvic fascia. JAMA 21:1701–1710
Word BH, Montgomery HA, Baden WF et al (1992) Vaginal approach to anterior paravaginal repair: Alternative techniques. In: Baden WF, Walker T (eds) Surgical repair of vaginal defects. JB Lippincott, Philadelphia, p 201
Young SB, Daman JJ, Bony LG (2001) Vaginal paravaginal repair: 1-year outcomes. Am J Obstet Gynecol 185:1360–1366
Zaccharin RF (1977) A Chinese anatomy–the supporting tissues of the Chinese and Occidental female compared and contrasted. Aust NZ J Obstet Gynaec 17:1–11
Zaccharin RF (1980) Pulsion enterocele: Review of functional anatomy of the pelvic floor. Obstet Gynecol 55:135–140
Zaccharin RF (1985) Abdomino-perineal repair of large pulsion enterocele. In: Zaccharin RF (ed) Pelvic floor anatomy and the surgery of pulsion enterocele. Springer, New York Vienna Heidelberg Berlin, pp 135–155
Zivkovic F, Tamussino K, Ralph G, Schied G, Auer-Grumbach M (1996) Long-term effects of vaginal dissection on the innervation of the striated urethral sphincter. Obstet Gynecol 87:257–260

Further Reading

Farrell SA, Dempsey T, Geldenhuys L (2001) Histologic examination of "fascia" used in colporrhaphy. Obstet Gynecol 98:794–798
Gauruder-Burmester A, Koutouzidou P, Rohne J, Gronewold M, Tunn R (2007) Follow-up after polypropylene mesh repair of anterior and posterior compartments in patients with recurrent prolapse. Int Urogynecol J Pelvic Floor Dysfunct 18:1059–1064
Singh K, Reid WM, Berger LA (2001) Assessment and grading of pelvic organ prolapse by use of dynamic magnetic resonance imaging. Am J Obstet Gynecol 185:71–77

5.2 Urinary Incontinence: Clinical and Surgical Considerations

JAN-PAUL ROOVERS and MATTHIAS OELKE

CONTENTS

5.2.1 Introduction

Urinary incontinence is a prevalent disorder that occurs more commonly in subjects with pelvic support disorders. Conditions affecting bladder control can be divided into problems affecting proper storage and those of normal bladder emptying as mentioned in one of the previous chapters on urodynamic testing. This chapter focuses primarily on problems of bladder storage that result in loss of urinary control. The epidemiology, clinical evaluation, and treatment options for urinary incontinence are discussed.

5.2.1.1 Definition

Urinary incontinence has been defined by the International Continence Society (ICS) as: "involuntary loss of urine which is objectively demonstrable and a social or hygienic problem" (ABRAMS et al. 2002). The ICS definition includes three separate and important concepts:

J.-P. ROOVERS, MD, PhD
Department of Obstetrics and Gynecology, Academic Medical Center, University of Amsterdam, Meibergdreef 9, 1105 AZ Amsterdam, The Netherlands
M. OELKE, MD, FEBU
Department of Urology, Medical School Hanover, University of Hanover, Carl-Neuberg-Strasse 1, 30625 Hanover, Germany

- The loss of urine is not voluntary.
- Urine loss must be demonstrable on objective testing, such as cystometry or cough testing.
- The incontinence must be perceived by the patient as a social or hygienic problem.

The definitions of incontinence are important to consider, as the studies regarding outcomes often use different definitions for urinary incontinence. Variations in definitions occur because there are different amounts of urine lost, frequency of these events and how the incontinence events impact the individual. In addition to the ICS definition of urinary incontinence, an important concept is that the term urinary incontinence denotes three different meanings:

- A symptom: subjective involuntary urine loss.
- A sign: objective demonstration of urine loss.
- A condition: the pathophysiology underlying incontinence by clinical or urodynamic techniques.

5.2.1.2 Epidemiology

5.2.1.2.1 Prevalence of Urinary Incontinence

While not a life-threatening condition, urinary incontinence is exceptionally common. Several reviews summarize the epidemiology of urinary incontinence. More than 40% of women over 40 are estimated to experience urinary incontinence (van der Vaart et al. 2000; Burgioe et al. 1991). A marked increase in the rate of urinary incontinence among individuals who are institutionalized is also seen, reaching as high as 72% (Toba et al. 2008). It has been shown that the prevalence of urinary incontinence increases with the age (Malmsten et al. 1997). Stress incontinence is more common overall as compared to urge incontinence, although urge incontinence is more prevalent in elder subjects. Overall, women are twice as likely to experience incontinence as men, but this ratio is actually much higher in women aged 25–64 years (Bump and Norton 1998).

Among women, increasing parity is associated with increasing rates of urinary incontinence (Schulman et al. 1997). The epidemiologic studies are limited by the lack of consistent definitions regarding urinary incontinence. As mentioned above, there is a variation in the definitions regarding frequency of urine loss, volume of urine loss, as well as bothersome symptoms resulting from the loss. Several studies show that the prevalence rate for symptoms of urinary incontinence is high, but that the portion of subjects that is bothered by this symptom is low (Hunskaar et al. 2000). One study showed that men were more likely to seek medical help for urinary incontinence than women, despite having a lower overall prevalence rate (Roberts et al. 1998). The prevalence of urinary incontinence has also been shown to be related to racial differences as is reflected by the higher prevalence in white women than black women (Kim et al. 2005).

Prevalence rates for surgical treatment of stress urinary incontinence provide another way to look at the concept of how bothersome the problem is to the individual. If it were bothersome enough that the subject opted for surgical treatment, one would assume that it is a considerable burden for them. Olsen and colleagues investigated the prevalence of surgical treatment for women with incontinence or pelvic organ prolapse (Olsen et al. 1997). They estimated that the risk of a woman undergoing a single operation for prolapse or urinary incontinence by age 80 years was 11.1%. Furthermore, 29.2% of the patients required more than one surgical repair for prolapse or urinary incontinence.

5.2.1.2.2 Risk Factors for Urinary Incontinence

Risk factors have to be established from well-designed epidemiological studies, which unfortunately are scarce. Most trials provide only cross-sectional and not longitudinal data on urinary incontinence; therefore, cross-sectional studies can only provide correlations, but cannot demonstrate cause-effect mechanisms. Identification of risk factors for urinary incontinence has the potential advantage that specific patient behavior, situations, or treatments can be avoided in order to prevent urinary incontinence.

Accepted risk factors for female stress urinary incontinence are increased age, elevated body-mass index (obesity), parity, pregnancy, and childbirth (Hunskaar et al. 2000). Factors related to obstetric injury during childbirth are older age at first delivery, epidural anesthesia, midline episiotomy, forceps, or vacuum extraction, suturing after perineal laceration, and birth weight (Persson et al. 2000). Cesarean section significantly reduces the risk of urinary incontinence when compared to vaginal delivery (odds ratio 1.7), but the risk of becoming incontinent after cesarean section is still significantly higher when compared to women not giving birth (odds ratio 1.5) (Rortveit et al. 2003). White women have a higher chance to develop stress urinary incontinence than black women (Brown et al. 1999). Other factors are also hypothesized to produce stress urinary incontinence, but epidemiological studies reveal heterogeneous results regarding these suggested factors, including hysterectomy, menopause, pelvic organ prolapse, and cigarette smoking. The key risk factors for male stress urinary incontinence are prostate operations (transurethral resection, open prostatectomy, radical prostatectomy, or radical cystoprostectomy). This suggests that the prostate itself is part of the continence mechanism in men.

Risk factors for urge urinary incontinence in both genders are cerebral stroke, cognitive impairment, impaired mobility, constipation, decreased fluid intake, depression, and prolonged bed wetting in childhood (Foldsprang and Momsen 1994). Furthermore, stress urinary incontinence operations might trigger de novo detrusor overactivity, and urge urinary incontinence (see Sect. 5.2.5.2); de novo detrusor overactivity appears after Marshal-Marchetti-Krantz vesico-urethropexy in ~40%, Burch colposuspension ~17%, facial slings ~17%, needle suspension ~6%, and tension-free vaginal tapes ~10%. Drugs can also cause or aggravate stress or urge urinary incontinence. Evidence for drug-induced stress urinary incontinence exists for a variety of medications, including α-blockers, anti-psychotics, and benzodiazepines; evidence for drug-induced urge incontinence exists for direct and indirect parasympathomimetics, antidepressants, serotonin agonists, and hormonal replacement; evidence for overflow incontinence exists for muscarinic receptor antagonists (anticholinergics), anti-Parkinson agents, and β-blockers (Tsakiris et al. 2008). Based on their receptor-binding or working mechanisms, many other drug classes are potentially able to influence the function of bladder or urinary sphincters as well; however, no hard evidence exists for drug classes other than the ones listed above.

5.2.2 Continence Mechanisms

The following mechanisms are believed to contribute to female urinary continence ("stress continence control system") (Oelke and Roovers 2008; DeLancey and Ashton-Miller 2004):

- Smooth and striated muscle cells in and around the urethra close the urethral lumen (active sphincteric system).
- The length of the urethra and urethral wall tension (collagen and elastic fibers, mucosa and submucosal cushion of blood vessels in the urethral wall) guarantee additional positive pressure in the urethra in the resting position (passive sphincteric system or urethral wall factor) (Zinner et al. 1980).
- Pressure transmission from the abdominal cavity to the proximal urethra (passive pressure transmission) (Enhörning 1961).
- Activation of the coughing reflex via the pudendal nerve leads to a fast contraction of the urethral rhabdomyosphincter and pelvic floor before and during vesical pressure increases (active pressure transmission) (Enhörning 1961; Kamo et al. 2004).
- Posterior urethral wall support by fibro-muscular tissue of the anterior vaginal wall and the tendinous arch of the pelvic fascia (hammock system) (DeLancey 1994).
- Ventral kinking of the urethra during contraction of the levator ani muscle, longitudinal muscle of the anus, and the hammock-muscle pulls the vagina and bladder base back and downwards and presses the urethra against the pubic bone (integral theory) (Petros and Ulmsten 1990).

5.2.3 Types of Urinary Incontinence

There are five different types of urinary incontinence.

5.2.3.1 Stress Urinary Incontinence

According to the International Continence Society, stress incontinence is defined as the involuntary loss of urine during increased abdominal pressure. Stress urinary incontinence can be due to a poorly functioning urethral sphincter muscle, termed "intrinsic sphincter deficiency" (ISD), or due to hypermobility of the bladder neck, implying loss of the active supports (neurological innervation and pelvic floor muscles) and/or connective tissue supports (passive supports). While it is common to artificially categorize the two conditions into separate entities, most subjects suffering from stress incontinence have a combination of both.

5.2.3.2 Urge Urinary Incontinence

Urge urinary incontinence is the complaint of involuntary urinary leakage accompanied or immediately preceded by urgency (complaint of a sudden compelling desire to void that is difficult or impossible to defer) and often associated with urinary frequency [complaint of frequent voiding during day time (=pollakisuria, >7 voids/day) or night time (=nocturia, >1 void/night)] (Abrams 2002). The corresponding urodynamic observation is detrusor overactivity incontinence, which is defined as urinary leakage due to involuntary detrusor contraction during the bladder-filling phase. Involuntary detrusor contractions produce a rise of intravesical pressure, which leads to urinary leakage when urethral pressure is exceeded. Urgency is the most bothersome urinary symptom that affects the quality of life most substantially.

Detrusor overactivity should be qualified as primary (=idiopathic) detrusor overactivity when no cause of involuntary detrusor contractions can be defined or secondary detrusor overactivity when a plausible cause of involuntary detrusor contractions is found. Secondary detrusor overactivity might appear in patients with urinary tract infection, bladder stones, bladder tumors, bladder catheters, or other foreign bodies in the bladder. Less frequent causes are bladder perforations due to transvaginal tapes (TVT procedure, Fig. 52.1) or non-absorbable sutures after pelvic operations (e.g., colposuspension, see Sect. 52.5). Detrusor overactivity in patients with urge urinary incontinence is therefore always caused by bladder abnormalities and distinguished from detrusor overactivity caused by neurological diseases (see Sect. 5.2.3.4, neurogenic urinary incontinence).

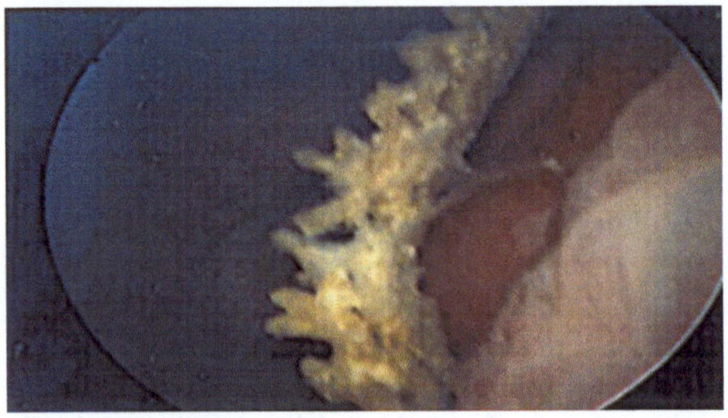

Fig. 5.2.1. Bladder perforation due to TVT procedure

5.2.3.3 Overflow Incontinence

Overflow incontinence refers to incontinence due to an over-distended bladder usually associated with a relatively hypotonic detrusor muscle. In this circumstance, the patient may leak because of increased abdominal pressure forcing urine out of the over-distended bladder or because of small detrusor contractions causing continuous small amounts of leakage, even at rest (detrusor overactivity with impaired contractility).

5.2.3.4 Neurogenic Urinary Incontinence

The term neurogenic incontinence is used when a patient has a relevant neurological disease and urinary incontinence. Urinary incontinence appears if patients have urinary sphincter paralysis and/or detrusor overactivity (Abrams 2002). Involuntary detrusor contractions in these patients are classified as neurogenic detrusor overactivity and, if these detrusor contractions are associated with urinary incontinence, as neurogenic detrusor overactivity incontinence.

Involuntary detrusor contractions in patients with neurological diseases are caused by decreased supraspinal nerve stimulation of the micturition center in the sacral spinal cord (S_2–S_4). During the bladder filling phase in healthy individuals, the neurons in the lateral horn of the grey matter of the sacral spinal cord continuously stimulate the detrusor via parasympathetic nerves (pelvic splanchnic nerves), the neurotransmitter acetylcholine, and muscarinic receptors on the detrusor cells, but, however, are inhibited by descending neurons of the supraspinal urinary centers in the pontine area, midbrain, and cerebral cortex via the neurotransmitters dopamine, GABA, serotonin, noradrenaline, and glutamate (de Groat 1998; Michel et al. 2005). In patients with neurological diseases, varying amounts of nerve cells or descending axons of the supraspinal urinary centers are damaged, which causes reduced inhibitory input on the neurons in the sacral micturition center leading to continuous stimulation of the detrusor cells and detrusor overactivity. Parkinson's disease, multiple sclerosis, cerebral infarction, cerebral trauma, or spinal cord injury are frequently and a transverse lesion of the spinal cord above the sacral micturition center is always associated with detrusor overactivity. Patients with Parkinson's disease have a chance of detrusor overactivity of 45–98%, depending on their disease stage. Detrusor overactivity is the first symptom of the disease in approximately 10% of patients with multiple sclerosis. Patients usually complain about urgency when afferent neurons and bladder sensation are intact; in cases of afferent nerve damage and diminished bladder sensation, the patient does not have the feeling of urgency anymore (e.g., transverse lesion of the spinal cord).

Neurogenic stress urinary incontinence appears when nerves innervating the urinary sphincter are damaged. The external urinary sphincter is innervated by motor neurons in the anterior grey matter of the sacral spinal cord (S_2–S_4), whose signals are transmitted via the pudendal nerves, acetylcholine, and nicotine receptors to the skeletal muscle (rhabdomyosphincter). Urinary sphincter paralysis decreases urethral pressure and leads to intermittent or continuous urinary leakage, depending on the residual function of the urethral sphincters.

An isolated damage of nerve cells that inhibits the micturition center in the sacral spinal cord or innervates the urethral sphincter is untypical for most of the neurological diseases. More frequently, other neurons are affected as well, causing a broad range of bladder and urinary sphincter dysfunctions (Fig. 52.2). Urodynamic investigations can clarify these changes in the bladder filling and voiding phase (e.g., reduced bladder compliance, detrusor-sphincter dyssynergia, functional bladder outlet obstruction with post-void residual urine, and stress urinary incontinence).

5.2.3.5 Extra-Urethral Incontinence

Extra-urethral incontinence refers to urine loss that occurs from sites other than the urethra meatus. Examples include genitourinary fistulas (vesicovaginal, uterovaginal, ureterovaginal, and urethrovaginal fistulae) as well as ectopic ureter. Presenting symptoms usually include continuous leakage throughout the day and night without correlation to stress or urge symptoms. The incontinence is often the result of a surgical complication, and this is established by history. The other common cause of fistulae is from obstetric trauma, although this is a much more significant problem in underdeveloped countries. Fistulas have also been

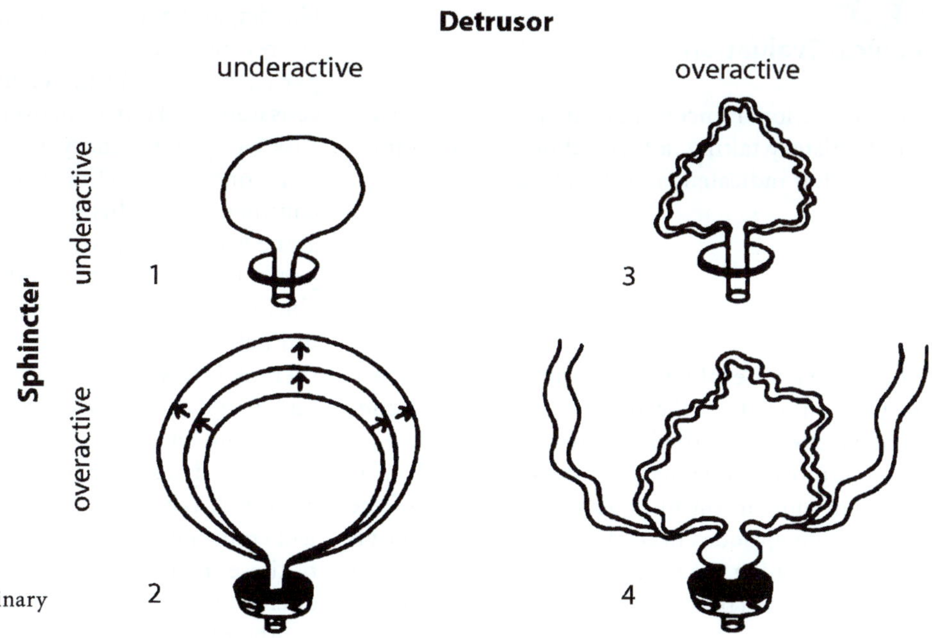

Fig. 5.2.2. Bladder and urinary sphincter dysfunctions

described in patients who forgot to visit a doctor for a check-up of a vaginal pessary used to treat genital prolapse.

The diagnosis of fistula is usually confirmed on vaginal examination of the vagina. Vesicovaginal fistulae may be diagnosed with a tampon placed in the vagina and retrograde instillation of methylene blue or indigo carmine into the bladder via a catheter. The patient ambulates for 30 min, and if blue dye stains the cranial part of the tampon, a vesicovaginal or vesicouterine fistula is suspected. If the test is negative, a similar test can be performed, but with administration of oral pyridium or intravenous indigo carmine to look for staining of the tampon with orange or blue, respectively. In the setting of a negative test for a fistula, staining with the second test is consistent with an ureterovaginal fistula. Diagnosis can be supplemented with cystoscopy, retrograde cystography, voiding cystourethrography, and intravenous pyelography. Hysterosalpingography is useful to establish the diagnosis of a vesicouterine fistula, which might occur following cesarean section.

Treatment of small fistulae may be conservative by a transurethral catheter for the duration of 3 months. In most cases, surgical correction will be performed with reported successful repair rates in the range of 67–100%.

5.2.4 Clinical Evaluation

The evaluation of incontinent subjects relies on accurate history taking, a focused physical examination, and, if indicated, additional tests.

5.2.4.1 Patient History

The history for evaluation of urinary incontinence focuses on whether the individual's primary concern is due to insufficient urethral resistance or due to an overactive detrusor muscle or both. It is especially important to establish the timing of the incontinent episodes in relationship to other activities. Establishing the timing and frequency of these episodes is often best determined by a bladder diary (see next page).

Patients who leak at night are more likely to have a detrusor-related problem or fistula, whereas those who leak only while ambulatory are more likely to have stress incontinence. It is also important to assess the impact of the problem on the patient's quality of life. Questions about pad usage, restriction of exercises, or other activities, including coitus, help to determine the impact of incontinence on the patient.

Questions about incontinence of stool or flatus should be addressed, as the prevalence of combined urinary and anal incontinence has been reported to be as high as 31% (Jackson et al. 1997). Also, the presence of other defecation symptoms should be assessed. These symptoms include: constipation, painful defecation, incomplete evacuation, digital evacuation, sensation of anal blockage, difficult emptying, and soiling. Attention is paid to the presence of prolapse symptoms. Finally, sexual function is assessed, and attention is paid to the presence of urinary incontinence during intercourse.

The past medical history should be explored, including conditions that limit mobility, neurologic function, and normal comprehension. Prior bladder problems, such as recurrent urinary tract infections, stones, or malignancy, are addressed. Co-existing conditions, such as congestive heart failure, diabetes or back problems, should be noted. Congestive heart failure and the resultant dependent peripheral edema may lead to nocturia as the third-spaced fluids return to circulation when the individual is recumbent at night. Prior pelvic surgeries, including hysterectomy, bladder, and bowel surgeries, are reviewed. Obstetrical reviews are also reviewed to determine vaginal parity, the largest birth weight, and whether or not forceps were used during delivery (see also Sect. 5.2.1.2.2 Risk factors for urinary incontinence).

In one series, clinical diagnosis of urinary incontinence with history and physical examination alone was accurate in only 65% of cases when compared to an urodynamic diagnosis. As mentioned above, when the treatment plan is conservative, it is unlikely that harm could be inflicted when empiric therapy is based on history if the post-void residual and urinalysis are negative.

A complete list of all prescription and non-prescription drugs that the patient is taking should be obtained. Table 5.2.1 lists drugs that significantly affect continence. When appropriate, discontinuation of these medications or substitution of appropriate alternative medications will often cure or significantly improve urinary incontinence.

Table 5.2.1. Commonly used drugs that can influence bladder function

Drug	Side effect
Antidepressants, antipsychotica, sedatives/hypnotics	Sedation, retention (overflow)
Diuretics	Frequency, urgency (OAB)
Caffeine	Frequency, urgency (OAB)
Anticholinergics	Retention (overflow)
Alcohol	Sedation, frequency (OAB)
Narcotics	Retention, constipation, sedation (OAB and overflow)
Alpha-adrenergic blockers	Decreased urethral tone (stress incontinence)

5.2.4.2 Validated Questionnaires

There are several validated disease-specific quality-of-life questionnaires to determine the quality of life related to micturition. The Urogenital Distress Inventory (UDI) comprises 19 questions to assess the presence and experiences both of micturition and prolapse symptoms (Shumaker et al. 1994). The Incontinence Impact Questionnaire (IIQ) comprises 30 questions to assess the effects of these symptoms on life quality, including effects on emotional health, physical activity, travel, daily living activities, sexual activity, and sleep. Short forms of both the UDI and IIQ have been developed that include only six and seven questions, respectively (Uebersax et al. 1995). The clinical value of validated questionnaires is that they can consistently assess micturition and prolapse symptoms and the activity limitations they cause. Furthermore, they are used in studies to quantify the effects of interventions.

5.2.4.3 Physical Examination

Patients are examined in the supine position with a filled bladder, meaning that the bladder is filled to a volume of at least 300 ml, but ideally so that the patients have an urge to void. If the bladder capacity does not allow such volume, the bladder diary can be helpful to determine what volume reflects a filled bladder.

A targeted clinical examination includes an examination of the back, abdomen, pelvis, rectum, and distal extremities. In the back examination, evidence of paraspinal tenderness, costovertrebal angle tenderness, asymmetry, or surgical scars can be investigated. Unlike the back examination, the abdominal examination is obligatory and focuses on whether there are masses, suprapubic tenderness, or surgical scars. On pelvic examination, the urethral meatus is inspected for irritation of prolapse of the mucosa. The bladder neck is assessed during maximal staining to assess the presence of excessive mobility of the urethra. Hypermobility can be assessed by performing a Q-tip test (see additional tests). In each examination, it is important to assess whether a genital prolapse is also present. Ideally, this part of the examination is performed using a Sims' speculum, allowing assessment of each vaginal compartment separately. The pelvic organ prolapse quantification (POP-Q) score is the scoring system of genital prolapse that has been advised by the International Continence Society (ICS) (Bump et al. 1996). The POP-Q system allows a quantified measurement of the anterior, middle, and posterior vaginal compartment, the diameter of the genital hiatus, the length of the perineal body, and the total vaginal length. This system has been shown to be reproducible, takes only 30 s, and is helpful to document the effects of prolapse surgery on the anatomical abnormalities involved. During the examination, the presence of vaginal atrophy is documented. Rectal examination is performed to assess normal sphincter tone and integrity. The patient is asked to squeeze, and both the squeezing pressure and duration are recorded. A normal sphincter tone and ability to contract the levator ani suggest an intact innervation to the pelvic floor though sacral roots S2–4. Distal extremity examination focuses on normal innervation and sensory dermatomes for the sacral nerve roots.

5.2.4.4 Additional Tests

- **Assessment of post-void residual volume**
  Measurement of post-void residual bladder volume should be performed in all patients presenting with urinary incontinence. Assessment can be done by bladder scan, ultrasound, or catheter-

ization. An estimation of residual bladder volume can also be made by abdominal palpation and percussion or by X-ray (Hilton and Stanton 1981). There is no agreement on the cut-off value to consider the residual volume as abnormal. Most publications use a cut-off value of 100–150 ml, although ideally residual bladder volume should not exceed 50 ml. Whereas inadequate emptying of the bladder may result in overflow incontinence, there is evidence that residual bladder volume in continent and incontinent women is similar (Diokno et al. 1988).

- **Urine analysis**
  Urine analysis is recommended to be performed in all patients. This analysis should minimally include a dipstick to test for the presence of blood, glucose, and leucocytes in urine. Although the exact relation between urinary tract infection and incontinence is not completely understood, it has been shown that symptomatic urinary tract infection is more common in incontinent than continent women (Rekers et al. 1992; Yarnell et al. 1982). A study comparing urodynamic evaluation before and after treatment of bacteriuria showed that both stress incontinence and urge incontinence might disappear (Bergman and Bhatia 1985).
- **Stress provocation test**
  If stress incontinence is suspected, a provocative stress test may be performed by asking the patient to cough vigorously while the examiner observes for urine loss from the urethra (Fischer et al. 1986). There is no consensus about the bladder volume at which the cough test has to be performed. A stress provocation test in supine position with a standard bladder volume of 200 ml has the best sensitivity to predict stress incontinence with multi-channel urodynamics as reference test (Hsu et al. 1999). The Bonney test is similar to the stress provocation test, except the bladder neck is lifted slightly with a finger or instrument inserted into the vagina while the bladder stress is applied. This checks to see if incontinence is the result of hypermobility of the bladder neck, but may obstruct the urethra, so its interpretation is unpredictable.
  The Marshall-Marchetti-Krantz test has been advocated as an adjunct to the stress provocation test. After a positive stress test, the index and middle fingers of the examiner's hand are pressed against the anterior vaginal wall, without pressing the urethra. The stress test is repeated, and if no leakage occurs this time, the Marshall-Marchetti-Krantz test is defined as positive. A positive Marshall-Marchetti-Krantz test has been taken as an indication that the patient will benefit from surgery. However, it has been stated that the urethrta is obstructed during the Bonney test and that the test may have a positive result irrespective the type of incontinence (Migliorini and Glenning 1987). A better prediction of successful surgery may be when a positive stress provocation test becomes negative with a vaginal pessary (Bhatia and Bergman 1985).
- **Urodynamic investigation**
  See Chapter 4.7.3
- **Bladder diary**
  The 24- to 48-h bladder diary provides a useful record of urinary frequency, average voiding volume, frequency of voiding, and frequency and nature of incontinent episodes, as well as type and volume of fluid intake (Bailey 1990). Patients are asked to collect and measure their urine output in a measuring cup for 24 or 48 h. The diary enables the physician to make helpful suggestions regarding the type and amount of fluid intake. For example, patients with significant nocturia may benefit from decreasing fluid intake after their evening meal or those that have frequency associated with excessive fluid ingestion can moderate their intake.
  It has been shown in a study performed by Larsson that there is a large overlap in frequency/volume charts between women with detrusor instability and healthy volunteers. No correlation was found in this study between data of the frequency/volume chart and cytometry. It was concluded that although the bladder diary may not be a tool with differential diagnostic capabilities, it offers a quantitative measure of the symptomatic degree of motor urgency and can be used to measure the effect of treatment (Larsson et al. 1991).
- **Q-tip test**
  During the Q-tip test a sterile swab is lubricated with sterile gel and under sterile conditions inserted in the urethra. It is first inserted with the tip in the bladder and then withdrawn until resistance of the tip is met at the bladder neck. During a Q-tip test the angle of the urethra with the horizontal plane is measured at rest and with Valsalva by inserting a Q-tip in the urethra (Karram and Bhatia 1988). The test is considered positive if the angle of excursion is 30 degrees or more. This test helps to diagnose urethral hyper-mobility, which is believed to respond well to surgical correction (Bakas et al. 2002). It is important to realize that

such an observation does not confirm that the patient's incontinence is due solely to a motility problem. Many women have hypermobility of the bladder neck without incontinence.

- **Cystoscopy**
  Cystoscopy is especially valuable in the diagnostic workup of patients with urge incontinence. Abnormalities in the bladder such as stones, foreign bodies or tumors can be diagnosed and sometimes immediately removed. A bladder washout (cytology of a sample of the salt solution used during cystoscopy) is helpful to rule out malignancies of the bladder.

5.2.4.5 Imaging

In patients with urinary incontinence the initial management includes no imaging evaluation, except for assessing the post-void residual urine using ultrasonography. However, if initial therapy fails then specialized management is required.

Imaging studies of the upper urinary tract are indicated in the following cases: (1) neurogenic urinary incontinence with high risk of renal damage, (2) chronic retention with incontinence, (3) untreated severe urogenital prolapse, and (4) suspicion of extra-urethral urinary incontinence by upper urinary tract anomaly. The choice of the imaging method (X-ray, ultrasound, CT, MRI, or isotope scanning) and their sequence depends on the clinical question and their availability, possibly preferring the least invasive and considering their cost effectiveness (Artibani and Cerruto 2005).

Ultrasound imaging of the bladder is able to detect some of the causes of secondary detrusor overactivity (e.g., bladder stones or papillary bladder tumors, Figs. 5.2.3 and 5.2.4) and should therefore be performed in all patients with suspicion of urge urinary incontinence. Patients might even have two or more causes for detrusor overactivity incontinence at the same time (e.g., bladder tumor in a patient with Parkinson's disease), which underlines the importance of a systematic assessment in all patients even when the cause of urinary incontinence seems to be obvious after initial investigation.

Magnetic resonance imaging or computer tomography can visualize disease-specific changes in the central nervous system such as substantia nigra defects in patients with Parkinson's disease, plaques in patients with multiple sclerosis, cerebral lesions

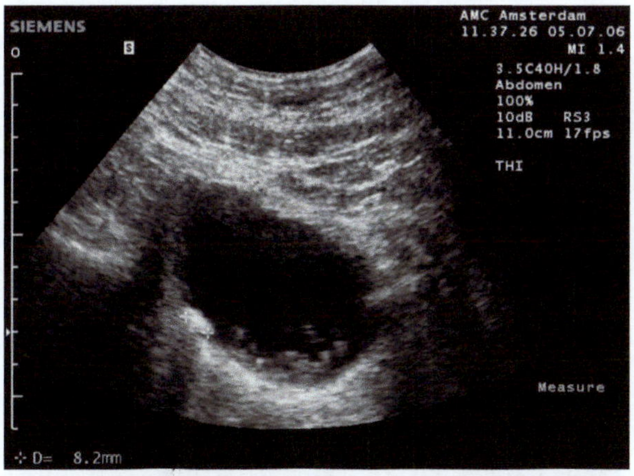

Fig. 5.2.3. Bladder stones

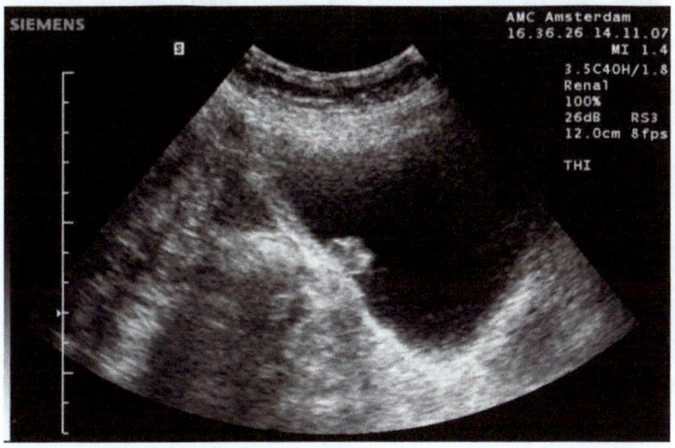

Fig. 5.2.4. Papillary bladder tumors

after cerebro-vascular accidents, brain tumors, and bone or spinal cord abnormalities in patients with myelodysplasia due to spina bifida. Ultrasound or X-ray imaging of the urinary tract is not able to visualize the cause of urinary incontinence in these patients, but might detect the consequences of neurogenic bladder dysfunction, such as hydronephrosis due to low bladder compliance, detrusor wall thickening due to detrusor-sphincter dyssynergia, vesico-ureteral reflux (Fig. 52.5), or postvoid residual urine. Ultrasound imaging should be done regularly in all patients with neurogenic bladder dysfunction in order to assess the current status of the lower and upper urinary tract. Hydronephrosis due to low bladder compliance is beside recurrent upper urinary tract infection one of the most frequent causes of renal insufficiency in these patients (Singhal and Mathew 1999). Early detection of hydronephrosis and adequate therapy can prevent renal insufficiency and dialysis (Ahmad and Granitsiotis 2007).

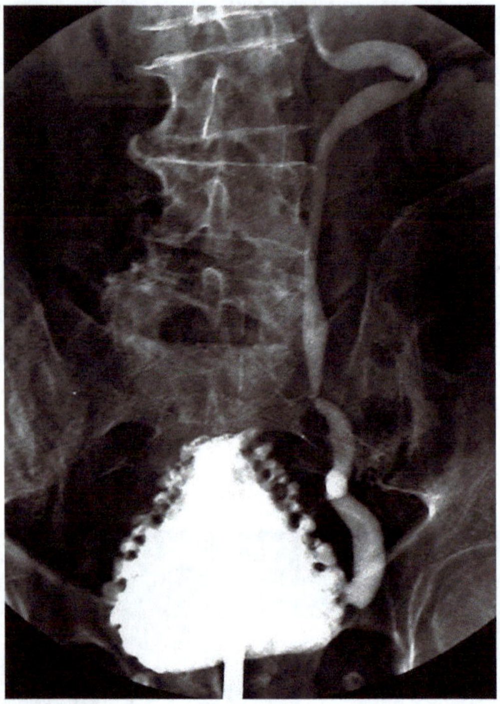

Fig. 5.2.5. Vesico-ureteral reflux

5.2.5 Treatment of Stress Incontinence

5.2.5.1 Conservative Treatment

5.2.5.1.1 Habit Training

Habit training is prescribed to assess an individual's normal voiding pattern. It is generally used for institutionalized subjects who have cognitive or functional impairments contributing to their incontinence. This therapy is more successful in patients with urge incontinence than in patients with stress incontinence, as prompted or timed voiding may allow for bladder emptying before the bladder involuntary contracts. Patients who have the symptom of stress incontinence due to overflow incontinence may benefit from behavior therapy.

5.2.5.1.2 Mechanical Devices

Mechanical devices to treat urinary incontinence can be divided into three categories: (1) intraurethral devices, (2) vaginal support devices, and (3) extraurethral devices. The main working mechanism of these devices is that they support the bladder neck, thus preventing the effect of hypermobility of the bladder neck. The intraurethral devices have a median corrected cure/improved rate of 43%, with a high rate of urinary tract infections (Vierhout and Lose 1997). These are primarily devices that are inserted into the urethra and secured in place with a balloon, similar to a Foley catheter balloon. They are disposable, and after each void, a new one is inserted. Vaginal devices include tampons, contraceptive diaphragms, bladder neck prosthetic devices, and pessaries. Mean corrected cured /improved rates are 63% for several different devices (Vierhout and Lose 1997). Side effects include vaginal discharge, pelvic pressure, and sexual symptoms.

The last category includes urethral occlusive devices for women that are applied by the patient. One type uses a suction cap that is squeezed and fitted over the urethral meatus. Silicone gel helps maintain the seal, and it is removed for voiding (Moore et al. 1999). Another device is a pad applied over the urethral meatus that seals the urethra.

5.2.5.1.3 Specialized Pelvic Physiotherapy

5.2.5.1.3.1 Pelvic Floor Muscle Training

Pelvic floor muscle training (PFMT) for the management of urinary incontinence was popularized by Arnold Kegel (1894–1981). PFMT has principally been recommended in the management of stress and mixed urinary incontinence, but has increasingly become part of the conservative treatment program offered to women with urge urinary incontinence.

For stress urinary incontinence, the aims of PFMT are to improve pelvic organ support (particularly of the bladder, bladder neck, and urethra) and increase intra-urethral pressure during exertion. The rationale that PFMT is effective in the treatment of stress incontinence is that (1) patients learn the use of a well-timed, fast and strong voluntary pelvic floor muscle contraction before and during the exertion, (2) pelvic floor muscle strength will be increased, and (3) pelvic floor muscle contraction will be facilitated through abdominal muscle contraction. This rationale was supported by the findings of a small randomized controlled trial, demonstrating that the use of a well-timed voluntary pelvic floor muscle contraction (called "the knack") could reduce leakage with coughing (Miller et al. 1998).

The Cochrane analysis on pelvic floor muscle training concludes that PFMT seems to be better than no treatment, placebo drug, or inactive control treatments for women with stress, urge, or mixed incontinence (Hay-Smith and Dumoulin 2006). The trials included in this meta-analysis suggested that the treatment effect might only be greater in women with stress incontinence who tended to be younger (in their 40s and 50s) and have participated in a supervised PFMT program for at least 3 months.

5.2.5.1.3.2 *Biofeedback Therapy*

Biofeedback therapy uses an electronic device to help individuals having difficulty identifying the levator ani muscles. Biofeedback therapy is recommended for treatment of stress incontinence, urge incontinence, and mixed incontinence. During biofeedback therapy, a special tampon-shaped sensor is inserted in the vagina or rectum, and a second sensor is placed on the abdomen. These sensors detect electrical signals from the pelvic floor muscles. The patients contracts and relaxes the pelvic floor muscles as told by the physiotherapist. The electric signals from the pelvic floor muscles are displayed on a computer screen. A small randomized controlled trial suggested that adding biofeedback therapy to PFMT resulted in better outcome as compared to PFMT only (Glavind et al. 1996). However, this was not confirmed by a larger trial conducted in the United States (Goode et al. 2003).

5.2.5.1.4 *Drug Treatment*

The serotonin (5-hydroxytryptamine [5-HT]) and noradrenalin (NA) reuptake inhibitor duloxetine is currently the only widely approved pharmacological treatment option for women with stress urinary incontinence (SUI). The rationale for employing duloxetine in SUI is based on the role of 5-HT and NA in the neurological control of the lower urinary tract. Animal studies have shown that duloxetine increases the concentration of 5-HT and NA in the sacral spinal cord, thereby facilitating an increased activity of the external urethral sphincter (rhabdosphincter) and preventing urine leakage during the storage phase of the micturition cycle (Thor and Katofiasc 1995). Importantly, 5-HT and NA exert only a modulating effect as they are not able to directly excite motor neurons. Glutamate is the key descending neurotransmitter and can be considered as the 'on/off' switch for micturition. In the absence of glutamate, no rhabdosphincter activity is observed, irrespective of the presence of 5-HT and NA. Hence, duloxetine enhances sphincter activity during urine storage when glutamate is released, but allows complete relaxation of the rhabdosphincter once glutamate release is inhibited during the voiding phase (Oelke et al. 2006).

The efficacy of duloxetine for treating women with SUI, as shown in several double-blind, placebo-controlled randomized clinical trials, has suggested a similar mode of action, although no direct evidence for this pathway in humans was available until recently (Dmochowski et al. 2003; Millard et al. 2004; Norton et al. 2002). Two recent studies provide support for duloxetine's mechanism of action in humans. Duloxetine was shown to have a significant effect on the excitability of pudendal motor neurons and on sphincter contractility in healthy women (Boy et al. 2006; Bump et al. 2004). In contrast, no relevant effect was observed on urethral resting tone. Another study reported important increases in Valsalva leak point pressure and in the rhabdosphincter electrical activity at rest and with coughing in women with SUI who responded to duloxetine. These studies support the hypothesis that duloxetine in women with SUI enhances urethral closure through neuromodulation of the rhabdosphincter.

5.2.5.2 Surgical Therapy

Surgical treatment should be considered when conservative measures fail. For the management of stress incontinence, hundreds of operations have been described. Before the introduction of the mid-urethral sling, it has been the trend that the surgical approach should depend upon whether the urodynamic diagnosis was bladder neck hypermobility or intrinsic sphincter deficiency (see Table 5.2.1). However, it has been shown that midurethral slings have good surgical outcome independent of the urodynamic diagnosis.

5.2.5.2.1 Anterior Colporraphy

Originally anterior colporraphy has been described as correcting stress incontinence. Comparative studies have shown that the long-term results of this procedure generate poor results (Bergman and Elia 1995). Therefore, this technique is reserved for the treatment of anterior vaginal wall prolapse.

5.2.5.2.2 Needle Urethropexy

During needle urethropexy a needle is passed bilaterally alongside the bladder neck from the abdominal approach through the space of Retzius. Sutures at the bladder neck are brought back through the space of Retzius and attached to the abdominal wall. Several modifications have been described, for example by Stamey, Pereyra, and Raz. As long-term results are poor, these techniques will rarely be performed nowadays.

5.2.5.2.3 Abdominal Retropubic Urethropexy (Colposuspension)

Until the end of the previous century, open retropubic urethopexy was the standard care in patients with hypermobility of the bladder neck. There are two common approaches: the Burch colposuspension and the Marshall-Marchetti-Krantz procedure. During both techniques the space of Retzius is dissected by an abdominal approach to reach the bladder neck. For the Burch operation, two or three permanent sutures are placed at each side of the bladder neck and anchored to Cooper's ligament on the ipsi-lateral side (see Fig. 5.2.6). During the

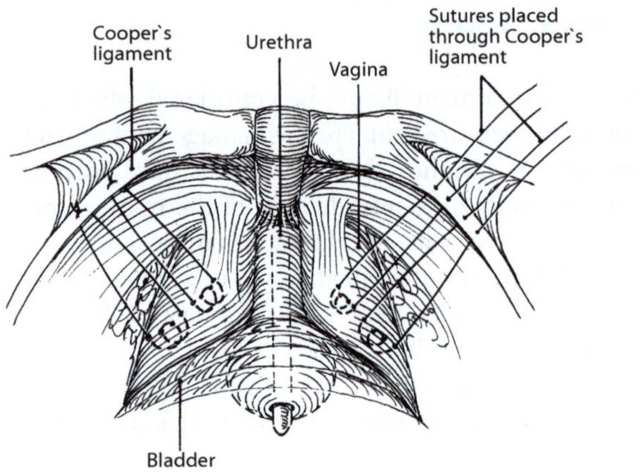

Fig. 5.2.6. Burch retropubic urethropexy. Bilateral pairs of permanent sutures are placed in the paravaginal fascia to support the anterior vaginal wall at the level of the bladder neck. Each suture is anchored to Cooper's ligament on the ipsilateral side (with permission, Chen and Horbach 1997)

Marshall-Marchetti-Krantz procedure, one to three pairs of non-absorbable sutures are placed at the bladder neck and sutured to the cartilage at the symphysis pubis.

The Burch colposuspension is the surgical technique with the longest documented follow-up (Kjølhede 2005). In randomized compared trials, it has been proven to be superior as compared to anterior colporraphy and needle suspension (Bergman and Elia 1995). The disadvantage of this technique is that the abdominal approach generates more morbidity. Hematoma may occur in the area of the paravaginal veins at the space of Retzius, particularly in association with dissection of the wrong tissue plane. Radiological imaging can assist in ruling out complications of a hematoma, abscess, or ureteral or bladder injury. Additionally, imaging can assist in ruling out osteitis pubis or osteomyelitis as a complication of the Marshall-Marchetti-Krantz procedure (Lentz 1995).

5.2.5.2.4 Suburethral Sling

The suburethral sling has traditionally been the operation of choice for the treatment of intrinsic sphincter deficiency and recurrent stress incontinence after a primary operation. Various materials have been utilized to perform a sling procedure, including autologous or heterologous fascial grafts from the rectus abdominus muscle or fascia lata. Cadaveric fascia lata allograft has also been used, but the results were very poor (Soergel et al. 2001).

The sling can be secured to the rectus abdominus fascia, Cooper's ligament, or the pubic bone itself by bone anchors (Bent and McLennan 1998). The pubovaginal sling uses a suture attached to each end of the sling to suspend it to the rectus sheath until it heals in place to the back of the pubic bone. The difference with the minimally invasive slings is that the sling is wrapped around the urethra. During a minimally invasive sling procedure a mesh is placed without tension under the midurethra. Since the introduction of the minimally invasive sling, the traditional sling is seldom performed for primary cases, but remains in use for recurrence.

5.2.5.2.5 Minimally Invasive Midurethral Sling

Minimally invasive midurethral slings have changed the way many surgeons treat stress urinary incontinence. Many of these midurethral sling procedures can be performed under local anesthesia with short operative times and minimal dissection. The tension-free vaginal tape (TVT) was one of the first widely available retropubic (RP) midurethral slings. During this procedure a synthetic polypropylene mesh is positioned at the midurethra via a vaginal incision of approximately 1 cm. This mesh is then directed under the symphysis pubis via a large curved needle to two small incisions in the abdominal wall. The mesh is adjusted so that it does not transport any force to the urethra. It does not need to be sutured as the mesh stays in place due to friction of the surrounding tissues once the protective plastic sleeve covering the tape is removed.

Randomized controlled trials have shown that, as compared to Burch colposuspension, TVT is equally effective. When costs are taken into consideration, TVT appears to be more cost efficient (Ward and Hilton 2002; Manca et al. 2007). Complication rates range from 1% to 7% and include bladder and other organ perforation, bleeding, voiding dysfunction, and de novo irritating voiding symptoms (Karram 2003).

More recently, the transobturator (TO) approach was developed in an attempt to further minimize associated morbidity. During the TO approach the midurethral tape is also inserted by a midurethral vaginal incision of about 1 cm, but instead of being placed retropubically, the mesh is passed through the obturator foramen by long curved needles. During the TO approach, the mesh exits at both sides just lateral of the groin (Fig. 5.2.7, with permission of Elsevier), whereas during the RP approach, the mesh exits the abdominal wall just above the level of the pubic bone. Randomized controlled trials show similar results for the RP and TO approach (Sung et al. 2007). However, the TO approach is associated with fewer complications as it avoids the area of the bladder and the space of Retzius (Sung et al. 2007).

5.2.5.2.6 Urethral Bulking Agents

In the presence of intrinsic sphincter deficiency without urethral hypermobility, bulking agents are a surgical option. A urethral injection is performed into the submucosa of the bladder neck and can be performed as a transurethral injection via a cystourethroscope or as a peri-urethral injection using a needle adjacent to the urethra. Several agents have been used, including bovine collagen, polytetrafluoroethylene, silicone, pyrolytic carbon-coated zirconium oxide beads, and autologous fat or chondrocytes. Whereas the risk of complications is low, the success rates are also lower than with many of the other procedures with an overall long-term cure rate reported as 20–30%, but with another 50–60% of subjects noting marked improvement (Bent and McLennan 1998). Repeated injections frequently have to be performed as many injectables tend to migrate. A specific problem is the development of overactive bladder symptoms due to migration to the bladder neck. Freedom from complications, especially in the elderly, makes this a useful technique in selected patients.

5.2.5.2.7 Artificial Urethral Sphincter

Artificial urethral sphincters are indicated in case other surgical procedures fail. Another indication is to treat men with post-prostatectomy urinary

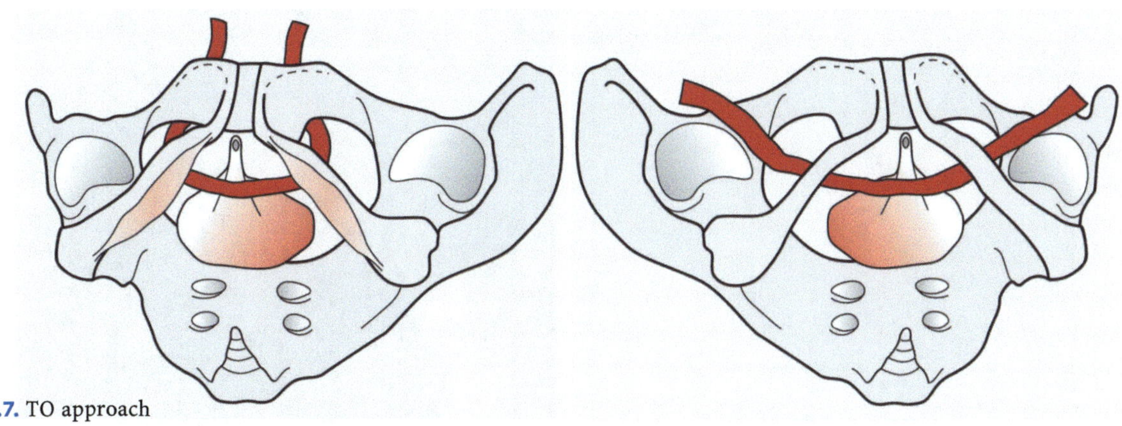

Fig. 5.2.7. TO approach

stress incontinence. An artificial sphincter is placed around the urethra, and a reservoir allows the sphincter to be inflated to maintain continence, and then deflated to allow emptying (Fig. 5.2.8). Success rates for the treatment of post-prostatectomy subjects are approximately 80%, but re-operation rates approach 50% for the treatment of complications, including infection and malfunction (Clemens et al. 2001). A review of 207 women treated with an artificial sphincter for intrinsic sphincter deficiency without mobility showed success in 88.7% with a re-operation of 5.9% (Costa et al. 2001).

5.2.6 Treatment of Urge or Neurogenic Urinary Incontinence

If the assessment of the patient revealed a plausible cause of urge urinary incontinence (secondary urge urinary incontinence), a causal treatment is the first choice. For example, if infection is found, incontinence will often disappear after antibiotic treatment of cystitis. Similarly disintegration and removal of bladder stones, transurethral resection of bladder

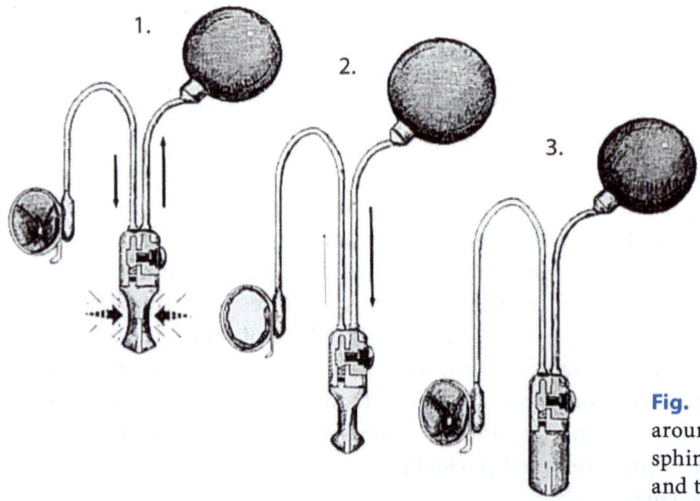

Fig. 5.2.8. An artificial sphincter is placed around the urethra, and a reservoir allows the sphincter to be inflated to maintain continence, and then deflated to allow emptying

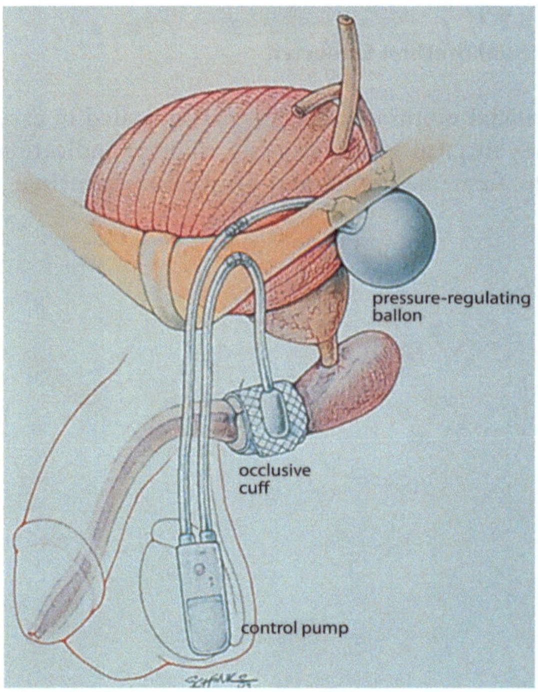

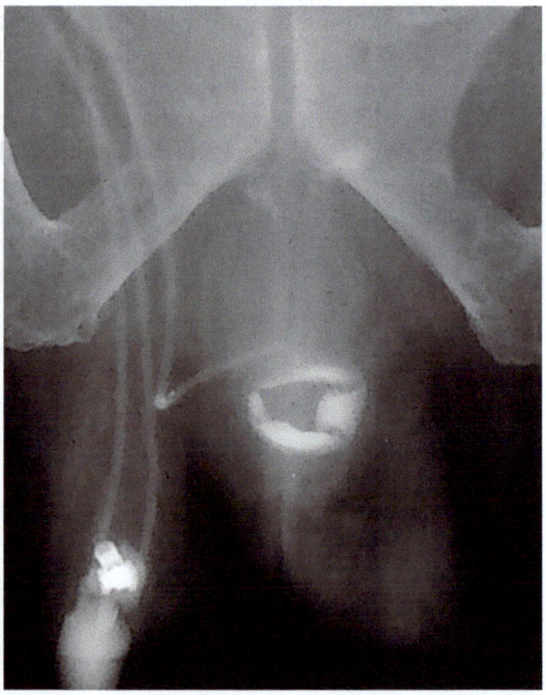

tumors, removal of foreign bodies in the bladder, etc., can prove effective.

The same strategy is applied to patients with neurogenic urinary incontinence if a causal therapy is available (e.g., L-DOPA treatment of Parkinson's patients). In patients with idiopathic urge urinary incontinence, neurogenic urinary incontinence due to detrusor overactivity without therapy directed at the specific cause or in those patients in whom causal therapy was not successful, symptomatic treatment is indicated. In patients with neurogenic urinary incontinence due to sphincter paralysis, stress urinary incontinence therapies might be applied (see Sect. 5.2.5). Treatment should always start with conservative methods and should only proceed with surgery if conservative methods have failed or had serious or bothersome side effects.

Most of the described conservative and surgical treatment options are well investigated. Cochrane collaboration meta-analyses are available for most of the conservative therapies (bladder training, pelvic floor muscle training, and oral medical treatment) and for botulinum toxin injections. Therefore, these treatment recommendations have the highest level of evidence (level 1a according to the Oxford classification). Randomized, placebo-controlled trials (level 1b according to the Oxford classification) are available for most of the other conservative and some of the operative therapies.

5.2.6.1 Conservative Treatment

All conservative treatment options can be used alone or in combination. Efficacy data are available for the mono-therapies, but combination treatment is expected to be more efficacious. Side effects are less frequent and less severe than with surgical treatments.

5.2.6.1.1 Behavior Therapy

Behavioral changes to avoid urinary leakage and increase the time between the voids should be an integral part treatment for urge urinary incontinence. Fluid intake and urine production have a linear relationship in men and women with undisturbed renal function. Abnormal drinking behavior with a high amount of fluid intake might be responsible for pollakisuria and even urinary incontinence. Fluid restriction before leaving the house or sleeping reduces urine production during this time and decreases bothersome urgency, frequency, or incontinence. However, fluid restriction should only be utilized temporarily, and the patient should keep drinking for about 1½ to 2 l within 24 h.

All drugs that cause detrusor overactivity and/or reduce urethral resistance are potentially able to cause or aggravate urinary incontinence. A recently written article demonstrated that direct or indirect parasympathomimetics, anti-depressants, serotonin-noradrenaline reuptake inhibitors, and hormonal replacement therapies (estrogens ± progestin) can cause detrusor overactivity (Tsakiris et al. 2008). Reduction of the dosage or change of the drug class might help avoiding or reducing incontinence episodes. Diuretic drugs for treatment of arterial hypertension can cause large, sudden effluxes of urine into the bladder that might trigger involuntary detrusor contractions (Diokno et al. 1991). Therefore, diuretics should not be used when a bathroom is unavailable or urgency, frequency, or incontinence is strictly unwarranted (e.g., before outside activities or at night). Diuretics should be changed to other drug classes, if possible. Caffeine or artificial sweeteners are implicated in causing and deteriorating detrusor overactivity and therefore should be reduced or avoided (Cartwright et al. 2007); caffeine-free coffee might be used instead.

5.2.6.1.2 Bladder Training

This conservative treatment modality, sometimes also classified as bladder drill or bladder re-training, contains three basic components: (1) patient information about bladder function and continence mechanisms, (2) scheduled voiding with fixed or flexible voiding intervals, and (3) positive reinforcement in order to give patients psychological support and encouragement (Fantl et al. 1991). The mechanism of action remains unclear, but may act via an increase of bladder capacity. Bladder training can be applied to patients who are physically and mentally fit and motivated. A voiding chart helps patients to realize their voiding frequency and encourages them to proceed with this conservative therapy approach. Bladder training can be combined with cognitive distraction techniques. A meta-analysis of bladder training trials was performed by the Cochrane collaboration showing that bladder training was more effective than no bladder training. Furthermore, the patients' perception of cure, quality of life, and side effects were in favor of bladder training when compared to anticholinergic treatment (oxybutynin, imipramine, or flavoxate), and bladder training was equally effective compared to pelvic floor muscle training with biofeedback (Wallace et al. 2004).

5.2.6.1.3 Pelvic Floor Muscle Training

Pelvic floor muscle training aims to improve pelvic organ support, increase intraurethral pressure during exertion or urgency, and intensify reflex inhibition of detrusor contractions. The training program consists of (1) well-timed, fast, and strong voluntary pelvic floor muscle contraction before and during exertion or urgency to increase the strength of the pelvic floor, (2) pelvic floor muscle endurance training, and (3) facilitation of pelvic floor muscle contraction through abdominal muscle contraction (Bø 2004). Pelvic floor muscle training is an active treatment and needs the active participation of the patient; therefore, the patient has to be motivated and physically fit to perform the program. Before treatment, the patient should be instructed about the pelvic floor anatomy, pelvic floor function, treatment program, and therapy goal. During treatment, the effects should be controlled by a physiotherapist or nurse practitioner. Pelvic floor exercises need to be performed for at least 2 months before significant effects can be expected. Pelvic floor muscle training was originally used to treat stress urinary incontinence, but showed favorable effects in patients with urge or mixed incontinence as well. A meta-analysis by the Cochrane collaboration demonstrated that pelvic floor muscle training can cure or improve urge urinary incontinence with a likelihood ratio of more than 2 compared to inactive treatments (Hay-Smith and Dumoulin 2006). However, pelvic floor muscle exercises are more effective in patients with stress urinary incontinence, especially in young patients and those who perform the pelvic floor muscle training more than 3 months.

5.2.6.1.4 Neurostimulation

Squeezing of the penile glans has been shown to suppress detrusor contractions by mechanical stimulation of the dorsal penile nerve, which is the most superficial branch of the pudendal nerve (Kondo et al. 1982). During neurostimulation, nerves and muscles are directly stimulated by electrical current, hereby influencing the activity of the bladder and urethral sphincters (van der Balken et al. 2004). The exact working mechanism is still unknown, but stimulation of pudendal nerves with consecutive stimulation of sympathetic hypogastric inhibitory neurons or central inhibition of pelvic parasympathomimetic excitatory neurons is most likely responsible for the favorable effects of neurostimulation (Lindström et al. 1983). Electrical stimulation seems to be more efficacious than mechanical stimulation. Electrical current should be administered close to the pudendal nerves in order to achieve neurostimulation; transvaginal, transrectal, penile, or clitoral stimulation is suitable for this purpose. Neurostimulation needs to be performed for a long period to achieve significant clinical effects and, after stopping the therapy, symptomatic relapse occurs frequently. Electrical stimuli might be painful in patients with normal sensation and, therefore, the patient has to be motivated to proceed with this treatment. However, neurostimulation is a viable treatment option for patients with neurogenic detrusor overactivity and impaired sensation of the lower abdomen.

5.2.6.1.5 Peripheral Neuromodulation

Neuromodulation is defined as the physiological process in which the influence of the activity in one neural pathway modulates the pre-existing activity in another via synaptic interaction (Craggs and McFarlane 1999). In other words, neurostimulation influences bladder function directly and neuromodulation indirectly. Somehow contradictory is the fact that most neuromodulation procedures contain the word "stimulation," which is incorrect when considered as the proposed working mechanism, but correct when one considers that electrical current has to be applied to stimulate one system in order to modulate the other. Peripheral application of electrical current leads to central inhibition of the bladder and suppression of detrusor overactivity. Furthermore, neuromodulation may lead to reorganization of the neuronal systems that control the bladder centrally and peripherally as well as to restoration of normal reflex patterns (Fall 1984). Peripheral neuromodulation can be performed by stimulation of the suprapubic skin or S2/S3 dermatome (percutaneous electrical nerve stimulation, TENS), thigh muscle, or tibial nerve (percutaneous tibial nerve stimulation, PTNS). Urodynamic studies revealed a decrease of detrusor overactivity and an increase of bladder capacity. A randomized, crossover study of patients with detrusor overactivity that were treated with TENS or the muscarinic receptor antagonist oxybutinin showed efficacy in favor of oxybutinin (Soomro et al. 2001). Nevertheless, peripheral neuromodulation is a viable treatment option for patients who prefer this treatment approach or are not suitable for other treatments.

5.2.6.1.6 Medical Treatment

Muscarinic receptors on the surface of detrusor cells mediate detrusor contractions after acetylcholine stimulation. In the human bladder wall, only muscarinic receptors type M_2 and M_3 are expressed, of which M_3 receptors are exclusively responsible for detrusor contraction in healthy individuals. However, M_2 receptors also mediate detrusor contractions in patients with neurogenic bladder dysfunction. Muscarinic receptor antagonists (anticholinergics) are drugs that block type M_2 and M_3 receptors and prevent or decrease involuntary detrusor contractions. Darifenacin, fesoterodine, oxybutynin, propiverin, solifenacin, tolterodine, and trospium chloride are registered drugs for oral use in adults (Table 5.2.2). Other drugs (e.g., tricyclic antidepressants or calcium channel blockers) have limited use these days for the oral treatment of urge or neurogenic urinary incontinence due to the unspecific inhibition of receptors and poor efficacy. All anticholinergic drugs increase bladder capacity and compliance and decrease urgency, frequency, and urinary incontinence significantly. Urge urinary incontinence episodes disappear in approximately 50% of patients, and subjective improvement is achieved in approximately 75% of patients. A Cochrane collaboration meta-analysis compared anticholinergic drugs with placebo and demonstrated that all anticholinergic drugs are equally effective, and all muscarinic receptor antagonists are significantly better in improving symptoms when compared to placebo (Nabi et al. 2006). A second Cochrane collaboration meta-analysis compared anticholinergic drugs with other non-medical therapies (bladder training, behavior therapy) and concluded that objective improvement was more common in patients with anticholinergic drugs, and the combination of anticholinergic drugs with bladder training was more effective than bladder training alone (Alhasso et al. 2006). Anticholinergic side effects are dry mouth, tachycardia, hypertension, constipation, blurred vision, fatigue, queasiness, vomiting, or confusion. All side effects occur significantly more frequently compared to placebo (Nabi et al. 2006).

Table 5.2.2. Registered anticholinergic drugs for the oral treatment of overactive bladder in children and adults. The dosages refer to adult Caucasians

Drug	Recommended daily dosage
Darifenacin	1×7.5–15 mg
Fesoterodine	1×4–8 mg
Oxybutynin	2–4×5 mg
	1×10 mg
Propiverin	2–4×15 mg
	1×30 mg
Solifenacin	1×5–10 mg
Tolterodine	2×1–2 mg
	1×4 mg
Trospium chloride	3×5–15 mg

Installation of drugs into the bladder (e.g., oxybutynin, capsaicin, and resiniferatoxin) is feasible for patients who are already on or are willing to perform intermittent self-catheterization. The efficacy of the drug can be increased due to the use of a higher dosage (oxybutynin until 0.7 mg/kg body weight/day), and systemic side effects can be avoided. Capsaicin and resiniferatoxin do not have an official registration yet, and therefore legal and reimbursement problems might appear.

5.2.6.2 Surgical Treatment

Operations should only be considered when conservative methods have failed or had serious or bothersome side effects. The patient needs to have an adequate performance status because surgery requires anesthesia, which might cause serious side effects itself. Transurethral procedures are performed while rinsing the bladder in order to allow good vision. In patients with neurogenic bladder dysfunction, rapid bladder filling, filling the bladder with cold rinsing fluid, or overdistension of the bladder might cause autonomic dysregulation, which results in hypotension or even cardiac arrest. Furthermore, adequate positioning of the patient for surgery is essential for achieving the treatment goal. Some patients with bone malformations are difficult to position adequately and therefore have to be excluded from certain procedures. While considering operations one has to bear in mind that patients from Third World countries do not have the opportunity or money to have repeated surgery, readjustments, catheters, or other supporting devices.

5.2.6.2.1 Botulinum Toxin Injections

The neurotoxin of the gram-positive, anaerobic bacterium Clostridium botulinum can be injected through a cystoscope and needle into the detrusor and causes irreversible blockage of acetylcholine release at the neuromuscular junction. This chemodenervation lasts approximately 6–12 months; the paralytic effects diminish after sprouting of the terminal nerve endings and re-innervation. Therefore, periodical re-injections are necessary to maintain the effects. Botulinum toxin should be injected in all parts of the bladder to allow equal distribution of the neurotoxin; 15–30 injection sites are usually sufficient to cover all parts of the bladder. Of the seven sub-types of botulinum toxins, only types A and type B are commercially available. There are differences in the biological activities among these products, and therefore different dosages have to be injected for different products. Furthermore, treatment of neurogenic detrusor overactivity needs a higher dosage than treatment of idiopathic detrusor overactivity. Botulinum toxin injections show excellent effects by increasing bladder capacity, bladder compliance, and the quality of life of the treated patients, decreasing urgency, frequency, and the amount of involuntary detrusor contractions as well as reducing urinary leakage (Schurch et al. 2005). A meta-analysis of the Cochrane collaboration confirmed superior effects compared to placebo or resiniferatoxin (Duthie et al. 2007). Botulinum toxin for the treatment of neurogenic detrusor overactivity is officially registered only in Switzerland (2007).

5.2.6.2.2 Sacral Neuromodulation

Sacral neuromodulation is an operative procedure in which an electrode is implanted in the sacral foramen S_3 unilaterally or bilaterally. The electrode is connected with an impulse generator that is positioned subcutaneously in the buttock or ventral abdominal wall (Fig. 5.2.9). The impulse generator is battery driven and sends electrical impulses continuously to the sacral nerves, suppressing involuntary detrusor contractions via afferent pudendal nerve stimulation and central inhibitory pathway activation. However, the exact working mechanism is still under discussion (van der Pal et al. 2006). Approximately 30% of patients who were therapy-resistant to conservative treatment modalities respond to sacral neuromodulation; therefore, test stimulations with temporarily and percutaneously implanted electrodes and an external impulse generator are used to evaluate treatment effects. Implantation of a permanent device (InterStim® system, Medtronic) is likely to be successful if the voiding frequency or incontinence episodes have decreased by at least 50% during the test stimulation. The treatment effect during test stimulation and after permanent placement is dependent on the position of the sacral electrodes. Therefore, X-ray imaging is routinely performed to control the position of the electrode(s) after placement (Figs. 5.2.10 and 5.2.11). More than 75% of the patients in whom the InterStim® system was implanted report a significant reduction of urgency, frequency, and urinary incontinence after the implantation (Grünewald and Jonas 2000). After 5 years, 68% of patients with urge incontinence and 56% of patients with urgency and frequency still had successful outcomes (van Kerrebroeck et al. 2007).

5.2.6.2.3 Bladder Augmentation

All different types of bladder augmentations aim to increase bladder capacity, reduce intravesical pressure, and equalize intravesical pressure during involuntary detrusor contractions. The two main types of bladder augmentations are autoaugmentation and intestinal augmentation. During the operation of both types of augmentations, the patient lies in the supine position, and the bladder is exposed via a median or transverse laparatomy.

- During autoaugmentation, the detrusor of the anterior bladder wall and bladder dome is split until the mucosa, which, however, has to remain intact. After several weeks, a bladder diverticulum forms at this place. The wall of the diverticulum only consists of bladder mucosa that is unable to contract during voluntary or involuntary detrusor contractions. During detrusor contractions,

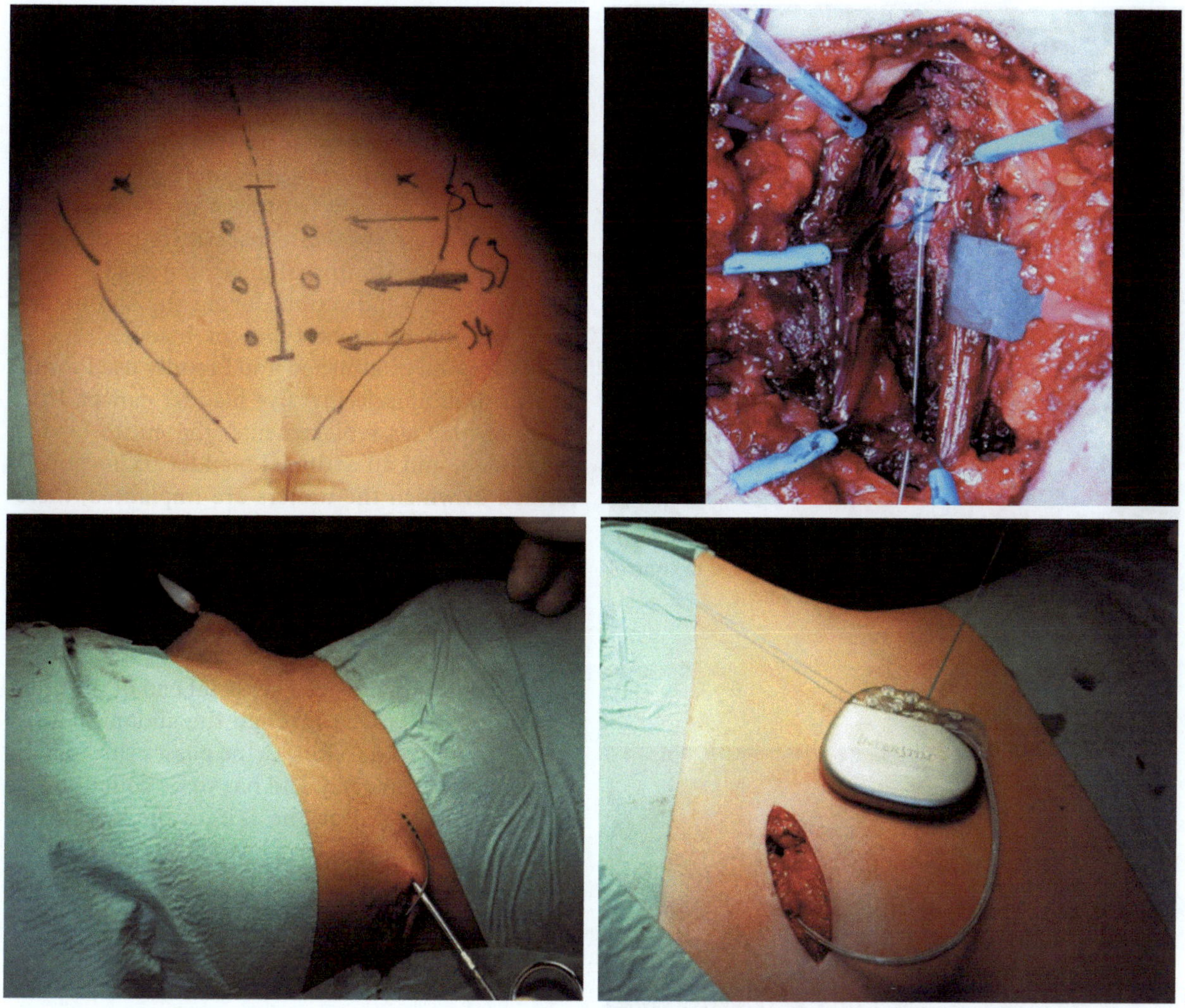

a b c d

Fig. 5.2.9a–d. The electrode is connected with an impulse generator that is positioned subcutaneously in the buttock or ventral abdominal wall

the intravesical pressure remains stable due to the windkessel effect of the diverticulum wherein the diverticulum expands to relieve pressure during bladder contractions that occur in the absence of urethral relaxation.

- During intestinal augmentation, the entire bladder wall is split in a vertical fashion, reaching from the trigone of the posterior bladder wall until the bladder neck of the anterior wall (clam cystoplasty). An anti-mesenterially detubularized segment of the small or large intestine is sutured into the gap of the split bladder wall. As a result, a bladder diverticulum forms at this place. The wall of the bladder diverticulum consists of the intestinal wall, which is not able to contract during voluntary or involuntary detrusor contractions. Furthermore, partial denervation of the bladder during clam cystoplasty is also responsible for suppression of detrusor overactivity.

Success rates in terms of treatment of urinary incontinence and reduction of intravesical pressure vary between 50–85%. Intestinal augmentation seems to have higher success rates, most probably due to the additional effect of partial denervation. Up to 45% of the patients with a bladder augmentation need to perform intermittent self-catheterization due to the high amount of postvoid residual urine. The diverticulum can be imaged with X-ray after transurethral or suprapubic filling of the bladder with contrast media (Fig. 5.2.12).

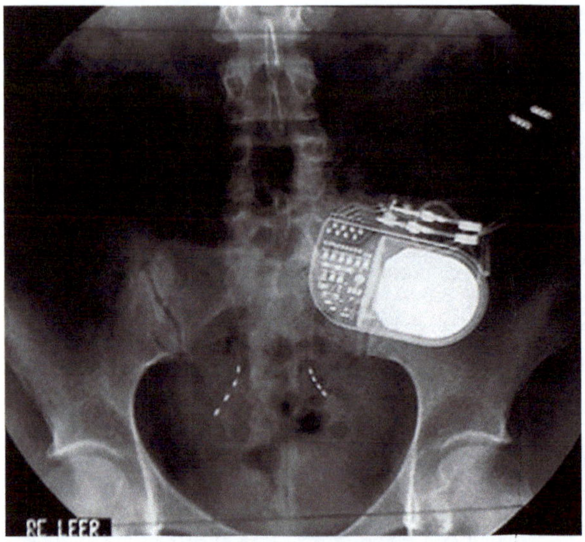

Fig. 5.2.10. X-ray imaging is routinely performed to control the position of the electrode(s) after placement

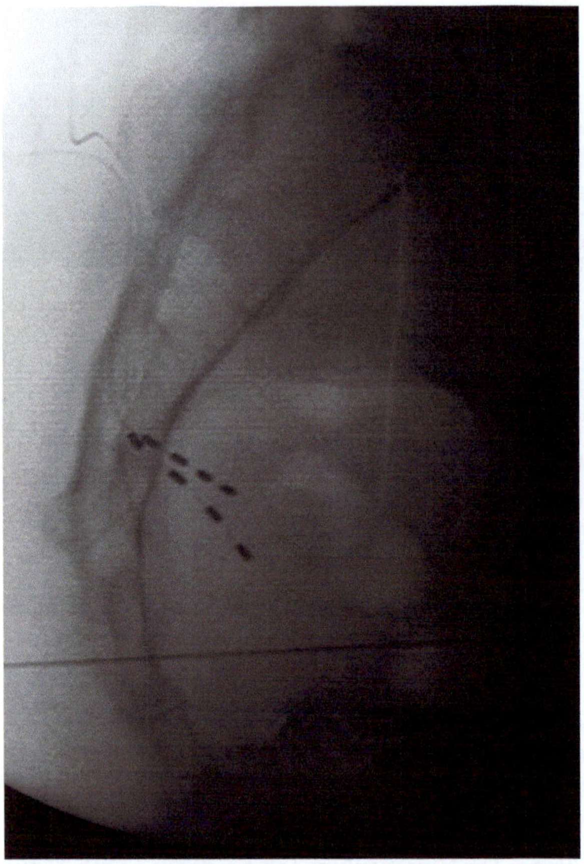

Fig. 5.2.11. X-ray imaging is routinely performed to control the position of the electrode(s) after placement

5.2.6.2.4 Bladder Replacement–Urinary Diversion

If all conservative or less invasive operative treatment strategies have failed to treat urinary incontinence successfully, bladder replacement is the last option. With new treatment methods and increasing efficacy of other conservative or operative treatments, urinary diversion seldom has been performed for this indication during the last decade. However, the different types of bladder replacements are well established and broadly used for the treatment of muscle-invasive bladder cancer. In all types of bladder replacements, the entire bladder is resected, and an artificial bladder of intestine is formed in which the ureters are implanted; therefore, the smooth muscle of the bladder, the producer of detrusor overactivity, is removed. The three main types of bladder replacements are:

- Conduits: a segment of colon or ileum is taken from the intestinal and the ureters are sutured into the proximal end. The distal end of the intestinal tube is guided through the abdominal wall and sutured to the skin. Urine passes through the conduit continuously and has to be collected in a bag that is pasted on the skin at the level of the conduit opening.
- Heterotopic neobladders: after removal of the bladder, a neobladder (pouch) is formed of ileum and/or colon. The neobladder is located in a

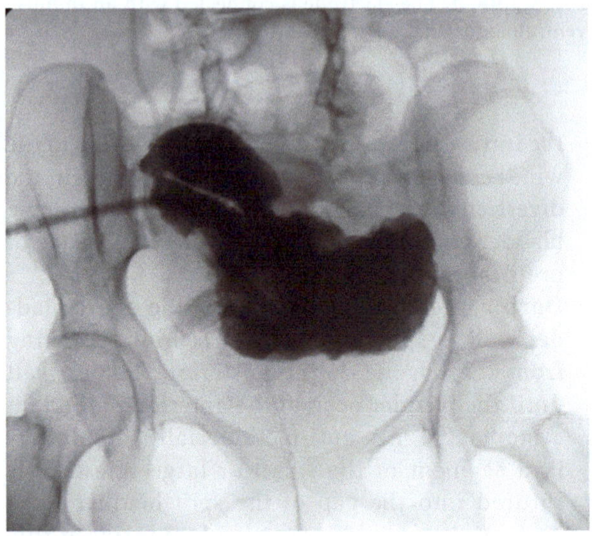

Fig. 5.2.12. The diverticulum can be imaged with X-ray after transurethral or suprapubic filling of the bladder with contrast media

position outside of the bladder bed (heterotopic, suprapubic urinary diversion), and a tube to the skin is created with the help of small intestine or the vermiform appendix; this tube usually ends in the umbilicus. The different types of heterotopic neobladders use a variable amount of small and/or large intestine; examples are the Mainz I or Kock pouches. The patients have to catheterize themselves several times per day via the navel-neobladder tube. A special type of heterotopic neobladder is the Mainz II pouch, which is created by plication of recto-sigmoid colon and implantation of the ureters in an anti-refluxive fashion; the patient empties urine during defecation.

- Orthotopic neobladders: the bladder can be removed with (supra-trigonal orthotopic neobladder) or without the trigone (infra-trigonal orthotopic neobladder). A neobladder is formed with the small and/or large intestine and sutured on the trigone or urethral stump. Therefore, the neobladder is positioned in the old bladder bed (orthotopic); examples are the Hautmann, Studer, or hemi-Kock pouches. Patients empty their neobladder by urethral sphincter relaxation and straining or by self-catheterization.

Conduits or heterotopic neobladders are also used to treat stress urinary incontinence. However, orthotopic neobladders are not suitable for the treatment of stress urinary incontinence because the patient would continue to lose urine due to the insufficient urethral closure mechanism. All types of urinary diversions have the disadvantage that, beside the full range of intraoperative complications, urine is reabsorbed by the intestinal mucosa, which might cause metabolic problems. A fibrotic stenosis at the uretero-intestinal anastomosis or at the skin level might cause hydronephrosis and renal insufficiency. Stone formation in hetero- or orthotopic neobladders might cause hematuria, chronic infection, or hydronephrosis. If the distal ileum was used, malabsorption of vitamin B_{12} can occur, which might cause megaloblastic anemia several years after the operation. Chronic contact of urine on the mucosa of the intestinal segment might also cause chronic inflammation (pouchitis) or even colorectal carcinoma.

References

Abrams P, Cardozo L, Fall M et al (2002) The standardisation of terminology of lower urinary tract function: report from the standardisation sub-committee of the International Continence Society. Neurourol Urodyn 21:167–178

Ahmad I, Granitsiotis P (2007) Urological follow-up of adult spina bifida patients. Neurourol Urodyn 26:978–980

Alhasso AA, McKinlay J, Patrick K, Steward L (2006) Anticholinergic drugs versus non-drug active therapies for overactive bladder syndrome in adults. Cochrane database for systematic reviews, issue 4. Art No: CD003193. DOI: 10.1002/14651858.CD003193.pub3

Artibani W, Cerruto MA (2005) The role of imaging in urinary incontinence. BJU Int 95:699–703

Bailey R (1990) How much information can be obtained from frequency/volume charts. Neurourol Urodyn 9:382–383

Bakas P, Liapis A, Creatsas G (2002) Q-tip test and tension-free vaginal tape in the management of female patients with genuine stress incontinence. Gynecol Obstet Ivest 53:170–173

Bent AE, McLennan M (1998) Surgical management of urinary incontinence. Obstet Gynecol Clin North Am 25:883–906

Bergman A, Bhatia NN (1985) Urodynamics: effect of urinary tract infection on urethral and bladder function. Obstet Gynecol 66:366–371

Bergman A, Elia G (1995) Three surgical procedures for genuine stress incontinence. Five-year follow-up of a prospective randomized study. Am J Obstet Gynecol 173:66–71

Bhatia NN, Bergman A (1985) Pessary test in women with urinary incontinence. Obstet Gynecol 65:220–226

Bø K (2004) Pelvic floor muscle training is effective in treatment of female stress urinary incontinence, but how does it work? Int Urogyn J Pelvic Floor Dysfunc 15:76–84

Boy S, Reitz A, Wirth B et al (2006) Facilitatory neuromodulative effect of duloxetine on pudendal motor neurons controlling the urethral pressure: a functional urodynamic study in healthy women. Eur Urol 50:119–125

Brown J, Grady D, Ouslander J et al (1999) Prevalence of urinary incontinence and associated risk factors in postmenopausal women. Obstet Gynecol 94:66–70

Bump RC, Norton PA (1998) Epidemiology and natural history of pelvic floor dysfunction. Obstet Gynecol Clin North Am 25:723–746

Bump RC, Mattiasson A, Bø K et al (1996) The standardization of terminology of female pelvic organ prolapse and pelvic floor dysfunction. Am J Obstet Gynecol 175:10–17

Bump RC, Benson JT, Yalcin I, Zhao YD, Peng G (2004) Biomechanical and electrophsiological effects of duloxetine in women with stress urinary incontinence. www.continet.org/publications/2004/PDF/0269.PDF

Burgio KL, Matthews KA, Engel BT (1991) Prevalence, incidence and correlates of urinary incontinence in healthy, middle-aged women. J Urol 146:1255–1259

Cartwright R, Srikrishna S, Cardozo L, Gonzalez J (2007) Does diet Coke cause overactive bladder? A 4-week crossover trial, investigating the effect of carbonated soft drinks on overactive bladder symptoms in normal volunteers. Neurourol Urodyn 26:626–627

Clemens JQ, Schuster TG, Konnak JW, McGuire EJ, Faerber GJ (2001) Revision rate after artificial urinary sphincter

implantation for incontinence after radical prostatectomy: actuarial analysis. J Urol 166:1372–1375
Costa P, Mottet N, Rabut B, Thuret R, Ben Naoum K, Wagner L (2001) The use of an artificial urinary sphincter in women with type III incontinence and a negative Marshall test. J Urol 165:1172–1176
Craggs M, McFarlane J (1999) Neuromodulation of the lower urinary tract. Exp Physiol 84:149–160
de Groat WC (1998) Anatomy of the central neural pathways controlling the lower urinary tract. Eur Urol 1:2–5
DeLancey JOL (1994) Structural support of the urethra as it relates to stress urinary incontinence: the hammock hypothesis. Am J Obstet Gynecol 170:1713–1720
DeLancey JOL, Ashton-Miller JA (2004) Pathophysiology of adult urinary incontinence. Gastroenterology 126 (Suppl 1):S23–S32
Diokno AC, Brown MB, Brock BM, Herzog AR, Normolle DP (1988) Clinical and cystometric characteristics of continent and incontinent on institutionalized elderly. J Urol 140:567–571
Diokno AC, Brown MD, Herzog AR (1991) Relationship between use of diuretics and continence status in the elderly. Urology 38:3 9–42
Dmochowski R, Miklos JR, Norton PA et al (2003) Duloxetine versus placebo for the treatment of North American women with stress urinary incontinence. J Urol 170 (4 Pt 1):1259–1263
Duthie J, Wilson DI, Herbison GP, Wilson D (2007) Botulinum toxin injections for adults with overactive bladder syndrome. Cochrane database for systematic reviews, issue 3. Art no: CD005493. DOI: 10.1002/14651858.CD005493.pub2
Enhörning G (1961) Simultaneous recording of intravesical and intraurethral pressure. Acta Chir Scand 276:1–68
Fall M (1984) Does electrostimulation cure urinary incontinence? J Urol 131:664–667
Fantl A, Wyman JF, McClish DK et al (1991) Efficacy of bladder training in older women with urinary incontinence. JAMA 265:609–613
Fischer, Rasmussen W, Hansen RI, Stage P (1986) Predictive values of diagnostic tests in the evaluation of female urinary stress incontinence. Acta Obstet Gynecol Scand 159:145–149
Foldsprang A, Mommsen S (1994) Adult female urinary incontinence and childhood bedwetting. J Urol 152:85–88
Glavind K, Nøhr SB, Walter S (1996) Biofeedback and physiotherapy versus physiotherapy alone in the treatment of genuine stress urinary incontinence. Int Urogynecol J 7:339–343
Goode PS, Burgio KL, Locher JL et al (2003) Effect of behavioral training with or without pelvic floor electrical stimulation on stress incontinence in women: a randomized controlled trial. JAMA 290:345–352
Grünewald V, Jonas U (2000) Neurostimulation for lower urinary tract voiding problems. Curr Urol Rep 1:199–203
Hay-Smith EJ, Dumoulin C (2006) Pelvic floor muscle training versus no treatment, or inactive control treatments, for urinary incontinence in women. Cochrane Database Syst Rev, issue 1. Art no. CD005654. DOI: 10.1002/14651858.CD005654
Hilton P, Stanton SL (1981) Algorithmic method for assessing urinary incontinence in elderly women. Br Med J 282:940–942
Hsu TK, Rackley RR, Appell RA (1999) The supine stress test: A simple method to detect intrinsic urethral sphincter dysfunction. J Urol 162:460–463
Hunskaar S, Arnold EP, Burgio K, Diokno AC, Herzog AR, Mallett VT (2000) Epidemiology and natural history of urinary incontinence. Int Urogyn J Pelvic Floor Dysfunc 11:301–319
Jackson SL, Weber AM, Hull TL, Mitchinson AR, Walters MD (1997) Fecal incontinence in women with urinary incontinence and pelvic organ prolapse. Obstet Gynecol 89:423–427
Kamo I, Cannon TW, Conway DA (2004) The role of bladder-to-urethral reflexes in urinary continence mechanisms in rats. Am J Physiol Renal Physiol 287:F434–F441
Karram M, Segal JL, Vassallo BJ, Kleeman SD (2003) Complications and untoward effect of the tension-free vaginal tape procedure. Obstet Gynecol 101:929–932
Karram MM, Bhatia NN (1988) The Q-tip test: standardization of the technique and its interpretation in women with urinary incontinence. Obstet Gynecol 71:807–811
Kim S, Harvey MA, Johnston S (2005) A review of the epidemiology and pathophysiology of pelvic floor dysfunction: do racial differences matter? J Obstet Gynaecol Can 27:251–259
Kjølhede P (2005) Long-term efficacy of Burch colposuspension: a 14-year follow-up study. Acta Obstet Gynecol Scand 84:767–772
Kondo A, Otani T, Takita T (1982) Suppression of bladder instability by penile squeeze. Br J Urol 54:360–362
Larsson G, Abrams P, Victor A (1991) The frequency/volume chart in detrusor instability. Neurourol Urodyn 10:533–543
Lentz SS (1995) Osteitis pubis: a review. Obstet Gynecol Surv 50:310–315
Lindström S, Fall M, Carlsson CA, Erlandson BE (1983) The neurophysiological basis of bladder inhibition in response to intravaginal electrical stimulation. J Urol 129:405–410
Malmsten UG, Milsom I, Molander U, Norlén LJ (1997) Urinary incontinence and lower urinary tract symptoms: an epidemiological study of men aged 45 to 99 years. J Urol 158:1733–1737
Manca A, Sculpher MJ, Ward K, Hilton P (2007) A cost-utility analysis of tension-free vaginal tape versus colposuspension for primary urodynamic stress incontinence. Br J Obstet Gynecol 3 110:255–262
Michel MC, Oelke M, Pieters SL (2005) The neuro-urological connection. Eur Urol (Suppl) 4:18–29
Migliorini GD, Glenning PP (1987) Bonney's test, fact or fiction? Br J Obstet Gynecol 94:157–159
Millard RJ, Moore K, Rencken R, Yalcin I, Bump RC (2004) Duloxetine Urinary Incontinence Study Group. Duloxetine vs placebo in the treatment of stress urinary incontinence: a four-continent randomized clinical trial. BJU Int 93:311–318
Miller JM, Ashton-Miller JA, DeLancey JO (1998) A pelvic muscle precontraction can reduce cough-related urine loss in selected women with mild SUI. J Am Geriatr Soc 46:870–874
Moore KH, Simons A, Dowell C, Bryant C, Prashar S (1999) Efficacy and user acceptability of the urethral occlusive device in women with urinary incontinence. J Urol 162:464–468

Nabi G, Cody JD, Ellis G, Herbison P, Hay-Smith J (2006) Anticholinergic drugs versus placebo for overactive bladder syndrome in adults. Cochrane Database Syst Rev, issue 4. Art no. CD003781. DOI: 10.1002/14651858.CD003781.pub2

Norton PA, Zinner NR, Yalcin I, Bump RC (2002) Duloxetine Urinary Incontinence Study Group. Duloxetine versus placebo in the treatment of stress urinary incontinence. Am J Obstet Gynecol 187:40–48

Oelke M, Roovers JP (2008) Continence: bladder neck vs mid-urethra. In: Badlani G, Davila GW, Michel MC, de la Rosette JJ (eds) Continence: current concepts and treatment strategies. Springer, London

Oelke M, Roovers JP, Michel MC (2006) Safety and tolerability of duloxetine in women with stress urinary incontinence. Brit J Obstet Gynecol 113 (Suppl 1):22–26

Olsen AL, Smith VJ, Bergstrom JO, Colling JC, Clark AL (1997) Epidemiology of surgically managed pelvic organ prolapse and urinary incontinence. Obstet Gynecol 98:501–506

Persson J, Wolner-Hansse P, Rydhstroem H (2000) Obstetric risk factors for stress urinary incontinence: a population-based study. Obstet Gynecol 96:440–445

Petros PE, Ulmsten U (1990) An integral theory of female urinary incontinence. Experimental and clinical considerations. Acta Obstet Gynecol Scand 153:7–31

Rekers H, Drogendijk AC, Valkenburg HA, Riphagen F (1992) The menopause, urinary incontinence and other symptoms of the genito-urinary tract. Maturitas 15:101–111

Roberts RO, Jacobsen SJ, Rhodes T et al (1998) Urinary incontinence in a community-based cohort: prevalence and healthcare seeking. J Am Geriatr Soc 46:467–472

Rortveit G, Daltveit AM, Hannestad YS et al (2003) Urinary incontinence after vaginal delivery or cesarean section. N Engl J Med 348: 900–907

Schulman C, Claes H, Matthijs J (1997) Urinary incontinence in Belgium: a population-based epidemiological survey. Eur Urol 32:315–320

Schurch B, de Seze M, Denys P et al (2005) Botulinum toxin type A is a safe and effective treatment for neurogenic urinary incontinence: results of a single treatment, randomized, placebo-controlled 6-month study. J Urol 174:196–200

Shumaker SA, Wyman JF, Uebersax JS, McClish D, Fanti JA (1994) Health related quality of life measures for women with urinary incontinence; The Urogenital Distress Inventory and the Incontinence Impact Questionnaire. Quality Life Res 3:291–306

Singhal B, Mathew KM (1999) Factors affecting mortality and morbidity in adult spina bifida. Eur J Pediatr Surg 9:31–32

Soergel TM, Shott S, Heit M (2001) Poor surgical outcomes after fascia lata allograft slings. Int Urogynecol J 12:247–253

Soomro NA, Khadra MH, Robson W, Neal DE (2001) A cross-over randomized trial of transcutaneous electrical nerve stimulation and oxybutinin in patients with detrusor instability. J Urol 166:146–149

Sung VW, Schleinitz MD, Rardin CR, Ward RM, Myers DL (2007) Comparison of retropubic vs transobturator approach to midurethral slings: a systematic review and meta-analysis. Am J Obstet Gynecol 197:3–11

Thor KB, Katofiasc MA (1995) Effects of duloxetine, a combined serotonin and norepinephrine reuptake inhibitor, on central neural control of lower urinary tract function in the chloralose-anesthetized female cat. J Pharmacol Exp Ther 274:1014–1024

Toba K, Ouchi Y, Orimo H et al (2008) Urinary incontinence in elderly inpatients in Japan: a comparison between general and geriatric hospitals. Aging 8:47–54

Tsakiris P, Oelke M, Michel MC (2008) Drug-induced urinary incontinence. Drugs Discovery Today: in press

Uebersax JS, Wyman JF, Shumaker SA, McClish DK, Fantl JA (1995) Short forms to assess life quality and symptom distress for urinary incontinence in women: The Incontinence Impact Questionnaire and the Urogenital Distress Inventory. Neurourol Urodyn 14:131–139

van der Balken MR, Vergunst H, Bemelmans BL (2004) The use of electrical devices for the treatment of bladder dysfunction: a review of methods. J Urol 172:846–851

van der Pal F, Heesakkers JP, Bemelmans BL (2006) Current opinion on the working mechanisms of neuromodulation in the treatment of lower urinary tract dysfunction. Curr Opin Urol 16:261–267

van der Vaart CH, de Leeuw JR, Roovers JP, Heintz AP (2000) De invloed van urine-incontinentie op de kwaliteit van leven bij thuiswonende Nederlandse vrouwen van 45–70 jaar. Ned Tijdschr Geneeskd 144:894–897

van Kerrebroeck PE, van Voskuilen AC, Heesakkers JP et al (2007) Results of sacral neuromodulation therapy for urinary voiding dysfunction: outcomes of a prospective, worldwide clinical study. J Urol 178:2029–2034

Vierhout ME, Lose G (1997) Preventive vaginal and intra-urethral devices in the treatment of female urinary stress incontinence. Curr Opin Obstet Gynecol 9:325–328

Wallace SA, Roe B, Williams K, Palmer M (2004) Bladder training for urinary incontinence in adults. Cochrane Database Syst Rev, issue 1. Art no. CD001308. DOI: 10.1002/14651558. CD001308.pub2

Ward K, Hilton P (2002) United Kingdom and Ireland Tension-free Vaginal Tape Trial Group. Prospective multicentre randomised trial of tension-free vaginal tape and colposuspension as primary treatment for stress incontinence. BMJ 325:67–70

Yarnell JW, Voyle GJ, Sweetnam PM, Milbank J, Richards CJ, Stephenson TP (1982) Factors associated with urinary incontinence in women. J Epidemiol Community Health 36:58–63

Zinner NR, Sterling AM, Ritter RC (1980) Role of inner urethral softness and urinary continence. Urology 16:115–117

Coloproctological Dysfunction

6.1 Constipation and Prolapse

Steve Halligan

CONTENTS

6.1.1 Introduction

Constipation is a symptom that we all have experienced at some time or another. While the vast majority of patients with constipation need no specialist medical investigation, the radiological investigation of severely affected patients has attracted considerable attention over recent years. This has happened in tandem with the parallel development of techniques for physiologic assessment and a greater understanding of the pathophysiology of the condition. Ultimately, despite this wealth of research, the role of imaging remains controversial. This chapter will define the role of evacuation proctography in the investigation of severely constipated patients and will stress the importance of a balanced interpretation that takes account of both structural and functional imaging findings in these individuals.

S. Halligan, MD, FRCR, MRCP
Professor of Gastrointestinal Radiology, Department of Specialist X-Ray, University College Hospital, 235 Euston Road, London, NW1 2BU, UK

6.1.2 Constipation

Constipation is the 'diseases of diseases' (Whorton 2000). The belief that constipation predisposes to "internal putrefaction" has been widely held since at least the 16th century BC (Ebbell 1937). By the beginning of the 19th century, there was a general medical consensus that constipation was the foremost disease of civilisation, a universal affliction of the industrialised societies. This concept was buttressed by the discovery that bacteria cause infection, thereby proving that "the colon was a sewage pit teeming with bacteria, a cesspit that, in patients with constipation, was not being regularly emptied" (Whorton 2000). Such concepts led directly to the notion of "autointoxication" – that the constipated patient was slowly and inevitably poisoning himself. The constipated patient, Charles Bouchard declared, "is always working towards his own destruction; he makes continual attempts at suicide by intoxication" (Bouchard 1906). The inevitable culmination of such theories is undoubtedly best expressed by the surgeon Arbuthnot Lane who, in the early 20th century, advocated colectomy as the cure-all for practically any disease you might care to mention (Lane 1913). Even in the 21st century, the notion of anto-intoxication remains alive and well; colonic irrigationists are enjoying thriving business despite no substantial evidence that their "therapy" is beneficial.

What is constipation? While all of us are familiar with the term, it should be borne in mind that it merely describes a symptom and so means different things to different people. Furthermore, because of the private nature of defaecation, what passes for normal bowel habit is particularly subjective and infrequently discussed. For example, there is considerable individual variation in response when people are asked to define constipation (Sandler and

Drossman 1987). Some will concentrate on bowel frequency, whilst others will be more concerned with ease of defecation, for example stool size and consistency, and the need for prolonged straining. Indeed, most people have more than one definition. Because of this, it is generally accepted that a satisfactory definition of constipation must include concepts of both infrequent defecation and difficult evacuation. While a globally valid definition of constipation probably remains elusive, the following is broadly applicable: infrequent stools defined by less than three per week and/or difficult evacuation defined by forceful straining for more than 25 per cent of the total time spent in the lavatory (Drossman 1994).

Chronic constipation is very common. It has been estimated that one in five apparently healthy middle-aged adults have symptoms suggesting functional constipation (Talley et al. 1993). In 1989 it was estimated that there were approximately 2.5 million physician consultations for constipation each year in the USA (Johanson et al. 1989). The economic impact is also considerable; a 1987 study estimated that cathartics were prescribed for 3 million people yearly in the USA, with over 200 million dollars spent on laxatives (Sandler et al. 1987). Furthermore, a study of severely constipated patients found that three-quarters had taken time off work because of their affliction, with one-fifth losing their job (Preston and Lennard-Jones 1986). As noted already, constipation is very common, and the vast majority of sufferers never visit a doctor for help: Population-based studies have revealed a high prevalence amongst those not seeking health care. Nevertheless, as a group those individuals who do consult a doctor tend to have worse symptoms and, as a consequence, probably real cause for complaint (Heaton et al. 1991).

A physical sign can be elicited on clinical examination, but a subjective experience or symptom is much more difficult to prove. Interestingly, while doctors usually accept patients' claims that they are constipated, patients are notoriously inaccurate when asked to define their own bowel frequency (Chaussade et al. 1989). In extreme cases some patients will deny the passage of stool in the face of objective evidence (obtained via transit studies) to the contrary (Hinton et al. 1969)! A study of 224 patients referred with complaints of severe constipation documented normal investigations in 49 (22%), with daily stools in 24 (11%) (Rex et al. 1992). It is important therefore to seek objective evidence of constipation rather than merely relying on the patient's historical account and subjective experience (Probert et al. 1994). For example, while infrequent defecation and small hard stools both imply slow colonic transit, an objective measure of this may be achieved by a simple test that documents the passage of ingested markers through the gut (Evans and Lennard-Jones 1992). It is clearly inappropriate to investigate all patients presenting with symptoms of constipation, even if this were economically feasible. The physician's role is to determine those whose symptoms are considered severe enough to warrant further investigation. Generally, severe constipation is three times more frequent in women, and the most severely affected patients are practically always female; in one series of patients whose constipation was severe enough for colectomy to be considered, all were women (Kamm et al. 1988).

It should be remembered that the primary aim of investigation is to sort patients into groups that are defined by the most prominent functional abnormality (e.g., slow transit, difficult evacuation), which will help to guide subsequent treatment. However, the treatment options for severe constipation are presently limited, and investigation may achieve little else other than to confirm symptom severity. It must be appreciated that this is not a field where there is any final histological arbiter. Functional disorders are difficult to analyze. Interpretation must be cautious and referenced to developments in related fields of diagnosis.

6.1.3 Investigation

Causes of constipation are myriad (Table 6.1.1). Indeed, the possibilities range from rare congenital abnormalities to carcinoma of the colon. Because the vast majority of cases are merely related to lifestyle and diet, a sensible approach to clinical investigation must be adopted. As stated above, further investigation is only warranted in those with severe symptoms or those where a sinister underlying cause could be responsible. 'Change in bowel habit' is a common symptom precipitating referral, especially in older patients where the worry is that a carcinoma might be present. Carcinoma, however, usually results in a change from constipation to diarrhoea rather than vice versa, and sinister symptoms such as anaemia

Table 6.1. Causes of constipation

Simple constipation	
Dietary:	Inadequate fibre
Lifestyle:	Repressed defecatory urge
Secondary constipation	
Congenital:	Hirschsprung's disease, idiopathic megarectum/megacolon
Mechanical:	Carcinoma
Drugs:	E.g., analgesics, antidepressants
Metabolic:	E.g., diabetic neuropathy, chronic renal failure
Endocrine:	E.g., hypothyroidism, hypercalcaemia
Neurological:	Multiple sclerosis, spinal trauma, autonomic neuropathy,
Parkinson's disease	
Psychological:	E.g., depression, anorexia
Idiopathic slow transit constipation	
Evacuation disorder	
Functional:	Anismus, ineffective straining, solitary rectal ulcer syndrome
Structural:	Rectocele, descending perineum
Constipation predominant irritable bowel syndrome	

and rectal bleeding may also be present. Where an underlying carcinoma is a real clinical possibility, patients require flexible sigmoidoscopy in the first instance or a total large bowel investigation if symptoms suggest a right-sided tumour, usually via barium enema, CT colonography or colonoscopy.

Symptoms of a carcinoma are usually relatively short-lived, whereas most patients will complain of chronic symptoms. Most of those who consult a doctor will respond to simple dietary measures once an underlying cause has been excluded if necessary. This leaves a group of patients who have severe symptoms of constipation, but in whom simple measures have been ineffective. Buried within these will be a small, but significant number of younger patients who have been markedly constipated all of their lives; this raises the possibility of a congenital disorder. In these patients abdominal palpation may reveal a hugely loaded colon, often with abdominal distension. In such instances, a simple water-soluble enema is all that is required to diagnose or exclude a congenital abnormality, with the emphasis on a lateral view of the contrast-filled rectum. There are three possibilities: Hirschsprung's disease, congenital megarectum or congenital megacolon. All three are defined by gross rectal dilatation, usually defined by a transverse measurement of 6 cm or more at the sacral promontory (Gladman et al. 2007; Preston et al. 1985). In the case of Hirschsprung's disease, there will be a relatively narrowed segment interposed between the dilated rectum and the anus, representing the contracted distal aganglionic segment, which can be of variable length (Fig. 6.1.1). In contrast, dilatation extends right down to the level of the pelvic floor/anorectal junction in patients with megarectum and megacolon. Distinction between the latter two depends on the sigmoid colon, which is of normal calibre in congenital megarectum (Fig. 61.2), but also dilated in those with congenital megacolon (Gattuso and Kamm 1997). Studies of colonic transit and rectal evacuation are unwarranted in any of these patients since the diagnosis is made by contrast studies. It should be noted that imaging is superior to physiological testing for diagnosis because the rectoanal inhibitory reflex (anal sphincter relaxation as a response to rectal distension) – the absence of which is used to diagnose Hirschsprung's disease – may be impossible to elicit in patients with megarectum simply because the balloon used is not large enough to distend the abnormal rectum.

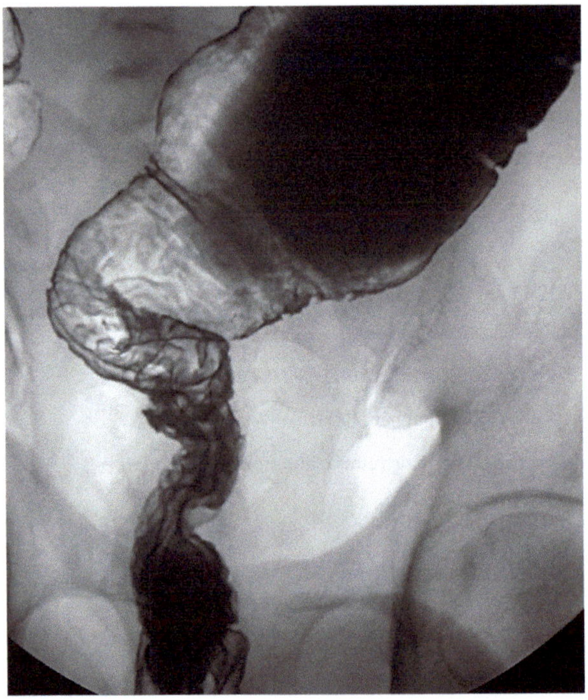

Fig. 6.1.1. Water-soluble enema in a 46-year-old man reveals a dilated proximal rectum with distal short segment, diagnosing Hirschsprung's disease

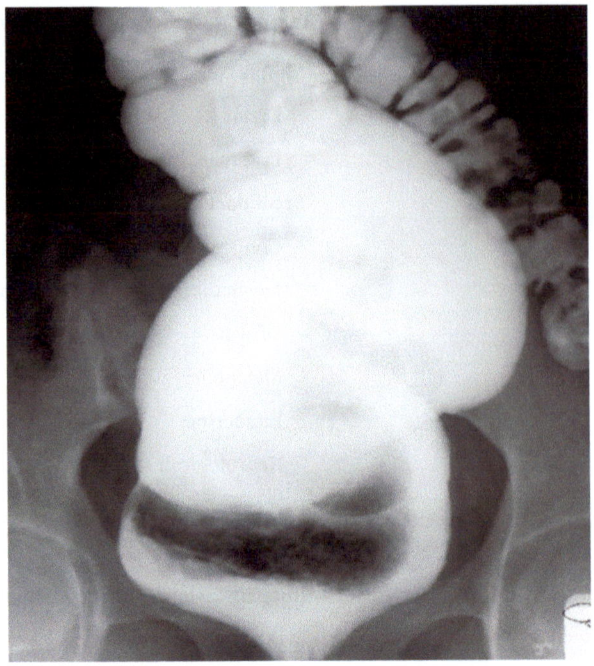

Fig. 6.1.2. Water-soluble enema in a 20-year-old man reveals a hugely dilated rectum that extends right down to the pelvic floor. There is no short segment, and the sigmoid colon is of normal calibre, suggesting the diagnosis is idiopathic megarectum

However, the majority of patients presenting with severe constipation have no readily identifiable 'organic' cause, and it seems reasonable to classify these on the basis of their functional disturbance. This is achieved by a combination of anorectal physiology testing, transit studies (Chap. 48) and evacuation proctography (Chap. 41). There are then a variety of possibilities; patients will be found to have slow colonic transit, abnormalities of rectal evacuation or a combination of both. Transit studies and their interpretation are detailed in Chapter 48. Patients who solely exhibit slow colonic transit are likely to be suffering from "idiopathic slow transit constipation" (Preston and Lennard-Jones 1986). These individuals are almost exclusively young women and additionally suffer constitutional symptoms and abdominal bloating together with a dramatically reduced stool frequency. There is some evidence that the underlying abnormality is not merely confined to the colon, but is more generalised. For example, many exhibit abnormal antroduodenal manometry (Glia and Lindberg 1998). The underling disorder remains obscure, but is likely to be related to a generalised sensory and autonomic neuropathy (Knowles et al. 1999), which might explain why colectomy so often fails to ameliorate symptoms (Bernini et al. 1998).

In other patients, the predominant characteristic may be difficult defecation: i.e., the patient cannot empty their rectum or they have to strain forcefully and for prolonged periods in order to do so, or they experience feelings of incomplete evacuation after stool passage. Most constipated patients with predominantly rectal symptoms probably experience a combination of all of these, a symptom complex termed "outlet obstruction" or "obstructed defecation". Obstructed defecation has been estimated to affect 7% of the adult Western population (D'Hoore and Penninckx 2003).

While classification of patients into those with colonic inertia and those with rectal outlet obstruction is now considered simplistic, it remains clinically convenient, and for this reason transit studies and evacuation proctography are frequently requested together. To further complicate matters, slow colonic transit and abnormal rectal evacuation frequently co-exist. For example, a study of 14 women suffering from idiopathic slow transit constipation found that they also had decreased rectal sensory perception when compared to controls, and few were able to pass a simulated stool (Read et al. 1986). Perhaps this interrelationship should not be surprising since, intuitively, transit and rectal evacuation ought to be related; if they were not, then stool delivered to the rectum at a normal rate in patients with isolated obstructed defecation would cause a megarectum within days! Supporting an interrelationship, normal volunteers who consciously suppress the urge to defecate show a dramatic slowing of proximal colonic transit within 1 week (Klauser et al. 1990). The situation is analogous to the 'ileocaecal brake', where increased delivery of intestinal contents to the caecum slows proximal small bowel transit. Furthermore, this relationship implies that treatment should be directed at normalising rectal evacuation in any patient who demonstrates both slow transit and impaired voiding, since the former could merely be a normal physiological response to the latter. Moreover, this approach also suggests that an assessment of rectal evacuation is probably the single most important test in severely constipated patients since it most precisely characterises the primary abnormality (Read 1989).

In many patients all investigations will be entirely normal, and this raises the possibility that the irritable bowel syndrome is responsible. Although irritable bowel is defined by the Rome criteria (Thompson et al. 1989), which centre on abdominal pain and change in bowel habit, there are constipation-predominant subgroups (Prior et al. 1990). Interestingly, many have heightened sensitivity to rectal distension, which might explain sensations of incomplete evacuation in those who complain of constipation (Prior et al. 1990).

6.1.4 Evacuation Proctography and Constipation

Constipation is the commonest reason to request evacuation proctography, although pelvic pain, prolapse (either rectal or otherwise) and anal incontinence may occasionally be other indications. For the reasons described above, the main aim of evacuation proctography is to characterise rectal evacuation; is it normal or not? Evacuation proctography will usually be of most use in those patients whose symptoms suggest 'obstructed defecation'.

Generally, proctographic findings may be broadly divided into two groups: abnormalities of rectal and pelvic floor configuration, and functional abnormalities of rectal emptying. Any competent proctographic report should incorporate an assessment of both of these. The overall picture is complicated by the fact that structural and functional rectal abnormalities usually co-exist, and it is therefore difficult to determine which one is the primary cause of the patient's symptoms, if either. Luckily, there are only a few possibilities: structural rectal abnormalities may be broadly grouped into prolapse, rectocele and pelvic floor descent, and functional abnormality generally means an inability to empty the rectum rapidly and completely, whatever its configuration. These possibilities are considered in the paragraphs below.

6.1.4.1 Rectal Prolapse

Rectal prolapse may be external or internal. External rectal prolapse is circumferential and tends to be "complete" – i.e. all of the rectal wall layers are involved. In essence, the rectum is extruded through the anus. In contrast, circumferential prolapse, which remains confined to the rectal ampulla or which only enters the anal canal, is termed intussusception (intra-rectal and intra-anal intussusception, respectively). Intussusception may involve all rectal wall layers or only involve the mucosa and its immediate subjacent layers. The term intussusception implies a circumferential process; when the phenomenon is confined to the anterior rectal wall, it is more correctly termed 'anterior mucosal prolapse'.

Complete rectal prolapse clearly needs surgical treatment. Diagnosis is usually not difficult, although evacuation proctography is occasionally necessary if the prolapse is very intermittent and cannot be demonstrated on the examination couch. The introduction of evacuation proctography facilitated the diagnosis of rectal prolapse and, furthermore, the dynamic nature of the examination meant that its mechanism could be studied directly for the first time. Cineradiographic studies revealed that rectal prolapse developed from a circumferential intussusception 6 to 8 cm from the anal verge (Broden and Snellman 1968), and it rapidly became clear that prolapse was frequently retained within the rectum, lending support to the concept of internal intussusception, first described in 1903 (Tuttle 1903). Whilst clinical diagnosis of intussusception relies on direct proctoscopy while the patient strains, the introduction of evacuation proctography meant that accurate diagnosis of intussusception, including subtle forms, was now possible.

Proctographic intussusception has been divided into a seven-point scale (Shorvon et al. 1989), but there is probably no practical need for such a detailed scoring system. It is easier to divide intussusception merely into high and low grades, which is an attempt to define whether it is abnormal or not, especially since intussusception is known to occur frequently in asymptomatic individuals. Low-grade intussusception is defined by a thin circumferential ring that originates in the rectal ampulla when emptying commences and travels towards the ano-rectal junction as voiding continues (Fig. 6.1.3). Importantly, it remains confined to the rectum. High-grade intussusception also develops in the same way and also remains confined within the rectum, but in this case the prolapsing folds are much thicker, bulkier and capacious (Fig. 6.1.4). Although it is possible to measure the thickness of prolapsing folds in order to differentiate between high- and low-grade intussusception, with 3 mm being the usually quoted threshold, it is difficult to measure such structures precisely and, in any event, such measurement is rarely clinically necessary: With experience, an accurate diagnosis can be made simply by inspecting the radiological images.

It is worth remembering that the rectum has to empty for intussusception to be revealed. Intussusception is most frequently and best visualised at the end of evacuation when the rectum is empty, and this is when it should be graded: If the apex of the prolapsing folds enters the anal canal then this is termed intra-anal intussusception, which is classed as a high-grade phenomenon (Fig. 6.1.5). Intra-anal intussusception is recognised by anal canal splaying as a consequence of the folds entering the canal. However, this may not always be most visible in the conventional lateral view because the rectal folds are coronal. Consequently, it may be worthwhile asking the subject to strain while proctography is performed in the anterior-posterior position, a position where the intussusception is most visible (McGee and Bartram 1993). Complete rectal prolapse is diagnosed when the full thickness of the rectal wall is extruded through the anal canal (Fig. 6.1.6). Care

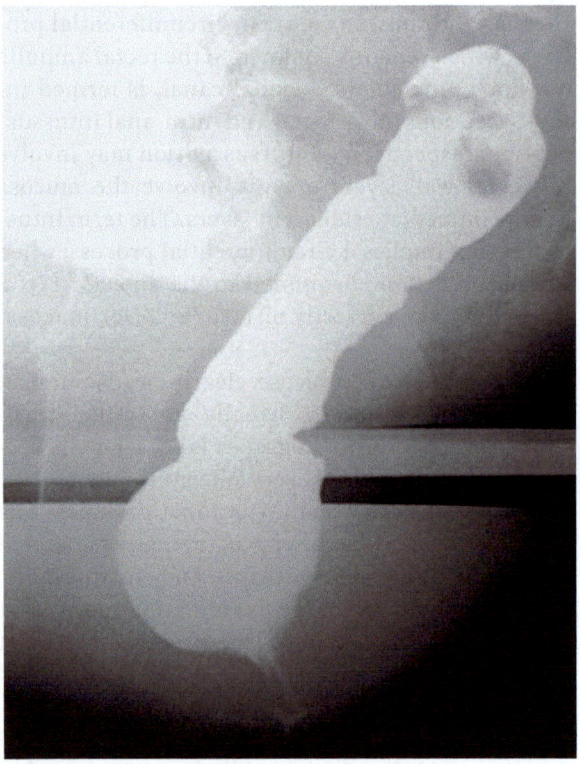

Fig. 6.1.3. In this case, lateral proctography reveals circumferential rectal infolding during evacuation, diagnosing intussusception. The folds remain high in the rectum and are not particularly thick. Such low-grade intussusception is a common finding

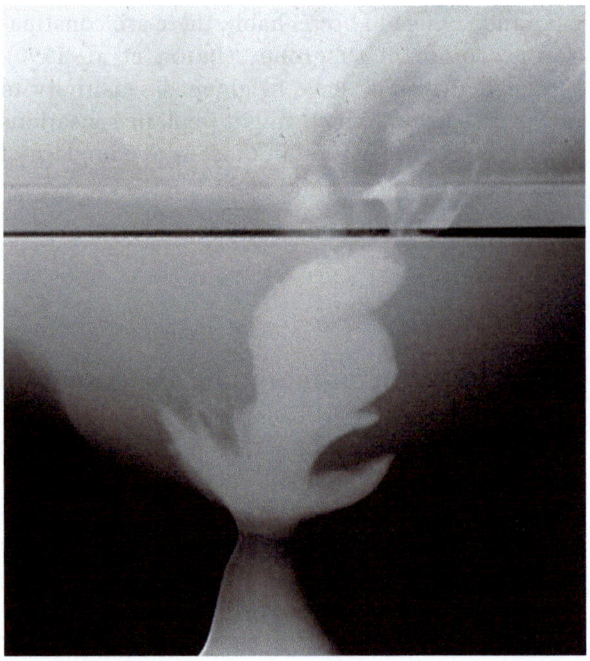

Fig. 6.1.4. Lateral proctography reveals circumferential rectal infolding during evacuation. The folds are thick and prominent and travel towards the distal rectum, typical of high-grade intussusception

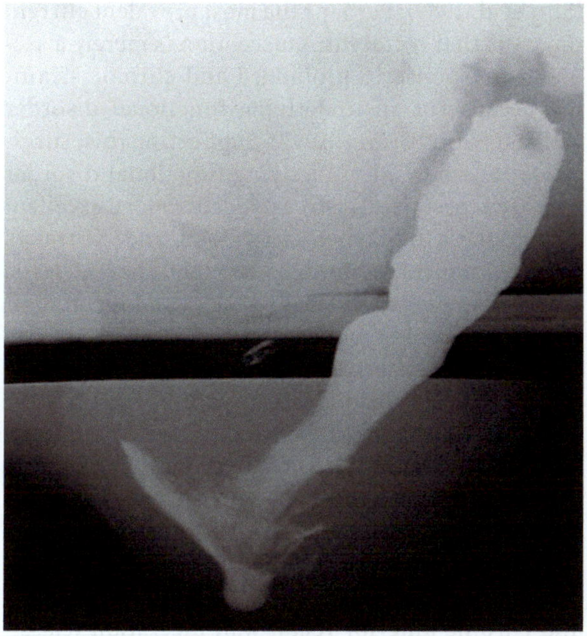

Fig. 6.1.5. The apex of the prolapsing folds enters the anal canal in this patient, diagnosing intraanal intussusception

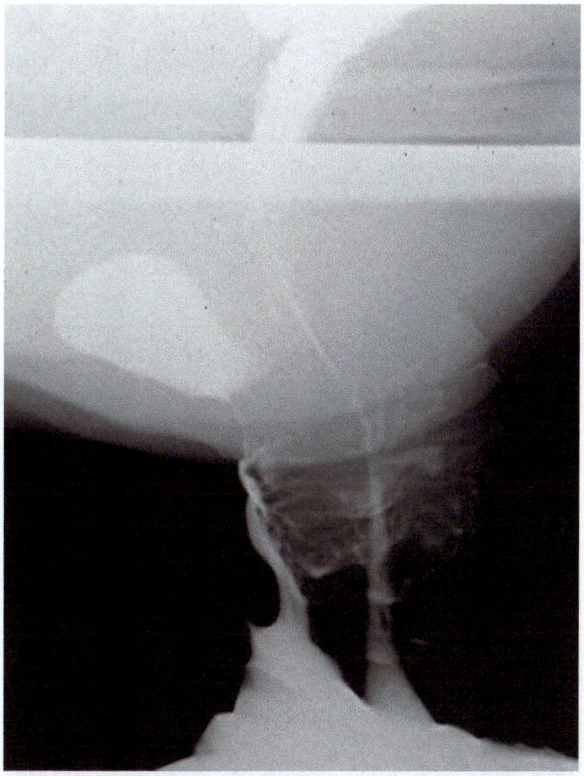

Fig. 6.1.6. Lateral proctography shows complete rectal prolapse, evidenced by extrusion of all rectal wall layers through the anus. There is also retained contrast within a rectocele

should be taken not to confuse this with the eversion of the anal margin that sometimes accompanies forceful straining. Anterior mucosal prolapse is diagnosed when only the anterior rectal wall appears to be infolding during rectal evacuation (Fig. 6.1.7); it is commonly seen in association with a rectocele and most likely represents collapse of the rectocele as it empties.

An association between intussusception and constipation has long been recognised, with several authors hypothesising that the prolapsing folds obstruct the rectal lumen and are thus the cause of incomplete evacuation (Ihre 1990). Because of this, proctographic diagnosis of intussusception has attracted considerable attention. Moreover, the clear implication is that once diagnosed, surgical obliteration of the prolapse will ameliorate symptoms (Hoffman et al. 1984). However, while some authors report excellent symptomatic results following surgery (Johansson et al. 1985; Liberman et al. 2000), others have had less success despite proof that the prolapse has been cured (Halligan et al. 1995; Christiansen et al. 1992; Orrom et al. 1991). The fact that intussusception can be demonstrated in asymptomatic volunteers casts some doubt on whether it is the primary cause of symptoms: Shorvon and co-workers (1989) found proctographic intussusception in 22 (50%) of 44 normal volunteers. While it is commonly believed that intussusception obstructs evacuation, this phenomenon is rarely seen in practice, and there is little evidence to support the supposition that the rectum is mechanically occluded by the prolapsing folds (Halligan et al. 1996). A proctographic study of patients with intussusception found that some patients with intussusception evacuated slowly, while others did not, but that this had no impact on the incidence of evacuatory symptoms (Dvorkin et al. 2005a). The authors concluded that subclassification of intussusception was of little clinical significance and that selection for surgery solely on the basis of proctographic appearances was illogical. In another study the same authors noted that intussusception occurring in symptomatic patients is of higher grade than that documented in asymptomatic controls (Dvorkin et al. 2005b). Other authors have found no relationship between proctographic features of intussusception and symptoms of constipation (Karlbom et al. 2004). It seems most likely to the author that high-grade intussusception is an epiphenomenon produced by forceful straining that then engenders an enhanced sensation of

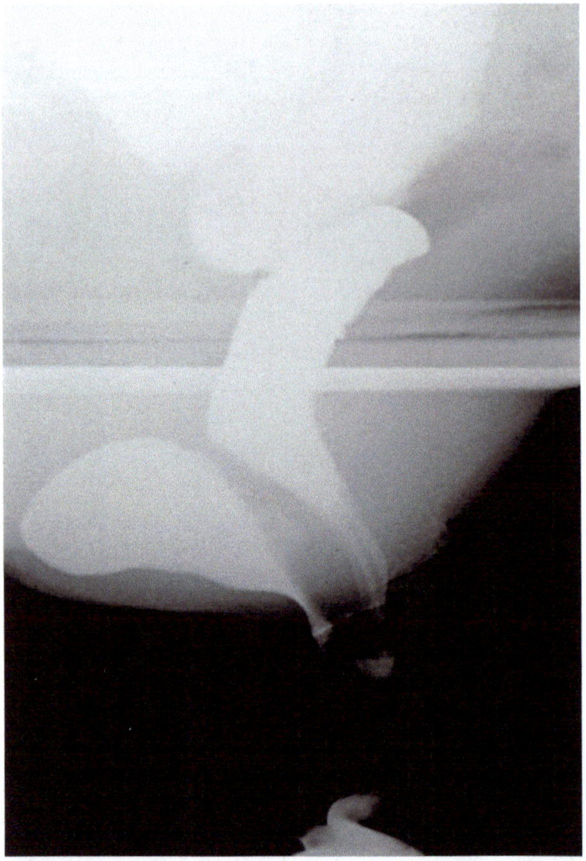

Fig. 6.1.7. In this woman the anterior rectal wall has prolapsed into the anal canal towards the end of evacuation. Note that the process is confined to the anterior rectal wall and is not circumferential so that the diagnosis is anterior mucosal prolapse rather than intussusception. Note that the prolapse also walls off contrast within a rectocele

incomplete evacuation, but does not in itself cause mechanical rectal blockage.

Much of this uncertainty may be explained by the fact that the mechanism of intussusception remains poorly understood in most cases. Some believe that intussusception inevitably progresses to complete rectal prolapse given enough time (Hoffman et al. 1984), whereas others suggest that longitudinal studies show no such progression (Mellgren et al. 1997). This raises the possibility that complete rectal prolapse and intussusception are different syndromes. It has also been suggested that rectal hypersensitivity, which encourages the subject to void small volumes repeatedly, in combination with a weak sphincter mechanism provides the ideal conditions for prolapse into the anal canal, and that this is the mechanism for all forms of rectal prolapse (Sun et al. 1989). Perhaps the most prevalent current theory is that rectal intussusception is merely a secondary response to prolonged and chronic straining because of an underlying functional disorder (Eu and Seow-Choen 1997). Supporting this, surgical series where an underlying functional disorder has been preoperatively excluded report excellent symptomatic outcomes (van Tets and Kuijpers 1995). Moreover, symptoms thought characteristic of intussusception, such as perineal and rectal digitation, are now known to be strongly associated with functional disorders.

The solitary rectal ulcer syndrome is a well-recognised clinical entity that describes a combination of rectal prolapse and functional abnormality of evacuation (Morio et al. 2005). The condition is characterised by repeated fruitless straining, often accompanied by the passage of blood and mucus. Proctoscopy usually reveals rectal inflammation and chronic anterior rectal wall ulceration (classically a "solitary ulcer") that is accompanied by specific histopathological changes within the prolapsing mucosa (Halligan et al. 1995), similar to those that are present in prolapsing bowel mucosa at other sites (prolapsing stomas, for example). Although the precise aetiology remains obscure, it is widely believed that ulceration is a direct result of mucosal ischaemia secondary to repeated straining (Womack et al. 1987). Proctographic abnormalities are common and many patients exhibit high-grade rectal intussusception or complete rectal prolapse (Fig. 6.1.8), in addition to prolonged and incomplete evacuation (Halligan et al. 1995). Endosonographic studies of the internal anal sphincter have also shown that this structure is abnormally thickened in patients with solitary rectal ulcer and that this finding may be predictive of high-grade rectal intussusception (Marshall et al. 2002). While treatment in the past was usually directed at surgical obliteration of the intussusception, contemporary treatment is more conservative and directed towards measures to ameliorate straining (Rao et al. 2006), although patients with complete rectal prolapse will usually require surgery to correct this.

6.1.4.2 Pelvic Floor Descent

By relating the position of the anorectal junction to a landmark, such as the ischial tuberosities or commode seat, proctography provides a simple method

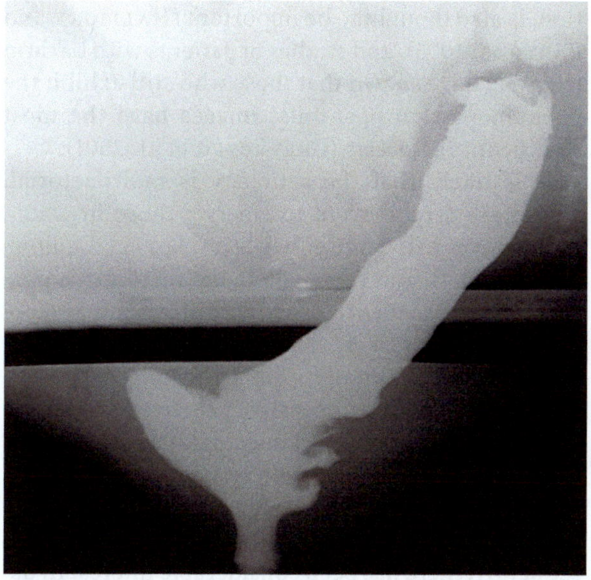

Fig. 6.1.8. Proctography shows rectal intussusception in this woman known to have solitary rectal ulcer syndrome (SRUS)

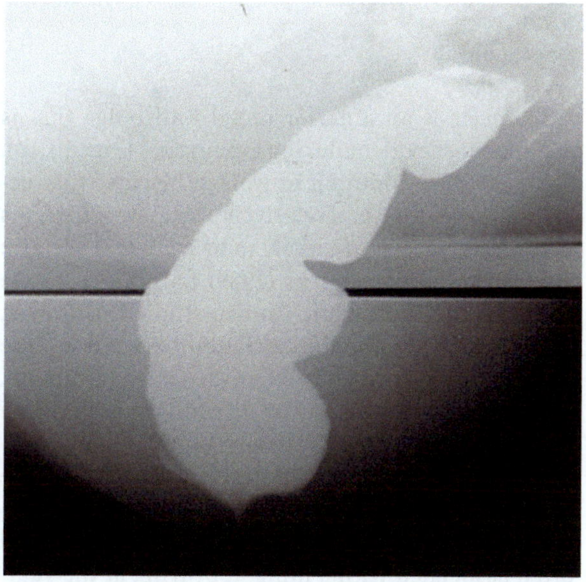

Fig. 6.1.9. Lateral proctography shows gross pelvic floor descent at rest, evidenced by the distance of the anorectal junction below the commode seat

to determine the position of the pelvic floor at rest and how far it descends during evacuation. It is generally accepted that proctography provides the most accurate estimate of pelvic floor position and descent because clinical methods using a perineometer measure movement of the anal verge during maximum straining and not to the point of anal canal opening (Oettle et al. 1985). Parks et al. (1966) described a clinical syndrome where the main finding was excessive pelvic floor descent, defined as more than 3–4 cm, coupled with a low resting level of more than 3 cm below the pubococcygeal line (Fig. 6.1.9). Of a series of 100 consecutive patients attending a rectal clinic, 12 displayed these characteristics, 10 of whom (83%) strained excessively at stool compared with only 20 (23%) of the remaining 88. Because of this, Parks suggested the underlying abnormality was likely due to irreparable pudendal nerve traction neuropathy as a consequence of chronic stretching (Parks et al. 1966). It has been estimated that the pudendal nerves may be stretched by as much as 20% over time (Henry et al. 1982).

It is clear is that excessive pelvic floor descent is frequently found in patients referred for evacuation proctography (Skomorowka et al. 1988) and is often seen in combination with perineal ballooning, rectocele, intussusception and impaired evacuation. Furthermore, there is no doubt that straining stresses the pudendal nerves; a study of asymptomatic individuals found that voluntary excessive straining temporarily slowed pudendal nerve latency when measured immediately afterwards (Engel and Kamm 1993). However, whether the pelvic floor ballooning that accompanies the syndrome is responsible for symptoms of constipation is uncertain. Indeed, many patients with pudendal neuropathy and pelvic floor descent are incontinent. In an attempt to explain this, it has been suggested that chronic straining, precipitated by an underlying functional disorder, causes pudendal neuropathy, the ultimate expression of which is sphincter denervation and subsequent incontinence (Henry et al. 1982). The pelvic floor may also be weakened by childbirth, which can also cause perineal descent. Thus, the finding probably reflects a multifactorial spectrum of pelvic floor injury rather than indicating a specific syndrome or aetiology. Supporting this, a prospective proctographic study of 213 patients found no correlation between pudendal neuropathy and perineal descent (Jorge et al. 1993). Surgery directed specifically at restoration of normal pelvic floor configuration is highly contentious and unlikely to be helpful, but behavioural therapy may help selected patients (Harewood et al. 1999).

6.1.4.3
Rectocele

A rectocele is an anterior rectal wall bulge that is usually most evident during evacuation (Fig. 6.1.10). Rectoceles are common in women because the rectovaginal septum is a relatively weak structure. As a result, rectoceles are likely to be a normal variant: Shorvon and co-workers (1989) found a rectocele in 96% of asymptomatic women studied. However, there is an undoubted association between a large rectocele and difficult rectal evacuation, although, like intussusception, it is difficult to determine whether the rectocele is the primary cause of problems. Patients, almost exclusively women, describe a specific constellation of symptoms: the urge to defecate is normal, but voiding is obstructed and often associated with a lump appearing at the vaginal introitus. Proctography is frequently requested for diagnosis, and a large rectocele may be defined as one deeper than 4 cm (Kelvin et al. 1992). It is frequently believed that the need to digitally manipulate the rectocele in order to facilitate emptying signifies functional significance (Halligan and Bartram 1995), e.g., by digitating the vagina in order to support the rectovaginal septum. Similarly, inability to fully empty the rectocele, evidenced by contrast retention within it at the end of evacuation, is also thought to be important (Halligan and Bartram 1995), and studies of patients with barium trapping have shown that those who still exhibit the phenomenon on post-toilet images have the most significant rectoceles (Greenberg et al. 2001).

It is likely that the aetiology is multifactorial. Two main groups seem to emerge: those in whom the rectovaginal septum has been damaged following childbirth and those where the rectocele is possibly the consequence of chronic straining at stool (the latter most likely due to a functional disorder of evacuation). Surgery aims to restore rectovaginal support, and postoperative proctography is able to demonstrate technical success in most patients (Loder et al. 1996). However, symptomatic failure is common (Arnold et al. 1990), possibly because any underlying functional disorder is not treated. Consequently, there has been considerable interest in using proctography not only for diagnosis, for which it is the gold-standard test, but also to predict symptomatic outcome. This has not been simple, and the results are confusing. For example, whilst some have found proctographic contrast retention within the rectocele to reliably predict good symptomatic outcome (Murthy et al. 1996), others have not: a study of 74 patients found no relationship between the size of the rectocele and ability to evacuate, and surgical outcome (van Dam et al. 2000). It seems likely that

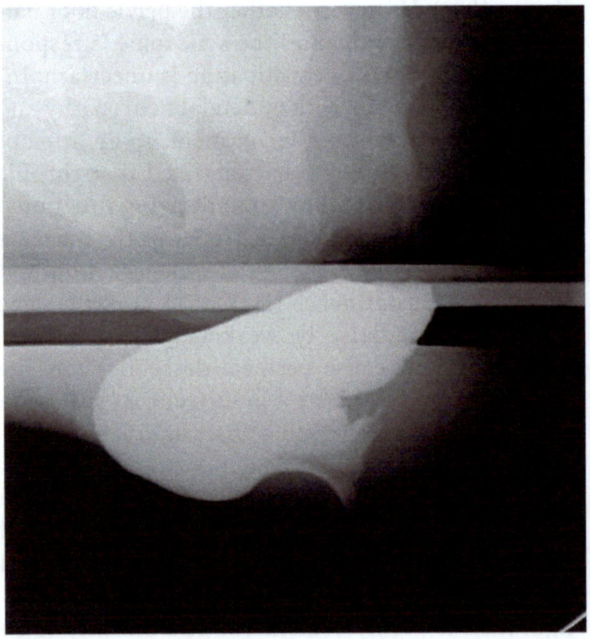
a

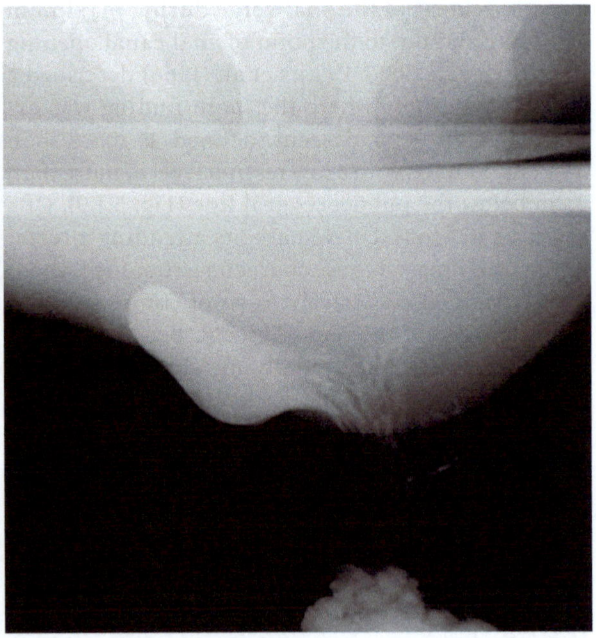
b

Fig. 6.1.10a,b. Proctography during evacuation reveals a large anterior rectocoele in this woman. Contrast is retained in the rectocoele after evacuation: "barium trapping"

outcome is confounded by the presence or absence of an underlying functional disorder, which is often neglected once attention has been drawn towards a large rectocele. For example, a study of 41 patients with difficult evacuation initially ascribed to rectocele found underlying functional disorder in 29 (71%) (Johansson et al. 1992). Supporting this, surgery is successful if a functional disorder has been excluded preoperatively (Tjandra et al. 1999). Indeed, behavioural therapy (biofeedback) alone may ameliorate symptoms (Mimura et al. 2000). Because rectoceles are commonest in middle-aged women, a plethora of other factors may contribute to symptoms, in addition to the size of the rectocele itself (Laarhoven et al. 1999). A recently introduced operation, stapled transanal rectal resection (the STARR procedure), treats rectoceles and intussusception by using a circular stapling device that permits trans-anal excision of redundant mucosa (Grassi et al. 2005). Again, the presence of a preoperative functional disorder seems to predict the persistence of symptoms postoperatively (Pechlivanides et al. 2007).

It should also be noted that rectoceles might also rarely be posterior in position (Fig. 6.1.11). However, in contrast to the anterior type, these are not due to a midline weakness. Rather, imaging in the frontal plane reveals that they are literalised to one side of the pelvic floor and are actually due to rectal herniation through the levator plate musculature (Halligan 1994). Thus, a more correct term is probably 'posterior perineal hernia'. In contrast to anterior rectocele, men are equally as affected, and the aetiology is most likely chronic straining (Cavallo et al. 1993) or sometimes a penetrating injury to the levator plate itself.

6.1.4.4 Functional Disorder

Ever since evacuation proctography first visualised the dynamics of rectal evacuation, there has been an understandable focus on perceived abnormalities of rectal configuration, with many investigators believing that these are responsible for obstructive symptoms. However, despite that fact that constipation is often defined as an inability to evacuate, proctographic estimates of the rate and completeness of

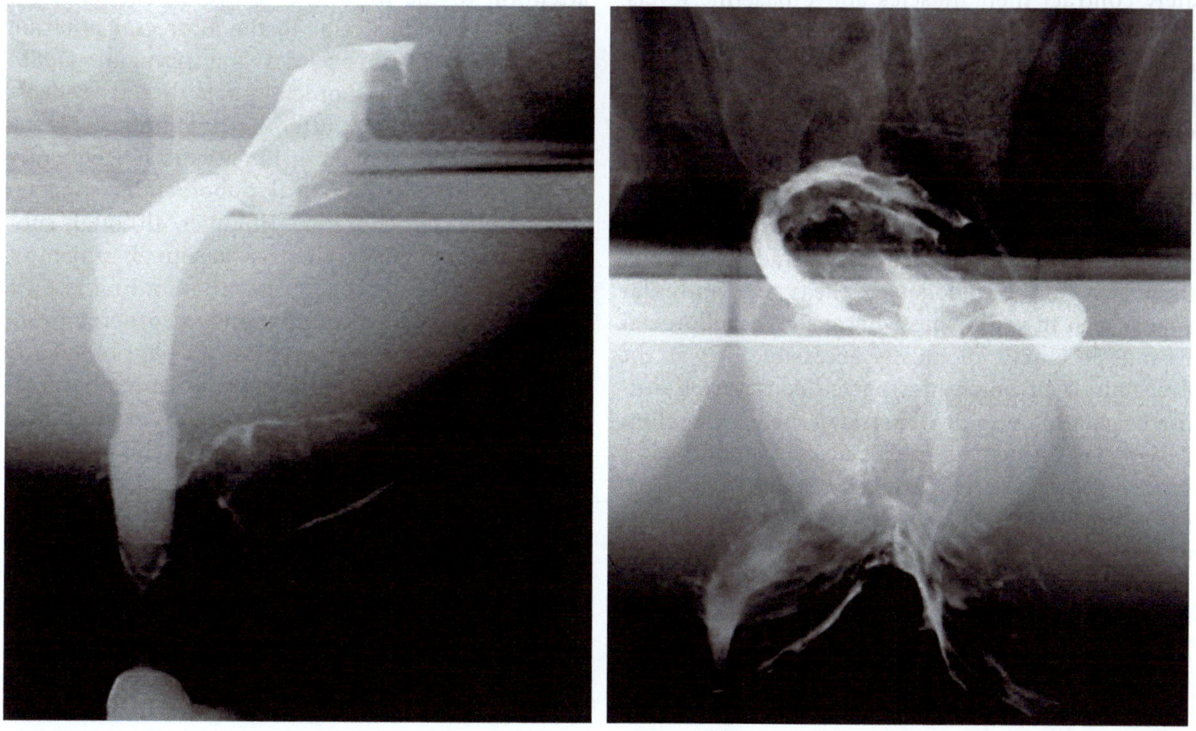

a b

Fig. 6.1.11a,b. Posterior perineal hernia or "posterior rectocele". The lateral proctogram during evacuation suggests a well-defined posterior rectal wall bulge in this 50-year-old man. Screening in the AP position during straining reveals that the bulge is a left-sided posterior perineal hernia rectal evacuation have received surprisingly little attention, especially in the earlier literature. Rectal evacuation is a functional event, requiring coordination between voluntary and involuntary nervous pathways, and smooth and striated muscles. It has long been recognised that some patients experience difficulties with rectal evacuation simply because of an inability to coordinate this necessarily complex series of events. Given this, the configuration the rectum adopts when emptying may be irrelevant if the patient can empty without effort. Conversely, abnormalities of rectal configuration actually can occur secondary to prolonged and chronic straining rather than as the primary cause of constipation.

Some patients cannot void without inappropriate effort. This is often attributed to hard and bulky stools, but some patients cannot evacuate their rectum even when it is only full of fluid (Alstrup et al. 1997). Why is this? Normally, striated pelvic floor musculature is in a state of tonic contraction, and in normal subjects this contraction is inhibited during defecation so that the pelvic floor relaxes to allow stool passage. Simultaneous electromyography of pelvic floor musculature in constipated patients has shown that some fail to relax their pelvic floor when attempting to evacuate. Indeed, many inappropriately contract their muscles above baseline levels: a study of 15 constipated women revealed that the puborectalis and external sphincter muscles contracted forcefully when the subject attempted to evacuate a rectal balloon, thereby preventing evacuation (Preston and Lennard-Jones 1985). There is therefore no primary structural abnormality as such; rather there is a disorder of functional integration. This syndrome has been termed "anismus" because it may be analogous to the type of muscular spasm seen in vaginismus. Because the puborectalis muscle is physiologically accessible, it was the first muscle in which unexpected contraction during evacuation was demonstrated, hence the alternative terms such as "non-relaxing puborectalis syndrome" (Fleshman et al. 1992) and "paradoxical puborectalis contraction syndrome" (Jones et al. 1987). Indeed, Wasserman (1964) first noticed the role of this muscle in constipation in 1968 and named it "puborectalis syndrome". However, it is increasingly recognised that the problem is unlikely to be confined to a single muscle, and a more general term such as "pelvic floor incoordination" may be preferable since it does not identify any particular muscular group or necessarily imply inappropriate contraction (Halligan and Bartram 1998). The latter is important because some patients fail to relax while straining, whereas others simply do not strain and so fail to generate adequate intrarectal pressure for evacuation to occur (Halligan et al. 1995). In any event, the cause is a functional disorder, and the end result is the same: failure to evacuate. The aetiology remains obscure, but anismus is likely to be a learned inappropriate response. For example, there is an association with pelvic surgery and previous sexual abuse (Leroi 1995). Although anismus can be found in both normal and incontinent patients (Jones et al. 1987), and may disappear when investigations are made away from the hospital environment (Duthie and Bartolo 1992), there is a clear association with constipation, and the diagnosis is worthwhile, not least because pelvic floor behavioural therapy using biofeedback has been very successful (Bleijenberg and Kuijpers 1987). This approach also avoids surgical treatment of secondary phenomena such as rectocele where this is unnecessary.

Because the puborectalis was the first muscle implicated, diagnosis has historically focussed on demonstrating inappropriate puborectalis contraction during attempted evacuation. Using evacuation proctography for diagnosis, workers have drawn attention to the finding of a prominent puborectal impression posterior to the anorectal junction (Fig. 6.1.12). Kuijpers and Bleijenberg (1986) suggested that the anorectal angle directly reflects puborectalis activity after finding failure of the anorectal angle to open in 12 patients subsequently found to have paradoxical puborectalis contraction on electromyography. However, although subsequently frequently cited as a sign of anismus, more recent evidence suggests this finding is only weakly associated with functional disorder: a proctographic study of 24 patients with physiologically proven anismus found that a prominent puborectal impression and acute anorectal angle configuration during attempted evacuation was unable to differentiate patients from asymptomatic control subjects (Halligan et al. 1995). Supporting this observation, simultaneous proctography and puborectal electromyography reveal no correlation between muscular activity and anorectal junction configuration (Thorpe et al. 1993).

Instead, the major proctographic difference between patients with and without anismus is intuitively obvious; patients with anismus cannot easily empty their rectum. Evacuation studies in normal volunteers show that they can empty their rectum

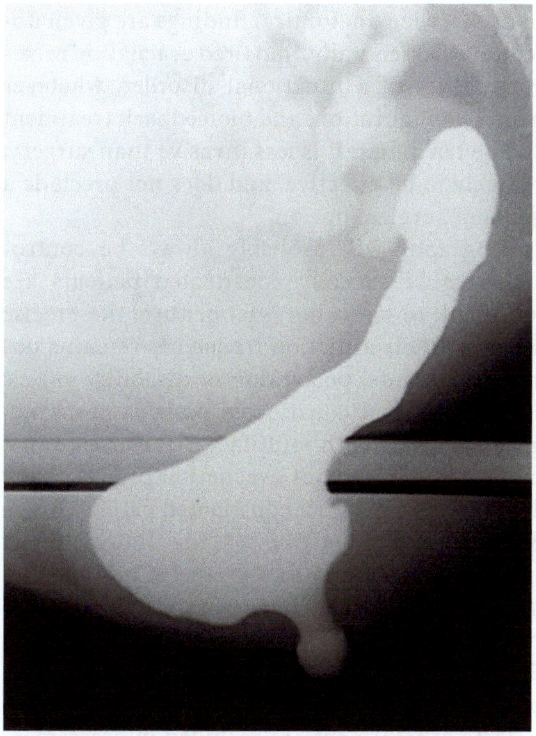

Fig. 6.1.12. Evacuation was very prolonged in this woman, suggesting anismus. Note the posterior rectal wall impression, presumed to be due to paradoxical puborectalis contraction

rapidly and completely (Kamm et al. 1989), whereas, in complete contrast, patients with anismus exhibit prolonged and incomplete evacuation, or indeed no evacuation at all. The rate and completeness of rectal evacuation are easily determined using evacuation proctography (Halligan et al. 1994), and it seems sensible to base a proctographic diagnosis of anismus on these. Using these criteria, Halligan and co-workers (1995) found abnormally prolonged and/or incomplete contrast evacuation during proctography in 20 of 24 patients (83%), whereas all controls evacuated rapidly and completely. Furthermore, anorectal angle measurements were non-specific and not predictive. Moreover, when the authors applied their findings prospectively to a continuous, unselected group of constipated patients, the positive predictive value of impaired proctographic evacuation for subsequent diagnosis of anismus by physiological criteria was in excess of 90% (Halligan et al. 2001). Using 120 cc of rectal contrast, evacuation times greater than 30 s predict functional disorder with precision (Halligan et al. 2001). The time taken to initiate anal canal opening and the rate of evacuation are more sensitive for diagnosis than the amount of contrast ultimately voided because most patients, even those with severe anismus, will eventually empty their rectum fully if given enough time to do so and if they can strain forcefully enough. Proctography is equally as good as electromyography for diagnosis of anismus (Jorge et al. 1993). There have also been attempts to use proctography to determine who will benefit from subsequent biofeedback therapy, and these data imply that those with moderate symptoms do better than those who are severely affected (McKee et al. 1999).

Anismus is characterised by chronic, excessive, prolonged straining, a practice that probably weakens the pelvic floor and encourages pelvic floor descent, intussusception and prolapse. Because of this, patients with anismus often have associated structural pelvic floor abnormalities by the time they come to be investigated (Fig. 6.1.13). It is highly likely that many surgical disappointments happen because an underlying diagnosis of anismus was neglected preoperatively. For example, a study of 41 patients whose constipation had been ascribed to rectocele found underlying anismus in 29 (71%) (Johansson et al. 1992), while another study found anismus in 34 (60%) of 56 (Mellgren et al. 1998). The same may apply to intussusception; a proctographic study of patients treated for intussusception found that symptoms persisted if there was an underlying functional disorder (Orrom et al. 1991). Furthermore, a study of patients with solitary rectal ulcer syndrome found that preoperative proctographic features of impaired evacuation predicted persistent postoperative symptoms in the face of objective evidence that the prolapse itself had been successfully treated (Halligan et al. 1995). These studies suggest that intussusception in some patients may merely be an epiphenomenon. When prolonged and incomplete contrast evacuation is encountered during proctography, a diagnosis of functional pelvic floor incoordination should be considered, whatever the rectal configuration adopted. Supporting this, a proctographic study of 58 constipated patients found that the only significant difference from controls was a prolongation of evacuation time and failure to fully empty the rectum, clearly suggesting that functional measurements of emptying are more important than changes in rectal configuration (Turnbull et al. 1988). It also seems that abnormalities of rectal configuration occurring secondary to incoordination do not prejudice the success of subsequent behavioural therapy (Lau et al. 2000).

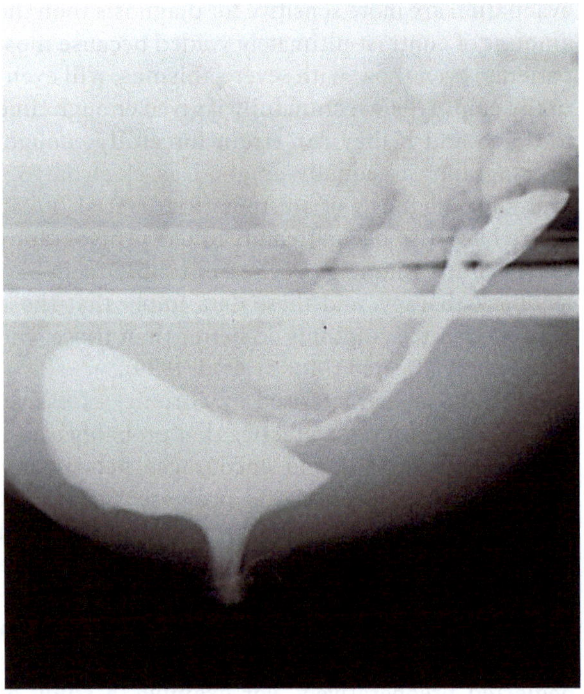

Fig. 6.1.13. Evacuation proctography in this 39-year-old woman reveals a large rectocoele, pelvic floor descent and ballooning, and enterocele. However, evacuation was prolonged and subsequent physiological testing found anismus, raising the possibility that the structural abnormalities demonstrated by imaging merely reflect functional disorder

6.1.5 Summary

Although evacuation proctography has been practiced widely for several years, its clinical relevance continues to be debated. While no one would argue against the pivotal role of endosonography for characterising the cause of anal incontinence, the positioning of proctography is less certain. Much of this uncertainty derives from the excessive attention that has been devoted to the detailed and complex anatomical measurements that are possible during the procedure, but which are ultimately unhelpful. Any rectal configuration occurring during emptying, other than that of a symmetrically collapsing tube, has been considered abnormal in the face of evidence to the contrary. The main value of proctography lies with its ability to simultaneously diagnose both structural and functional abnormalities and to determine which is most likely to be relevant in each individual case. Problems with interpretation most often occur when anatomical findings are given undue emphasis. Generally, impaired evacuation raises the possibility of a functional disorder, whatever the rectal configuration, and biofeedback treatment should be tried first: It is less invasive than surgery, more likely to be effective, and does not preclude a subsequent surgical option.

Proctography will probably always be controversial because severely constipated patients are very difficult to treat, not least because the precise aetiology of their affliction frequently remains obscure and patients' perception of disability varies. It is inevitable that constipated patients are a heterogeneous group with multifactorial causes. What is the value, therefore, of evacuation proctography to clinicians faced with a constipated patient? Some workers have attempted to assess the clinical impact of proctography (Hiltunen et al. 1994; Ott et al. 1994), but these studies have attracted fierce criticism from advocates of the technique (Kelvin et al. 1995; Halligan 1995). Evaluation of imaging techniques is fraught with difficulty, especially when the effects of treatment are included in assessment of outcomes and so confound the results. This especially disadvantages proctography, because constipation treatment for functional disorders is so often ineffective.

As stated in the introduction to this chapter, the main role of proctography is to place patients into clinically defined groups, and the utility of proctography may be better assessed via its impact on clinical decision making. With this in mind, a prospective study of 50 consecutive patients referred for evacuation proctography sought to determine the effect of imaging on clinical understanding and management: Using a pre- and post-intervention design, the authors found that evacuation proctography had considerable diagnostic and therapeutic effect and significantly increased the diagnostic confidence of referring physicians (Harvey et al. 1999). Indeed, 44 of 47 (94%) requesting clinicians generally found proctography to be of 'major' or 'moderate' benefit to their clinical decision making (Harvey et al. 1999).

Presently, there is a trend towards expanding the basic proctographic examination to encompass the entire pelvic floor (Kelvin and Maglinte 1997), an approach that probably has most appeal to the urogynaecologic patient (Lienemann et al. 1997) and which is discussed in detail in Chapter 4.1. Dynamic pelvic MR imaging (Chap. 4.2) has also been specifically employed to image constipated patients (Healey et al. 1997). Ultimately, for the reasons described above, evaluation of rectal evacuation will remain central to meaningful clinical assessment. Although this can be performed in the supine position, it is often a difficult and messy procedure, and few investigators have access to the more practical vertical configuration machines (Schoenberger et al. 1998). It is also clear that, like conventional proctography, MR imaging also reveals supposed abnormalities in asymptomatic subjects (Goh et al. 2000). While MR imaging undoubtedly warrants further investigation, the anatomical possibilities offered should not detract from the diagnosis of underlying functional problems in the constipated patient.

References

Alstrup N, Ronholt C, Fu C, Rasmussen O, Sorensen M, Christiansen J (1997) Viscous fluid expulsion in the evaluation of the constipated patient. Dis Colon Rectum40:580–584

Arnold MW, Stewart WR, Aguilar PS (1990) Rectocele repair: 4 years experience. Dis Colon Rectum 33:684–687

Bernini A, Madoff RD, Lowry AC, Spencer MP, Gemlo BT, Jensen LL, Wong WD (1998) Should patients with combined colonic inertia and nonrelaxing pelvic floor undergo subtotal colectomy? Dis Colon Rectum 41:1363–1366

Bleijenberg G, Kuijpers HC (1987) Treatment of the spastic pelvic floor syndrome with biofeedback. Dis Colon Rectum 30:108–111

Bouchard C (1906) Lectures on auto-intoxication in disease or self-poisoning of the individual. Philadelphia: Davis pp. 15

Broden B, Snellman B (1968) Procidentia of the rectum studied with cineradiography: a contribution to the discussion of the causative mechanism. Dis Colon Rectum 11:330–347

Cavallo G, Salzano A, Grassi R, de Lillo ML (1993) Functional intraperineal pouch of rectal wall (posterior rectocele). Dis Colon Rectum 36:179–181

Chaussade S, Khyari A, Roche H et al (1989) Determination of total and segmental colonic transit time in constipated patients: results in 91 patients with a new simplified method. Dig Dis Sci 34:1168–1172

Christiansen J, Zhu BW, Rasmussen OO, Sorensen M (1992) Internal rectal intussusception: results of surgical repair. Dis Colon Rectum 35:1026–1029

D'Hoore A, Penninckx F (2003) Obstructed defecation. Colorectal Dis 5:280–287

Drossman DA (1994) Idiopathic constipation: definition, epidemiology and behavioural aspects. In: Kamm M, Lennard-Jones J, eds. Constipation. Petersfield: Wrightson Biomedical p. 11–17

Duthie GS, Bartolo DC (1992) Anismus: the cause of constipation? World J Surg 16:831–835

Dvorkin LS, Knowles CH, Scott SM, Williams NS, Lunniss PJ (2005a) Rectal intussusception: characterization of symptomatology. Dis Colon Rectum 48:824–831

Dvorkin LS, Gladman MA, Epstein J, Scott SM, Williams NS, Lunniss PJ (2005b) Rectal intussusception in symptomatic patients is different from that in asymptomatic volunteers. Br J Surg 92:866–872

Ebbell BB (1937) The papyrus Ebers. Copenhagen: Levin and Munksgaard p. 30–32

Engel AF, Kamm MA (1994) The acute effect of straining on pelvic floor neurological function. Int J Colorect Dis 9:8–12

Eu KW, Seow-Choen F (1997) Functional problems in adult rectal prolapse and controversies in surgical management. Br J Surg 84:904–911

Evans RC, Kamm MA, Hinton JM, Lennard-Jones JE (1992) The normal range and a simple diagram for recording whole gut transit time. Int J Colorect Dis 7:15–17

Fleshman JW, Dreznik Z, Cohen E, Fry RD, Kodner IJ (1992) Balloon expulsion test facilitates diagnosis of pelvic floor outlet obstruction due to nonrelaxing puborectalis muscle. Dis Colon Rectum 35:1019–1025

Gattuso JM, Kamm MA (1997) Clinical features of idiopathic megarectum and idiopathic megacolon. Gut 41:93–99

Gladman MA, Dvorkin LS, Scott SM, Lunniss PJ, Williams NS (2007) A novel technique to identify patients with megarectum. Dis Colon Rectum 50:621–629

Glia A, Lindberg G (1998) Antroduodenal manometry findings in patients with slow-transit constipation. Scand J Gastroenterol 33:55–62

Goh V, Halligan S, Kaplan G, Healy JC, Bartram CI (2000) Dynamic MR imaging of the pelvic floor in asymptomatic subjects. AJR 174:661–666

Grassi R, Romano S, Micera O, Fioroni C, Boller B (2005) Radiographic findings of post-operative double stapled trans anal rectal resection (STARR) in patient with obstructed defecation syndrome (ODS). Eur J Radiol 53:410–416

Greenberg T, Kelvin FM, Maglinte DD (2001) Barium trapping in rectoceles: are we trapped by the wrong definition? Abdom Imaging 26:587–590

Halligan S (1994) Posterior perineal hernia or posterior rectocoele? Clin Radiol 49:219

Halligan S (1995) The benefits or otherwise of evacuation proctography. Abdom Imaging 20:280

Halligan S, McGee S, Bartram CI (1994) Quantification of evacuation proctography. Dis Colon Rectum 37:1151–1154

Halligan S, Bartram CI (1995) Is barium trapping in rectocoeles significant? Dis Colon Rectum 38:764–768

Halligan S, Bartram CI (1996) Is digitation associated with proctographic abnormality? Int J Colorect Dis 11:167–171

Halligan S, Bartram CI (1998) Anismus: Fact or fiction? Dis Colon Rectum 41:1070–1071

Halligan S, Nicholls RJ, Bartram CI (1995) Proctographic changes following rectopexy for solitary rectal ulcer syndrome and preoperative predictive factors for a successful outcome. Br J Surg 82:314–317

Halligan S, Nicholls RJ, Bartram CI (1995) Evacuation proctography in patients with solitary rectal ulcer syndrome: anatomic abnormalities and frequency of impaired emptying and prolapse. AJR 164:91–95

Halligan S, Thomas J, Bartram CI (1995) Intrarectal pressures and balloon expulsion related to evacuation proctography. Gut 31:100–104

Halligan S, Bartram CI, Park HY, Kamm MA (1995) The proctographic features of anismus. Radiology 197:679–682

Halligan S, Bartram C, Hall C, Wingate J (1996) Enterocele revealed by simultaneous evacuation proctography and peritoneography: does "defecation block" exist? AJR 167:461–466

Halligan S, Malouf A, Bartram CI, Marshall MM, Hollings N, Kamm MA (2001) Predictive value of impaired proctographic evacuation for diagnosis of anismus. AJR 177:633–636

Harewood GC, Coulie B, Camilleri M, Rath-Harvey D, Pemberton JH (1999) Descending perineum syndrome: audit of clinical and laboratory features and outcome of pelvic floor retraining. Am J Gastroenterol 94:126–130

Harvey C, Halligan S, Bartram CI, Hollings N, Shadev A, Kingston K (1999) Evacuation Proctography: A prospective study of diagnostic and therapeutic impact. Radiology 211:223–227

Heaton KW, Ghosh S, Braddon FEM (1991) How bad are the symptoms and bowel dysfunction of patients with the irritable bowel syndrome? A prospective controlled study with emphasis on stool form. Gut 32:73–79

Healy JC, Halligan S, Reznek RH, Watson S, Bartram CI, Kamm MA, Phillips RKS, Armstrong P (1997) Dynamic magnetic resonance imaging of the pelvic floor in patients with obstructed defecation. Br J Surg 84:1555–1558

Henry MM, Parks AG, Swash M (1982) The pelvic floor in the descending perineum syndrome. Br J Surg 69:470–472

Hiltunen KM, Kolehmainen H, Matikainen M (1994) Does defaecography help in diagnosis and clinical decision making in defecation disorders? Abdom Imaging 19:355–358

Hinton JM, Lennard-Jones JE, Young AC (1969) A new method for studying gut transit times using radio-opaque markers. Gut 10:842–847

Hoffman MJ, Kodner IJ, Fry RD (1984) Internal intussusception of the rectum: Diagnosis and surgical management. Dis Colon Rectum 27:435–441

Ihre T (1990) Intussusception of the rectum and the solitary rectal ulcer syndrome. Ann Med 22:419–423

Johanson JF, Sonnenberg A, Koch TR (1989) Clinical epidemiology of chronic constipation. J Clin Gastroenterol 11:525–536

Johansson C, Nilsson BY, Holmstrom B, Dolk A, Mellgren A (1992) Association between rectocele and paradoxical sphincter response. Dis Colon Rectum 35:503–509

Johansson CJ, Ihre T, Ahlback SO (1985) Disturbances in the defecation mechanism with special reference to intussusception of the rectum. Dis Colon Rectum 28:920–924

Jones PN, Lubowski DZ, Swash M, Henry MM (1987) Is paradoxical contraction of puborectalis muscle of functional importance? Dis Colon Rectum 30:667–670

Jorge JMN, Wexner SD, Ehrenpreis ED, Nogueras JJ, Jagelman DG (1993) Does perineal descent correlate with pudendal neuropathy? Dis Colon Rectum 36:475–483

Jorge JM, Wexner SD, Ger GC, Salanga VD, Nogueras JJ, Jagelman DG (1993) Cinedefecography and electromyography in the diagnosis of nonrelaxing puborectalis syndrome. Dis Colon Rectum 36:668–676

Kamm MA, Hawley PR, Lennard-Jones JE (1988) Outcome of colectomy for severe idiopathic constipation. Gut 29:969–973

Kamm MA, Bartram CI, Lennard-Jones JE (1989) Rectodynamics–Quantifying rectal evacuation. Int J Colorect Dis 4:161–163

Karlbom U, Graf W, Nilsson S, Påhlman L (2004) The accuracy of clinical examination in the diagnosis of rectal intussusception. Dis Colon Rectum 47:1533–1538

Kelvin FM, Maglinte DDT, Hornback JA, Benson JT (1992) Pelvic prolapse: assessment with evacuation proctography (defecography). Radiology 184:547–551

Kelvin FM, Maglinte DDT, Benson JT, Pittman JS (1995) Re: The role of defecography in clinical practice. Abdom Imaging 20:279–280

Kelvin FM, Maglinte DDT (1997) Dynamic cystoproctography of female pelvic floor defects and their interrelationships. AJR 169:769–774

Klauser AG, Voderholzer WA, Heinrich CA, Schindlbeck NE, Muller-Lissner SA (1990) Behavioural modification of colonic function: can constipation be learned? Dig Dis Sci 35:1271–1275

Knowles CH, Scott SM, Wellmer A, Misra VP, Pilot MA, Williams NS, Anand P (1999) Sensory and autonomic neuropathy in patients with idiopathic slow transit constipation. Br J Surg 86:54–60

Kuijpers HC, Bleijenberg G (1986) The spastic pelvic floor syndrome: A cause of constipation. Dis Colon Rectum 28:669–672

Kuijpers HC, Bleijenberg G, de Morree H (1986) The spastic pelvic floor syndrome. Large bowel outlet obstruction caused by pelvic floor dysfunction–a radiological study. Int J Colorect Dis 1:44–48

Lane WA (1913) An address on chronic intestinal stasis. BMJ ii:1126

Laarhoven CJHM, Kamm MA, Bartram CI, Halligan S, Hawley PR, Phillips RKS (1999) Relationship between anatomic and symptomatic long-term results after rectocele repair for impaired defecation. Dis Colon Rectum 42:204–211

Lau CW, Heymen S, Alabaz O, Iroatulam AJ, Wexner SD (2000) Prognostic significance of rectocele, intussusception and abnormal perineal descent in biofeedback treatment for constipated patients with paradoxical puborectalis contraction. Dis Colon Rectum 43:478–482

Leroi AM (1995) Anismus as a marker of sexual abuse: consequences of abuse on anorectal motility. Dig Dis Sci 40:1411–1416

Liberman H, Hughes C, Dippolito (2000) Evaluation and outcome of the Delorme procedure in the treatment of rectal outlet obstruction. Dis Colon Rectum 43:188–192

Lienemann A, Anthuber C, Baron A, Kohz P, Reiser M (1997) Dynamic MR colpocystorectography assessing pelvic floor descent. Eur Radiol 7:1309–1317

Loder P, Watson S, Halligan S, Bartram CI, Phillips RKS (1996) Transperineal repair of symptomatic rectocoele with marlex mesh: A clinical, physiological and radiological assessment of treatment. J Am Coll Surg 183:257–261

Marshall M, Halligan S, Fotheringham T, Bartram C, Nicholls RJ (2002) Predictive value of internal anal sphincter thickness for diagnosis of rectal intussusception in patients with solitary rectal ulcer syndrome. Br J Surg 89:1281–1285

McKee RF, McEnroe L, Anderson JH, Finlay IG (1999) Identification of patients likely to benefit from biofeedback for outlet obstruction constipation. Br J Surg 86:355–359

McGee SG, Bartram CI (1993) Intra-anal intussusception: diagnosis by posteroanterior stress proctography. Abdom Imaging 2:136–140
Mellgren A, Schultz I, Johansson C, Dolk A (1997) Internal rectal intussusception seldom develops into total rectal prolapse. Dis Colon Rectum 40:817–820
Mellgren A, Lopez A, Schultz I, Anzen B (1998) Rectocele is associated with paradoxical anal sphincter reaction. Int J Colorect Dis 13:13–16
Mimura T, Roy AJ, Storrie JB, Kamm MA (2000) Treatment of impaired defecation associated with rectocele by behavioural retraining (biofeedback). Dis Colon Rectum 43:1267–1272
Morio O, Meurette G, Desfourneaux V, D'Halluin PN, Bretagne JF, Siproudhis L (2005) Anorectal physiology in solitary ulcer syndrome: a case-matched series. Dis Colon Rectum 48:1917–1922
Murthy VK, Orkin BA, Smith LE, Glassman LM (1996) Excellent outcome using selective criteria for rectocele repair. Dis Colon Rectum 39:374–378
Oettle GJ, Roe AM, Bartolo DC, Mortensen NJ (1985) What is the best way of measuring perineal descent? A comparison of radiographic and clinical methods. Br J Surg 72:999–1001
Orrom WJ, Bartolo DCC, Miller R, Mortensen NJ, Roe AM (1991) Rectopexy is an ineffective treatment for obstructed defecation. Dis Colon Rectum 34:41–46
Ott DJ, Donati DL, Kerr RM, Chen MYM (1994) Defecography: results in 55 patients and impact on clinical management. Abdom Imaging 9:349–354
Parks AG, Porter NH, Hardcastle JD (1966) The syndrome of the descending perineum. Proc R Soc Med 59:477–482
Pechlivanides G, Tsiaoussis J, Athanasakis E, Zervakis N, Gouvas N, Zacharioudakis G, Xynos E (2007) Stapled transanal rectal resection (STARR) to reverse the anatomic disorders of pelvic floor dyssynergia. World J Surg 31:1329–1335
Preston DM, Lennard-Jones JE, Thomas BM (1985) Towards a radiologic definition of idiopathic megacolon. Gastrointest Radiol 10:167–169
Preston DM, Lennard-Jones JE (1985) Anismus in chronic constipation. Dig Dis Sci 30:413–418
Preston DM, Lennard-Jones JE (1886) Severe chronic constipation of young women: idiopathic slow transit constipation. Gut 27:41–48
Prior A, Maxton DG, Whorwell JP (1990) Anorectal manometry in irritable bowel syndrome: differences between diarrhoea and constipation predominant subjects. Gut 31:458–462
Probert CSJ, Emmett PM, Cripps HA, Heaton KW (1994) Evidence for the ambiguity of the term constipation: the role of the irritable bowel syndrome. Gut 35:1455–1458
Rao SS, Ozturk R, De Ocampo S, Stessman M (2006) Pathophysiology and role of biofeedback therapy in solitary rectal ulcer syndrome. Am J Gastroenterol 101:613–618
Read NW (1989) Tests of anorectal function: Summary and conclusions. In: Read NW, ed. Gastrointestinal motility: which test? Wrightson Biomedical Ltd. p. 277–282
Read NW, Timms JM, Bannister JJ, Donnelly TC, Read MG (1986) Impairment of defecation in young women with severe constipation. Gastroenterology 90:53–60
Rex DR, Lappas JC, Goutet RC, Madura JA (1992) Selection of constipated subjects as subtotal colectomy candidates. J Clin Gastroenterol 15:212–217
Sandler RS, Drossman DA (1987) Bowel habits in young adults not seeking health care. Dig Dis Sci 32:841–845
Schoenberger AW, Debatin JF, Guldenschuh I, Hany TF, Steiner P, Krestin GP (1998) Dynamic MR defecography with a superconducting, open-configuration MR system. Radiology 206:641–646
Shorvon PJ, McHugh S, Diamant NE, Somers S, Stevenson GW (1989) Defecography in normal volunteers: results and implications. Gut 30:1737–1749
Skomorowska E, Hegedus V, Christiansen J (1988) Evaluation of perineal descent by defaecography. Int J Colorect Dis 3:191–194
Sun WM, Read NW, Donnelly TC, Bannister JJ, Shorthouse AJ (1989) A common pathophysiology for full thickness rectal prolapse, anterior mucosal prolapse and solitary rectal ulcer. Br J Surg 76:290–295
Talley NJ, Weaver AL, Zinmeister AR, Melton LJ (1993) Functional constipation and outlet delay: A population based study. Gastroenterology 105:781–790
van Tets WF, Kuijpers JHC (1995) Internal rectal intussusception–fact or fancy? Dis Colon Rectum 38:1080–1083
Thompson WG, Dotevall G, Drossman DA, Heaton KW, Kruis W (1989) Irritable bowel syndrome: guidelines for the diagnosis. Gastroenterol Int 2:92–95
Thorpe AC, Williams NS, Badenoch DF, Blandy JP, Grahn MF (1993) Simultaneous electromyographic proctography and cystometrography. Br J Surg 80:115–120
Tjandra JJ, Ooi BS, Tang CL, Dwyer P, Carey M (1999) Transanal repair of rectocele corrects obstructed defecation if it is not associated with anismus. Dis Colon Rectum 42:1544–1550
Turnbull GK, Bartram CI, Lennard-Jones JE (1988) Radiologic studies of rectal evacuation in adults with idiopathic constipation. Dis Colon Rectum 31:190–197
Tuttle JP (1903) A treatise on the diseases of the anus, rectum and pelvic colon. Appleton, New York and London p. 961
van Dam JH, Hop WC, Schouten WR (2000) Analysis of patients with poor outcome of rectocele repair. Dis Colon Rectum 43:1556–1560
Wasserman IF (1964) Puborectalis syndrome (rectal stenosis due to anorectal spasm). Dis Colon Rectum 7:87–98
Whorton J (2000) Civilisation and the colon: constipation as the "diseases of diseases." BMJ 321:1586–1589
Womack NR, Williams NS, Holmfield JH, Morrison JF (1987) Pressure and prolapse: the cause of the solitary rectal ulcer syndrome. Gut 28:1228–1233

Coloproctological Dysfunction

6

6.2 Investigation of Fecal Incontinence

ADIL E. BHARUCHA

CONTENTS

6.2.1 Introduction

Fecal incontinence (FI) is generally caused by altered bowel habit, predominantly diarrhoea, with or without pelvic floor dysfunction. Appropriate testing for diseases causing FI (e.g., spinal imaging for patients with suspected spinal cord lesions) should be guided by the clinical features. Similarly, changes in bowel habit should be investigated using conventional techniques (e.g., endoscopy, serological testing for celiac sprue, stool studies, breath tests for carbohydrate intolerance etc) dependent on the patient's age and the clinical presentation.

This chapter will focus on the assessment of those anorectal functions responsible for maintaining continence. There is considerable evidence that investigations of anorectal structure and function complement but do not replace thorough clinical assessment in the evaluation and management of FI. Anal manometry, assessment of rectal sensation, and endoanal imaging, either by ultrasound or MRI, are useful initial investigations in most ambulatory patients with significant symptoms (BHARUCHA 2003). Additional tests, e.g., anal sphincter electromyography (EMG), evaluation of pelvic floor motion by dynamic MRI or barium defecography, and assessment of rectal compliance and sensation by a barostat are also useful for understanding the pathophysiology in selected patients with FI (BHARUCHA et al. 2005a).

A. E. BHARUCHA, MD, MBBS
Professor of Medicine, Clinical Enteric Neuroscience Translational & Epidemiological Research Program, Mayo Clinic, College of Medicine, 200 First Street SW, Rochester, MN 55905, USA

6.2.2 Tests of Function

6.2.2.1 Anal Manometry

Measurement

Anal manometry is best conducted in a laboratory with the necessary technical and interpretative expertise. At a minimum, anal resting and squeeze pressure, and the recto-anal inhibitory reflex should be assessed during manometry (Fig. 6.2.1), (Sect. 4.8.3). Recto-anal pressure changes during straining, stimulating defecation, should also be assessed when an evacuation disorder is suspected. Indeed, in one series, 18% of patients with fecal incontinence also had features of a rectal evacuation

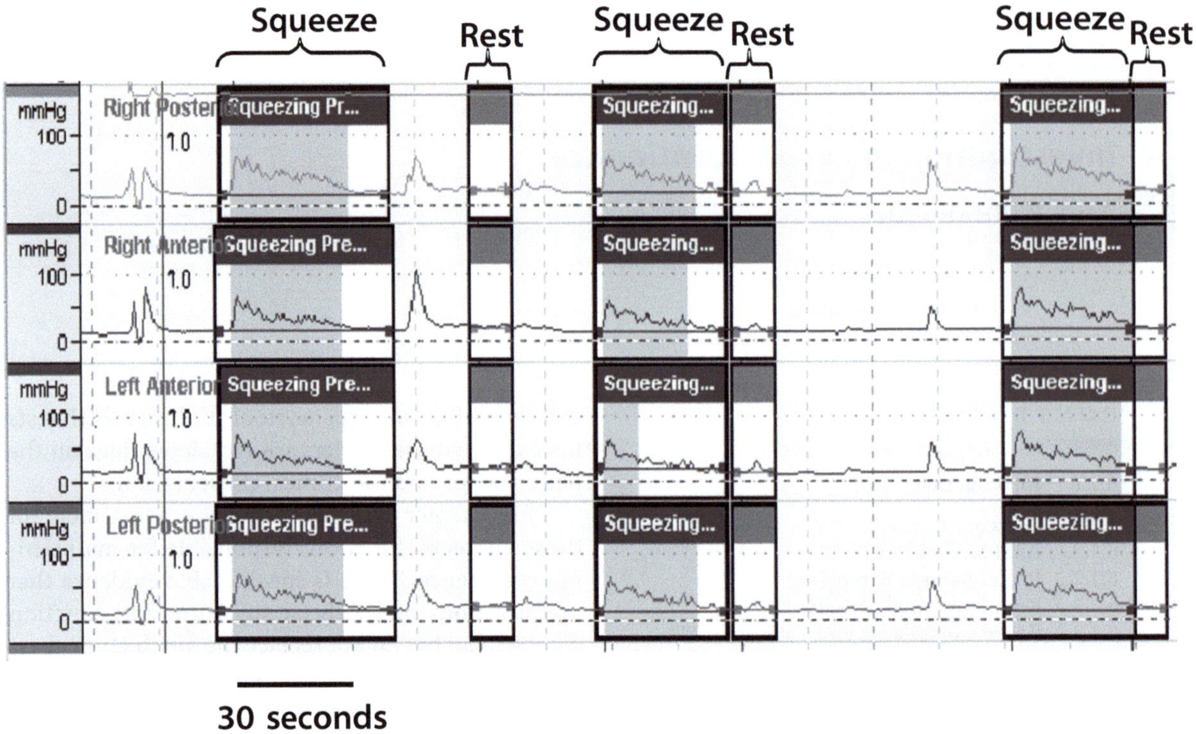

Fig. 6.2.1. Anal sphincter pressures assessed on 3 separate occasions by 4 circumferentially oriented transducers stationed at 1 cm from the anal verge; transducers were located in separate quadrants. The maximum squeeze pressure is the highest pressure recorded by all 4 transducers during one of 3 maneuvers; the average squeeze pressure is calculated by averaging pressures across all 4 maneuvers. In this example, resting and squeeze pressures were comparable in all 4 quadrants. (Reproduced with permission from Bharucha (2004) Outcome measures for fecal incontinence: Anorectal structure and function. Gastroenterology 126:S90–S98)

disorder (Bharucha et al. 2005a). Techniques for conducting and analyzing anorectal manometry are not standardized, and have been discussed in detail elsewhere (Rao et al. 2002; Bharucha et al. 2004) (Sect. 4.8.3). Salient considerations are as follows:

a) *Recording System.* The manometric catheter assembly includes a rectal balloon and pressure transducers located in the anal canal. Water-perfused sensors are considerably cheaper and are probably comparable to solid-state manometry for measuring anal pressures. With the advent of anal endosonography, vector manometry is no longer used for identifying anal sphincter defects. High-resolution manometry uses closely-spaced solid-state sensors to simultaneously measure circumferential pressures in the rectum and throughout the anal canal, obviating the need to perform a station pull-through manoeuvre, which is relatively cumbersome and time consuming. This technique permits 16 circumferential channels to be positioned at one level to provide measurements that are not affected by circumferential asymmetry (Fig. 6.2.2). Anal pressures measured by high-resolution manometry have been significantly correlated to traditional manometry (Jones et al. 2007). However, normal values for anal pressures measured by high resolution manometry are unavailable and further studies are necessary to determine if high-resolution manometry is superior to conventional manometry for understanding rectoanal dysfunctions.
b) *Measurement Technique.* As described in Section 4.8.3, with traditional (i.e., not high resolution) catheters, anal resting, and squeeze pressures are measured while the transducer is gradually withdrawn in 0.5 or 1-cm steps from the anal verge to the rectum. Pressures are measured when the transducer is stationary; the station pull-through procedure avoids the artefact induced by reflex anal sphincter contraction during a rapid pull-through procedure. Anal pressures should preferably be calculated by averaging all four quad-

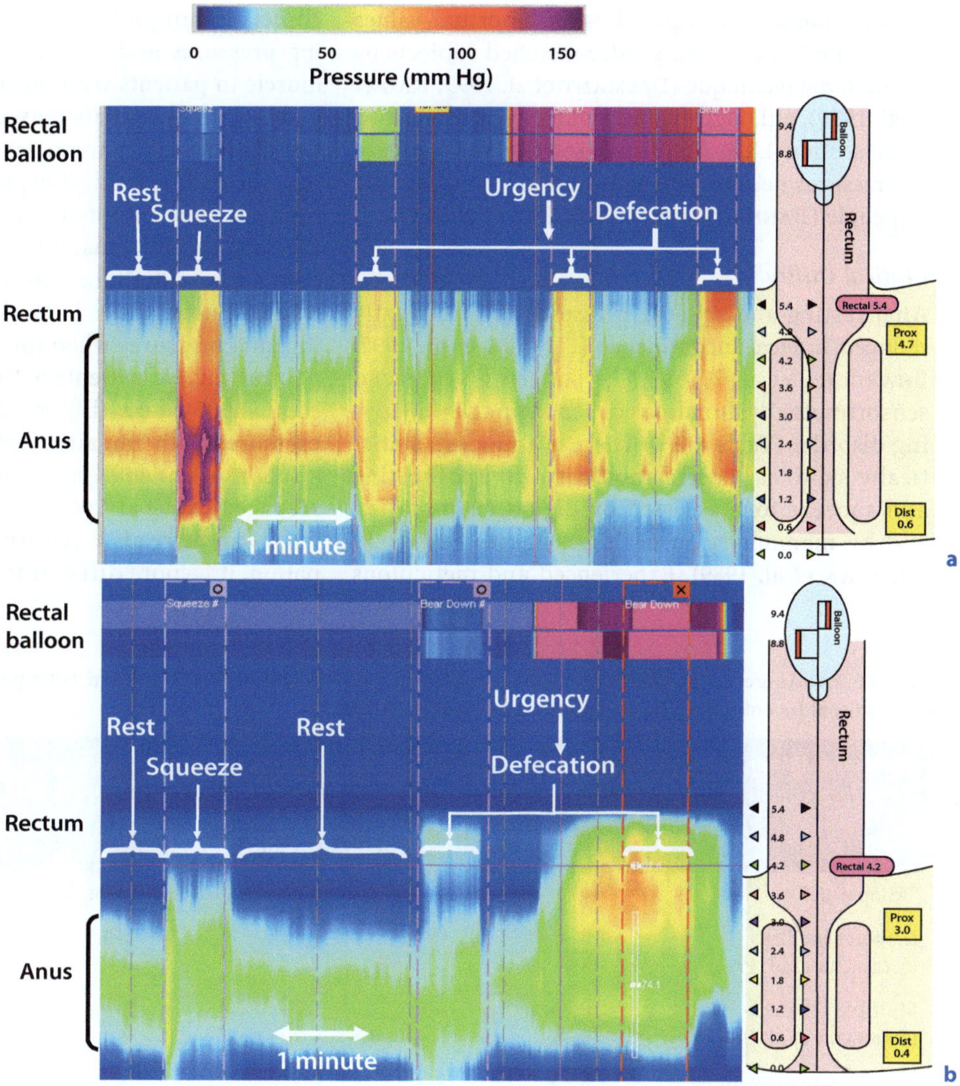

Fig. 6.2.2a,b. Comparison of anal pressures at rest, during squeeze, and during simulated evacuation recorded by high resolution manometry in a healthy subject (**a**) and a woman with fecal incontinence (**b**). Each figure depicts pressures recorded by 12 sensors. The far right cartoon shows these sensors, 10 of which are evenly distributed in the distal rectum and anal canal at 0.6 cm intervals, and 2 of which are located in the more proximally located rectal balloon. Each panel shows only 1 (of 3) squeeze manoeuvres for clarity and 3 (**a**) or 2 (**b**) manoeuvres with simulated defecation. a shows normal anal resting (68 mmHg) and squeeze pressures (127 mmHg); the squeeze response was sustained for 20 seconds. Defecatory mechanisms were assessed during 3 maneuvers with the rectal balloon inflated to 0, 50 mL, and 100 mL, with this subject reporting urgency after the 50 mL distension. Consequently, it is during only the 3rd maneuver that the rectal pressure (107 mmHg) was higher than the anal pressure (79 mmHg), providing the gradient necessary for rectal evacuation. In the patient with fecal incontinence (**b**), the anal canal was shorter (2.6 cm) and anal resting (50 mmHg) and squeeze pressures (58 mmHg) were lower. There was a positive recto-anal pressure gradient during defecation

rants to account for anal sphincter asymmetry. Variations in patient effort also need to be taken into account. Resting pressures are probably less susceptible to artefact than are squeeze pressures. Squeeze pressure should be measured by asking patients to squeeze (i.e., contract) the sphincter for at least 30 seconds, and to average pressure over this duration. Defecation is normally accompanied by increased intra-rectal pressure and anal relaxation (Rao and Patel 1997).

c) *Normal ranges.* Since anal pressures are affected by age, gender, and technique, measurements ideally should be compared against normal values obtained in age- and gender-matched subjects by the same technique (DIAMANT et al. 1999; RAO et al. 1999), although typical values are as described in section 4.8.3. Both anal resting and squeeze pressures decline with age, even in asymptomatic people (BANNISTER et al. 1987; FOX et al. 2006).

Clinical Utility

Anal resting and squeeze pressures are frequently reduced in fecal incontinence (FI) (SUN et al. 1992; BHARUCHA et al. 2005a). The pattern of anorectal sensorimotor dysfunctions depends on the underlying disorder (Table 6.2.1). There is a modest, statistically significant correlation between anal resting and squeeze tone assessed by digital examination and by manometry in healthy subjects and in FI (HALLAN et al. 1989). Experienced and meticulous clinicians can probably accurately gauge anal resting pressures and contraction of the puborectalis muscle in patients with normal or markedly abnormal (i.e., reduced or increased) function. Some question therefore, if manometry is necessary. However, in addition to quantifying pressures as a continuous rather than a discrete (i.e., normal, reduced, or increased) variable, manometry is probably more accurate than a digital examination for (i) identifying minor abnormalities in anal pressures, (ii) measuring anal pressures when the clinical examination is painful, e.g., in patients with an anal fissure (JONES et al. 2005), and (iii) identifying increased anal pressures with impaired sphincteric relaxation in a subset of patients, predominantly men, with fecal seepage (RAO et al. 2004b). Though the puborectalis "lift" can be readily discerned by a clinical examination, it is more difficult to appreciate contraction

Table 6.2.1. Anorectal Sensori-Motor Disturbances in Fecal Incontinence. Reprinted with permission from BHARUCHA (2003) Fecal Incontinence. Gastroenterology 124(6):1672–1685

Etiological Factor	Anal sphincter pressure	Threshold for internal sphincter relaxation	Threshold for external sphincter contraction	Rectal sensation[a]	Rectal compliance	Pelvic floor function
"Idiopathic"	↓	↓	↓	↓ or ↑	↓	↓
Diabetes mellitus (CARUANA et al. 1991)	R ↓; S ↓	↔	↑	↓↓	↔	NA
Multiple sclerosis (CARUANA et al. 1991)	R ↔; S ↓↓	↓	↑	↓↓	↔	NA
Elderly patients with fecal impaction and incontinence (READ and ABOUZEKRY 1986)	R ↔; S ↔	↓	↑	↓	NA	↓
Acute radiation proctitis (YEOH et al. 1998)	R ↓; S ↓	NA	NA	↔	↓	NA
Chronic radiation injury (VARMA et al. 1985)	NA	NA	NA	↑	↓	NA
Ulcerative colitis (DENIS et al. 1979; RAO et al. 1987)	S ↓ incontinent patients	↓ (active colitis only)	NA	↑ (active colitis only)	↓ (active colitis only)	NA
Spinal cord injury – high spinal lesion, i.e. T12 or higher (SUN et al. 1990a)	R ↔; S ↓	↓	↔	↓	↓	NA
Low spinal lesion, i.e. below T12	R ↓; S ↓	↔	↓	↓	↔	NA

Information pertains to patients with underlying disease and fecal incontinence.
↑ = Increased; ↓ = decreased; ↔ = no change; R = resting, S = squeeze sphincter pressure, NA = not available
[a] Rectal sensation expressed as volume thresholds for perception; ↑ sensation indicates volume threshold for perception was lower compared to normals

of the external sphincter. Moreover, because anal pressures decline with age even in asymptomatic subjects, it can be challenging to gauge if anal tone is normal or reduced in older people by a digital examination alone. However, even among patients with weak or normal anal pressures, additional factors (e.g., diarrhoea, disturbances of rectal compliance and/or sensation) may also contribute to FI. The effects of biofeedback therapy on anal resting and squeeze pressures are reported to be small and inconsistent and do not correlate with symptom improvement (Bharucha 2004).

Anorectal testing may also reveal features of a functional rectal evacuation disorder, i.e., impaired relaxation or paradoxical contraction of the anal sphincter (i.e., dyssynergia) or inadequate augmentation of rectal pressure (i.e., inadequate propulsive forces) during simulated evacuation (Rao et al. 1998). However, it is important to recognize that anorectal manometry is conducted in the horizontal position. In addition, because expulsion efforts do not mimic the recto-colonic coordination or stool delivery present in normal defecation, manometry may over diagnose dyssynergia. Moreover, the anal sphincter or puborectalis may not relax during defecation in up to 20% of asymptomatic subjects (Voderholzer et al. 1997).

6.2.2.2 Rectal Balloon Expulsion

Measurement

The rectal balloon expulsion test can be conducted in a physician's office. The patient's ability to expel a water-filled balloon while seated on a commode in a private setting is assessed. Normal expulsion occurs within 60 seconds. The balloon may be inflated by a fixed volume, typically 50 mL (Rao et al. 2002), or alternatively until the patient experiences the desire to defecate (Minguez et al. 2004). The test may also be conducted in the left lateral decubitus position, wherein a rectal balloon is connected over a pulley to weights, which provide external traction when necessary to facilitate rectal balloon expulsion. (Barnes and Lennard-Jones 1985; Bharucha et al. 2005b). In the author's laboratory, subjects with normal rectoanal expulsion can expel the balloon spontaneously or aided by external traction of up to 100 gm. Patients with pelvic floor dysfunction require more external traction to expel a rectal balloon.

Clinical Utility

The balloon expulsion test is a useful screening test for a functional defecation disorder, but it does not define the mechanism of disordered evacuation (Minguez et al. 2004). Because the balloon may not mimic the patients' stool, patients with convincing symptoms together with manometric and radiological evidence of a functional defecation disorder may have normal balloon expulsion. Conversely, a normal balloon expulsion study does not always exclude a functional defecation disorder (Rao et al. 2004a).

6.2.2.3 Rectal and Anal Sensation

Measurement

(See also Sect. 4.8.4, 4.8.5). Most anorectal laboratories assess rectal sensation by progressively distending a latex balloon manually. Research studies and some clinical laboratories assess rectal sensation by distending a polyethylene balloon with a barostat. Thresholds for first perception, desire to defecate, and severe urgency are measured during distension (Whitehead and Palsson 1998). Because age (Bannister et al. 1987; Fox et al. 2006), and the rate and pattern of distension affect rectal perception (Sun et al. 1990c), results from different laboratories may not be comparable. Table 6.2.2 lists studies in which rectal sensory thresholds were studied in > 20 asymptomatic subjects and in which 95% confidence intervals for sensory thresholds could be estimated. These data indicate that 95% confidence intervals for sensory thresholds in asymptomatic subjects are relatively wide. A barostat permits more controlled distension compared to manual techniques. Moreover, balloon pressure and volume can be measured during distension, thereby assessing pressure/volume relationships (Law et al. 2001; Bharucha et al. 2001). Anal sensation is assessed by determining the threshold for perception of an electrical stimulus or temperature change in the anal canal (Salvioli et al. 2001). Assessments of anal temperature sensation are of uncertain significance and are largely investigational.

Clinical Utility

Thresholds for rectal sensation may be normal, reduced, or increased in FI (Sun et al. 1992; Bharucha et al. 2005a). When rectal sensation is reduced, stool may leak before the external sphincter contracts (Buser and Miner 1986; Sun et al. 1990b). Sensory

Table 6.2.2. Rectal Sensory Thresholds Measured by a Latex Balloon. Reproduced with permission from Bharucha (2006a) Update of tests of colon and rectal structure and function. J Clin Gastroenterol 40(2):96–103

First Author	Number (Age range)	Method of Inflation	Mean (95% CI) Thresholds in mL for women
Bannister (Bannister et al. 1987)	48 younger (19–55 years) and 37 elderly subjects (66–87 years)	Manual inflation by air in 50 mL increments with 1 minute rest in between increments	[a]FS – ~100% by 100 mL DD – 100% by 175 mL
Ryhammer (Ryhammer et al. 1997)	75 women (20–83 years)	Inflated with water @ 50 mL/minute by a pump.	FS – 71 (24, 213) DD – 117 (47, 294) Urge – 170 (78, 371)
Rao (Rao et al. 1999)	45 subjects (20–70 years)	Manual inflation by 10, 20, 30, 40, 60, 80, 110, 140, 170, 200, 240, 280, and 320 mL air for 1 minute with 2 minutes rest in between inflations	FS – 19 (15, 23) DD – 103 (83, 123) Urge – 173 (150, 196) MTV – 230 (205, 255)
Sloots (Sloots et al. 2000)	28 subjects (age 22–67 years)	Inflated with water @ 50 mL/minute by a pump[b]	[a]FS – 102 (75, 129) Urg – 159 (126, 191) MTV – 239 (202, 276)
Bharucha (Bharucha et al. 2005b)	41 subjects (age 23–69 years)	Manual inflation with air @ 20 mL/5 seconds.	FS – 46 (14, 87) DD – 89 (38, 172) Urg – 166 (90, 300)

Abbreviations – FS – first sensation; DD – Desire to defecate; Urg – Rectal urgency; MTV – Maximum tolerated volume
a These are thresholds for all subjects (i.e., men and women) in this study
[b] Rectal sensation was also assessed by a barostat in this study

retraining can restore coordinated contraction of the external sphincter and improve fecal continence (Wald and Tunuguntla 1984; Buser and Miner 1986). However patients require at least some rectal perception to benefit from sensory retraining. In uncontrolled studies, preserved rectal sensation before biofeedback therapy and improved sensation after biofeedback therapy predicted improved continence (Chiarioni et al. 2002). Conversely, some incontinent patients have exaggerated rectal sensation, perhaps resulting from rectal hypersensitivity and/or reduced rectal capacity (Sect. 6.2.2.4) (Bharucha et al. 2005a).

6.2.2.4 Rectal Compliance and Capacity

Measurement

Compliance is measured by assessing rectal pressure-volume relationships, either by manually inflating a latex balloon inside the rectum with air or water or by distending a highly compliant polyethylene balloon with a barostat (Fig. 6.2.3). The barostat technique is preferable because the rate of distension is controlled and because a polyethylene balloon is infinitely compliant. Patients are examined in a semi-prone position to reduce pelvic hydrostatic pressure. An initial or "conditioning" distension ensures that subsequent measurements of rectal compliance and sensory thresholds are reproducible. Pressure-volume relationships reflect passive properties (i.e., connective tissue), muscle tone (i.e., "static" properties), and phasic responses to distension (i.e., "dynamic" properties). It is unclear if pressure-volume relationships are affected by structures extrinsic to the rectum. When balloon pressure and volume are allowed to equilibrate at intervening steps, the contractile response induced by distension subsides. Under these circumstances, compliance (i.e., passive properties and tone) can be characterized. The pressure-volume ratio at different distension thresholds is an incomplete index of "compliance" compared to the entire pressure-volume curve.

Clinical Utility

Reduced compliance may cause symptoms of rectal urgency and frequent defecation in diarrhoea-predominant irritable bowel syndrome, ulcerative

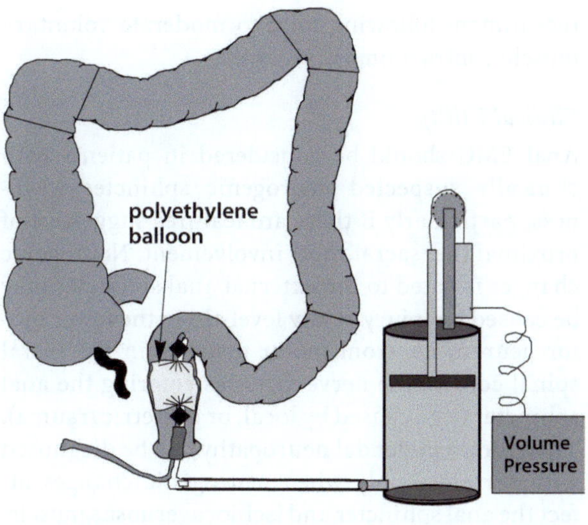

Fig. 6.2.3. A rectal barostat assembly. A highly compliant polyethylene balloon is inflated by a barostat, which monitors intra-balloon pressure and volume. (Reproduced with permission from BHARUCHA (2004) Outcome measures for fecal incontinence: Anorectal structure and function. Gastroenterology 126:S90–S98)

colitis, or radiation injury. The rectal capacity, (i.e., the balloon volume at the maximum imposed pressure), is also reduced in a subset of women with idiopathic FI (BHARUCHA et al. 2005a; ANDREWS et al. 2007). Moreover, reduced rectal capacity was associated with the symptom of urgency and with rectal hypersensitivity in FI (Fig. 6.2.4) (BHARUCHA et al. 2005a; DEUTEKOM et al. 2007). This association between reduced rectal capacity or compliance and rectal hypersensitivity has been confirmed by other studies (CHAN et al. 2005; SIPROUDHIS et al. 2005). Reduced rectal adaptation to distension is particularly significant for patients with FI and normal anal pressures (SIPROUDHIS et al. 1999).

6.2.2.5 Pudendal Nerve Terminal Motor Latency (PNTML)

Measurement

(Sect. 4.8.3.3). PNTML are used to identify pudendal nerve injury and to ascertain if anal sphincter weakness is attributable to pudendal nerve injury, anal sphincter injury, or both (DIAMANT et al. 1999). The index finger is covered by a glove containing stimulating and recording electrodes that stimulate the

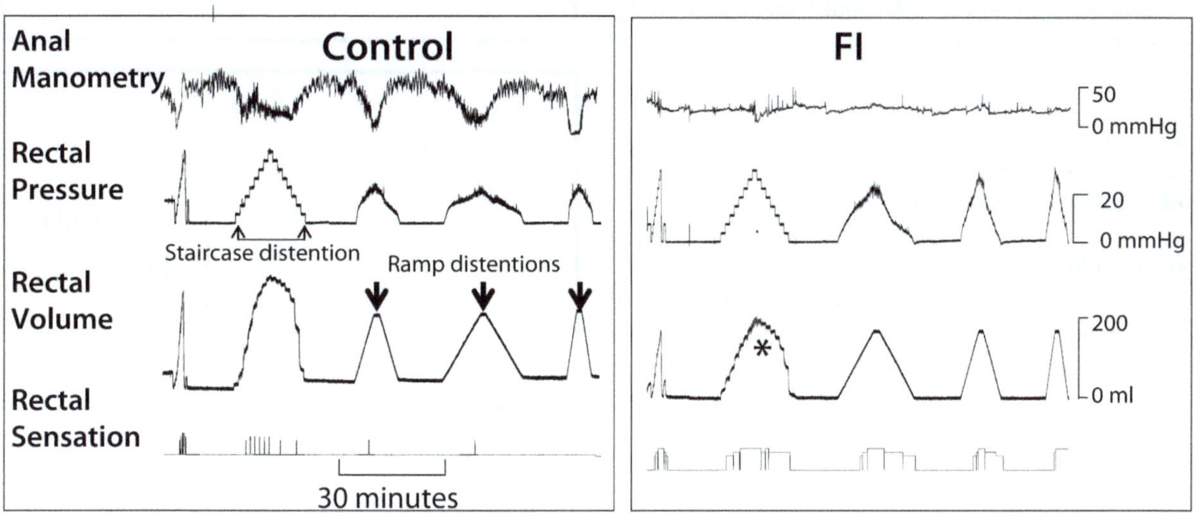

Fig. 6.2.4. Anorectal motility and symptoms during rectal distension in a control subject (left panel) and in FI (right panel). Features in FI include (i) smaller rectal capacity [i.e., maximum rectal volume (*)] and lower compliance (i.e., rate of change in volume) during staircase distension; (ii) higher rectal pressures during ramp distensions from 0–200 mL at 50, 25, and 100 mL/minute (indicated by *arrows*); and (iii) rectal hypersensitivity. During rectal distensions, the patient with FI pressed the event marker at lower rectal pressures and/or volumes and kept the event marker pressed for longer durations, indicating more prolonged sensation. Also, observe lower anal resting pressure and less anal relaxation during rectal distension in FI. (ANDREWS et al. (2007) Rectal sensorimotor dysfunction in women with fecal incontinence. Am J Physiol Gastrointest Liver Physiol 292:G282–289, used with permission)

nerve as the nerve travels around the pelvic brim. Measuring the shortest latency between stimulus delivery and recording is critically dependent on ensuring that the examining finger in close proximity to the nerve. In theory, delayed latencies indicate pudendal neuropathy.

Clinical Utility

Initial studies suggested that patients with pudendal neuropathy do not fare as well as patients without neuropathy after surgical repair of sphincter defects. However, the utility of PNTML to ascertain pudendal neuropathy has been challenged on several grounds. Since PNTML measures only the fastest conducting fibers in the pudendal nerve, nerve latencies may be normal even if only a few normally conducting fibers remain (under diagnosis). Normative data for this test are also inadequate. The reproducibility of the test between different examiners, or on different days, is unknown. The sensitivity and specificity of the test are uncertain (in one study, approximately 50% of patients with prolonged PNTML had normal anal canal squeeze pressures) (Wexner et al. 1991). In contrast to earlier studies, more recent studies suggest the test does not predict improvement, or the lack of improvement, after surgical repair of anal sphincter defects (Malouf et al. 2000). A position statement issued by the American Gastroenterological Association (AGA) recommended that PNTML should not be used in the evaluation of FI (Diamant et al. 1999).

6.2.2.6 Needle Electromyography (EMG) of the External Sphincter

Introduction

(Section 4.8.3.2) EMG provides a sensitive measure of denervation (fibrillation potentials) and can usually identify myopathic damage (small polyphasic motor unit potentials), neurogenic damage (large polyphasic motor unit potentials), or mixed injury (Fig. 6.2.5).

Methods

Each side of the external anal sphincter (EAS) is examined with 1 or 2 concentric needle insertions (Bharucha et al. 2005a). The puborectalis muscle is examined by inserting a needle in the midline between the anus and tip of the coccyx, passing it through the EAS and into the deeper puborectalis. Insertional activity at rest, motor unit potential amplitude and duration, percent polyphasia, and recruitment following mild to moderate voluntary muscle contraction are assessed.

Clinical Utility

Anal EMG should be considered in patients with clinically suspected neurogenic sphincter weakness, particularly if there are features suggestive of proximal (i.e. sacral root) involvement. Neurogenic changes isolated to the external anal sphincter may be caused by injury at any level along the lower motor neuron, i.e. from motor neurons in the sacral spinal cord to the nerve fascicles entering the anal sphincter (e.g., caused by local, or obstetric trauma). Therefore, a pudendal neuropathy can be diagnosed with certainty only when neurogenic changes affect the anal sphincter and ischiocavernosus muscle. Needle EMG of the puborectalis can be used to distinguish disorders that affect this muscle and the

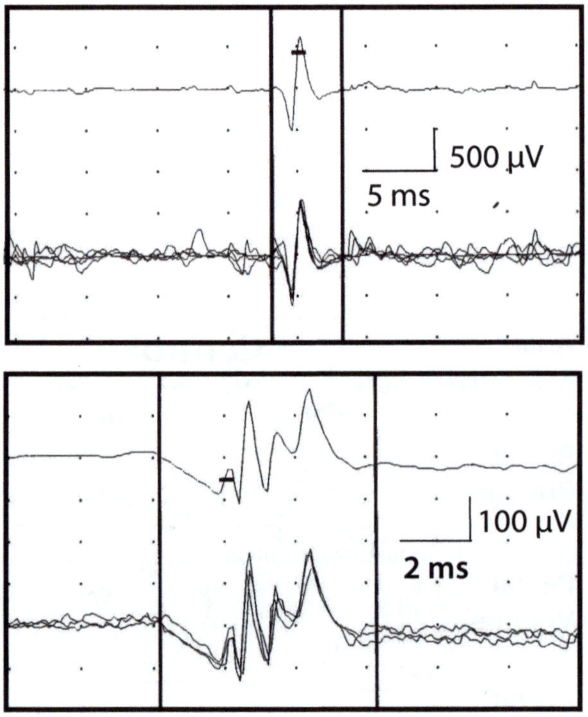

Fig. 6.2.5. Representative examples of a normal motor unit (*upper panel*) and an abnormal motor unit (*lower panel*). The upper panel depicts an average of several superimposed similar motor units, which are shown in the lower panel. In contrast to the normal motor unit, the polyphasic motor unit, recorded in a patient with fecal incontinence, is larger, longer, and has more phases, indicative of neurogenic injury. Reprint with permission from Bharucha (2006a) Update of Tests of Colon and Rectal Structure and Function. J Clin Gastroenterol 40(2):96–103. (Reproduced with permission from Bharucha (2006) Update of tests of colon and rectal structure and function. J Clin Gastroenterol 40(2)96–103)

external sphincter muscle selectively or in combination (Bartolo et al. 1983). When performed by an experienced professional, EMG is not associated with severe discomfort. However the utility of anal EMG versus an alternative approach (i.e., imaging the lumbosacral spinal cord) needs to be assessed. Anal EMG predicted the response to sacral nerve stimulation in FI (Altomare et al. 2004).

6.2.3 Tests of Structure

6.2.3.1 Endoanal Ultrasound (EUS)

Introduction

Endoanal ultrasound is widely used to identify anal sphincter injury (i.e., defects, scars, or atrophy) and anal fistulae. The technique is filly described in Chapter 4.4.

Clinical Utility

EUS identifies anal sphincter thinning and defects which are often clinically unrecognized and may be amenable to surgical repair (Stoker et al. 2001) (Fig. 6.2.6). Whereas endoanal ultrasound reliably identifies anatomic defects or thinning of the internal sphincter, interpretation of external sphincter images is much more subjective, operator-dependent, and confounded by normal anatomical variations in the external sphincter (Bartram and Sultan 1995). Substantial interobserver variability has been reported. Both the external sphincter and perirectal fat are echogenic and may be indistinguishable, which can preclude accurate characterization of external sphincter thickness and identification of external sphincter atrophy. As described in Chapter 4.4, the asymmetry of the external sphincter – often in the upper anal canal and particularly in women needs to be recognized so as not to impair discrimination of normal variation from sphincter defects.

6.2.4 Tests of Structure and Function

6.2.4.1 Dynamic Proctography (Defecography)

Introduction

During dynamic proctography, anorectal anatomy and pelvic floor motion are recorded with the patient at rest, coughing, squeezing, and straining to expel barium from the rectum. The anorectal angle and position of the anorectal junction are tracked during these manoeuvres as well as retention and evacuation of contrast material (Fig. 6.2.7). (The technique is fully described in Chap. 4, Sect. 4.1.2).

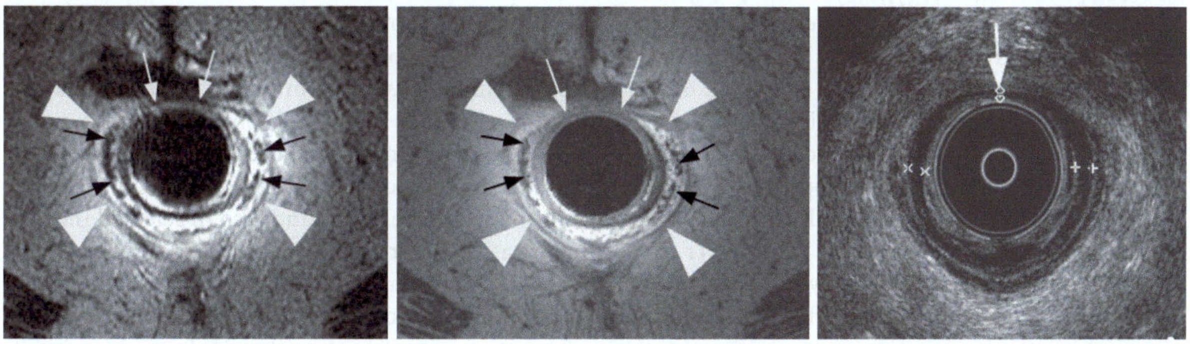

Fig. 6.2.6. Endoanal fast spin-echo T2-weighted (*left panel*) and spin-echo T1-weighted (*center panel*) MR images demonstrate marked atrophy of the external anal sphincter (arrowheads) in a 75-year-old incontinent patient, making the internal anal longitudinal muscle prominent (*black arrows*). Corresponding endoanal ultrasound images (*right panel*) identified patchy thinning of the internal sphincter also seen on the MR images (*white arrows*), but not external sphincter atrophy. (Reproduced with permission from Bharucha et al. (2005) Relationship between symptoms and disordered continence mechanisms in women with idiopathic fecal incontinence. Gut 54:546–555)

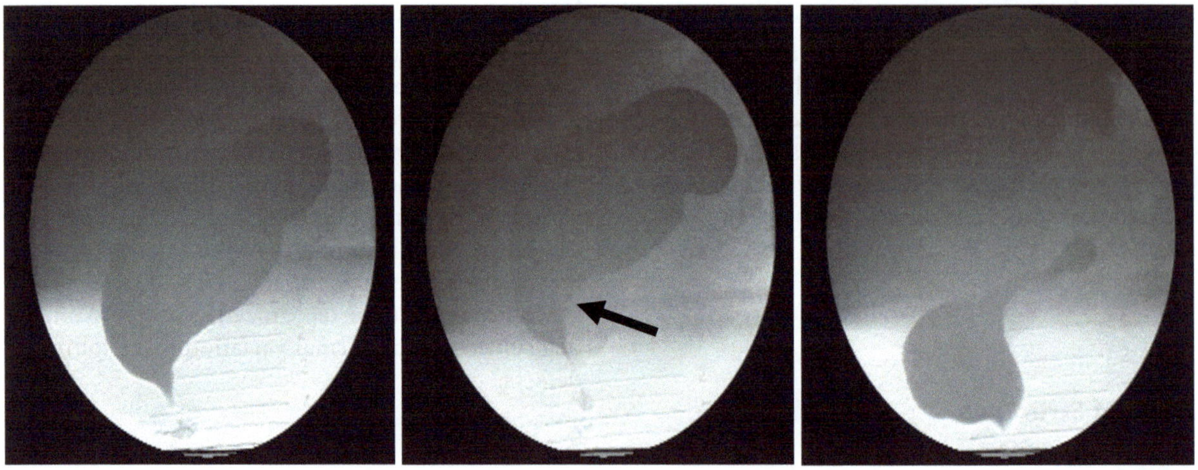

Fig. 6.2.7. Anorectal images at rest, squeeze, and evacuation in a patient with symptoms of difficult defecation. During squeeze, the puborectalis indentation (*black arrow*) was more prominent and the anorectal junction was elevated by 2 cm. Perineal motion was measured by markings on the commode at 1 cm intervals. Evacuation was associated with reduced perineal descent (1 cm), a rectocoele, and incomplete relaxation of the puborectalis/anal sphincters, which resulted in inability to expel rectal barium despite prolonged straining. (Reproduced with permission from Bharucha (2006) Update of tests of colon and rectal structure and function. J Clin Gastroenterol 40(2):96–103)

Methods

The methods for conducting and in particular interpreting evacuation proctography are incompletely standardized (Diamant et al. 1999). Though the test is generally conducted with liquid barium, a thick barium paste (Anatrast™, E-Z-EM, Westbury, NY) is probably preferable to liquid barium, particularly for incontinent patients. Anorectal descent is measured with reference to the pubococcygeal line. However, because the bony landmarks of this line (i.e., pubis, sacrococcygeal junction) may not be visualized in the same image as the anorectum, anorectal descent during manoeuvres is often measured with reference to the commode (see Sect. 4.1.3.1). Thus, the inter-observer reproducibility for defecography is good for some (e.g., rectococele, enterocoele) findings but may be suboptimal for others (e.g., intussusceptions, anorectal angle measurements, puborectalis impression) (Diamant et al. 1999; Dobben et al. 2005), partly because there is no consensus on whether the rectal axis should be drawn through the anterior, central, or posterior wall.

Clinical Utility

Prior to dynamic MR imaging, dynamic proctography was the only modality for identifying excessive perineal descent, internal rectal intussusceptions, rectoceles, sigmoidoceles, or enteroceles; puborectalis dysfunction during squeeze and evacuation can also be characterized (Shorvon et al. 1989; Agachan et al. 1996) (Chap. 6.1) Clinical use of evacuation proctography to assess evacuation disorders is however variable amongst different institutions across the world perhaps because the technique is partially standardized, and in some instances radiologists are not particularly enthusiastic about doing the test. In experienced hands anorectal manometry and balloon expulsion generally suffice to diagnose or exclude a functional disorder of defecation. Despite some limitations, dynamic proctography may be useful when the results of routine diagnostic tests (i.e., anal manometry, rectal balloon expulsion) are inconsistent, or conflict with the clinical diagnosis in constipated patients, and also in selected incontinent patients, particularly prior to surgery. Dynamic proctography may be particularly useful when there is a high index of suspicion for excessive perineal descent, a significant rectocele (e.g., in patients who splint the vagina to facilitate rectal emptying), an enterocele, or internal rectal intussusceptions. These findings may also help educate patients about the nature of the disorder and reinforce the need for treatment (e.g., pelvic floor retraining).

6.2.4.2 Pelvic MRI

Anatomy and Physiology

Pelvic MRI is the only imaging modality that can visualize both anal sphincter anatomy and global pelvic floor motion (anterior, middle, and posterior compartments) in real-time without radiation exposure (FLETCHER et al. 2003). This topic is detailed in Chapter 4.2; only salient points will be repeated here.

Methods

The sphincters can be imaged by an endoanal coil or by phased-array imaging. Pelvic floor motion can be visualized by dynamic imaging (i.e., image acquisition every 1.4 to 2 seconds) in the desired cross-sectional plane while patients squeeze their pelvic floor muscles, evacuate ultrasound gel from the rectum, and do a Valsalva maneuver. The exam can be performed using conventional, closed-configuration MR systems, as there is little difference in the detection of clinically relevant findings between supine MR and seated MR using open-configuration magnets, excluding rectal intussusceptions (BERTSCHINGER et al. 2002).

Clinical Utility

Although there is disagreement about which technique is superior for evaluating the internal anal sphincter, in experienced hands MR is equivalent to, or better than ultrasound for assessing the external sphincter (MALOUF et al. 2001). Endoanal MRI, but not EUS revealed external sphincter atrophy, in 20% of women with idiopathic FI but not in asymptomatic, age-matched controls (BHARUCHA et al. 2005a). In another study, 60% of patients with FI had some atrophy of the external sphincter and 20% had significant atrophy (TERRA et al. 2006). External sphincter atrophy was associated with age, female gender, and weaker maximal squeeze pressures. The clinical significance of external sphincter atrophy is unclear, it may predict patients who are less likely to fare well after repair of external sphincter defects (BRIEL et al. 1999; DOBBEN et al. 2007). Endoanal MRI also may reveal puborectalis atrophy in FI (BHARUCHA et al. 2005a).

Dynamic MR imaging provides an appreciation of global pelvic floor motion visualizing the bladder and genital organs as well as the rectum. Dynamic MRI avoids some of the limitations of barium defecography when assessing pelvic floor motion (DIAMANT et al. 1999) and is also useful in selected patients with fecal incontinence, e.g., in patients clinically suspected to have increased perineal descent or a rectocele (STOKER et al. 2001). Dynamic MRI is probably more accurate than a clinical examination for quantifying perineal descent (BHARUCHA et al. 2005b).

6.2.5 Anorectal Testing: Utility and Caveats

Several studies have shown that anorectal testing is useful in patients with FI (LIBERMAN et al. 2001). It may provide additional diagnostic information over and above clinical assessment in 19% to 98% of patients (Tables 6.2.3 and 6.2.4), and influences and specifically alters the management plan in 75–84% and 10–19% respectively. These studies evaluated the utility of anal manometry, endoanal ultrasound, and pudendal nerve terminal motor latency but did not assess the utility of MRI nor anal sphincter electromyography in FI.

However, there are several caveats to diagnostic testing in FI.

Firstly, these tests are not widely available and are most useful when they are conducted using appropriate techniques and interpreted in full clinical context. For example, there are several nuances to conducting and interpreting anal pressures measured by manometry. Because anal pressures are affected by age, gender, and the measurement technique, they should be compared against normal values obtained in age- and gender-matched subjects by the same technique (DIAMANT et al. 1999). The interpretation of ultrasound images of the anal sphincter can be challenging because the normal external anal sphincter may be asymmetric, limiting identification of sphincter defects.

Secondly, the range of diagnostic testing should be individualized and guided by a variety of factors i.e., the patient's age, symptom severity, bowel habit, response to conservative measures (e.g., regulation of bowel habits by anti-diarrhoeal agents), and planned therapeutic interventions.

Thirdly, most patients with FI tolerate anorectal testing reasonably well. A recent study evaluated pain, embarrassment, discomfort, and anxiety by separate 5-point Likert scales ranging from 1 (i.e., "none") to 5 (i.e., "extreme") in 211 patients with fecal inconti-

Table 6.2.3. Assessment of Anorectal Functions by Clinical Assessment and Diagnostic Testing. Reprinted with permission from Bharucha (2006) Anorectal manometry and imaging are necessary in patients with fecal incontinence. [Editorial] Am J Gastroenterol 101(12):2679–2681

Parameter	Clinical Examination vs Diagnostic Testing
Anal Resting and Squeeze Pressures	Manometry is more precise than a clinical examination (Hallan et al. 1989)
Anal Structural Injury	Imaging is more sensitive than a clinical exam for identifying sphincter defects and can also characterize location and nature (e.g., defect, atrophy) of sphincter injury
Neurogenic sphincter injury	Location and severity only identifiable by anal EMG
Rectal sensation and compliance	Can be assessed by rectal balloon distention only
Pelvic floor motion	Clinical assessment is reasonably correlated to pelvic MRI (Bharucha et al. 2005b)

Table 6.2.4. Impact of Diagnostic Testing on Management in Fecal Incontinence. Reprinted with permission from Bharucha (2006) Anorectal manometry and imaging are necessary in patients with fecal incontinence. [Editorial] Am J Gastroenterol 101(12):2679–2681

Finding	Impact on Management
Normal Anal Pressure	Underscores importance of other factors (e.g., abnormal rectal sensation, diarrhea) to FI
External anal sphincter defect	May be amenable to surgical repair
Neurogenic injury to anal sphincter	May guide the decision to repair sphincter defects
Reduced rectal sensation	Can be restored by biofeedback therapy, thereby restoring FI

nence (Deutekom et al. 2006). For all 3 tests (i.e., defecography, MRI, and combined anorectal tests [i.e., manometry, pudendal nerve terminal motor latency, rectal capacity and sensation]), the reported burden of testing was low, with average scores in the 1 to 2 range for all 4 items. There was statistically significant differences in the rated burden between MRI, which had the lowest average score, and defecography, which had the highest score, although this was small and of uncertain clinical significance.

Fourthly, because the therapeutic options for fecal incontinence are in general limited to regulation of bowel habit, pelvic floor retraining, and surgery, it may be premature at the current time to assess the impact of diagnostic testing on management. In the conventional paradigm for many diseases (e.g., chest pain, deep venous thrombosis), diagnostic testing is primarily justified by its potential impact on mortality and management. It is challenging to justify a role for diagnostic testing in FI on these grounds alone given the options for managing FI are limited and continue to evolve. For example, the utility of repairing small anal sphincter defects in FI, particularly those discovered several years after vaginal delivery is questionable given recent studies suggest that fecal continence deteriorates over time after surgical repair of sphincter defects (Cheung and Wald 2004). Newer approaches (e.g., sacral nerve stimulation) for managing fecal incontinence are being studied (Andrews and Bharucha 2005) and may enjoy greater success. Nonetheless, diagnostic testing may provide important information that guides clinical management (Table 6.2.4). Moreover, an improved understanding of the pathophysiology of the condition may help patients cope with this often devastating symptom. These issues are important because one in five women with fecal incontinence report the symptom has a moderate or severe impact on quality of life (Bharucha et al. 2005c). While < 10% of all women with FI discussed the symptom with a physician in the past year, 84% of women with severe FI had consulted a physician for this symptom (Bharucha et al. 2005c), justifying the decision to test women who ask for help. In other diseases (e.g., coronary artery disease), diagnostic testing may reduce anxiety and uncertainty regarding the condition (Mushlin et al. 2005). However, there is no information on the impact of diagnostic testing on patients' perceptions of their illness in FI.

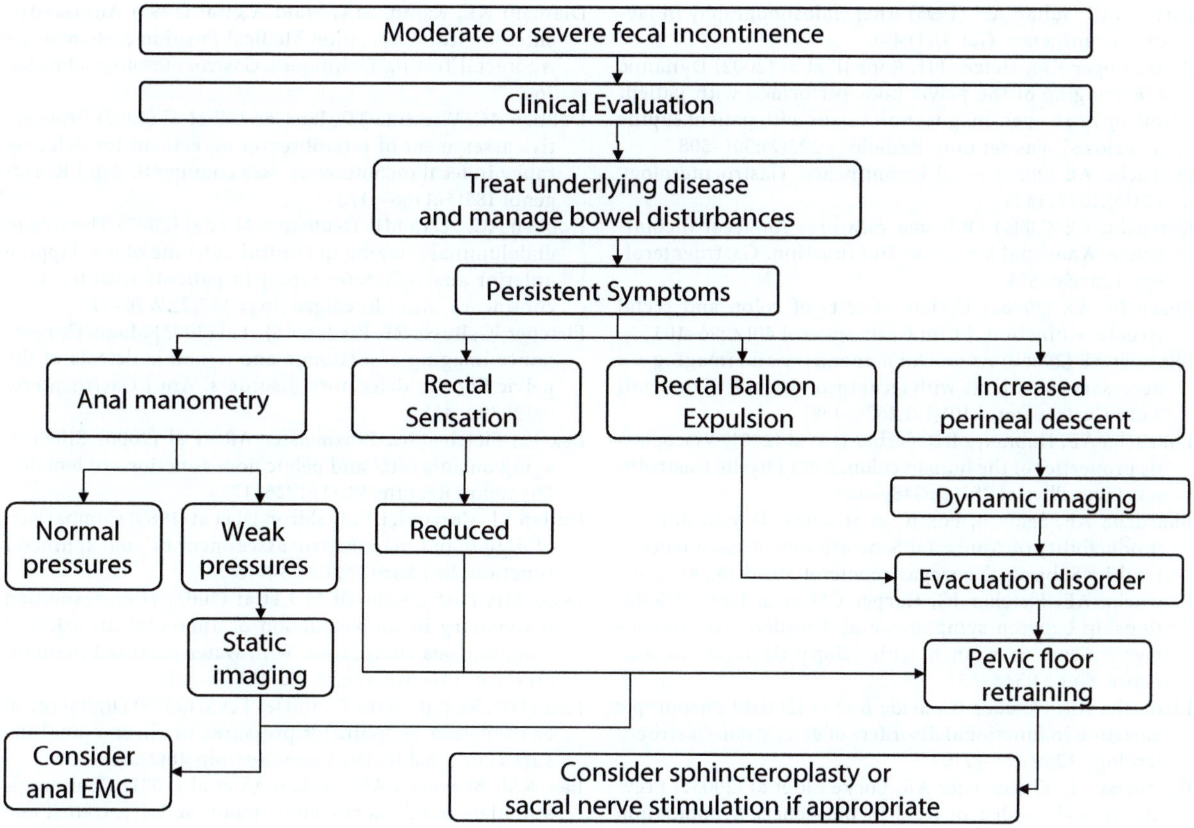

Fig. 6.2.8. Simplified algorithm for managing fecal incontinence. The investigations are guided by the clinical features and the response to conservative measures, particularly management of bowel disturbance. Thereafter, further measures (e.g., pelvic floor retraining) may be necessary

6.2.6 Summary

Carefully performed diagnostic testing is useful for understanding the pathophysiology and facilitating the management of FI. Test results should be interpreted together with the clinical features (i.e., age, symptom severity, bowel habits, and response to conservative measures). The indications and modalities for testing will continue to evolve.

Acknowledgments

This work was supported in part by USPHS NIH Grants R01 HD41129 and DK-68055.

References

Agachan F, Pfeifer J, Wexner SD et al (1996) Defecography and proctography. Results of 744 patients. Dis Colon Rectum 39(8):899–905

Altomare DF, Rinaldi M, Petrolino M et al (2004) Reliability of electrophysiologic anal tests in predicting the outcome of sacral nerve modulation for fecal incontinence. Dis Colon Rectum 47(6):853–857

Andrews C, Bharucha AE (2005) The etiology, assessment, and treatment of fecal incontinence. Nat Clin Pract Gastroenterol Hepatol 2(11):516–525

Andrews C, Bharucha AE, Camilleri M et al (2007) Rectal sensorimotor dysfunction in women with fecal incontinence. Am J Physiol Gastrointest Liver Physiol 292(1):G282–289

Bannister JJ, Abouzekry L, Read NW (1987) Effect of aging on anorectal function. Gut 28(3):353–357

Barnes PR, Lennard-Jones JE (1985) Balloon expulsion from the rectum in constipation of different types. Gut 26(10):1049–1052

Bartolo DC, Jarratt JA, Read MG et al (1983) The role of partial denervation of the puborectalis in idiopathic faecal incontinence. Br J Surg 70(11):664–667

Bartram CI, Sultan AH (1995) Anal endosonography in faecal incontinence. Gut 37(1):4–6
Bertschinger KM, Hetzer FH, Roos JE et al (2002) Dynamic MR imaging of the pelvic floor performed with patient sitting in an open-magnet unit versus with patient supine in a closed-magnet unit. Radiology 223(2):501–508
Bharucha AE (2003) Fecal incontinence. Gastroenterology 124(6):1672–1685
Bharucha AE (2004) Outcome measures for fecal incontinence: Anorectal structure and function. Gastroenterology 126:S90–S98
Bharucha AE (2006a) Update of tests of colon and rectal structure function. J Clin Gastroenterol 40(2):96–103
Bharuch AE (2006b) Anorectal manometry and imaging are necessary in patients with fecal incontinence. (Editorial) Am J Gastroenterol 101(12):2679–2681
Bharucha AE, Hubmayr RD, Ferber IJ et al (2001) Viscoelastic properties of the human colon. Am J Physiol Gastrointest Liver Physiol 281(2):G459–466
Bharucha AE, Seide B, Fox JC et al (2004) Day-to-day Reproducibility of Anorectal Sensorimotor Assessments in Healthy Subjects. Neurogastroenterol Motil 16:241–250
Bharucha AE, Fletcher JG, Harper CM et al (2005a) Relationship between symptoms and disordered continence mechanisms in women with idiopathic fecal incontinence. Gut 54:546–555
Bharucha AE, Fletcher JG, Seide B et al (2005b) Phenotypic variation in functional disorders of defecation. Gastroenterology 128:1199–1210
Bharucha AE, Zinsmeister AR, Locke ER et al (2005c) Prevalence and burden of fecal incontinence: A population based study in women. Gastroenterology 129:42–49
Briel JW, Stoker J, Rociu E et al (1999) External anal sphincter atrophy on endoanal magnetic resonance imaging adversely affects continence after sphincteroplasty. Br J Surg 86(10):1322–1327
Buser WD, Miner BP (1986) Delayed rectal sensation with fecal incontinence. Successful treatment using anorectal manometry. Gastroenterology 91(5):1186–1191
Caruana BJ, Wald A, Hinds JP et al (1991) Anorectal sensory and motor function in neurogenic fecal incontinence. Comparison between multiple sclerosis and diabetes mellitus. Gastroenterology 100(2):465–470
Chan CL, Lunniss PJ, Wang D et al (2005) Rectal sensorimotor dysfunction in patients with urge faecal incontinence: evidence from prolonged manometric studies. Gut 54(9):1263–1272
Cheung O, Wald A (2004) Review article: the management of pelvic floor disorders. Aliment Pharmacol Ther 19(5):481–495
Chiarioni G, Bassotti G, Stanganini S et al (2002) Sensory retraining is key to biofeedback therapy for formed stool fecal incontinence. Am J Gastroenterol 97(1):109–117
Denis P, Colin R, Galmiche JP et al (1979) Elastic properties of the rectal wall in normal adults and in the patients with ulcerative colitis. Gastroenterology 77(1):45–48
Deutekom M, Terra MP, Dobben AC et al (2006) Patients‘ perception of tests in the assessment of faecal incontinence. Br J Radiol 79(938):94–100
Deutekom M, Dobben AC, Terra MP et al (2007) Clinical presentation of fecal incontinence and anorectal function: what is the relationship? Am J Gastroenterol 102(2):351–361
Diamant NE, Kamm MA, Wald A et al (1999) Am Gastroenterological Association Medical Position Statement on Anorectal Testing Techniques. Gastroenterology 116:732–760
Dobben AC, Wiersma TG, Janssen LW et al (2005) Prospective assessment of interobserver agreement for defecography in fecal incontinence. [see comment]. Am J Roentgenol 185(5):1166–1172
Dobben AC, Terra MP, Deutekom M et al (2007) The role of endoluminal imaging in clinical outcome of overlapping anterior anal sphincter repair in patients with fecal incontinence. Am J Roentgenology 189(2):W70–77
Fletcher JG, Busse RF, Riederer SJ et al (2003) Magnetic resonance imaging of anatomic and dynamic defects of the pelvic floor in defecatory disorders. Am J Gastroenterol 98(2):399–411
Fox JC, Fletcher JG, Zinsmeister AR et al (2006) Effect of aging on anorectal and pelvic floor functions in females. Dis Colon Rectum 49(11):1726–1735
Hallan RI, Marzouk DE, Waldron DJ et al (1989) Comparison of digital and manometric assessment of anal sphincter function. Br J Surg 76(9):973–975
Jones MP, Post J, Crowell MD et al (2007) High-resolution manometry in the evaluation of anorectal disorders: a simultaneous comparison with water-perfused manometry. Am J Gastroenterol 102(4):850–855
Jones OM, Ramalingam T, Lindsey I et al (2005) Digital rectal examination of sphincter pressures in chronic anal fissure is unreliable. Dis Colon Rectum 48(2):349–352
Law NM, Bharucha AE, Undale AS et al (2001) Cholinergic stimulation enhances colonic motor activity, transit and sensation in humans. Am J Physiol Gastrointest Liver Physiol 281(5):G1228–G1237
Liberman H, Faria J, Ternent CA et al (2001) A prospective evaluation of the value of anorectal physiology in the management of fecal incontinence. Dis Colon Rectum 44(11):1567–1574
Malouf AJ, Norton CS, Engel AF et al (2000) Long-term results of overlapping anterior anal-sphincter repair for obstetric trauma. Lancet 355(9200):260–265
Malouf AJ, Halligan S, Williams AB et al (2001) Prospective assessment of interobserver agreement for endoanal MRI in fecal incontinence. Abdom Imaging 26(1):76–78
Minguez M, Herreros B, Sanchiz V et al (2004) Predictive value of the balloon expulsion test for excluding the diagnosis of pelvic floor dyssynergia in constipation. Gastroenterology 126(1):57–62
Mushlin AI, Kern LM, Paris M et al (2005) The value of diagnostic information to patients with chest pain suggestive of coronary artery disease. [see comment]. Med Decis Making 25(2):149–157
Rao SS, Patel RS (1997) How useful are manometric tests of anorectal function in the management of defecation disorders? Am J Gastroenterol 92(3):469–475
Rao SS, Read NW, Davison PA et al (1987) Anorectal sensitivity and responses to rectal distention in patients with ulcerative colitis. Gastroenterology 93(6):1270–1275
Rao SS, Welcher KD, Leistikow JS (1998) Obstructive defecation: a failure of rectoanal coordination. Am J Gastroenterol 93(7):1042–1050
Rao SS, Hatfield R, Soffer E et al (1999) Manometric tests of anorectal function in healthy adults. Am J Gastroenterol 94(3):773–783

Rao SS, Azpiroz F, Diamant N et al (2002) Minimum standards of anorectal manometry. Neurogastroenterol Motil. 14(5):553–559

Rao SS, Mudipalli RS, Stessman M et al (2004a) Investigation of the utility of colorectal function tests and Rome II criteria in dyssynergic defecation (Anismus). Neurogastroenterol Motil 16(5):589–596

Rao SS, Ozturk R, Stessman M et al (2004b) Investigation of the pathophysiology of fecal seepage. Am J Gastroenterol 99(11):2204–2209

Read NW, Abouzekry L (1986) Why do patients with faecal impaction have faecal incontinence. Gut 27(3):283–287

Ryhammer AM, Laurberg S, Bek KM (1997) Age and anorectal sensibility in normal women. Scand J Gastroenterol 32(3):278–284

Salvioli B, Bharucha AE, Rath-Harvey D et al (2001) Rectal compliance, capacity and rectoanal sensation in fecal incontinence. Am J Gastroenterol 96(7):2158–2168

Shorvon PJ, McHugh S, Diamant NE et al (1989) Defecography in normal volunteers: results and implications. Gut 30(12):1737–1749

Siproudhis L, Bellissant E, Pagenault M et al (1999) Fecal incontinence with normal anal canal pressures: where is the pitfall? Am J Gastroenterol 94(6):1556–1563

Siproudhis L, El Abkari M, El Alaoui M et al (2005) Low rectal volumes in patients suffering from fecal incontinence: what does it mean? Aliment Pharmacol Ther 22(10):989–996

Sloots CE, Felt-Bersma RJ, Cuesta MA et al (2000) Rectal visceral sensitivity in healthy volunteers: influences of gender, age and methods. Neurogastroenterol Motil 12(4):361–368

Stoker J, Halligan S, Bartram CI (2001) Pelvic floor imaging. Radiology 218(3):621–641

Sun WM, Read NW, Donnelly TC (1990a) Anorectal function in incontinent patients with cerebrospinal disease. Gastroenterology 99(5):1372–1379

Sun WM, Read NW, Miner TB (1990b) Relation between rectal sensation and anal function in normal subjects and patients with faecal incontinence. Gut 31(9):1056–1061

Sun WM, Read NW, Prior A et al (1990c) Sensory and motor responses to rectal distention vary according to rate and pattern of balloon inflation. Gastroenterology 99(4):1008–1015

Sun WM, Donnelly TC, Read NW (1992) Utility of a combined test of anorectal manometry, electromyography, and sensation in determining the mechanism of "idiopathic" faecal incontinence. Gut 33(6):807–813

Terra MP, Deutekom M, Beets-Tan TG et al (2006) Relationship between external anal sphincter atrophy at endoanal magnetic resonance imaging and clinical, functional, and anatomic characteristics in patients with fecal incontinence. Dis Colon Rectum 49(5):668–678

Varma JS, Smith AN, Busuttil A et al (1985) Correlation of clinical and manometric abnormalities of rectal function following chronic radiation injury. Br J Surg 72(11):875–878

Voderholzer WA, Neuhaus DA, Klauser AG et al (1997) Paradoxical sphincter contraction is rarely indicative of anismus. Gut 41(2):258–262

Wald A, Tunuguntla AK (1984) Anorectal sensorimotor dysfunction in fecal incontinence and diabetes mellitus. Modification with biofeedback therapy. N Engl J Med 310(20):1282–1287

Wexner SD, Marchetti F, Salanga VD et al (1991) Neurophysiologic assessment of the anal sphincters. Dis Colon Rectum 34(7):606–612

Whitehead WE, Palsson OS (1998) Is rectal pain sensitivity a biological marker for irritable bowel syndrome: psychological influences on pain perception. Gastroenterology 115(5):1263–1271

Yeoh EK, Russo A, Botten R et al (1998) Acute effects of therapeutic irradiation for prostatic carcinoma on anorectal function. Gut 43(1):123–127

Coloproctological Dysfunction

6

6.3 Surgical Management of Fecal Incontinence

Steven D. Wexner and Sherief Shawki

CONTENTS

6.3.1 Introduction

Fecal incontinence is the inability to have control of gas or stool evacuation and inability to defer the act of defecation until a socially proper time and place. Intact musculature including the puborectalis and internal and external anal sphincters are prerequisites for fecal control, as is a functioning nerve supply to these muscles. Other factors contributing to fecal continence include stool consistency, rectal sensitivity and capacity, and an intact anorectal sampling reflex. Any impairment to one or more of these factors can result in fecal incontinence.

Although very devastating, it is socially stigmatized, and therefore it may be underreported and perhaps underestimated. A community-based survey among nearly 7,000 person showed that 2.2% suffered from fecal incontinence (Nelson et al. 1995), although a subsequent meta-analysis revealed a rate of 11–15% (Macmillan et al. 2004).

Fecal incontinence is considered the second leading cause for nursing home placement, as up to 45% of nursing home residents are estimated to have some form of fecal incontinence (Whitehead et al. 2001). In addition to its social burden, fecal incontinence imposes an economic impact on the health-care system. This problem was emphasized in 1999 when Mellgren et al. studied long-term costs of fecal incontinence among 63 patients. During this study period, the average overall charges per patient were $17,166, and the total charges were $559,341.

S. D. Wexner, MD, FACS, FRCS, FRCS(Ed)
Chairman, Department of Colorectal Surgery, Chief of Staff, Cleveland Clinic Florida, 2950 Cleveland Clinic Boulevard, Weston, FL 33331, USA

S. Shawki, MD
Research Fellow, Department of Colorectal Surgery, Cleveland Clinic Florida, 2950 Cleveland Clinic Boulevard, Weston, FL 33331, USA

Assessment of fecal incontinence severity, and thereby the need for treatment and the subsequent outcome of the mode of treatment used, requires a scoring system. Browning and Parks (1983) introduced one of the first fecal incontinence scoring systems. Although it was simple and assessed continence condition for solid and liquid stool, as well as flatus, this scoring system did not take in account the degree and frequency of incontinence. These two important factors were considered in the scoring system devised by Miller et al. (1988) and was modified later by Pescatori et al. (1992); the maximum score was six and did not consider the frequency of stool lost.

Another scoring system was used in multiple studies evaluating the effect of dynamic graciloplasty in the management of fecal incontinence. This Quantified Continence Scale scoring system assessed only liquid and solid incontinence in terms of frequency (Williams et al. 1991; Baeten et al. 1995). American Medical Systems developed a scoring system for assessment of artificial bowel sphincter. This scoring system involved evaluation of the consistency and frequency – ranging from "never" to "several times a day" (including six degrees of different frequencies) – of lost stool as well as lifestyle alteration. It is highly complex and ranges from 0–120.

Among the numerous scoring systems for fecal incontinence, the Cleveland Clinic Florida Fecal Incontinence Score (CCF-FI), more commonly known as the Wexner score, is by far the most popular and most widely used validated scoring system (Jorge and Wexner 1993) (Table 6.3.1). The fecal incontinence measures the frequency of incontinence to gas, liquid and solid stool, lifestyle alteration and finally the use of protective pads. Each of these variables is given a scale of 0–4: a total score of 0 = normal control and a score of 20 = complete incontinence. This scoring system has been validated by many studies; one of these validating studies showed that a score of 9 correlates with significant fecal incontinence that affects quality of life, and it can be considered as an indication for surgical interference (Rothbarth et al. 2001).

Vaizey's score, a minor modification of the Wexner score, was introduced in 1999 (Table 6.3.2). This score combined components of the previous scores using the Wexner score as the basis for their modifications, but added an additional category for urgency. These modifications took into consideration three main factors. Wearing a pad may not be an index of incontinence severity so much as a personal estimate that may vary from one patient to another, hence its weight is reduced in the new scale. Usage of antidiarrheal medications is considered as part of the whole management plane, and failure with/without these medication matters. Finally, they considered fecal urgency, defined as the inability to defer the bowel movement long enough until proper timing, without overt fecal incontinence, as a valuable factor in the whole assessment of the fecal incontinence patient condition. However, the addition of ability to defer defecation more than 15 min did not take into consideration stool consistency, which could be an influencing factor; this item was given the highest weight (Vaizey et al. 1999).

Table 6.3.1. Wexner fecal incontinence scoring system (Jorge and Wexner 1993)

Type of incontinence	Frequency				
	Never	Rarely	Sometimes	Usually	Always
Solid	0	1	2	3	4
Liquid	0	1	2	3	4
Gas	0	1	2	3	4
Wears pad	0	1	2	3	4
Lifestyle alteration	0	1	2	3	4

Never, 0; rarely, < 1/month; sometimes, < 1/week, > 1/month; usually, < 1/day, > 1/week; always, > 1/day. 0, perfect; 20, complete incontinence

6.3.2 Etiology

Anal sphincter defects and pudendal nerve injury can occur during vaginal delivery and are by far the most common causes of fecal incontinence (Table 6.3.3), consequently making this problem more prevalent in women (Madoff et al. 1992).

Obstetric-related trauma is a main contributing factor. Third-degree perineal tear, forceps delivery, primiparous delivery, birth weight over 4 kg and occipito-posterior position at delivery are all factors associated with obstetric-related anal sphincter trauma and subsequent fecal incontinence (Bannister et al. 1987). Injury occurs after midline and lateral episiotomies in 12% and 2% of delivering

Table 6.3.2. Vaizey's score (Vaizey et al. 1999)

	Never	Rarely	Sometimes	Weekly	Daily
Incontinence for solid stool	0	1	2	3	4
Incontinence for liquid stool	0	1	2	3	4
Incontinence for gas	0	1	2	3	4
Alteration in lifestyle	0	1	2	3	4
				No	Yes
Need to wear a pad or plug				0	2
Taking constipating medicines				0	2
Lack of ability to defer defecation for 15 min				0	4

Never, no episodes in the past 4 weeks; rarely, 1 episode in the past 4 weeks; sometimes, > 1 episode in the past 4 weeks, but < 1 a week; weekly, 1 or more episodes a week, but < 1 a day; daily, 1 or more episodes a day. Minimum score = 0 = perfect continence; maximum score = 24 = totally incontinent. Perhaps because of the ease of the Wexner score, it remains much more widely cited than the Vaizey score (Google Scholar.com 20 January 2008)

Table 6.3.3. Causes of fecal incontinence (% estimated based upon literature review)

Sphincter abnormality (most common; about 80–90%)	Congenital problems	Inadequate rectal sensation (< 5%)
Sphincter defects	Spina bifida	Neurologic conditions
• Obstetric injury	Imperforate anus	• Cerebrovascular accidents
○ Third- or fourth-degree tears	Myelomeningocele	• Dementia
○ Forceps injury	**Inadequate rectal/reservoir capacity/compliance (<5%)**	• Multiple sclerosis
○ Episiotomy	Inflammatory bowel disease	• Brain/spinal cord injuries
Anorectal surgery	Pelvic radiotherapy	• Neoplasms
• Fistula surgery	Pelvic sepsis	**Overflow incontinence (< 5%)**
• Dilatation injury	Neorectum (sphincter-saving operations)	Fecal impaction
• Sphincterotomy	Low anterior resection	Encopresis
• Hemorrhoidectomy	Colonic J-pouch anal anastomosis	Psychotropic drugs
Other trauma	Colo-anal anastomosis	**Altered stool consistency/diarrheal conditions (< 5%)**
Denervation problems (mostly as confounding factor; 20–35%)	Ileorectal anastomosis	Irritable bowel syndrome
Primary	Ileal J-pouch anal anastomosis	Inflammatory bowel disease
• Pudendal neuropathy	Collagen vascular disease	Laxative abuse
• Chronic straining	• Scleroderma	Malabsorption syndrome
• Descending perineal syndrome	• Amyloidosis	Short gut syndrome
• Vaginal deliveries	• Dermatomyositis	Radiation enteritis
Secondary	Rectal ischemia	**Miscellaneous**
• Spinal cord and pelvic floor nerves		Aging
• Diabetic neuropathy		Rectal prolapse

women, respectively (Sultan et al. 1994). Another common confounding factor is pudendal nerve neuropathy, which eventually results in a shorter anal canal, lower pressures and increased sphincter fiber content; furthermore, a successful outcome is less likely to be achieved (Snooks et al. 1990). Although not as frequently implied as obstetric injury, anorectal surgery, including division of the anal sphincters during surgery for fistula in ano, can lead to fecal incontinence (Parks et al. 1976).

It has been shown that limited simple division of an "acceptable" portion of the sphincter muscles in a low anal fistula can be accompanied by varying degrees of impairment of fecal control in up to 34% of patients (Sainio and Husa 1985; Shouler et al. 1986). The internal sphincter might be injured by forceful dilatation during certain procedures, such as Lord's operation for treatment of hemorrhoids. This injury might affect the ability of fecal control either in temporary or permanent ways. This finding is especially true in patients who are predisposed to and/or had some preoperative impairment due to generalized weakness of the pelvic floor, perineal descent and/or pudendal neuropathy (MacDonald et al. 1992).

Denervation of the sphincters may be idiopathic. Idiopathic incontinence is more common in multiparous women, although other factors, such as nerve entrapment, rectoanal intussusception, descending perineum syndrome and habitual straining at during evacuation, have all been implied. Fecal incontinence may also result from peripheral neuropathies due to diabetes mellitus, multiple neurofibromatosis and multiple sclerosis.

6.3.3 Clinical Approach

6.3.3.1 History

Thorough history is an important step during patient assessment, including information about the frequency, duration and severity of incontinence, whether to solid or liquid stool and/or gas, and the impact on quality of life, should be obtained. A detailed review of other related systems, such as neurologic and gastrointestinal problems as well as obstetric and gynecologic history, should be carefully undertaken. Past surgical history, including bowel resections and especially history of anorectal surgical procedures, should be detailed.

Pseudo-incontinence should be distinguished from true incontinence; pseudo-incontinence occurs when patients with normal anal sphincters are aware of the desire to defecate, but cannot withhold the act. This problem can be caused by a non-compliant rectum secondary to inflammatory proctitis, radiation proctitis or presence of a neo-rectum (following restorative proctectomy or proctocolectomy). Incontinence can be due to diarrhea or very soft stool and may be secondary to dietary habits, irritable bowel syndrome, diverticular disease, or inflammatory bowel disease. Some patients may be totally unaware of the passage of stool as sensory loss may be associated with rectal prolapse or neuropathy and can be either primary or secondary. Alternatively, the patient might be aware of an impending accident, but cannot prevent it. This type of incontinence is usually due to motor dysfunction, which is usually seen in sphincteric injury, but intact innervation. However, many patients with incontinence have multifactorial etiology attributable to both.

6.3.3.2 Physical Examination

Anorectal examination includes inspection of the perineum for any pathology, such as fistula, piles, skin excoriation, anal opening (tight or patulous), perineal descent and scars. Digital anorectal examination is important to assess resting and squeezing tones, and the presence of any muscle disruption. Anal inspection and digital rectal examination can give accurate information about internal and external anal sphincter function, but are inaccurate for determining external anal sphincter defects <90 degrees (Dobben et al. 2007a). Anoscopy is always used in anorectal examination to exclude hemorrhoids, fistulas and fissures.

6.3.4 Investigation

6.3.4.1 Physiologic Studies

A series of tests is used to assess the different facets of fecal control. Anorectal manometry gives an idea about the anal sphincters' resting and squeezing pressures, rectal capacity, as well as rectoanal inhibitory reflex, information that reflects muscle function, rectal compliance and the sampling mechanism. Resting pressure is produced mainly by the internal anal sphincter (IAS), which is a smooth muscle in a state of continuous involuntary contraction providing a natural barrier to the involuntary loss of stool. This barrier is normally between 50 and 70 mmHg.

Squeeze pressure results from the voluntary contraction of the EAS and puborectalis muscle, which elevates the intra-anal pressure to reach two to three times its baseline values (100 to 180 m mHg). Also the EAS undergoes reflex contraction in response to rectal distension, increased intra-abdominal pressure and posture alteration, which is a very important mechanism in preventing leakage during activities such as coughing or lifting (Parks et al. 1962). About 50–85% of the resting tone is produced by the internal anal sphincter; the external anal sphincter is responsible for 25–30%, which is important to eliminate the need for constant voluntary attention to the sphincters. Finally, anal cushion expansion shares the remaining 5–15% of pressure, which seems to be essential for perfect anal control (Gibbons et al. 1986; Jorge and Wexner 1997).

The high pressure zone represents the effectively functional part of the anal canal in patients with fecal incontinence. It is that part of the anal canal in which the pressures are greater than half of the maximum pressure at rest. These parameters show abnormally lowered and diminished recordings during manometry that accordingly should be improved after surgical intervention aiming at regaining higher pressures and creating a new high pressure zone to restore anal control function.

The Recto-anal inhibitory reflex results from the transient contraction of the external anal sphincter followed by relaxation of the internal anal sphincter as a result of distal rectal distension. It is believed that this "sampling" reflex helps the recognition and discrimination of rectal contents, whether solid, liquid stool or gas, and thereby gives the person a signal about needing to go to the restroom, whether urgent or not. This reflex is mediated via a reflex arch at the spinal level. It is lost in diseases and conditions that involve neuropathies and resection of distal mucosa.

Rectal compliance is the change in rectal pressure in response to any change in volume. When the call of defecation is to be deferred, rectal contents have to be contained. Thus, the smaller change in pressure to a larger change in volume reflects the elastic characteristics of the rectal wall, thereby reducing the pressure and urge for defecation. This feature is lost with inflammatory bowel disease and conditions where a neo-rectum is created, such as colonic J-pouch for low rectal cancer and Ileal J-pouch for mucosal ulcerative colitis. Defecography, does not have an essential role in the preoperative evaluation of fecal incontinence other than documenting the inability to hold rectal contents and the occurrence of premature leaks (Smith and Blatchford 2006).

Electrophysiological studies include electromyography, which helps map the anal sphincter, and the pudendal nerve terminal motor latency test to evaluate the integrity of the pudendal nerve. Whereas the usefulness and practicality of anorectal physiologic studies has been questioned (Hallan et al. 1989), endoanal ultrasound is definitely an important tool in the assessment of fecal incontinence. However, electromyography and ultrasonography are complimentary evaluations.

An electromyography can be performed with a needle electrode, an anal plug or surface electrodes. It can be performed as either a concentric-needle or single-fiber study. The most common and most accurate method for assessment of fecal incontinence is the concentric-needle exam. This study tends to show functional defects, whereas an ultrasonography is only used for revealing structural defects therefor the two studies are complimentary. As an example, an ultrasonography will often reveal anterior-based abnormality, which could be a scar or a defect, whereas an electromyography would discern whether or not that particular area has neurological activity and if so whether the activity is normal or abnormal. It is perhaps easier to think of the two examinations in an analogous fashion:the EMG is like the microscopic evaluation and the ultrasound is like the macroscopic evaluation of a pathology specimen. The important adjunct to the EMG is of course the baseline for future assessment, which is of great prognostic significance when contemplating surgery.

6.3.4.1.1 Imaging

Endoanal ultrasound is widely available and is reasonably accurate. More recently, endoanal MRI was introduced. In a prospective comparative study of 237 patients, endoanal ultrasound and endoanal

MRI were comparable in the detection of external sphincter defects (Dobben et al. 2007b). In a multicentric study, 200 patients with fecal incontinence with a mean Vaizey (modified Wexner) score of 18 were evaluated with endoanal MRI for an external sphincter condition by radiologists blinded to their functional state. It was found that MRI was highly sensitive in detecting EAS atrophy; in addition, it was noted that the more atrophy detected in MRI, the poorer were the functional results of the sphincter in terms of squeeze pressures, suggesting that in this way endoanal MRI would help in better patient selection with subsequent better outcome (Terra et al. 2006a).

Imaging also has an important role in postoperative assessment as it gives an idea about the technical outcome, which when correlated with clinical outcome can provide complimentary parameters that help determine the efficacy of the surgical treatment implemented and, in case of failure, helps make the decision whether to undertake a re-do operation or another surgical alternative. Dobben et al. (2007c) showed that endoluminal imaging can be effectively used in postoperative assessment regarding tissue at overlap and residual defects following sphincteroplasty, as well as preoperatively for detection of external sphincter muscle atrophy. They evaluated 30 patients suffering from fecal incontinence due to external sphincter defects. This assessment included pre- and postoperative endoanal ultrasound (EUS) and endoluminal magnetic resonance (EMRI) associated with functional assessment using the Vaizey (modified Wexner) score. They found that both two-dimensional endoanal ultrasonography and endoanal MR imaging were comparable and accurate in detecting sphincter defects and assessing the structural integrity, respectively; thereby, the latter was more useful in evaluating sphincter thickness and atrophy, while the former was effective in the assessment of residual external sphincter defects.

Another study done by the same group showed that external phased-array MRI and endoanal MRI are both comparable in detecting external anal sphincter atrophy and consequently proper patient selection for surgical repair. However, there were both inter- and intra-observer variability among the evaluating radiologists; they concluded that both techniques are helpful and can be included in the evaluation; however, the availability of the technique and experience level cannot be overemphasized in order to obtain accurate results (Terra et al. 2006b). Finally, as endoanal ultrasound is widely available and cheaper, this technique is the method of choice. Endoanal MRI, when available, gives information about the external sphincter muscle, which might play a role in patient selection and have a predictive value for the outcome of anterior anal repair (Briel et al. 1999; Terra et al. 2006a; Dobben 2007c).

6.3.5 Management of Fecal Incontinence

6.3.5.1 Conservative Management

Conservative management of fecal incontinence involves dietary modification with fiber. Medications such as bulking agents, including natural and synthetic fiber, render soft/liquid forms of stool into a more formed solid state to help control. This therapy is especially effective in pseudo-incontinence where the problem is mainly due to altered stool consistency, such as chronic diarrheal conditions, rather than muscular problems. Constipating agents could be used in the same way when the cause of incontinence is more likely due to a motility problem such as irritable bowel syndrome (Ehrenpreis et al. 2007).

Biofeedback trains patients to know how to use their sphincters more effectively. There are many different methods of providing biofeedback, including the use of electromyography, intra- or peri-anal sensors, manometry and intrarectal balloon systems. The main theme is to encourage the patient to feel and recognize the anal contraction by giving them a real-time visual picture, in the form of a curve or diagram, representing their contraction in any of the methods used.

6.3.5.2 Surgical Management of Fecal Incontinence

Surgical management can be divided into four categories (Table 6.3.4). The first type of operation includes repair of existing muscle and/or scar. These methods include direct central apposition, overlapping central repair, post anal repair and total pelvic flow repair. The common denominator of these operations is that preexisting muscle is either brought together, overlapped, imbricated or plicated. The second surgical option includes either augmentation or substitution of the anal sphincter muscles. These options include graciloplasty, which is a neuromuscular stimulation, and artificial bowel sphincter. A third category is sacral nerve stimulation, which includes device implantation meant to enhance the efficacy of an existing central complex. A newer fourth group of therapies includes local anatomic alteration and encompasses injectable therapies and radiotherapy treatment.

Table 6.3.4. Management of fecal incontinence

Conservative
Dietary
• Increase fiber intake
• Bulking agents
Pharmacological
• Supplementing fibers
• Motility-altering agents
Biofeedback
Surgical intervention
Defects
• Sphincter repair
○ Direct apposition
○ Overlapping sphincteroplasty + internal sphincter imbrication
Intact sphincters
• Injectables
○ Carbon beads
○ Silicone
○ Polytetrafluoroethylene (PTFE)
Controlled energy delivery, therapy for treatment of fecal incontinence (SECCA)
• Sacral nerve stimulation (± sphincter defect)
End stages
• Muscle transfer
• Artificial bowel sphincter
Diversion
• Colostomy
• Ileostomy

6.3.5.3 Sphincter Repair

Traditionally, surgical management of fecal incontinence has included the techniques of the levator muscle imbrication posterior to the anal canal or both posterior and anterior to the anal canal as described by Keighley (1984). Unfortunately neither of these techniques has an overwhelmingly high success rate or a particularly long durability, and accordingly, neither of these techniques is routinely being performed at the present time. The most recent North American series was undertaken by Maxwell, Wexner and colleagues and described a success rate of 35% (Browning and Parks 1983; Briel and Schouten 1995; Korsgen et al. 1997; Matsuoka et al. 2000).

Sphincteroplasty is the most common surgical procedure encountered in the management of fecal incontinence. It is considered in patients who have an isolated sphincter defect as the residual muscle still retains its functional ability.

Direct apposition involves the mobilization of the external sphincter, excision of the scar and suturing the muscle in an end-to-end fashion. It was associated with a 40% incidence of failure attributed to suture disruption, and it was abandoned. The technique was modified later to excise the scar tissue, and the muscle ends were overlapped rather than apposed (Parks and McPartlin 1971). Slade et al. (1977) further modified the technique to include the scar tissue in the overlap instead of excising it.

6.3.5.4 Overlapping Anterior Sphincteroplasty

This method is the most commonly used technique for repair of anterior sphincter defects.

6.3.5.4.1 Technique

Following a full mechanical and oral and parenteral antibiotics preparation, the patient is positioned in the prone jackknife position under general endotracheal anesthesia. A 120° anterolateral incision is made; dissection is undertaken until entering the ischiorectal fossae on each side where the healthy parts of the external anal sphincter on both sides of the defect are identified as well as the scar tissue, which is divided in the midline. Division is followed by further dissection to separate the external sphincter from the internal one along the intersphincteric groove. Additional imbrication of the internal anal sphincter associated with approximation of the levator muscle is undertaken prior to performance of the external sphincter overlap.

In this procedure the overlapped scar tissue gives tissue bulk in which the sutures can take hold, augments the sphincter size, restores the high pressure zone and re-creates a perineal body in female patients (Fig. 6.3.1). Wexner et al. (1991) and Fleshman et al. (1991) showed that if anal sphincter length is restored along with enough anal pressure, this provides an appropriate high pressure zone reflected as improved functional outcomes in terms of continence.

Creation of a diverting stoma for this procedure is considered unnecessary by most authors. Also, food intake restriction after the procedure with or without constipating agents has not been proved to improve the outcome (Ctercteko et al. 1988; Fleshman et al. 1991). Overlapping sphincteroplasty achieves an overall accepted outcome ranging between 47% and 89%, at a mean follow-up of less than 3 years, with a wound infection rate ranging from 0–24%. Good pudendal nerve terminal motor latency was found to correlate with more successful outcomes (Wexner et al. 1991).

Unfortunately long-term follow-up has shown that overlapping sphincteroplasty reveals very disappointing results of less than 50%, and in fact "perfect" control has been reported in less than 15% of patients in a follow-up of over 5 to 10 years. Forty-nine patients were evaluated after overlapping sphincteroplasty with a mean follow-up of 6 years; 42% showed improved continence, and only 14% were completely continent (Halverson and Hull 2002) (Table 6.3.5).

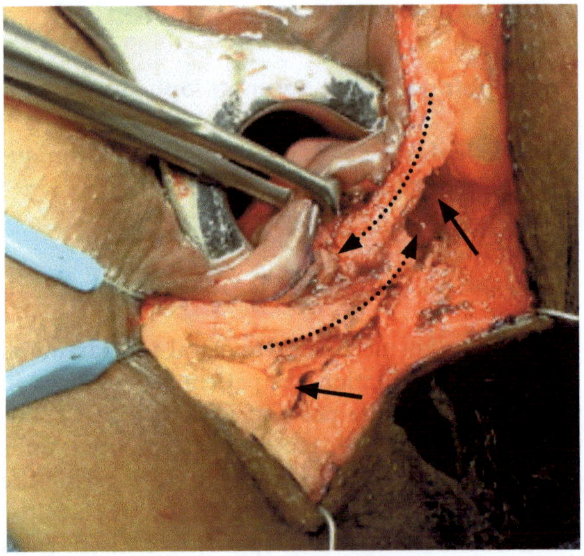

Fig. 6.3.1. External sphincter overlapped (*dotted arrows*). Solid arrows show both ischiorectal fossae

Table 6.3.5. Overlapping sphincteroplasty results

Author	Year	Number of cases	Rate of success
Short term: < 3-year follow-up			
Fang et al.	1984	79	89%
Engel et al.	1994	55	76%
Oliveira et al.	1996	55	71%
Sitzler et al.	1996	31	74%
Young et al.	1998	56	86%
Long term: 5–10-year follow-up			
Halverson and Hull	2002	49	42%
Barisic et al.	2006	65	74%
Grey et al.	2007	47	60%
Maslekars et al.	2007	72	80%

Long-term functional outcome after a minimum of 5 years following sphincter repair could be assessed in 38 patients. None was fully continent for both stool and flatus, and only four were totally continent for solid and liquid stool. However, 23 had an overall improved continence state (Malouf et al. 2000).

6.3.5.5 Artificial Bowel Sphincter

The artificial bowel sphincter is the modification of the American Medical Systems artificial urinary sphincter (Minneapolis, MN). It is potentially indicated in end-stage fecal incontinence where there is insufficient muscle available for repair, but sufficient perineal tissue to help prevent device extrusion. Such conditions may occur following surgical excision or traumatic injury of the anal sphincters. Patients with psychological instability, mental disorder or neuromuscular disease are not candidates for the procedure. Patients with perianal sepsis disease should not undergo this procedure; thus, patients suffering from severe cutaneous radiation damage perianal Crohn's disease or perianal infections should be excluded.

The device is composed of three components that are all connected in a liquid-filled tightly closed system. An inflatable cuff (the sphincter) is inserted around the anal canal. A pressure-regulating balloon is placed in the space of Retzius in the anterior abdominal wall and acts as a reservoir of the fluid. The pressure in the balloon should always be higher in this system. Finally, a control pump connects with both the cuff and the balloon via reinforced silicone tubing. The pump is situated in the subcutaneous layer of the scrotum or in the labus majorum in male and female patients, respectively.

6.3.5.5.1 Technique

The procedure should be performed under meticulous aseptic precautions and under cover of antibiotics as infection is the main morbidity and cause of failure of the artificial bowel sphincter. Two teams can work together, one working on inserting the balloon and the other team on inserting the pump and the cuff in the proper places. While the patient is in the lithotomy position, a tunnel is created around the anal canal through one anterior or two lateral perianal incisions. This tunnel is created by blunt dissection considering the size of the cuff as well as the depth of the tunnel to avoid future erosion. A suprapubic transverse incision is made; dissection is undertaken through the layers of the abdominal wall till the extraperitoneal space anterior to the urinary bladder where the pressure-regulating balloon is placed.

By means of tunneling, two tunnels are burrowed in the subcutaneous area, one from the balloon and the other from the cuff, and both aim towards the pump either situated in the scrotum or the labus majorum accordingly. Connections are placed properly to create a functioning closed system. All of the components are filled with radiopaque fluid to facilitate subsequent radiological assessment when needed. This step is followed by equilibrating the pressures in the system in such a way that the balloon is kept at a higher pressure, thus keeping the sphincter inflated with the fluid, thereby closing the anal canal and maintaining continence. When the patient has the call for defecation, s/he presses the pump several times to deflate the sphincter cuff, allowing the anal canal to open. The higher pressure in the balloon gradually refills the cuff, again closing the anal canal.

A multicenter, prospective cohort study assessed the safety and efficacy of artificial bowel sphincters in 112 incontinent patients (Mahieu et al. 1984). At the 1-year follow-up, 75 (67%) had a functional device, and 85% enjoyed significant improvement in continence and quality of life. Twenty-five percent experienced wound infection that mandated surgical intervention, and 41 patients had their artificial sphincters explanted (Fig. 6.3.2).

In a recent systematic review of the literature, at the end of the follow-up period, approximately 66% of patients had accepted the functional artificial bowel sphincter. In studies with long follow-up (mean, 5 years; range, 5–10 years), the explantation rate was almost 50%. Infection was the most common complication (22%) and the most common reason for further surgical intervention. Other reasons for surgical intervention include erosion, fecal impaction, non-healing perineal wound, pain or malfunction (leaks, migration or cuff rupture). In all studies, there has been clinically significant improvement in fecal incontinence scores and in quality of life (Mundy et al. 2004).

In general, although a substantial number of patients eventually lose their artificial bowel sphincters, it remains one of the important tools in managing end-stage fecal incontinence (Table 6.3.6). In

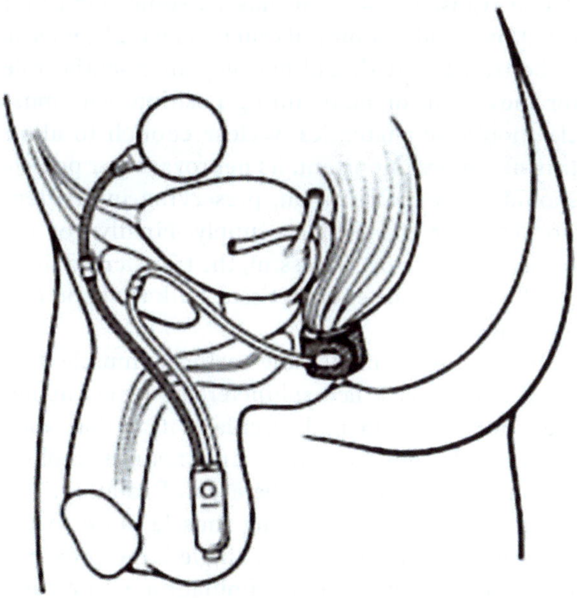

Fig. 6.3.2. Final position of an artificial bowel sphincter in a male (American Medical Systems, Minnetonka, MN)

Table 6.3.6. Artificial bowel sphincter results

Author	Year	N	Infection rate	Permanent explants	Re-implants	Overall success
Lehur et al.	2000	24	4%	4	4	83%
O'Brien et al.	2000	13	23%	3	0	77%
Wong et al.	2002	112	38%	34	7	67%
Ortiz et al.	2002	22	9%	7	2	68%
Devesa et al.	2002	53	21%	10	2	49%
Parker et al.	2003	37	34%	14	7	49%
Michot et al.	2003	25	12%	3	2*	80%
Casal et al.	2004	10	10%	1	2	90%

*Two patients were waiting for replacement at the time of publication

some instances, the major loss or major decline in the tissues requires a preliminary non-stimulated graciloplasty transposition to bulk the perineum and reduce the risk of erosion of the subsequently implanted cuff.

6.3.5.6 Muscle Transposition – Graciloplasty

Replacing the injured or dysfunctional sphincter muscle with another skeletal muscle is an acceptable option for end-stage fecal incontinence. In order to transfer a skeletal muscle, some important functional and anatomical criteria exist. The muscle to be transferred should not play an essential role for movement or maintaining position. The muscle should be anatomically close enough to allow transfer; more important, its neurovascular pedicle should allow mobilization, preserving intact, tension-free nerve and blood supply. Finally, for the transposition to be successful, the transferred muscle should provide enough tissue bulk (Person and Wexner 2005).

In the animal model, the sartorius muscle gave good results as a neo-sphincter; however, in humans it has a segmental vascularization that when transposed around the anal canal restricts mobilization and compromises the arch of rotation. The gluteus maximus is a strong muscle close to the rectum, but does not have a single large proximal nerve bundle amenable to stimulation. Chetwood (1902) reported the first use of the gluteus maximus as a neosphincter. This initial report was followed by several modifications (Pearl et al. 1991; Devesa et al. 1992) (Table 6.3.7). However, the muscle participates essentially in daily activities, such as running, climbing stairs and standing from the sitting position; hence, its transposition may result in compromising these important functions.

Table 6.3.7. Non-stimulated bilateral gluteoplasty series

Author	Year	Patients	Good results	Fair results
Schoemaker	1909	6	6	–
Bristom	1944	3	2	1
Prochiantz	1982	15	9	1
Hentz	1982	5	4	–
Chen and Zhang	1987	6	3	1
Pearl et al.	1991	7	4	2
Christiansen et al.	1995	7	0	3
Devesa et al.	1992	10	6	3
Devesa et al.	1997	17	9	1

In humans, the gracilis muscle, the most superficial adductor muscle, has minimal strength and range of motion; besides, its neurovascular bundle is proximal and has a consistent location, about four finger breadths downwards and outwards from the pubis. These factors enable the gracilis to be an appropriate choice for this operation.

Whereas the normal external sphincter contains about 80% type-I, slow-twitch, fatigue-resistant fibers and is thus able to maintain continuous contraction (KONSTEN et al. 1993), the gracilis, like all other skeletal muscles, has type-II, fast-twitch, nonfatigue-resistant fibers that are unable to maintain prolonged contraction. When the latter fibers are exposed to a continuous low-frequency electrical current, they eventually transform to the former fiber type (PETTE and VRBOVA 1992). The first graciloplasty was described by PICKRELL et al. in 1968 when the first stimulated graciloplasty was introduced (PERSON and WEXNER 2005). However, the concept of transforming fast fibers to slow fibers using a constant electric current was independently discovered at a later time (BAETEN et al. 1991; WILLIAMS et al. 1991).

6.3.5.6.1 Technique

The procedure is undertaken under general anesthesia with the patient in the lithotomy position and after administration of parenteral antibiotics.

6.3.5.7 Harvesting the Gracilis Muscle

This step is achieved through two incisions distributed on the medial aspect of the thigh along the gracilis muscle. The muscle is dissected distally through these incisions until its tendon proximal to the head of the tibia as well as proximally to its neurovascular bundle. The neurovascular bundle is generally situated four finger breadths below the ipsilateral pelvic ramus. In order to assure safety and to permit nerve stimulator use, the anesthesiologist avoids use of muscle-relaxing agents and especially paralysis.

The gracilis is left in the upper thigh incision waiting to be transposed after preparing its new bed around the anorectum. In approximately 5% to 10% of patients, the proximal arcade vessel is the only supply of the entire length of the gracilis muscle. Therefore, in a small number of patients, when the one to three perforated vessels entering the lateral aspect of the gracilis muscle are divided and the tendons are divided, the distal ⅓ to ⅔ of the muscle becomes devascularized. In these individuals, a vascular delay procedure is performed on the contralateral leg, leaving the tendon intact. Over the course of approximately the next 4 weeks, the muscle will become sufficiently vascularized through the single proximal arcade, and the surgeon can safely return to harvest and transpose the muscle at that time.

6.3.5.8 Preparing the New Position

Two circumanal lateral perianal incisions are made around the anal opening. A tunnel is then bluntly created around the anal canal with great caution not to injure the rectum, the vagina or the urethra. Another subcutaneous tunnel is formed subcutaneously to connect the newly created perianal bed with the upper thigh incision. The muscle is transferred to its new position and wrapped around the anal canal in a gamma (γ), alpha (α) or epsilon (ε) configuration. The next step is to fix the gracilis tendon by a non-absorbable suture in the contralateral ischial tuberosity or alternatively to the subcutaneous tissue or ipsilateral ischial tuberosity if the muscle is short.

6.3.5.9 Attaching the Electrical Source

The hardware is composed of a neurostimulator and electrodes. The two electrodes are inserted in the muscle bulk near the entrance of the supplying nerve, the obturator nerve, into the muscle. The neurostimulator is implanted in a subcutaneous pocket in the anterior abdominal wall in the pubic area, and through subcutaneous connections the electrodes are connected to the stimulator. Following the operation the conditioning phase starts; over 8 weeks a constant electrical current is applied on the neosphincter to allow fiber transformation. The patient is supplied with a magnet that, when applied on the neurostimulator, turns it off, allowing defecation, and when removed, the electrical current recurs, resulting in contraction of the neosphincter and closure of the anal canal.

In a multicenter trial by BAETEN et al. (2000) that included 115 patients who received a stimulating graciloplasty from 1993–1999, the success rate defined as a 50% decrease in frequency of incontinent episodes was achieved in 62% of patients who had no stoma at the time of operation at 1-year follow-up. At 18 and 24 months, these results were found in 55% and 56%, respectively, with 15% in this group experiencing complete continence and 42% experiencing 50% to 99% continence. In patients who had a stoma at the time of graciloplasty, the success rate was 37.5% at 1 year and rose to 62% at 18 months.

A systematic review showed that a considerable morbidity was associated with this procedure. The morbidity rate ranged up to 2.08 per patient with most common adverse events, including infection (28%), malfunctioning neurostimulator or electrodes (15%), and leg pain (13%). However patient satisfaction regarding continence as a measure of efficacy ranged from 42% to 85%.

Complications requiring surgical intervention and explantation of the device ranged from 0.14 to 1.07 per patient. Causes included erosion of the muscle into the anal canal, rectal perforation by enema, infections of the stimulator or electrodes, migration of the electrodes, battery failure, detachment of the tendon from the ischium, perianal abscess and/or fistula (Chapman et al. 2002).

Ortiz et al. (2003) compared the outcomes of dynamic graciloplasty and artificial bowel sphincters at a follow-up of 3 years. There were no significant differences in the complication rate, wound healing problems or explantation rates; however, the artificial bowel sphincter was found to be more effective in improving fecal incontinence (Table 6.3.8). Although stimulated graciloplasty is performed throughout the world, it is not available in the USA as the manufacturer never pursued FDA approval, which is unfortunate. There are certain groups of patients in whom insufficient perineal tissue exists without safe implantation of the artificial bowel sphincter, and sacral nerve stimulation will also not work. These patients would be best served by a stimulated graciloplasty, but unfortunately this procedure cannot be performed. As an alternative for patients in the US who have insufficient perineal tissue, a preliminary gracilis transposition followed by an artificial bowel sphincter should be considered.

Table 6.3.8. Stimulated-graciloplasty results

Author	Year	N	Overall morbidity %	Overall success %
Madoff et al.	1999	128	41%	66%
Baeten et al.	2000	123	74%	60%
Wexner et al.	2002	115	-	62%
Bresler et al.	2002	24	41.6%	79%
Rongen et al.	2003	200	61%	72%
Penninckx	2004	60	73%	75%
Thornton et al.	2004	38	75%	73%

6.3.5.10 Sacral Nerve Stimulation

The concept of using electric stimulation for improving poorly functioning pelvic organs was proposed about a century ago to treat urinary incontinence (In Person and Wexner 2005) and went through multiple phases, including transcutaneous stimulation, inserting electrodes into the vagina (Alexander et al. 1970) or rectum (Hopkinson 1972), implanting them directly into the pelvic organs (Caldwell et al. 1968) and finally, to avoid inserting foreign material in the pelvic organs, sacral nerve stimulators (Tanagho and Schmidt 1982), which were first used to treat urinary incontinence. It was subsequently noted that patients with both urinary and fecal incontinence treated with the sacral nerve stimulator for urinary incontinence also experienced improvement in fecal incontinence, which prompted investigating the implementation of sacral nerve stimulators in the management of fecal incontinence. In 1995, the first promising results on three patients were presented by Matzel et al. (1995); two gained perfect continence, and the third improved significantly.

6.3.5.11 Mechanism of Action

The pelvic floor and anorectal region receive both somatic as well as autonomic innervation. Direct branches from the sacral plexus (S2–S4) supply the levator ani and puborectalis with motor innervation. The inferior rectal nerve, a branch of the pudendal nerve, innervates the external anal sphincter. The superficial perineal nerve, another branch of the pudendal nerve, is responsible for sensory innervation. Autonomic innervation involves both the sympathetic and parasympathetic systems. The latter arises from the sacral plexus S2–S4. Thus, the continence mechanisms receive their controlling innervation, motor, sensory and autonomic, from the sacral plexus (Matzel et al. 1990).

It has been shown that electrical stimulation at that level results in stimulation of all the innervating components with subsequent modulation of nerve-musculature function; thereby, a malfunctioning pelvic floor musculature could be improved (Tanagho 1993). This finding is evidenced by the reduced rectal sensory threshold and improved expulsion time by its influence on the sensory pathways; however, the effect on the autonomic system results in increasing the resting anal pressure as well as rectal blood flow (Kenefick et al. 2003).

6.3.5.11.1 Technique

The initial process consists of three phases.

Stage One

The aim of this stage is to evaluate the probability of success in each patient prepared to receive a sacral nerve stimulator. The procedure is done while the patient is in the prone position, usually under local anesthesia, and without muscle relaxants. Under fluoroscopic guidance, needle electrodes are carefully placed into the dorsal foramina of S2, S3 and S4, trying to place the electrodes aligned with and close to the sacral nerve while leaving the foramina and entering the pelvis.

Each time an intermittent electric current is applied and the outcome checked. Normally, stimulation of S2 results in perineal muscle contraction and external rotation of the ipsilateral leg. Stimulation of S3 causes contraction of the external sphincter and levator ani associated with planter flexion of the first and second toes. Stimulation of S4 results in strong contraction of the external anal sphincter with no other musculature activity. This testing is done bilaterally, and accordingly, if a desired response is observed, the second stage is initiated.

Stage Two

As a direct continuum to a successful stage one, a temporary electrode is inserted, which subsequently if successful will remain as a permanent electrode in the last stage. In both options, the electrode is connected to an external temporary stimulator. This test period usually takes about 2 weeks. The external stimulator produces a continuous stimulation of a 15 Hz and a pulse width of 210 us, except for at defecation or urination. At the end of the 2 weeks, the patient is assessed for symptom improvement. Evaluation involves a bowel diary, fecal incontinence score, anorectal physiology testing and quality-of-life assessment.

Stage Three

The final phase of a successful evaluation is a permanent stimulator implantation in the subcutaneous tissue of the lower back. The same parameters used in the second stage are applied in stage three as well (Fig. 6.3.3). The patient is given a hand-held device by which he/she can activate/deactivate the stimulator and, more important, can modulate the amplitude of the currency.

Jarrett et al. (2004) concluded in their systematic review that a sacral nerve stimulator for fecal incontinence was extremely effective in improving continence and quality of life. It has also been shown that these effects are maintained for long periods of follow-up without significant deterioration. Thirteen percent (19 out of 149 patients) experienced

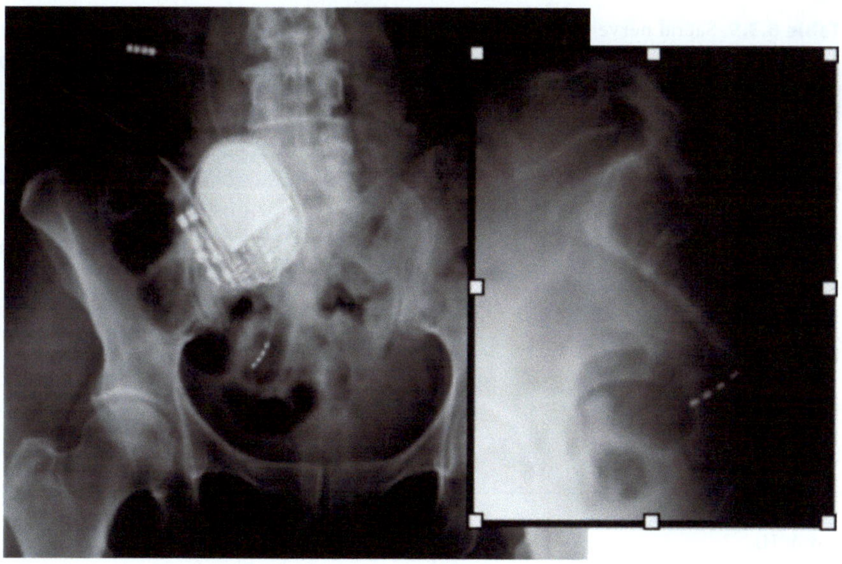

Fig. 6.3.3. Final position of the stimulator and electrodes (Medtronic Inc., Minneapolis, MN)

complications. Infection necessitating removal of the device occurred in three patients, seven patients needed replacement of leads, six patients felt pain at the site of implantation, and wound dehiscence occurred in only one patient.

The morbidity associated with sacral nerve stimulation is significantly less than the morbidity associated with either an artificial bowel sphincter or stimulated graciloplasty (Table 6.3.9). In large measure this vast improvement in the safety profile is due to the fact that none of the dissections and none of the implants are in close proximity to the anus. Moreover, the efficacy of the sacral nerve stimulation device far exceeds the efficacy of either the artificial bowel sphincter or graciloplasty. Specifically, the sacral nerve stimulator also improves sensation, whereas the artificial anal sphincter and graciloplasty "stimulated or non-stimulated" only serve as mechanical barriers to the passage of stool; hence, there is no augmentation of sensation with these other operations.

6.3.5.12 Injectable Bulking Agents for the Anal Sphincter

Injectable agents were initially used for treatment of female stress urinary incontinence. The idea was to physically augment the sphincter by the submucosal injection of bulking agents aiming to restore sphincter function. Glutaraldehyde cross-linked collagen (Monga et al. 1995), autologous fat (Haab et al. 1997) and carbon beads (Lightner et al. 2001) have been used for this purpose. Soon the concept was introduced to the colorectal field, and similar materials were used as bulking agents for the anal sphincters in patients with fecal incontinence (Shafik 1995; Kumar et al. 1998). Soon polytetrafluoroethylene (PTFE) (Teflon, Dupont, Wilmington, DE; Shafik 1993) and silicone (Malouf et al. 2001) were added to the injectable list.

The early results were promising; however, the fecal control effect over time declined either due to flattening or migration of these bulking agents that sometimes necessited subsequent further injection. Durasphere FI, initially designed for treating urinary stress incontinence, is another bulking agent composed of pyrolytic, carbon-coated, zirconium-oxide beads suspended in a water-based carrier gel containing B-glycan. These beads were designed to be non-migratory, non-absorbable and biocompatible. It is supplied as ready-prepared 1- or 3-ml sterile syringes ready for injection submucosally in the anal canal and distal rectum.

6.3.5.12.1 Technique

This procedure can be undertaken as an outpatient technique. Complete bowel preparation is not mandatory; however, a fleet enema might be helpful for cleaning the distal colon and rectum, thus providing a clean work environment. While the patient is on the examining table in the prone jackknife position, proper exposure of the anal canal is achieved by anoscopes. The bulking agent is subsequently in-

Table 6.3.9. Sacral nerve stimulation results

Author	Year	Number	Follow-up median (range) months	Improvement			
				Mean resting pressure	Mean squeeze pressure	Fecal incontinence score	
Ganio et al.	2001	16	15.5 (3–45)	37.7→49.1[b]	67.3→82.6[b]	Williams	4.1→1.25
Leroi et al.	2001	6	6	77→86[a]	56.5→60.8[a]	Urgency	4.8→2.3
Kenefick et al.	2002	15	24 (3–60)	35→49[a]	43→69[a]	FI episodes	11→0
Matzel et al.	2004	34	(5–60)	-	37.3→72.5[b]	FI episodes	16.4→2
Altomare et al.	2004	14	14 (6–48)	36.5→32[b]	72→62[b]	FI episodes	14→0.5
Jarret et al.	2004	46	12 (1–72)	46→49[a]	62→93[a]	Wexner	7.5→1
Rasmussen et al.	2004	37	6 (0–36)	42→33[a]	90→100[a]	Wexner	16→6

[a] cm H_2O
[b] mm Hg

jected in the submucosal area about 0.5–1 cm above the dentate line typically 45 degrees apart.

Weiss et al. (2002) prospectively applied this technique to ten patients (seven females) with a mean age of 64 years in an open-label pilot trial. These patients did not have sphincter defects and failed other non-surgical treatment options. Generally, 80% of patients improved after this procedure, with a significant reduction of Wexner score from 13 at baseline to 10 and 9.3 at 3 and 6 months after the procedure, respectively. This salutary effect was associated with improvement in fecal continence ability and quality-of-life assessment scores, proving that this procedure is easy to perform, well tolerable and offers improvement in fecal continence.

Another study included 18 patients with fecal incontinence. In this study the authors injected the material at the site of the sphincter defect, aiming at restoring the symmetry of the anal canal. With a mean follow-up of 28.5 months, the Wexner score decreased from a baseline of 11.89 to about 8 at 12 months ($P = 0.002$), with an associated improvement in quality of life. There was a significant correlation between the number of injected sites and the degree of improvement, with no attenuation of the effect over time (Davis et al. 2003).

The possible mechanism of action is to fill the area of the sphincter defect to restore the contour of the anal canal or bulking the intact sphincter and thus regaining the ability to close the anal canal at rest and during squeeze, respectively. Furthermore, the continuous formation of fibrosis around the injection sites may provide a satisfactory long-term effect.

6.3.5.13 Radiofrequency

The use of heat in medicine goes back thousands of years. The mechanism by which radiofrequency delivers heat energy to tissues depends on a high-frequency alternating current that flows between two electrodes – active and dispersive. This results in extremely rapid frictional movement of ions and thus heat generation in the tissue. As a result, collagen fibers in the heated tissues contract; furthermore, the subsequent healing and remodeling processes cause shortening and tightening of the tissues (Gustavson 1964). This mechanism has been effectively employed in the management of different conditions, including obstructive apnea syndrome (Powell et al. 1998), benign prostatic hyperplasia (Dawkins et al. 1997), joint capsule instability (Hecht et al. 1999) and gastroesophageal reflux disease (GERD) (Richards et al. 2001; Triadafilopoulos and Utley 2001; Triadafilopoulos et al. 2002).

Technology innovations resulted in modifying the technique into temperature-controlled radiofrequency heat delivering systems. By virtue of a continuous feedback mechanism, the temperature of treated tissues is monitored, and the heat energy delivery is controlled in order to keep the temperature within a normal range to avoid tissue burning. This method is also accompanied by a simultaneous cooling system. The modification showed effectiveness in treating GERD, the Stretta procedure, (Curon Medical, Inc., Sunnyvale, CA); a similar procedure based on the same concept, the Secca procedure, has evolved for treating fecal incontinence. The Secca system is composed of a central control device to monitor the temperature adjustments from one side and the function of the apparatus from the other side (Fig. 6.3.4). It has a four-channel radiofrequency generator and an anoscopic handpiece. This handpiece has four titanium needle electrodes; each electrode has temperature-sensitive sensors at the tip and base in order to continuously monitor the temperature of the tissue and mucosa.

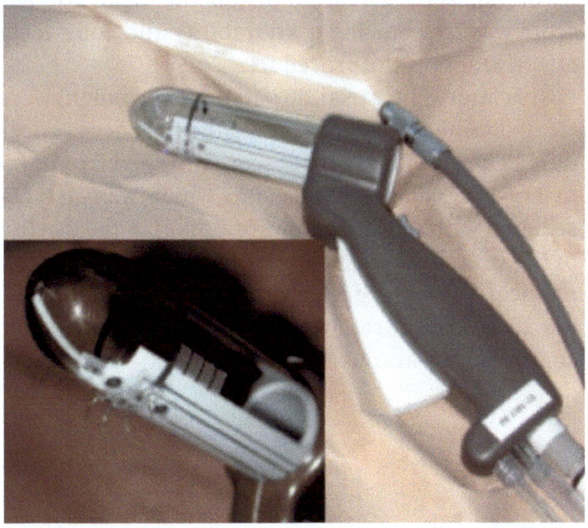

Fig. 6.3.4. Secca procedure. The anoscopic handle piece with the four titanium electrodes deployed (Curon Medical, Sunnyvale, CA, which declared bankruptcy on 15 October 2006)

6.3.5.13.1 Technique

The patient is placed in the prone Jackknife position; anesthesia can be either intravenous conscious sedation with local anesthesia or a general inhalational agent. Under direct vision, the handpiece is inserted into the anal canal so that the needle's line is at or just above the dentate line. Caution should always used, making sure that the cooling system is set up and functioning properly. The needles are deployed into the tissues, and the radiofrequency energy is delivered under the control and monitoring of the central module. Each needle receives and thereby delivers about 465 KHz, 2–5 W, for 90 s. With any increase in the tissue temperature beyond the pre-selected limit (85° C) or interruption in the cooling system, the power is automatically shut down. In this manner, each needle causes a thermal lesion in the anal sphincter; each set is composed of four lesions applied to the four quadrants and is repeated up to about 15 mm proximal to the dentate line in the anal canal, depending on the length of the anal canal, a piece of information obtained from the preoperative anal ultrasound.

The first pilot study (Takahashi et al. 2002) was carried out on ten female patients who under went the Secca procedure for fecal incontinence. Early results showed a reduction in the Wexner score from a mean of 13.5 at baseline to 5 after 12 months ($P<0.01$), with an associated improvement in quality of life. At the 2-year follow-up, the mean Wexner score was 7.3, showing the durability and long-term effectiveness of the procedure.

In a multicenter trial, 50 patients (43 women) were treated for fecal incontinence using the Secca procedure. The baseline Wexner score dropped from 14.5 to 11.1 at 6 months ($P<0.0001$), which was also associated with significant improvement in the quality of life (Efron et al. 2003). Unfortunately, the Curon medical company declared bankruptcy in November 2006, and the radiofrequency device is no longer commercially available.

6.3.6 Conclusion

Fecal incontinence is a very heterogeneous classification of a tremendously distressing and disabling physical disorder. The degree of incontinence must be considered in the context of the lifestyle and activity of the patient. For example, an elderly bedridden nursing home patient incontinent for liquid stool on an occasional basis has a vastly different implication than a young active professional incontinent for the same liquid stool on an occasional basis. In addition, daily incontinence of gas in someone who professionally lectures for a living might be vastly more distressing than a once per week episode of solid stools in a nursing home patient. Therefore, in order to quantify the severity of the incontinence, the Wexner incontinence score or an alternative scoring system should be used. If the patient's fecal incontinence score warrants investigation, then imaging studies are essential in order to help determine the best method of treatment. In general, a combination of anal ultrasonography or anal magnetic resonance imaging combined with pudendal nerve terminal motor latency assessment will form the cornerstone for therapeutic selection.

Much of the determination is based on whether or not an intact sphincter mechanism exists. If MRI and/or ultrasound reveal an anatomically intact sphincter, then anal electromyography can be used to determine the functionality of that sphincter. Sphincter defects are best repaired through an overlapping mechanism. However, because of the very poor long-term result, patients are counseled that the overlapping repair will form the first steps in the recovery and that at some subsequent date, either soon after the initial repair or in the future, additional therapy may be necessary. In patients without a defect or patients who after the defects have been repaired still continue to have a functionally poor sphincter mechanism, as well as in patients with a multifocal defect, other therapy should be selected. The range of these treatments is determined in large measure by the anatomy of the sphincter. For example, the patient with multifocal defects might be best served by either a graciloplasty or an artificial bowel sphincter, whereas the patient with an anatomically intact, but functionally unsatisfactory repair might be best served by sacral nerve stimulations or injectables. The algorithm shows the therapeutic determination again in large measure based on imaging results. The ultimate goal in these patients, regardless of therapy, is to restore normal or near normal bowel control at least to an acceptable level and avoid the ultimate alternative of a permanent stoma.

Algorithm 6.3.1. Strategy for managing fecal incontinence

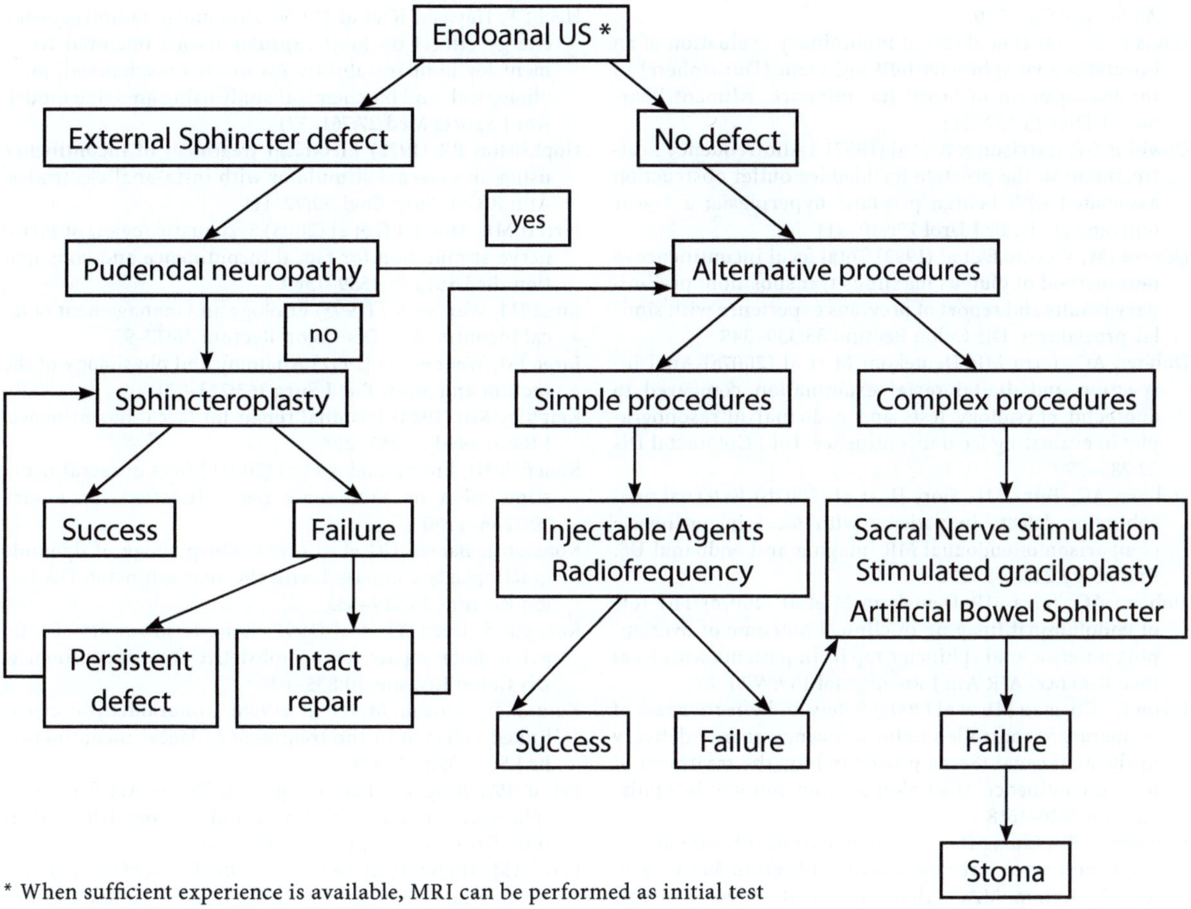

* When sufficient experience is available, MRI can be performed as initial test

References

Alexander S, Rowan D et al (1970) Treatment of urinary incontinence by electric pessary. A report of 18 patients. Br J Urol 42:184–190

Altomare DF, Rinaldi M, Petrolino M et al (2004) Permanent sacral nerve stimulation for fecal incontinence and associated urinary incontinence. Int J Colorectal Dis 19:203–209

Baeten CG, Konsten J et al (1991) Dynamic graciloplasty for treatment of faecal incontinence. Lancet 338:1163–1165

Baeten CG, Geerdes BP et al (1995) Anal dynamic graciloplasty in the treatment of intractable fecal incontinence. N Engl J Med 332:1600–1605

Baeten CG, Bailey HR et al (2000) Safety and efficacy of dynamic graciloplasty for fecal incontinence: report of a prospective, multicenter trial. Dynamic Graciloplasty Therapy Study Group. Dis Colon Rectum 43:743–751

Bannister JJ, Gibbons C et al (1987) Preservation of faecal continence during rises in intra-abdominal pressure: is there a role for the flap valve? Gut 28:1242–1245

Barisic GI, Krivokapic ZV, Makovic VA et al (2006) Outcome of overlapping sphincter anal sphincter repair after 3 months and after a mean of 80 month. Int J Colorectal Dis 21:52–56

Briel JW, Stoker et al (1999) External anal sphincter atrophy on endoanal MRI adversally effects continence after sphincteroplasty. Br J Surg 86:1322–1327

Bristom O (1944) Plastiches Erzatz des M. sphincter ani. Acta Chir Scand 90:431–448

Browning GG, Parks AG (1983) Postanal repair for neuropathic faecal incontinence: correlation of clinical result and anal canal pressures. Br J Surg 70:101–104

Caldwell KP, Cook PJ et al (1968) Stress incontinence in females: report on 31 cases treated by electrical implant. J Obstet Gynaecol Br Commonw 75:777–780

Casal E, San Ildefonso A, Carracedo R et al (2004) Artificial bowel sphincter in severe anal incontinence. Colorectal Dis 6:180–184

Chapman AE, Geerdes B et al (2002) Systematic review of dynamic graciloplasty in the treatment of faecal incontinence. Br J Surg 89:138–153

Chen YL, Zhang XH (1987) Reconstruction of rectal sphincter by transposition of gluteus muscle for fecal incontinence. J Pediatr Surg 22:62–64

Chetwood CH (1902) Plastic operation of the sphincter ani with report of a case. Med Rec 61:529

Christiansen J, Hansen CR, Rasmussen O (1995) Bilateral gluteus maximus transposition for anal incontinence. Br J Surg 82:903–905

Ctercteko GC, Fazio VW et al (1988) Anal sphincter repair: a report of 60 cases and review of the literature. Aust N Z J Surg 58:703–710

Davis K, Kumar D et al (2003) Preliminary evaluation of an injectable anal sphincter bulking agent (Durasphere) in the management of faecal incontinence. Aliment Pharmacol Ther 18:237–243

Dawkins GP, Harrison NW et al (1997) Radiofrequency heat-treatment to the prostate for bladder outlet obstruction associated with benign prostatic hyperplasia: a 4-year outcome study. Br J Urol 79:910–914

Devesa JM, Vicente E et al (1992) Total fecal incontinence–a new method of gluteus maximus transposition: preliminary results and report of previous experience with similar procedures. Dis Colon Rectum 35:339–349

Dobben AC, Terra MP, Deutekom M et al (2007a) Anal inspection and digital rectal examination compared to anorectal physiology tests and endoanal ultrasonography in evaluating fecal incontinence. Int J Colorectal Dis 22:783–790

Dobben AC, Terra MP, Slors JF et al (2007b) External anal sphincter defects in patients with fecal incontinence: comparison of endoanal MR imaging and endoanal US. Radiology 242:463–471

Dobben AC, Terra MP, Deutekom M et al (2007c) The role of endoluminal imaging in clinical outcome of overlapping anterior anal sphincter repair in patients with fecal incontinence. AJR Am J Roentgenol 189:W70–77

Efron JE, Corman ML et al (2003) Safety and effectiveness of temperature-controlled radio-frequency energy delivery to the anal canal (Secca procedure) for the treatment of fecal incontinence. Dis Colon Rectum 46:1606–1616; discussion 1616–1618

Ehrenpreis ED, Chang D et al (2007) Pharmacotherapy for fecal incontinence: a review. Dis Colon Rectum 50:641–649

Engel AF, Kamm MA, Sultan AH et al (1994) Anterior sphincter repair in patients with obstetric trauma. Br J Surg 160:637–640

Fang DT, Nivatvongs S, Vermeulen FD et al (1984) Overlapping sphincteroplasty for acquired fecal incontinence. Dis Colon Rectum 27:720–722

Fleshman JW, Peters WR et al (1991) Anal sphincter reconstruction: anterior overlapping muscle repair. Dis Colon Rectum 34:739–743

Ganio E, Ratto C, Masin A et al (2001) Neuromodulation for fecal incontinence: Outcome in 16 patients with definitive implant. The initial Italian Sacral Neuromodulation Group (GINS) experience. Dis Colon Rectum 44:965–970

Gibbons CP, Bannister JJ et al (1986) An analysis of anal sphincter pressure and anal compliance in normal subjects. Int J Colorectal Dis 1:231–237

Grey BR, Sheldon RR, Telford KJ, Kiff ES (2007) Anterior anal sphincter repair can be of long term benefit: a 12-year case cohort from a single surgeon. BMC Surg. 11:7–11

Gustavson KH (1964) On the chemistry of collagen. Fed Proc 23:613–617

Haab F, Zimmern PE et al (1997) Urinary stress incontinence due to intrinsic sphincteric deficiency: experience with fat and collagen periurethral injections. J Urol 157:1283–1286

Hallan RI, Marzouk DE et al (1989) Comparison of digital and manometric assessment of anal sphincter function. Br J Surg 76:973–975

Halverson AL, Hull TL (2002) Long-term outcome of overlapping anal sphincter repair. Dis Colon Rectum 45:345–348

Hecht P, Hayashi K et al (1999) Monopolar radiofrequency energy effects on joint capsular tissue: potential treatment for joint instability. An in vivo mechanical, morphological, and biochemical study using an ovine model. Am J Sports Med 27:761–771

Hopkinson BR (1972) Electrical treatment of incontinence using an external stimulator with intra-anal electrodes. Ann R Coll Surg Engl 50:92–111

Jarrett ME, Mowatt G et al (2004) Systematic review of sacral nerve stimulation for faecal incontinence and constipation. Br J Surg 91:1559–1569

Jorge JM, Wexner SD (1993) Etiology and management of fecal incontinence. Dis Colon Rectum 36:77–97

Jorge JM, Wexner SD (1997) Anatomy and physiology of the rectum and anus. Eur J Surg 163:723–731

Keighley MR (1984) Postanal repair for faecal incontinence. J R Soc Med 77:285–288

Kenefick NJ, Emmanuel A et al (2003) Effect of sacral nerve stimulation on autonomic nerve function. Br J Surg 90:1256–1260

Konsten J, Baeten CG et al (1993) Morphology of dynamic graciloplasty compared with the anal sphincter. Dis Colon Rectum 36:559–563

Korsgen S, Deen KI et al (1997) Long-term results of total pelvic floor repair for postobstetric fecal incontinence. Dis Colon Rectum 40:835–839

Kumar D, Benson MJ et al (1998) Glutaraldehyde cross-linked collagen in the treatment of faecal incontinence. Br J Surg 85:978–979

Lehur PA, Roig JV, Duinslaeger M (2000) Artificial anal sphincter: prospective clinica and manometric evaluation. Dis Colon Rectum 43:1100–1106

Leroi AM, Michot F, Grise P et al (2001) Effect of sacral nerve stimulation in patients with fecal and urinary incontinence. Dis Colon Rectum 44:779–789

Lightner D, Calvosa C et al (2001) A new injectable bulking agent for treatment of stress urinary incontinence: results of a multicenter, randomized, controlled, double-blind study of Durasphere. Urology 58:12–15

MacDonald A, Smith A et al (1992) Manual dilatation of the anus. Br J Surg 79:1381–1382

Macmillan AK, Merrie AE et al (2004) The prevalence of fecal incontinence in community-dwelling adults: a systematic review of the literature. Dis Colon Rectum 47:1341–1349

Madoff RD, Williams JG et al (1992) Fecal incontinence. N Engl J Med 326:1002–1007

Mahieu P, Pringot J et al (1984) Defecography: II. Contribution to the diagnosis of defecation disorders. Gastrointest Radiol 9:253–261

Malouf AJ, Norton CS et al (2000) Long-term results of overlapping anterior anal-sphincter repair for obstetric trauma. Lancet 355:260–265

Malouf AJ, Vaizey CJ et al (2001) Internal anal sphincter augmentation for fecal incontinence using injectable silicone biomaterial. Dis Colon Rectum 44:595–600

Maslekar S, Gardiner AB, Duthie GS (2007) Anterior anal sphincter repair for fecal incontinence: Good long-term results are possible. J Am Coll Surg 204:40–46

Matsuoka H, Mavrantonis C et al (2000) Postanal repair for fecal incontinence – is it worthwhile? Dis Colon Rectum 43:1561–1567

Matzel KE, Schmidt RA et al (1990) Neuroanatomy of the striated muscular anal continence mechanism. Implications for the use of neurostimulation. Dis Colon Rectum 33:666–673
Matzel KE, Stadelmaier U et al (1995) Electrical stimulation of sacral spinal nerves for treatment of faecal incontinence. Lancet 346:1124–1127
Mellgren A, Jensen LL et al (1999) Long-term cost of fecal incontinence secondary to obstetric injuries. Dis Colon Rectum 42:857–865; discussion 865–867
Michot F, Costaglioli B, Leroi AM et al (2003) Artificial anal sphincter in severe fecal incontinence: outcome of prospective experience with 37 patients in one institution. Ann Surg 237:52–56
Miller R, Bartolo DC et al (1988) Prospective study of conservative and operative treatment for faecal incontinence. Br J Surg 75:101–105
Monga AK, Robinson D et al (1995) Periurethral collagen injections for genuine stress incontinence: a 2-year follow-up. Br J Urol 76:156–160
Mundy L, Merlin TL et al (2004) Systematic review of safety and effectiveness of an artificial bowel sphincter for faecal incontinence. Br J Surg 91:665–672
Nelson R, Norton N et al (1995) Community-based prevalence of anal incontinence. JAMA 274:559–561
O'Brien PE, Skinner S (2000) Restoring control: the Acticon Neosphincter artificial bowel sphincter in the treatment of anal incontinence. Dis Colon Rectum 43:1213–1216
Oliviera L, Pfeifer J, Wexner SD (1996) Physiological and clinical outcome of anterior sphincteroplasty. Br J Surg 83:502–505
Ortiz H, Armendariz P et al (2003) Prospective study of artificial anal sphincter and dynamic graciloplasty for severe anal incontinence. Int J Colorectal Dis 18:349–354
Parker SC, Spencer MP, Madoff RD et al (2003) Artificial bowel sphincter: Long-term experience at a single institution. Dis Colon Rectum 46:722–729
Parks AG, McPartlin JF (1971) Late repair of injuries of the anal sphincter. Proc R Soc Med 64:1187–1189
Parks AG, Porter NH et al (1962) Experimental study of the reflex mechanism controlling the muscle of the pelvic floor. Dis Colon Rectum 5:407–414
Parks AG, Gordon PH et al (1976) A classification of fistula-in-ano. Br J Surg 63:1–12
Pearl RK, Prasad ML et al (1991) Bilateral gluteus maximus transposition for anal incontinence. Dis Colon Rectum 34:478–481
Person B, Wexner SD (2005) Advances in the surgical treatment of fecal incontinence. Surg Innov 12:7–21
Pescatori M, Anastasio G et al (1992) New grading and scoring for anal incontinence. Evaluation of 335 patients. Dis Colon Rectum 35:482–487
Penninckx F (2004) Belgian experience with dynamic graciloplasty for fecal incontinence. Br J Surg 91:872–878
Pette D, Vrbova G (1992) Adaptation of mammalian skeletal muscle fibers to chronic electrical stimulation. Rev Physiol Biochem Pharmacol 120:115–202
Powell NB, Riley RW et al (1998) Radiofrequency volumetric tissue reduction of the palate in subjects with sleep-disordered breathing. Chest 113:1163–1174
Prochiantz A, Gross P (1982) Gluteal myoplasty for sphincter replacement. Priciples, results and prospects. J Pediatr Surg 17:25–30
Rasmussen OO, Buntzen S, Sorensen M et al (2004) Sacral nerve stimulation in fecal incontinence. Dis Colon Rectum 47:1156–1158
Richards WO, Scholz S et al (2001) Initial experience with the Stretta procedure for the treatment of gastroesophageal reflux disease. J Laparoendosc Adv Surg Tech A 11:267–273
Rongen MJ, Uludag O, El Naggar K et al (2003) Long-term follow-up of dynamic graciloplasty for fecal incontinence. Dis Colon Rectum 46:716–721
Rothbarth J, Bemelman WA et al (2001) What is the impact of fecal incontinence on quality of life? Dis Colon Rectum 44:67–71
Sainio P, Husa A (1985) Fistula-in-ano. Clinical features and long-term results of surgery in 199 adults. Acta Chir Scand 151:169–176
Shafik A (1993) Polytetrafluoroethylene injection for the treatment of partial fecal incontinence. Int Surg 78:159–161
Shafik A (1995) Perianal injection of autologous fat for treatment of sphincteric incontinence. Dis Colon Rectum 38:583–587
Shouler PJ, Grimley RP et al (1986) Fistula-in-ano is usually simple to manage surgically. Int J Colorectal Dis 1:113–115
Sitzler PJ, Thompson JP (1996) Overlap repair of damaged anal sphincter. A single surgeon series. Dis Colon Rectum 39:1356–1360
Slade MS, Goldberg SM et al (1977) Sphincteroplasty for acquired anal incontinence. Dis Colon Rectum 20:33–35
Smith LE, Blatchford GJ (2006) Physiologic testing. The ASCRS textbook of colon and rectum surgery. Wolf BG, Fleshman JW, Beck DE, Pemberton JH, Wexner SD (eds) Springer Science+Business Media, LLC, New York, pp 40–56
Snooks SJ, Swash M et al (1990) Effect of vaginal delivery on the pelvic floor: a 5-year follow-up. Br J Surg 77:1358–1360
Sultan AH, Kamm MA et al (1994) Third degree obstetric anal sphincter tears: risk factors and outcome of primary repair. BMJ 308:887–891
Takahashi T, Garcia-Osogobio S et al (2002) Radio-frequency energy delivery to the anal canal for the treatment of fecal incontinence. Dis Colon Rectum 45:915–922
Tanagho EA (1993) Concepts of neuromodulation. Neurourol Urodyn 12:487–488
Tanagho EA, Schmidt RA (1982) Bladder pacemaker: scientific basis and clinical future. Urology 20:614–619
Terra MP, Deutekom M et al (2006a) Relationship between external anal sphincter atrophy at endoanal magnetic resonance imaging and clinical, functional, and anatomic characteristics in patients with fecal incontinence. Dis Colon Rectum 49:668–678
Terra MP, Beets-Tan RG et al (2006b) MRI in evaluating atrophy of the external anal sphincter in patients with fecal incontinence. AJR Am J Roentgenol 187:991–999
Thornton MJ, Kennedy ML, Lubowski DZ et al (2004) Long-term follow-up of dynamic graciloplasty for fecal incontinence. Colorectal Dis 6:470–476
Triadafilopoulos G, Utley DS (2001) Temperature-controlled radiofrequency energy delivery for gastroesophageal reflux disease: the Stretta procedure. J Laparoendosc Adv Surg Tech A 11:333–339

Triadafilopoulos G, DiBaise JK et al (2002) The Stretta procedure for the treatment of GERD: 6 and 12 month follow-up of the US open label trial. Gastrointest Endosc 55:149–156

Vaizey CJ, Carapeti E et al (1999) Prospective comparison of faecal incontinence grading systems. Gut 44:77–80

Weiss EG, Efron JE et al (2002) Submucosal injection of carbon coated beads is a successful and safe office based treatment for fecal incontinence. Dis Colon Rectum 45:46–47

Wexner SD, Marchetti F et al (1991) The role of sphincteroplasty for fecal incontinence reevaluated: a prospective physiologic and functional review. Dis Colon Rectum 34:22–30

Whitehead WE, Wald A et al (2001) Treatment options for fecal incontinence. Dis Colon Rectum 44:131–142; discussion 142–144

Williams NS, Patel J et al (1991) Development of an electrically stimulated neoanal sphincter. Lancet 338:1166–1169

Wong WD, Congliosi SM, Spencer MP et al (2002) The safety and efficacy of the artificial bowel sphincter for fecal incontinence: results from a multicentre cohort study. Dis Colon Rectum 45:1139–1153

Young CJ, Mathur MN, Eyers AA et al (1998) Successful overlapping anal sphincter repair: Relation to patient age, neuropathy, and colostomy formation. Dis Colon Rectum 41:344

Subject Index

G

H

I

K

L

M

N

O

P

V

W

List of Contributors

Paul Abrams, MD, FRCS
Professor of Urology
Bristol Urological Institute
Southmead Hospital
Bristol BS10 5NB
UK

Email: paul_abrams@bui.ac.uk

Clive I. Bartram, FRCS, FRCP, FRCR
Professor
Consultant Radiologist (Retired)
St Mark's Hospital
Princess Grace Hospital
Nottingham Place
London W1U 5NY
UK

Email: cibartram@gmail.com

Adil E. Bharucha, MBBS, MD
Professor of Medicine
Clinical Enteric Neuroscience Translational and Epidemiological Research Program
Mayo Clinic, College of Medicine
200 First Street SW
Rochester, MN 55905
USA

Email: bharucha.adil@mayo.edu

Annette C. de Bruijne-Dobben, PhD
Department of Radiology
Academic Medical Center
University of Amsterdam
Meibergdreef 9
1105 AZ Amsterdam
The Netherlands
and presently:
Senior advisor Knowledge Center
The Netherlands Health Care Inspectorate
St. Jacobsstraat 16
3511 BS Utrecht
The Netherlands

Email: ac.bruijne@igz.nl

John O. L. DeLancey, MD
Norman F. Miller Professor of Gynecology
Director, Pelvic Floor Research Group
Director, Fellowship in Female Pelvic Medicine and Reconstructive Surgery
L4000 Women's Hospital
University of Michigan
1500 E. Medical Center Drive
Ann Arbor, MI 48109-0276
USA

Email: delancey@umich.edu

Hans Peter Dietz, MD, PhD, FRANZCOG, DDU, CU
Associate Professor in Obstetrics and Gynaecology
Nepean Clinical School, University of Sydney
Nepean Hospital
Penrith NSW 2750
Australia

Email: hpdietz@bigpond.com

Anton V. Emmanuel, MD, BSc, FRCP
Director of GI Physiology Unit
University College Hospital
235 Euston Road
London NW1 2BU
UK

Email: a.emmanuel@ucl.ac.uk

Joel G. Fletcher, MD
Associate Professor of Radiology
Department of Radiology
Mayo Clinic
200 First Street SW
Rochester, MN 55905
USA

Email: fletcher.joel@mayo.edu

Douglass S. Hale, MD, FACOG, FACS
Director Female Pelvic Medicine
& Reconstructive Surgery Fellowship
Associate Clinical Professor
Indiana University/Methodist Hospital
1633 N Capitol Avenue, Suite 436
Indianapolis, IN 46202
USA

Email: dough22@aol.com

Steve Halligan, MD, MRCP, FRCR
Professor of Gastrointestinal Radiology
Department of Specialist X-Ray
University College Hospital
235 Euston Road
London NW1 2BU
UK

Email: s.halligan@ucl.ac.uk

Fadi Housami, MD, MRCS
Clinical Research Registrar
Bristol Urological Institute
Southmead Hospital
Bristol BS10 5NB
UK

Email: fhousami@bui.ac.uk

Matthias Oelke, MD, FEBU
Department of Urology
Medical School Hanover
University of Hanover
Carl-Neuberg-Strasse 1
30625 Hanover
Germany

Email: oelke.matthias@mh-hannover.de

Jan-Paul Roovers, MD, PhD
Department of Obstetrics and Gynecology
Academic Medical Center
University of Amsterdam
Meibergdreef 9
1105 AZ Amsterdam
The Netherlands

Email: j.p.roovers@amc.uva.nl

Sherief Shawki, MD
Research Fellow
Department of Colorectal Surgery
Cleveland Clinic Florida
2950 Cleveland Clinic Boulevard
Weston, FL 33331
USA

Email: shawkis@ccf.org

Hassan Siddiki, MD
Department of Radiology
Mayo Clinic
200 First Street SW
Rochester, MN 55905
USA

Email: siddiki.hassan@mayo.edu

Jaap Stoker, MD, PhD
Professor of Radiology
Department of Radiology
Academic Medical Center
University of Amsterdam
Meibergdreef 9
1105 AZ Amsterdam
The Netherlands

Email: j.stoker@amc.uva.nl

Stuart A. Taylor, MD, MRCP, FRCR
Senior Lecturer in Radiology
Department of Specialist X-Ray
University College Hospital
2F Podium, 235 Euston Road
London NW1 2BU
UK

Email: stuart.taylor@uclh.nhs.uk

Wolfgang H. Umek, MD
Associate Professor
Department of Obstetrics and Gynecology
Medical University of Vienna
Waehringer Guertel 18
1090 Vienna
Austria

Email: wolfgang.umek@gmail.com

David B. Vodušek, PhD
Professor of Neurology
Medical Faculty, University of Ljubljana
and
Medical Director
Division of Neurology, University Medical Centre
1525 Ljubljana
Slovenia

Email: david.vodusek@kclj.si

Christian Wallner, MSc
Department of Anatomy and Embryology
Academic Medical Center
University of Amsterdam
Meibergdreef 69–71
1105 BK Amsterdam
The Netherlands

Email: c.wallner@amc.uva.nl

Steven D. Wexner, MD, FACS, FRCS, FRCS(Ed)
Chairman, Department of Colorectal Surgery
Chief of Staff
Cleveland Clinic Florida
2950 Cleveland Clinic Boulevard
Weston, FL 33331
USA

Email: wexners@ccf.org

Medical Radiology Diagnostic Imaging and Radiation Oncology

Titles in the series already published

Diagnostic Imaging

Innovations in Diagnostic Imaging
Edited by J. H. Anderson

Radiology of the Upper Urinary Tract
Edited by Erich K. Lang

The Thymus - Diagnostic Imaging, Functions, and Pathologic Anatomy
Edited by E. Walter, E. Willich, W. R. Webb

Interventional Neuroradiology
Edited by A. Valavanis

Radiology of the Lower Urinary Tract
Edited by Erich K. Lang

Contrast-Enhanced MRI of the Breast
S. Heywang-Köbrunner, R. Beck

Spiral CT of the Chest
Edited by M. Rémy-Jardin, J. Rémy

Radiological Diagnosis of Breast Diseases
Edited by M. Friedrich, E. A. Sickles

Radiology of Trauma
Edited by M. Heller, A. Fink

Biliary Tract Radiology
Edited by P. Rossi. Co-edited by M. Brezi

Radiological Imaging of Sports Injuries
Edited by C. Masciocchi

Modern Imaging of the Alimentary Tube
Edited by A. R. Margulis

Diagnosis and Therapy of Spinal Tumors
Edited by P. R. Algra, J. Valk, J. J. Heimans

Interventional Magnetic Resonance Imaging
Edited by J. F. Debatin, G. Adam

Abdominal and Pelvic MRI
Edited by A. Heuck, M. Reiser

Orthopedic Imaging
Techniques and Applications
Edited by A. M. Davies, H. Pettersson

Radiology of the Female Pelvic Organs
Edited by E. K. Lang

Magnetic Resonance of the Heart and Great Vessels
Clinical Applications
Edited by J. Bogaert, A. J. Duerinckx, F. E. Rademakers

Modern Head and Neck Imaging
Edited by S. K. Mukherji, J. A. Castelijns

Radiological Imaging of Endocrine Diseases
Edited by J. N. Bruneton in collaboration with B. Padovani, M.-Y. Mourou

Radiology of the Pancreas
2nd Revised Edition
Edited by A. L. Baert. Co-edited by G. Delorme, L. Van Hoe

Trends in Contrast Media
Edited by H. S. Thomsen, R. N. Muller, R. F. Mattrey

Functional MRI
Edited by C. T. W. Moonen, P. A. Bandettini

Emergency Pediatric Radiology
Edited by H. Carty

Liver Malignancies
Diagnostic and Interventional Radiology
Edited by C. Bartolozzi, R. Lencioni

Spiral CT of the Abdomen
Edited by F. Terrier, M. Grossholz, C. D. Becker

Medical Imaging of the Spleen
Edited by A. M. De Schepper, F. Vanhoenacker

Radiology of Peripheral Vascular Diseases
Edited by E. Zeitler

Diagnostic Nuclear Medicine
Edited by C. Schiepers

Radiology of Blunt Trauma of the Chest
Edited by P. Schnyder, M. Wintermark

Portal Hypertension
Diagnostic Imaging and Imaging-Guided Therapy
Edited by P. Rossi. Co-edited by P. Ricci, L. Broglia

Virtual Endoscopy and Related 3D Techniques
Edited by P. Rogalla, J. Terwisscha van Scheltinga, B. Hamm

Recent Advances in Diagnostic Neuroradiology
Edited by Ph. Demaerel

Multislice CT
Edited by M. F. Reiser, M. Takahashi, M. Modic, R. Bruening

Pediatric Uroradiology
Edited by R. Fotter

Transfontanellar Doppler Imaging in Neonates
Edited by A. Couture, C. Veyrac

Radiology of AIDS
A Practical Approach
Edited by J. W. A. J. Reeders, P. C. Goodman

CT of the Peritoneum
Edited by A. Rossi, G. Rossi

Magnetic Resonance Angiography
2nd Revised Edition
Edited by I. P. Arlart, G. M. Bongartz, G. Marchal

Applications of Sonography in Head and Neck Pathology
Edited by J. N. Bruneton in collaboration with C. Raffaelli, O. Dassonville

3D Image Processing
Techniques and Clinical Applications
Edited by D. Caramella, C. Bartolozzi

Imaging of the Larynx
Edited by R. Hermans

Pediatric ENT Radiology
Edited by S. J. King, A. E. Boothroyd

Imaging of Orbital and Visual Pathway Pathology
Edited by W. S. Müller-Forell

Radiological Imaging of the Small Intestine
Edited by N. C. Gourtsoyiannis

Imaging of the Knee
Techniques and Applications
Edited by A. M. Davies, V. N. Cassar-Pullicino

Perinatal Imaging
From Ultrasound to MR Imaging
Edited by Fred E. Avni

Diagnostic and Interventional Radiology in Liver Transplantation
Edited by E. Bücheler, V. Nicolas, C. E. Broelsch, X. Rogiers, G. Krupski

Imaging of the Pancreas
Cystic and Rare Tumors
Edited by C. Procacci, A. J. Megibow

Imaging of the Foot & Ankle
Techniques and Applications
Edited by A. M. Davies, R. W. Whitehouse, J. P. R. Jenkins

Radiological Imaging of the Ureter
Edited by F. Joffre, Ph. Otal, M. Soulie

Radiology of the Petrous Bone
Edited by M. Lemmerling, S. S. Kollias

Imaging of the Shoulder
Techniques and Applications
Edited by A. M. Davies,J. Hodler

Interventional Radiology in Cancer
Edited by A. Adam, R. F. Dondelinger, P. R. Mueller

Imaging and Intervention in Abdominal Trauma
Edited by R. F. Dondelinger

Radiology of the Pharynx and the Esophagus
Edited by O. Ekberg

Radiological Imaging in Hematological Malignancies
Edited by A. Guermazi

Functional Imaging of the Chest
Edited by H.-U. Kauczor

Duplex and Color Doppler Imaging of the Venous System
Edited by G. H. Mostbeck

Multidetector-Row CT of the Thorax
Edited by U. J. Schoepf

Multislice CT
2nd Revised Edition
Edited by M. F. Reiser, M. Takahashi, M. Modic, C. R. Becker

Radiology and Imaging of the Colon
Edited by A. H. Chapman

Multidetector-Row CT Angiography
Edited by C. Catalano, R. Passariello

Focal Liver Lesions
Detection, Characterization, Ablation
Edited by R. Lencioni, D. Cioni, C. Bartolozzi

Imaging in Treatment Planning for Sinonasal Diseases
Edited by R. Maroldi, P. Nicolai

Clinical Cardiac MRI
With Interactive CD-ROM
Edited by J. Bogaert, S. Dymarkowski, A. M. Taylor

Dynamic Contrast-Enhanced Magnetic Resonance Imaging in Oncology
Edited by A. Jackson, D. L. Buckley, G. J. M. Parker

Contrast Media in Ultrasonography
Basic Principles and Clinical Applications
Edited by Emilio Quaia

Paediatric Musculoskeletal Disease
With an Emphasis on Ultrasound
Edited by D. Wilson

MR Imaging in White Matter Diseases of the Brain and Spinal Cord
Edited by M. Filippi, N. De Stefano, V. Dousset, J. C. McGowan

Imaging of the Hip & Bony Pelvis
Techniques and Applications
Edited by A. M. Davies, K. Johnson, R. W. Whitehouse

Imaging of Kidney Cancer
Edited by Ali Guermazi

Magnetic Resonance Imaging in Ischemic Stroke
Edited by R. von Kummer, T. Back

Diagnostic Nuclear Medicine
2nd Revised Edition
Edited by Christiaan Schiepers

Imaging of Occupational and Environmental Disorders of the Chest
Edited by P. A. Gevenois, P. De Vuyst

Virtual Colonoscopy
A Practical Guide
Edited by P. Lefere, S. Gryspeerdt

Contrast Media
Safety Issues and ESUR Guidelines
Edited by H. S. Thomsen

Head and Neck Cancer Imaging
Edited by R. Hermans

Vascular Embolotherapy
A Comprehensive Approach
Volume 1: *General Principles, Chest, Abdomen, and Great Vessels*
Edited by J. Golzarian. Co-edited by S. Sun, M. J. Sharafuddin

Vascular Embolotherapy
A Comprehensive Approach
Volume 2: *Oncology, Trauma, Gene Therapy, Vascular Malformations, and Neck*
Edited by J. Golzarian. Co-edited by S. Sun, M. J. Sharafuddin

Vascular Interventional Radiology
Current Evidence in Endovascular Surgery
Edited by M. G. Cowling

Ultrasound of the Gastrointestinal Tract
Edited by G. Maconi, G. Bianchi Porro

Parallel Imaging in Clinical MR Applications
Edited by S. O. Schoenberg, O. Dietrich, M. F. Reiser

MRI and CT of the Female Pelvis
Edited by B. Hamm, R. Forstner

Imaging of Orthopedic Sports Injuries
Edited by F. M. Vanhoenacker, M. Maas, J. L. Gielen

Ultrasound of the Musculoskeletal System
Edited by S. Bianchi, C. Martinoli

Clinical Functional MRI
Presurgical Functional Neuroimaging
Edited bei C. Stippich

Radiation Dose from Adult and Pediatric Multidetector Computed Tomography
Edited by D. Tack, P. A. Gevenois

Spinal Imaging
Diagnostic Imaging of the Spine and Spinal Cord
Edited by J. Van Goethem, L. van den Hauwe, P. M. Parizel

Computed Tomography of the Lung
A Pattern Approach
Edited by J. A. Verschakelen, W. De Wever

Imaging in Transplantation
Edited by A. Bankier

Radiological Imaging of the Neonatal Chest
2nd Revised Edition
Edited by V. Donoghue

Radiological Imaging of the Digestive Tract in Infants and Children
Edited by A. S. Devos, J. G. Blickman

Pediatric Chest Imaging
Chest Imaging in Infants and Children
2nd Revised Edition
Edited by J. Lucaya, J. L. Strife

Color Doppler US of the Penis
Edited by M. Bertolotto

Radiology of the Stomach and Duodenum
Edited by A. H. Freeman, E. Sala

Imaging in Pediatric Skeletal Trauma
Techniques and Applications
Edited by K. J. Johnson, E. Bache

Image Processing in Radiology
Current Applications
Edited by E. Neri, D. Caramella, C. Bartolozzi

Screening and Preventive Diagnosis with Radiological Imaging
Edited by M. F. Reiser, G. van Kaick, C. Fink, S. O. Schoenberg

Percutaneous Tumor Ablation in Medical Radiology
Edited by T. J. Vogl, T. K. Helmberger, M. G. Mack, M. F. Reiser

Liver Radioembolization with ^{90}Y Microspheres
Edited by J. I. Bilbao, M. F. Reiser

Pediatric Uroradiology
2nd Revised Edition
Edited by R. Fotter

Radiology of Osteoporosis
2nd Revised Edition
Edited by S. Grampp

Gastrointestinal Tract Sonography in Fetuses and Children
Edited by A. Couture, C. Baud, J. L. Ferran, M. Saguintaah, C. Veyrac

Intracranial Vascular Malformations and Aneurysms
2nd Revised Edition
Edited by M. Forsting, I. Wanke

High-Resolution Sonography of the Peripheral Nervous System
2nd Revised Edition
Edited by S. Peer, G. Bodner

Imaging Pelvic Floor Disorders
2th Revised Edition
Edited by J. Stoker, S. A. Taylor, J. O. L. DeLancey

Coronary Radiology
2th Revised Edition
Edited by M. Oudkerk, M. F. Reiser

Cardiothoracic Imaging with MDCT
2th Revised Edition
Edited by M. Rémy-Jardin, J. Rémy

Springer

RADIATION ONCOLOGY

Lung Cancer
Edited by C. W. Scarantino

Innovations in Radiation Oncology
Edited by H. R. Withers, L. J. Peters

Radiation Therapy of Head and Neck Cancer
Edited by G. E. Laramore

Gastrointestinal Cancer – Radiation Therapy
Edited by R. R. Dobelbower, Jr.

Radiation Exposure and Occupational Risks
Edited by E. Scherer, C. Streffer, K.-R. Trott

Interventional Radiation
Therapy Techniques – Brachytherapy
Edited by R. Sauer

Radiopathology of Organs and Tissues
Edited by E. Scherer, C. Streffer, K.-R. Trott

Concomitant Continuous Infusion
Chemotherapy and Radiation
Edited by M. Rotman, C. J. Rosenthal

Intraoperative Radiotherapy – Clinical Experiences and Results
Edited by F. A. Calvo, M. Santos, L. W. Brady

Interstitial and Intracavitary Thermoradiotherapy
Edited by M. H. Seegenschmiedt, R. Sauer

Non-Disseminated Breast Cancer
Controversial Issues in Management
Edited by G. H. Fletcher, S. H. Levitt

Current Topics in Clinical Radiobiology of Tumors
Edited by H.-P. Beck-Bornholdt

Practical Approaches to Cancer Invasion and Metastases
A Compendium of Radiation Oncologists' Responses to 40 Histories
Edited by A. R. Kagan with the Assistance of R. J. Steckel

Radiation Therapy in Pediatric Oncology
Edited by J. R. Cassady

Radiation Therapy Physics
Edited by A. R. Smith

Late Sequelae in Oncology
Edited by J. Dunst, R. Sauer

Mediastinal Tumors. Update 1995
Edited by D. E. Wood, C. R. Thomas, Jr.

Thermoradiotherapy and Thermochemotherapy
Volume 1:
Biology, Physiology, and Physics
Volume 2:
Clinical Applications
Edited by M. H. Seegenschmiedt, P. Fessenden, C. C. Vernon

Carcinoma of the Prostate
Innovations in Management
Edited by Z. Petrovich, L. Baert, L. W. Brady

Radiation Oncology of Gynecological Cancers
Edited by H. W. Vahrson

Carcinoma of the Bladder
Innovations in Management
Edited by Z. Petrovich, L. Baert, L. W. Brady

Blood Perfusion and Microenvironment of Human Tumors
Implications for Clinical Radiooncology
Edited by M. Molls, P. Vaupel

Radiation Therapy of Benign Diseases
A Clinical Guide
2nd Revised Edition
S. E. Order, S. S. Donaldson

Carcinoma of the Kidney and Testis, and Rare Urologic Malignancies
Innovations in Management
Edited by Z. Petrovich, L. Baert, L. W. Brady

Progress and Perspectives in the Treatment of Lung Cancer
Edited by P. Van Houtte, J. Klastersky, P. Rocmans

Combined Modality Therapy of Central Nervous System Tumors
Edited by Z. Petrovich, L. W. Brady, M. L. Apuzzo, M. Bamberg

Age-Related Macular Degeneration
Current Treatment Concepts
Edited by W. E. Alberti, G. Richard, R. H. Sagerman

Radiotherapy of Intraocular and Orbital Tumors
2nd Revised Edition
Edited by R. H. Sagerman, W. E. Alberti

Modification of Radiation Response
Cytokines, Growth Factors, and Other Biolgical Targets
Edited by C. Nieder, L. Milas, K. K. Ang

Radiation Oncology for Cure and Palliation
R. G. Parker, N. A. Janjan, M. T. Selch

Clinical Target Volumes in Conformal and Intensity Modulated Radiation Therapy
A Clinical Guide to Cancer Treatment
Edited by V. Grégoire, P. Scalliet, K. K. Ang

Advances in Radiation Oncology in Lung Cancer
Edited by B. Jeremić

New Technologies in Radiation Oncology
Edited by W. Schlegel, T. Bortfeld, A.-L. Grosu

Multimodal Concepts for Integration of Cytotoxic Drugs and Radiation Therapy
Edited by J. M. Brown, M. P. Mehta, C. Nieder

Technical Basis of Radiation Therapy
Practical Clinical Applications
4th Revised Edition
Edited by S. H. Levitt, J. A. Purdy, C. A. Perez, S. Vijayakumar

CURED I • LENT
Late Effects of Cancer Treatment on Normal Tissues
Edited by P. Rubin, L. S. Constine, L. B. Marks, P. Okunieff

Radiotherapy for Non-Malignant Disorders
Contemporary Concepts and Clinical Results
Edited by M. H. Seegenschmiedt, H.-B. Makoski, K.-R. Trott, L. W. Brady

CURED II • LENT
Cancer Survivorship Research and Education
Late Effects on Normal Tissues
Edited by P. Rubin, L. S. Constine, L. B. Marks, P. Okunieff

Radiation Oncology
An Evidence-Based Approach
2th Revised Edition
Edited by J. J. Lu, L. W. Brady

Primary Optic Nerve Sheath Meningioma
Edited by B. Jeremić, S. Pitz

Springer

MIX
Papier aus verantwortungsvollen Quellen
Paper from responsible sources
FSC® C105338

If you have any concerns about our products,
you can contact us on
ProductSafety@springernature.com

In case Publisher is established outside the EU,
the EU authorized representative is:
Springer Nature Customer Service Center GmbH
Europaplatz 3, 69115 Heidelberg, Germany

Printed by Libri Plureos GmbH
in Hamburg, Germany